PROGNOSIS
AND RISK
ASSESSMENT IN
CARDIOVASCULAR
DISEASE

PROGNOSIS AND RISK ASSESSMENT IN CARDIOVASCULAR DISEASE

Edited by

Amar S. Kapoor, M.D.

Associate Clinical Professor, Department of Medicine
University of California, Los Angeles
UCLA School of Medicine
Los Angeles, California
Director, Interventional Cardiology
St. Mary Medical Center
Long Beach, California

Bramah N. Singh, M.D., D. Phil.

Professor, Department of Medicine
University of California, Los Angeles
UCLA School of Medicine
Chief, Cardiology Section
West Los Angeles Veterans Administration Hospital
Los Angeles, California

Churchill Livingstone
New York, Edinburgh, London, Melbourne, Tokyo

About the cover

Life is represented by a rejuvenating ring of energy. The circles of life represent a balance
between positive forces and negative forces. Prognosis is a harmonious balance
between the ring of life energy and the circles of life.

Amar S. Kapoor

Library of Congress Cataloging-in-Publication Data

Prognosis and risk assessment in cardiovascular disease / edited by
  Amar S. Kapoor, Bramah N. Singh.
        p.   cm.
    Includes bibliographical references and index.
    ISBN 0-443-08768-7
    1. Cardiovascular system—Diseases—Prognosis. 2. Cardiovascular
system—Diseases—Risk factors.
    [DNLM: 1. Cardiovascular Diseases—diagnosis. 2. Prognosis.
3. Risk Factors.   WG 100 P964]
RC669.P74 1993
616.1'07—dc20
DNLM/DLC
for Library of Congress   92-49268
                                                                    CIP

Distributed in the United Kingdom by Churchill Livingstone, Robert Stevenson House, 1–3
Baxter's Place, Leith Walk, Edinburgh EH1 3AF, and by associated companies, branches, and
representatives throughout the world.

Accurate indications, adverse reactions, and dosage schedules for drugs are provided in this
book, but it is possible that they may change. The reader is urged to review the package
information data of the manufacturers of the medications mentioned.

The Publishers have made every effort to trace the copyright holders for borrowed material. If
they have inadvertently overlooked any, they will be pleased to make the necessary
arrangements at the first opportunity.

Copy Editor: *Paul Bernstein*
Production Designer: *Maryann King*
Production Supervisor: *Sharon Tuder*
Cover Design: *Paul Moran*

Printed in the United States of America

First published in 1993   7 6 5 4 3 2 1

To our colleagues who provide health care conscious of risk-benefit and survival analysis; to our wives, Narinder Kapoor and Roshni Singh; and to our children, Nimmi and Saabir Kapoor, and Pramil, Nalini, and Sanjiv Singh.

Contributors

Seth D. Bilazarian, M.D.
Instructor, Department of Cardiology, Boston University School of Medicine, Boston, Massachusetts

Bradford P. Blakeman, M.D.
Associate Professor, Department of Thoracic and Cardiovascular Surgery, Loyola University of Chicago Stritch School of Medicine, Maywood, Illinois

Sarana Boonbaichaiyapruck, M.D.
Interventional Cardiology Fellow, Cardiology Section, Hospital of the Good Samaritan, Los Angeles, California

Gregory L. Burke, M.D., M.S.
Associate Professor and Vice-Chairman, Department of Public Health Sciences, Bowman Gray School of Medicine of Wake Forest University, Winston-Salem, North Carolina

Lucien Campeau, M.D.
Emeritus Professor, Department of Medicine, University of Montreal Faculty of Medicine; Senior Cardiologist, Montreal Heart Institute, Montreal, Quebec, Canada

Jay N. Cohn, M.D.
Professor and Head, Cardiovascular Division, Department of Medicine, University of Minnesota Medical School—Minneapolis, Minneapolis, Minnesota

Peter J. Counihan, M.B., M.R.C.P.I.
Clinical Research Fellow, Department of Cardiological Sciences, St. George's Hospital Medical School, London, England

Michael H. Crawford, M.D.
Robert S. Flinn Professor and Chief, Division of Cardiology, Department of Internal Medicine, University of New Mexico School of Medicine, Albuquerque, New Mexico

William E. Curtis, M.D.
Fellow, Department of Surgery, Johns Hopkins University School of Medicine; Staff, Department of Surgery, The Johns Hopkins Hospital, Baltimore, Maryland

Michael de Buitleir, M.D.
Associate Professor, Department of Medicine, University of Wisconsin Medical
School; Co-Director, Cardiac Electrophysiology, Division of Cardiology, University
of Wisconsin Hospital, Madison, Wisconsin

Prakash C. Deedwania, M.D.
Clinical Professor, Department of Medicine, University of California, San Francisco,
School of Medicine, San Francisco, California; Chief, Cardiology Section, Veterans
Administration Medical Center, Fresno, California

Jack J. Farahi, M.D.
Senior Fellow, Cardiology Section, West Los Angeles Veterans Administration
Medical Center, Los Angeles, California

Manning Feinleib, M.D., Ph.D.
Director, National Center for Health Statistics, Centers for Disease Control,
Hyattsville, Maryland

Noble O. Fowler, M.D.
Professor Emeritus, Departments of Medicine and Pharmacology and Cell
Biophysics, University of Cincinnati College of Medicine; Staff, Division of
Cardiology, Department of Internal Medicine, University of Cincinnati Medical
Center, Cincinnati, Ohio

Therese Fuchs, M.D.
Assistant Professor, Department of Cardiology, Boston University School
of Medicine; Director, Electrophysiology Laboratory, Boston City Hospital,
Boston, Massachusetts

Timothy J. Gardner, M.D.
Professor, Department of Surgery, Johns Hopkins University School of Medicine;
Cardiac Surgeon, Cardiac Surgery Service, The Johns Hopkins Hospital, Baltimore,
Maryland

Richard F. Gillum, M.D.
Special Assistant for Cardiovascular Epidemiology, Office of Analysis and
Epidemiology, National Center for Health Statistics, Centers for Disease Control,
Hyattsville, Maryland

Anton P. M. Gorgels, M.D.
Associate Professor, Department of Cardiology, University Hospital of Limburg;
Cardiologist, University of Limburg, Maastricht, the Netherlands

Stuart W. Jamieson, M.B.
Professor and Head, Division of Cardiothoracic Surgery, Department of Surgery,
University of California, San Diego, School of Medicine, San Diego, California

Michael B. Jorgensen, M.D.
Staff Cardiologist, Cardiology Section, Kaiser Permanente Medical Center,
Los Angeles, California

Masoor Kamalesh, M.D.
Research Fellow, Institute for Prevention of Cardiovascular Disease,
Department of Medicine, Harvard Medical School; Cardiology Fellow, Division of
Cardiology, New England Deaconess Hospital, Boston, Massachusetts

Amar S. Kapoor, M.D.
Associate Clinical Professor, Department of Medicine, University of California,
Los Angeles, UCLA School of Medicine, Los Angeles, California; Director,
Interventional Cardiology, St. Mary Medical Center, Long Beach, California

Wishwa N. Kapoor, M.D.
Professor, Department of Medicine, University of Pittsburgh School of Medicine,
Pittsburgh, Pennsylvania

Sanjiv Kaul, M.D.
Associate Professor, Department of Medicine, University of Virginia School of
Medicine; Co-Director, Cardiac Imaging, University of Virginia Hospital,
Charlottesville, Virginia

David T. Kelly, M.B., Ch.B.
Scandrett Professor of Cardiology and Head, Department of Medicine, University of
Sydney; Director, Hallstrom Institute of Cardiology, Royal Prince Alfred Hospital,
Sydney, New South Wales, Australia

Nicholas T. Kouchoukos, M.D.
John M. Shoenberg Professor of Cardiovascular Surgery, Division of Cardiothoracic
Surgery, Department of Surgery, Washington University School of Medicine; Surgeon-
in-Chief, The Jewish Hospital of Saint Louis, Saint Louis, Missouri

Jolene M. Kriett, M.D.
Assistant Clinical Professor, Division of Cardiothoracic Surgery, Department of
Surgery, University of California, San Diego, School of Medicine, San Diego, California

Ole Lund, M.D.
Senior Surgical Resident and Registrar, Department of Thoracic and
Cardiovascular Surgery, Skejby Sygehus—Aarhus University Hospital,
Aarhus, Denmark

Jan Kyst Madsen, M.D., Ph.D.
Lecturer, University of Copenhagen; Senior Registrar, Cardiovascular
Laboratory, Department of Medicine B, Rigshospitalet, University Hospital,
Copenhagen, Denmark

Dennis T. Mangano, M.D., Ph.D.
Professor and Vice Chairman, Department of Anesthesia, University of California, San Francisco, School of Medicine, San Francisco, California

Teri A. Manolio, M.D., M.H.S.
Medical Officer, Division of Epidemiology and Clinical Applications, National Heart, Lung, and Blood Institute, National Institutes of Health, Bethesda, Maryland

John H. McAnulty, M.D.
Professor, Division of Cardiology, Department of Medicine, Oregon Health Sciences University School of Medicine, Portland, Oregon

Robert F. McCauley, M.D.
Medical Director, Respiratory Services, Internal Medicine Department, Humana Hospital West Anaheim, Anaheim, California

William J. McKenna, M.D.
Reader in Cardiology, Department of Cardiological Sciences, St. George's Hospital Medical School, London, England

Sally E. McNagny, M.D., M.P.H.
Assistant Professor, Division of General Internal Medicine, Department of Medicine, Emory University School of Medicine; Co-Director, Medical Walk-in Clinic, Grady Memorial Hospital, Atlanta, Georgia

Freny Vaghaiwalla Mody, M.D.
Assistant Professor in Residence, Department of Medicine, University of California, Los Angeles, UCLA School of Medicine; Staff Physician, Cardiology Section, West Los Angeles Veterans Administration Medical Center, Los Angeles, California

Fred Morady, M.D.
Professor, Department of Medicine, University of Michigan Medical School; Director, Cardiac Electrophysiology, Division of Cardiology, University of Michigan Medical Center, Ann Arbor, Michigan

Richard W. Nesto, M.D.
Assistant Professor, Department of Medicine, Harvard Medical School; Co-Director, Institute for Prevention of Cardiovascular Disease, New England Deaconess Hospital, Boston, Massachusetts

Robin M. Norris, M.D.
Honorary Professor, Division of Cardiovascular Therapeutics, Department of Pharmacology and Clinical Pharmacology, University of Auckland School of Medicine; Cardiologist, Coronary Care Unit, Green Lane Hospital, Auckland, New Zealand

Larry A. Osborn, M.D.
Associate Professor, Division of Cardiology, Department of Internal Medicine, University of New Mexico School of Medicine, Albuquerque, New Mexico

Roque Pifarré, M.D.
Professor and Chairman, Department of Thoracic and Cardiovascular Surgery, Loyola University of Chicago Stritch School of Medicine, Maywood, Illinois

Philip J. Podrid, M.D.
Associate Professor, Department of Cardiology, Boston University School of Medicine; Director, Arrhythmia Service, Section of Cardiology, University Hospital, Boston, Massachusetts

Thomas S. Rector, Ph.D.
Senior Research Associate, Cardiovascular Division, Department of Medicine, University of Minnesota Medical School—Minneapolis, Minneapolis, Minnesota

Eugene D. Robin, M.D.
Professor Emeritus, Departments of Medicine and Physiology, Stanford University School of Medicine, Stanford, California; Tsurai Indian Health Care Clinic, Trinidad, California

Luz-Maria Rodriguez, M.D.
Cardiologist, Department of Cardiology, University Hospital Maastricht, Maastricht, the Netherlands

Arthur Selzer, M.D., M.A.C.P.*
Professor, Department of Cardiology, University of California, San Francisco, School of Medicine; Co-Director, Training Program, Division of Cardiology, Pacific Presbyterian Medical Center, San Francisco, California

Bramah N. Singh, M.D., D. Phil.
Professor, Department of Medicine, University of California, Los Angeles, UCLA School of Medicine; Chief, Cardiology Section, West Los Angeles Veterans Administration Hospital, Los Angeles, California

Joep L. Smeets, M.D.
Director, Department of Electrophysiology, University Hospital Maastricht, Maastricht, the Netherlands

John A. Spittell, Jr., M.D.
Professor, Department of Medicine, Mayo Medical School; Consultant, Division of Cardiovascular Disease, Cardiovascular Department, Mayo Clinic, Rochester, Minnesota

* Deceased.

Peter C. Spittell, M.D.
Senior Associate Consultant, Division of Cardiovascular Disease, Cardiovascular
Department, Mayo Clinic, Rochester, Minnesota

Robert Stauffer, M.D.
Fellow, Cardiology Section, Kaiser Permanente Medical Center, Los Angeles,
California

R. Sudhir Sundaresan, M.D.
Assistant Professor, Division of Cardiothoracic Surgery, Department of Surgery,
Washington University School of Medicine, Saint Louis, Missouri

H. Robert Superko, M.D.
Medical Director, Cholesterol Research Center; Medical Research Scientist,
Lawrence Berkeley Laboratory, University of California, Berkeley,
Berkeley, California; Director, Institute for Progressive Atherosclerosis Management,
Sequoia Hospital, Redwood City, California

Pierre Théroux, M.D.
Associate Professor, University of Montreal; Director, Coronary Care Unit,
Montreal Heart Institute, Montreal, Quebec, Canada

Hein J. J. Wellens, M.D.
Professor and Chairman, Department of Cardiology, University Hospital of Limburg,
Maastricht, the Netherlands

Nanette Kass Wenger, M.D.
Professor, Division of Cardiology, Department of Medicine, Emory University
School of Medicine; Director, Cardiac Clinics, Grady Memorial Hospital, Atlanta,
Georgia

Harvey D. White, M.B., Ch.B.
Director, Coronary Care Unit, Specialist in Cardiovascular Research, Cardiology
Department, Green Lane Hospital, Auckland, New Zealand

Preface

In the past, the art of prognosis was in the hands of experienced clinicians who had developed a sense of the expected course of disease if no treatment had been applied. Against such a background, the effects of therapeutic interventions were evaluated with respect to the outcome in terms of symptom relief, quality of life, and mortality.

During the last few decades, there has been a bewilderingly rapid growth in the understanding of the pathophysiology of cardiovascular disease; there have been enormous advances in pharmacologic and invasive modalities of treatment; and there have been changes in the natural history of numerous cardiovascular disorders. Therefore, more than ever before, there is now a need for a detailed understanding of the natural history of cardiovascular disease and the impact of rapidly advancing therapeutic developments. The importance of the prognostic implications of individual disorders is further emphasized by the growing number of crucial clinical trials in the wake of such developments.

It is now possible to arrive at a very accurate diagnosis of most cardiovascular disorders through a combination of clinical resources and diagnostic procedures, both invasive and noninvasive. Precision in diagnosis and delivery of treatment aimed at altering the prognosis and improving the quality of life for the patient are central to the issue of treatment. The modality of therapy chosen will clearly depend on a detailed understanding of the prognosis of the individual disorder to be treated. It will also hinge on the risk as well as the cost of procedures used relative to the expected outcome that results from a particular form of therapy.

Prognosis and Risk Assessment in Cardiovascular Disease is designed to provide an authoritative source of current information for determining prognosis in major cardiovascular disease entities. The authors and co-authors who provide what are rapidly changing perspectives for various disorders are leaders in their specific areas. They have collated and distilled the material from landmark studies and clinical trials relative to their own experience as consultants in cardiovascular disease.

The book is presented in seven sections. The first section provides an overview of risk-benefit analysis, prevalence, incidence, and patterns of mortality in cardiovascular disease. There is a particular focus on the epidemiology and clinical relevance of major risk factors for the pathogenesis of coronary artery disease.

Section II is devoted to risk assessment in and prognosis of coronary artery disease syndromes; this section includes risk stratification for the patient surviving myocardial infarction. In clinical practice, coronary artery disease and its complications dominate contemporary adult cardiology and are responsible for the largest components of cardiovascular mortality and morbidity. For appropriate emphasis, 10 chapters are devoted to the different facets of the disease. Notably absent in this section is the effect of percutaneous transluminary angioplasty and related interventional approaches to myocardial revascularization; no meaningful data are available despite the very widespread use of these techniques in the treatment of coronary artery disease.

Section III deals with the natural history and timing of surgery and its impact on the prognosis of mitral and aortic valve disease. In Section IV, risk assessment and the prognosis of patients with heart failure, hypertrophic cardiomyopathy, and pericardial disease are discussed. This is followed by an in-depth analysis of conduction system abnormalities, arrhythmias, the difficult and frustrating problem of syncope, and sudden cardiac death, which remains a major therapeutic problem in the United States, where it accounts for no less than 400,000 cases a year. Section V, on atrial fibrillation, is designed to draw attention to the fact that atrial fibrillation not only is the most common arrhythmia that requires treatment, but also is not a benign arrhythmia; it accounts for considerable morbidity and mortality.

The penultimate section deals with the prognostic cardiovascular features of miscellaneous noncardiac disorders, and includes a chapter on the important issue of risk assessment in patients undergoing noncardiac surgery. The final section of this book deals with the impact of cardiovascular surgery on prognosis. Undoubtedly, cardiac surgery has been and remains one of the spectacular advances in cardiovascular medicine over the last 30 years. There has been continued innovation in techniques of cardiac surgery, preservation of the myocardium during surgery, postoperative care and, in cases of transplantation, major changes in immunosuppression and the control of rejection. All have had a profound impact on morbidity and mortality of major cardiovascular diseases. Various chapters in this section provide a current perspective and discuss future trends.

The information included in this book's discussion of prognosis in cardiovascular medicine is relevant to the clinical practice of the discipline. The book is designed to assist in the clinical decision-making process with respect to the choice of an appropriate therapeutic modality and the timing of a particular intervention. As they occur, future advances will need to be placed in perspective by stringently controlled clinical trials, many of which are ongoing.

We are indebted to all the contributors who delivered their manuscripts in a timely fashion and shared with us their enthusiasm for and excitement about such a book. We would also like to thank Avé McCracken, executive editor at Churchill Livingstone, and Paul Bernstein for their help, guidance, and encouragement during the preparation of this book.

Amar S. Kapoor, M.D.
Bramah N. Singh, M.D., D.Phil.

Contents

Section III: Risk Assessment and Prognosis of Valvular Heart Disease

Section I

RISK FACTORS AND PROGNOSIS

1

Risk-Benefit Analysis in Cardiovascular Disease

Eugene D. Robin
Robert F. McCauley

BACKGROUND

Sweeping changes are occurring both in the health care system and in societal perceptions of the role and value of medical care. These changes inevitably have a deep and growing impact on the practice of cardiology and cardiovascular surgery. One important change is that the public's high esteem for physicians has progressively eroded during the past 20 years.[1] Another is that the public is becoming increasingly educated with respect to both the capabilities and the limitations of individual physicians and of wide segments of general health care provision and various subspecialty expertise.

Paradoxically, with the growth of medical technology and science, the public's increased critical awareness of limitations is accompanied by increasing expectations of the benefits to be derived from medical care. The combination of increased scrutiny coupled with increased expectation commonly leads to disillusionment when increased expectations are not achieved.

There is a growing awareness within the medical profession and among the public of the soft, often shifting and frequently contradictory, nature of the data base and processes that determine the character of medical practice. There is also a growing recognition of the importance of prospective randomized controlled clinical trials (PRCCT) in assessing the benefits versus risks of various diagnostic and management modalities. But the total number of current management modalities that have been rigorously assessed is pitifully small. Even if the total includes modalities that have been shown to be effective by extensive empirical observations, say, the use of penicillin in the treatment of pneumococcal pneumonia, it appears that perhaps 10 to 20%[2] or less of current practice has been acceptably documented to be of benefit. (Incidentally, it would be interesting to estimate more accurately the percentage of acceptably documented practices, but this task has not been undertaken.)

Most physicians have not been adequately trained in clinical epidemiology and are unable to evaluate critically the management modalities that they use. Moreover, they are often unaware of the necessity for a critical risk-benefit analysis of their day-to-day management practices.

One result is wide geographic variations in the use of various modalities. These geographic variations occur both within the United States and internationally. Wennberg provided a particularly relevant series of analyses on the variations of the use of a variety of surgical treatments from region to region in the United States.[3] He concluded that the variations in frequency of use of many forms of surgical treatment express a difference in practice style and are not based on any firm scientific data.

A recent example of a striking international difference involves the treatment of thyrotoxicosis. A hypothetical 43-year-old woman would have been treated with radioactive iodine therapy by 79% of U.S. experts, by 22% of European experts, and by only 11% of Japanese clinicians. An antithyroid drug was the initial choice of 31% of American experts, 78% of European experts, and 88% of Japanese experts.[4] As the late development of thyroid cancer is at least a theoretical risk of radioactive thyroid therapy, it is easy to understand the reluctance of Japanese experts to use this form of treatment. Surgical thyroidectomy was the choice of a very small group of experts in the United States, Europe, and Japan. To the best of our knowledge, no prospective controlled randomized trial has provided rigorous data with which to select scientifically among the three alternative forms of treatment. No strictly validated form of treatment can account for these differences. Grave's disease in the United States, Europe, and Japan is presumably the same disease.

A variety of social forces shape and often dictate the utilization of various management modalities. One obvious force is money. Medicine during the past 25 years has undergone extensive commercialization. The income derived directly or indirectly from various procedures and treatments influences the frequency of use. Thus, the $2 billion per year spent for pulmonary artery catheters[5] is a potent force increasing its utilization (see below). Positron emission scanning (PET) is being promoted as a screening test for coronary artery disease. Does anyone doubt the key role of profit-making in motivating the promoters?

However, it is an oversimplification to regard money as the sole social driving force. Prestige, power, acclaim, tradition, and competition are also potent driving forces in our society. Medicine is by no means exempt. In a general way, medical systems are subject to the same forces that mold the rest of society. Risk-benefit perceptions in medicine are influenced by the same social forces that drive society generally.

GENERAL ELEMENTS OF MEDICAL RISK-BENEFIT ANALYSIS

It is important to emphasize that the objective of minimizing risks and maximizing benefits should be improved patient welfare rather than the surrogate criteria that are often employed.[6] The fact that a given agent may reduce atheromatous deposits in coronary arteries does not establish that the use of the agent will reduce the probability of an acute myocardial infarction either in individual patients or in the population.[7] This consideration leads to an important principle. Analyses of efficacy and safety of clinical interventions should be based on (patient or population) outcome analysis.

It also leads to a simple but useful definition of a medical risk. A medical risk is a potential effect of a medical intervention that adversely affects either the quantity of life or the quality of life, or both, for indi-

vidual patients or for populations of patients. A medical benefit is a potential effect of a medical intervention that improves either the quantity of life or the quality of life, or both.

It is important to recognize that risks and benefits are inextricably interwoven and that rational decision-making requires some estimate of a risk-benefit ratio. For example, as benefits become smaller and smaller, the risk-benefit ratio becomes larger and larger; when benefit is zero, the risk-benefit ratio is infinite. When the benefit is zero, no risk, however small, is justified. Unfortunately, in the absence of data obtained from prospective randomized controlled clinical trials, an accurate and quantitative estimate of the risk-benefit ratio for a given intervention is not possible.

In general, understanding or evaluating medical risks has been a long-neglected and underemphasized aspect of medicine. It is of interest that conventional syntheses of medical history focus on medical advances, thus giving the impression that medical history consists simply of an unbroken string of successes.

Clinical epidemiology has devised the terms *type 1* and *type 2 errors* to describe failures, in an effort to assess accurately the benefits of various medical modalities.[8] Only recently have the terms *type 3* and *type 4 errors* been devised to describe accurately failures to assess the risks of various medical interventions.[9]

Medical school curricula, postgraduate medical education, and, in particular, subspecialty medical training rarely emphasize the nature and frequency of medical risks. An important concept in understanding the nature of medical risks is the concept of excess mortality or excess morbidity related to medical intervention. This concept involves a quantitative estimate of the mortality or morbidity that may result from the use of a medical intervention whose net impact on patient outcome is deleterious. Operationally, the existence of excess mortality or morbidity can only be determined by an adequate controlled trial, so that the intrinsic mortality or morbidity of a given disease is estimated from the control group and subtracted from the mortality or morbidity found in the experimental (treated) group. Given the fact that patients may die or do poorly as a result of the natural life history of their disease, without a clinical trial, excess mortality or morbidity tends to be undetectable (unless the values are dramatic). For example, the dramatic excess mortality related to the use of the antiarrhythmic agents flecainide and encainide was not even suspected until the performance of an adequate clinical trial (see pp. 12–16).

Medicine as a whole is subject to the process of cultural lag. Cultural lag is the failure of one aspect of a cultural complex to keep pace with changes in social or scientific progress. Some patients are still being treated with specific antiarrhythmic drugs for innocent ventricular ectopy despite convincing evidence that the risk-benefit ratio involved may be sharply unfavorable.[10]

A major problem associated with the evaluation of risks involves the fact that overt complications frequently occur long (months to years) after the management modality has been used. For example, the carcinogenic effects of diethylstilbestrol (DES) used to "prevent" spontaneous abortions resulted in genital carcinoma to the offspring of the treated mothers.[11] The carcinogenic effects of low-level diagnostic x-rays require years to be manifested.[12]

Late complications of management modalities are usually not detected by even adequate PRCCTs. The negative effect of the invention must be dramatic and must involve large numbers before the risk becomes obvious.

IATROEPIDEMICS AND OTHER FORMS OF MEDICAL RISK

An *iatroepidemic* is a systematic preventable medical error introduced and widely practiced that produces harm or death to masses of patients. In brief, an iatroepidemic is a plague caused by physicians.

Analysis of iatroepidemics can be used as a probe to examine the prevalence, cause, and prevention of needless harm to patients and thus provide a useful tool for improving patient outcome. Almost no specialty in medicine, nor in all of medicine as a system, appears to be immune.[6,13–16]

Iatroepidemics differ from other causes of patient harm. Iatrogenic accidents are random individual accidents that affect patients during medical care that cause harm independent of the natural life history of their disease. These are random events. Examples include wrong doses of drugs given to patients and nosocomial infections introduced during medical care.

Iatroepidemics also differ from gross errors in physician judgment or gross defects in physician character. All three causes of medical error occur as more or less random, unpredictable events. The essential element of iatroepidemics is that they are not inevitable. They could—and should—be prevented. Iatroepidemics differ from medical progress in that the latter depends on data, ideas, approaches, and concepts not available at the time that a given medical intervention was introduced and implemented.

Did the failure to use thrombolytic therapy for acute myocardial infarction 20 years ago constitute an iatroepidemic? Of course not. The availability of effective thrombolytic agents depended on data and concepts that were not available at that time. By our

definition, the harm caused by a true iatroepidemic could have been anticipated and prevented at some point along the way.

BENEFITS VERSUS RISKS OF PROSPECTIVE RANDOMIZED CONTROLLED CLINICAL TRIALS

Accepting as axiomatic that PRCCTs provide the most valid approach to estimating benefits versus risks of medical practices, it is useful to analyze the benefits versus risks of PRCCTs themselves. One interesting characteristic of such trials is that the net risk benefit ratio of any trial depends on whether the modality being evaluated ultimately turns out to be effective. For specific modalities that turn out to be highly effective, a PRCCT could delay the use of beneficial treatments or tests in substantial numbers of patients. For specific modalities that have either little benefit or unacceptable risks, or both, the PRCCT should protect large numbers of patients from injury. In the present period, with a high rate of introduction of new technologies and medical science, it is probable that delays inherent in subjecting new approaches to PRCCT on balance act to improve patient outcome.

The major benefit of a PRCCT is simply this: it provides the most objective and rigorous approach for evaluating the management modalities in clinical practice. Thus, the trial provides the gold standard to evaluate medical interventions.

PRCCTs can provide a unique mechanism for uncovering medical risks that would otherwise not be detectable. Assume that a given drug is used to treat a disorder with significant given intrinsic mortality. The deaths of patients receiving the drug tend to be accepted as part of the natural history of the disease. By comparing the mortality in the placebo treated group with the mortality in the experimental group, excess mortality can be detected and quantitated. If the drug in question has a dramatic effect in increasing mortality, a PRCCT may not be required to detect excess mortality.

The control group in PRCCT can provide valuable insights into the natural life history of a given disease process. For example, the mortality per year of patients with ventricular premature beats not treated with antiarrhythmic agents provides useful data on the mortality of ventricular ectopy in the general population (see p. 14).

Clinical trials can provide rigorous data about the risks of various procedures, such as surgery or invasive diagnostic methods. Such trials can also provide rigorous data about the validity of noninvasive procedures. A clinical trial designed to study the efficacy of throm bolytic therapy in the treatment of pulmonary embolism provided convincing evidence about the dubious benefits of ventilation scanning in that disorder.[17]

The results of PRCCTs can provide clues concerning pathogenetic mechanisms. For example, it appears that patients with early cancer of the colon treated with megadoses of vitamin C have a shorter survival than colon cancer patients not receiving vitamin C.[18] If confirmed in a larger trial, the finding that vitamin C increases mortality in early colon cancer would provide an important lead concerning the metabolic requirements of cancer cells.

Potential errors associated with clinical trials are described along with potential risks, in this discussion. The rationale is that significant errors lead to incorrect conclusions, hence to incorrect management of patients. A number of potential risks and potential errors are associated with PRCCTs. One risk is that the subjects included in either the control group or the experimental group could be harmed. Assume that a given form of therapy ultimately proves effective. Clearly, the patients in the control group have been deprived of a beneficial form of treatment for a period of time. Assume that a given form of therapy is without benefit or ultimately has significant risks. In this case, the subjects in the experimental group have been exposed to the risks without the possibility of benefit. Neither physicians nor the general public are likely to appreciate the fact that volunteers participating in a clinical trial are performing acts of high social value and often, indeed, acts of heroism. Nor are their sacrifices generally acknowledged.

The use of invasive therapeutic procedures and diagnostic procedures involves the intrinsic risks of such procedures. The dangers of such risks are particularly troublesome when these procedures are performed solely to obtain data and have little to do with decision-making to benefit individual patients. For example, performing several coronary angiograms (per patient) to determine the impact of a given intervention on coronary artery disease carries the risk of death in 1/1,000 to 5/1,000 performed.[19] The occurrence of individual deaths during such clinical trials is a near-certain consequence.

Unfortunately, errors in the design, implementation, and interpretation of the results of PRCCT are common. The design of the study might not ensure that the patients being studied are typical of those encountered in the clinical setting. For example, the accuracy of cardiac Thallium scanning was evaluated in normals and in patients with mild coronary artery disease. Thallium scanning was found to be highly sensitive and specific in the evaluation of myocardial perfusion. Several years later, in a repeat study, when the population being tested included patients with well-established coronary artery disease with low ejection fractions and failing left ventricles, the specificity of the test was found to be about 50%, an unacceptably low value. This well-known error in experimental design is known as a comparison of "the sickest of the sick with the wellest of the well."[20]

CLINICAL TRIALS AND ERRORS

Trials are commonly designed without outcome analysis as the criterion to be evaluated. Outcome analysis asks the question: What is the impact of the given intervention on the length of survival or quality of life? Rather, surrogate criteria are used, often followed by unwarranted extrapolation of the results to presumed patient outcome.

A study investigates the effect of combined colestipol-niacin therapy on coronary atherosclerosis and coronary venous grafts.[7] Angiographic evidence of some reperfusion was found in about 14% of the lesions studied for 2 years. This is all very interesting scientifically, but the outcome question is whether fewer of these patients suffered myocardial infarction or death. The study provides no answer to the question "Did the patient (as opposed to the arteries) benefit from the treatment?" Incidentally, the risks of colestipol-niacin therapy were largely ignored. In a study by Rossouw and Rifkin[21] involving nicotinic acid, a reduction in coronary artery deaths but a significant increase in noncardiac deaths was found.

Implementation errors appear to be common. If the investigators reporting on a specific therapy have a preconceived bias about the probable usefulness of their therapy, then the results can be described in ways that favor that therapy. One hundred and five patients undergo extracranial-intracranial bypass for intracranial internal carotid artery stenosis.[22] Morbidity and mortality after surgery and during a mean follow-up of 54 months are reported. Seventy-three of 82 survivors had no further stroke or transient ischemic attack after surgery, an impressive positive result. A major focus of the study was the patency rate of the bypass itself, a surrogate criterion to be sure.

The fatal flaw in the report, however, is the absence of a control group. The authors, instead, compared their 105 patients to previously reported outcomes from medical therapy and thereby managed to make EC/IC appear effective in managing intracranial internal carotid artery stenosis. When a PRCCT was performed, it became obvious that the surgery was not effective; indeed, the net effect was patient harm.[23] Patients experiencing a TIA or stroke tend to improve afterwards, whether treated surgically or not. On close analysis of all patients from the same trial, it became clear that patients in both the operated and the unoperated groups improved. Patients who were spared surgery, however, improved faster. Thus, in the category of mortality, surgical treatment offered no benefit; in the category of functional improvement, surgical therapy caused net harm.[23A]

Extracranial-intracranial anastomosis for cerebrovascular disease is now largely discredited.

During the course of a clinical trial involving surgery in the experimental group, 22 of 401 patients (5.5%) selected at random to undergo the surgical procedure refused permission for the operation. However, these patients were counted in the statistical analysis as having undergone surgery.[24] In reality, they were either part of the control group or should properly have been omitted from the study. Obviously these patients were not exposed to the risks of surgery and thus the estimate of surgical complications was erroneously low.

If the outcome of the 22 patients was favorable, the surgery would have been considered more effective than was accurate. If the 22 patients fared worse than the experimental group, the experimental group actually did better than was estimated.

A common error committed in clinical trials conducted in hospitals or clinics is a difference in the level of care afforded the control versus the experimental group of patients. In some trials, the patients in the experimental group are monitored more carefully and thoughtfully than are the control patients. Often, however, the problem of integrating the care provided by the experimenters with the care provided by the physicians caring for the patients detracts from patient care. If the study is conducted in a double-blind fashion, such problems may be minimal.

Basic interpretive errors fall into two groups: errors involved with evaluating benefits and errors involved with evaluating risks. Type 1 errors are false-positive errors that assign statistical benefit to a given modality when such benefit does not exist. Type 2 errors are false-negative errors. The observed distinction is regarded as not significant (no benefit), whereas in reality a benefit exists. Type 2 errors can arise in circumstances in which n values are too small and a higher n value would be required to demonstrate statistically significant benefit. The terms type 1 and type 2 often are used qualitatively to connote false-positive and false-negative results arising from clinical trials.[8]

Type 3 errors are underestimates or represent a failure to detect the statistical risks of screening, diagnostic, preventive, or therapeutic interventions.[9] Type 3 errors generally fall into one of three categories.

Type 3A errors involve a failure to study adequate numbers of patients to detect risks. An example of a type 3A error is a recent randomized controlled clinical trial to evaluate the use of hyperbaric oxygen as a treatment of osteoradionecrosis of the mandible. The data show that the rate of successful treatment is higher in the (air-treated) control subjects than in the group treated with hyperbaric oxygen. However, the number of patients in each group is small, and the difference between the two groups is of borderline significance (Ingle R, Jr: personal communication). The problem is not trivial. If, indeed, there is risk with treatment, the issues are quite different than if there is no statistical evidence of efficacy. If hyperbaric oxygen in this disease impairs healing, the clinical use of hyperbaric oxygen in osteoradionecrosis should be interdicted. A significant group difference would also have important biologic (mechanistic) implications. It would suggest that hyperbaric oxygen may interfere with tissue healing by an unknown mechanism. Obviously a clinical trial with a higher n value is required to determine whether impaired wound healing is a reality.

Type 3B errors involve failures to look for or detect specific risks in an experimental versus a control group. For example, the use of pulmonary artery flow-directed catheters (Swan-Ganz) produces pathologic evidence of direct injury to the endocardium of the right ventricle in a high percentage of subjects: the battered endocardium syndrome.[25] Without suitable autopsies of an adequate number of control (no catheter) versus experimental (catheterized) subjects, the quantitative nature of this risk cannot be assessed. The use of the catheter is also associated with difficulties in interpretation of the data obtained by its use. In turn, interpretive errors can have a negative impact on patient outcome.[26] Failure to include these interpretive errors in an analysis of outcome will underestimate the true risks of the catheter.

Type 3C errors involve delayed risks in which the harm to subjects occurs months to years after the initial use of the modality. As a result, the risk-benefit ratio of the modality is seriously underestimated. For example, screening normal schoolchildren for scoliosis is widely practiced on an international basis and is mandated by law in some states in the United States. After an initial screening by physical examination, subjects with an apparent positive result undergo a series of radiographic examinations of the spine for verification of the diagnosis, for monitoring the rate of progression with time, and for monitoring the effects of various treatments by bracing or by surgery. The number of spinal radiographs involved can be very large. In one pilot study, an average of 46 films per treated patient were taken.[27] This is a population of young children known to be especially sensitive to the carcinogenic effects of low-level radiation. In a recent case control study women radiographed for scoliosis several decades before showed an increased incidence of breast cancer.[28] There is little question that within a 20- to 30-year period, an unknown number of patients will suffer an excess prevalence of leukemia and cancer of the breast, and the children of screened pregnant women will have birth defects as a result of screening. Because these complications are a delayed risk, they are not factored appropriately into the overall risk-benefit analysis of the value of screening for scoliosis.

Type 4 errors are those caused by an overestimate of risks leading to the abandonment of a given medical intervention. This type of error was previously called the "tomato" effect.[29] While a staple of the European diet during the sixteenth century, tomatoes were actively shunned in North America until the nineteenth century because practically everyone in North America "knew" that the tomato was poisonous. This "knowledge" obviously was based on an inadequate clinical trial.

During the late 1960s, the potential role of aspirin in preventing coronary thrombosis was anticipated. During the 1970s, hope dissipated because a number of inadequate clinical trials showed only a slightly beneficial effect, so that the risks of aspirin prophylaxis seemed to exceed the benefits.[30] It now appears that low-dose aspirin is effective in patients with overt atherosclerosis in preventing subsequent myocardial infarction or stroke. Low-dose aspirin also has a favorable risk-benefit ratio as prophylaxis against myocardial infarction in males 50 years of age or greater.[31] If so, the failure to use aspirin generally during the 1970s represents a type 4 error. It should be emphasized that type 3 errors appear to be much more frequent than type 4 errors. This stems, in part, from the failure of medicine to establish effective mechanisms for the rapid recognition and correction of errors.

A number of errors stem from the misuse of statistical methods. Selecting an incorrect or inappropriate statistical method for analyzing data appears to be common. One study suggests that approximately 75% of the statistical analyses provided in the medical literature are flawed.[32]

A common error is to perform subgroup analysis on the data obtained from a clinical trial in an effort to find significant statistical differences in some subgroups that will yield a positive, rather than a negative, result. As significance analyses are estimates of probability, it is usually possible to come up with some positive results simply on the basis of random chance. A study originally designed to determine the impact of cholesterol-lowering surgery on coronary artery disease finds that there is a statistically significant effect on some tests dealing with peripheral vascular disease. This is published as evidence that the surgery is effective. The fact that there is no significant difference in patients with respect to coronary artery disease and cerebrovascular disease is played down or ignored.[24]

A form of "significance boosting" involves the pooling of data from several independent studies, none of which shows a significant difference between controls and experimentals. This can be done in a primitive fashion by simple data pooling.[33] Or this can be attempted by a formal type of statistical analysis called meta analysis.[34] As probability calculations depend on the number of observations, significance boosting may provide a claim for efficacy that cannot otherwise be justified.

Two institutionalized cultural forms are conceptually similar to meta-analysis. One is the so-called consensus conference and the other expert policy statements on various aspects of medical management generated by a committee and issued under the sponsorship of various professional groups. In each, a group of "experts" convenes to consider a given area in medicine and to generate a statement that reflects the state of the art.

The use of such guides to management usually overlooks several important problems. Experts without adequate rigorous data are not experts at all. They are a group of humans expressing mere opinions. The summation of these opinions, therefore, pools not only experience, special knowledge, and careful reflection but also ignorance and prejudice. Whether this pooling produces an arithmetic or an exponential summation of ignorance and prejudice probably varies from one specific group to another. As a rule, such groups are usually benefit oriented and pay scant attention to the risks involved in a given intervention.

Consensus statements tend to be frozen in time. Once the statement is issued, little attention is given to revisions, even when new data make the original statement no longer tenable. Minority views and disagreements are not provided much, if any, weight. Without organized feedback, amends cannot be made for serious errors as they become apparent. Using consensus conferences or organizational edicts as guidelines for medical decision-making can place patients in jeopardy.

Occasionally those responsible for conducting clinical trials use a rather questionable approach for a study in which the statistical analysis reveals that the outcome in the experimental group is not statistically different from the outcome in the controls. However, the mean value is more favorable. The workers inflate the nonsignificant difference to the status of a positive result. The nonsignificant result is elevated to a favorable outcome in the discussion and summary section of the final publication that supports the intervention that has been studied. This is a common ploy in studies performed by groups that have a prior conviction that the intervention has a highly favorable risk-benefit ratio. It can be a useful method designed to soften the impact of having spent millions of dollars or of being responsible for the loss of some lives in performing a clinical trial that ultimately showed marginal results at best.

A common misuse of PRCCT is the inclusion of a promissory note in publications that pledges to organize such a trial in the future or at least emphasize the desirability of such a trial to test the clinical validity of whatever is claimed.

For example, in the heat of a journal exchange in 1988, an advocate of aggressive therapy for primary pulmonary hypertension states "We did not consider the therapy 'successful' but rather suggested that further studies evaluating the long-term effects are necessary before a decision concerning its utility are necessary and before a decission concerning its utility could be made. He [Dr. Robin] may be interested to know that several such studies (PRCCT) are underway or in development."[35] In 1992, the world is still waiting.

One problem is that adequate clinical trials require substantial expertise in design, implementation, and interpretation of PRCCT. In addition, substantial resources must be mobilized and expended. It is far easier to promise a trial than to carry a suitable trial through to its conclusion.

CLINICAL TRIALS AND ETHICS

A common objection to the organization of controlled clinical trials is that to conduct one is "unethical." The physicians involved in a given modality somehow know the risk-benefit ratio of a given modality is strongly favorable, and it would therefore be unethical to deprive the control group of the benefits of the modality so that a PRCCT could be performed. Some of the general characteristics of this dependence on ethics are instructive. It is not considered unethical to treat patients without adequate proof that such treatment is both safe and effective. The basis of such an approach represents an aberration of the old Cartesian dictum, *ego cogito ergo sum*: "I think, therefore I am."[36] These ethically driven physicians seem to feel *ego credo ergo sait*: "I believe, therefore it must be."

The ethical analysis frequently corresponds to a conclusion that is beneficial to the ethicist in terms of money or prestige, and so forth. Self-interest is, of course, not uncommonly a key determinant of ethical dogma.

Several examples illustrate the general point. American devotees of the use of hyperbaric oxygen for the treatment of various diseases are engaged in a soul-searching debate. Should they continue a PRCCT to test whether hyperbaric oxygen is efficacious in the treatment of carbon monoxide poisoning? To do so would be to deprive some patients of a life-saving form of treatment.[37] This profound concern with patient outcome occurs at a time when a carefully executed PRCCT trial in France has already demonstrated that hyperbaric oxygen treatment offers no benefit to carbon monoxide patients over those resulting from oxygen inhalation at ambient barometric pressure.[38]

According to one group of users of pulmonary artery flow-directed catheters[39]:

> Naturally, the question arises: Why has the randomized study not been done? The answer is obvious. Ethically, my colleagues and I do not want to deny the benefits of a PA catheter to a patient in a shock state. Until a safe, reliable, good technique is available and acceptable to the medical community, what should we do? Should we go back to the unreliable, inconsistent clinical examination techniques and change therapy randomly? Many physicians may be reluctant to do so or to wait for a prospective randomized trial.

As they believe that they somehow know that the catheter is needed, how can they in good conscience support an appropriate trial?

This reasoning is extended further by the pulmonary artery catheter group who, having established that 47% of the most highly trained catheter users cannot pass an examination dealing with its use and interpretations, urge a licensing process to weed out the users of a device whose safety and efficacy has by their admission not been adequately tested.[40] An editorialist commenting on the performance of those tested urges PRCCT for new technologies but not for the catheter itself.[41]

Several conclusions can be stated about the general desirability of PRCCT:

1. Only a small percentage of correct medical practice has been critically evaluated by PRCCT. This fact should lead to great humility about the secure basis of much of current medical practice.

2. There is a growing awareness among physicians that an adequate scientific base for medicine requires such trials. This is confirmed by the ever growing number of articles in the medical literature reporting such trials involving various aspects of medical practice.

3. PRCCT provided the most scientific and acceptable approach to determine the balance between risks and benefits of medical practice.

4. Like all other aspects of medical practice, PRCCTs are not free from risks, but the benefits exceed the risks, so that the risk-benefit ratio of PRCCTs is highly favorable.

5. Like all other aspects of medical science and medical practice, the design of such trials, the implementation of such trials, and above all the interpretations of the results of such trials require critical, unbiased and thoughtful evaluation.

These are contentious times. Therefore, it is not surprising that there are now self-serving obscurantist assaults on the general idea of PRCCTs. Such a recent article uses pseudophilosophical arguments to buttress the assault[42]; outcome analysis that seeks to determine the efficacy or safety of a given medical intervention is discredited as a form of utilitarianism.[42] This extrapolation suggests there is something magical about the job description of a physician that is divorced from efforts to improve either the quantity or the quality of life. John Stuart Mills, the founder of utilitarianism who proposed the goal "the greatest happiness of the greatest numbers," would spin in his grave at the philosophical vulgarization.

CURRENT IATROEPIDEMICS

The identification of current iatroepidemics is obviously more important than identification of those that occurred in the past. Doing something about current iatroepidemics should provide rapid improvements in patient outcome. Analyzing those that occurred in the past, while useful and educational, cannot undo harm that has already occurred.

The following analyses use a number of approaches that are not conventionally employed in medical risk-benefit analysis. Some understanding of these is also required for accurate risk assessment. These approaches include:

Contemporary Critical Medical History

In order to understand the causes and miscalculations that give rise to systematic medical errors, it is useful to review the temporal events and the thinking that gave rise to the systematic error. Such a review leans heavily on contemporaneous medical literature related to the given modality. For readers lacking extensive experience with historical analysis, some of its risks and benefits might be summarized.

An important benefit of analyzing contemporary medical history is that the analysis can provide insight into the thinking and data that gave rise to a given medical practice. Analyzing the background of the use of encainide/flecainide clearly shows the errors that led to multiple preventable deaths (see below). Such an analysis facilitates a process by which the nature and kind of errors can be used to prevent similar errors in the future. Contemporary medical history, if recorded, ensures that there is a record of what occurred at a given point in time. Such a record is particularly important for medical history, a discipline that until now has tended to emphasize past triumphs and to ignore past errors. Conventional medical history appropriately hails the introduction of insulin into the treatment of diabetes mellitus. One must return to long outdated medical literature to realize that arsenic salts were once used to treat diabetes.[42] It is no longer possible to determine the morbidity and mortality associated with that treatment.

A major benefit of contemporary historical analysis

is that much of history is never recorded and, with the passage of time, is simply lost. Much of contemporary history resembles the mythical tree in the forest that falls unobserved. Its falling has no impact on the future course of events.

The rhetorical question, "what will history say of a given form of practice?," more accurately should ask "what might history have said?" because there is substantial probability that the events surrounding that practice will be lost to recorded history. Conventional history as opposed to contemporary history is more prone to human prejudice. The written history of World War II would have been quite different if the Axis forces had won.

Contemporary history also has its risks. The passage of time can provide perspective and balance to an analysis of specific events. Contemporary medical history is probably more subject to analyst prejudice and bias.

In a superb contemporary history of ultrasound,[43] Oakley quoted various public figures on history as follows:

> In Ulysses, James Joyce wrote, "History is a nightmare from which I am trying to awake."[44] Thomas Carlyle said, "The history of the world is but the biography of greedy men."[45] Historian Edward Gibbon complained that history "[is] little more than the register of the crimes, follies, and misfortunes of mankind"[46] while Henry Ford, being a practical soul, simply described history as "bunk."[47] Finally, the German philosopher Hegel is said to have reflected sensibly: "What experience and history teach is this—that people and governments never have learned anything from history, or acted on principles deduced from it."[48]

These opinions may be overly pessimistic.

Despite its risks, we believe that contemporary historical analysis provides a useful insight into iatroepidemics. In particular, contemporary historical analysis can answer such questions as, "Was a given iatroepidemic preventable or not?" As a result, we have used contemporary critical historical analysis extensively.

Relationship of Prognosis To Risk-Benefit Analysis

A fundamental medical decision involves the relation between the risks of a disease versus the risks of a medical intervention. This ancient problem was recognized by Hippocrates, when he stated that "desperate diseases require desperate measures."[49] Unfortunately many modern intensivists do not recognize the converse: "nondesperate diseases require nondesperate measures."

A modern extension of the Hippocratic dictum is that translation of a given risk-benefit ratio into medical management requires an accurate estimate of the risks of nontreatment or nonmanagement. Given, for example, an infection like HIV with a bleak prognosis, the use of relatively untested therapies even with high toxicity is rational. Using similar hazardous agents to treat self-limited infections is, of course, not rational. As a result, a given risk-benefit ratio characterizing a given test or treatment may lead to different decisions for one disease as compared with another disease.

It is not generally recognized that current estimates of prognosis are often based on empirical, anecdotal, unreliable, impressionistic data. As a result, widely accepted estimates of prognosis may be grossly erroneous. This in turn may lead to interventions that are, so to speak, "worse than the disease" to be treated or prevented. Errors in the evaluation of prognosis can be positive (more years survival estimated than accurate) or negative (fewer years survival than estimated).

There are, of course, intrinsic difficulties in establishing an accurate statistical prognosis for a given disease state for groups of patients or a specific estimate for individual patients. There may be considerable variations between the onset of a given disease and the time the illness is diagnosed. Patients presenting themselves to academic centers may have far-advanced disease and the milder variant of the same disease may not impact on conventional estimates of prognosis. There may be considerable changes in prognosis with time or treatment, or both. Since 1977, the mortality of bronchial asthma has increased progressively (see p. 26). The prognosis for the disease now is slightly but significantly worse than 15 years ago.[50] As a result of such problems, there are major errors in current estimates of prognosis.

There are at least two approaches to improve accuracy of prognosis estimates. One is to use the control (placebo) group in a PRCCT to estimate the untreated natural life history of a given disease. The second approach is to organize prospective ongoing, long-term clinical studies of untreated patients using the same precautions involving homogeneity of patient selection as those used in conventional PRCCT of various therapies or tests. Such studies have major difficulties because it may be required to withhold therapy from patients, an unacceptable practice if the therapy has substantial efficacy.

The bottom lines are that (1) medical estimates of prognosis even as a range of values are frequently inaccurate, (2) cardiologists should attempt to evaluate critically prognostic estimates that they use in guiding therapy, and (3) approaches to improving the accuracy of prognostic estimates should be more widely used.

Social Anthropology and Archeology

It is generally unappreciated that many forms of medical management are rooted in similar approaches by primitive societies. Understanding the re-

lationship of a given intervention to its anthropologic antecedents may clarify current understanding of the practice. Primitive societies had and have a belief in the value of positive magic and negative magic (taboo). Positive magic consists of a rite or practice to improve the probability of a favorable outcome; in medical terms, that is to improve efficacy or reduce risks or both.[51] Negative magic consists of avoidance of certain practices to improve efficacy and/or reduce risks. Cholesterol avoidance, for example, can be analyzed usefully as a form of negative magic (see below).

Sociological Factors

The form of a given society and its norms of social behavior can have profound effects on specific forms of medical behavior. For example, our society emphasizes the importance of economic rewards. It is not surprising that much of current medical practice is driven by commercial pressures. An example is the proposal to introduce positron emission tomography (PET) scanning for coronary artery disease. There is essentially no evidence that the use of PET scanning will improve survival from coronary artery disease. It is clear, however, that screening the normal population will generate large sums of money.

Legal-Medical Interactions

The legal system, especially the processes making up tort (personal injury) law, can have profound effects on the forms that medical practice takes. Physicians frequently ascribe current tendencies to overtest or overtreat to "defensive medicine," practices designed to avoid lawsuits.

Analysis of Cultural Lag, Cultural Arrest, and Cultural Regression

Cultural lag is the failure of social systems to keep pace with advances in science. Fourteen years ago, substantial doubts about ventilation scanning in the diagnosis of pulmonary embolism were raised.[52] Eight years ago, it was demonstrated that ventilation lung scans lack adequate specificity for acceptable management of the diagnosis of pulmonary embolism in most patients.[53] Despite yet another recent demonstration of this fact,[54] ventilation scanning continues to be widely practiced.

Cultural arrest is the failure of a social system to change despite the existence of overwhelming objective evidence that a given practice does not conform to reality. For example, an impression survives that accumulation of data on patients, independent of the impact of data on patient outcome, is firmly rooted in cardiology.[55] Cultural regression is the process of using approaches that contradict current scientific information. As a result of cultural lag, cultural arrest, and cultural regression, medicine is exceedingly slow in correcting errors, even mass errors. Limitations of our own knowledge will not permit the application of all these approaches to each of the iatroepidemics described herein.

CURRENT IATROEPIDEMICS INVOLVING CARDIOVASCULAR DISEASE

In some of the examples that follow, the data are available with which to categorize the sequence of events indubitably as an iatroepidemic. In other examples, the identification of a management modality as an iatroepidemic involves a subjective judgment on our part.

Encainide-Flecainide Disaster

The administration of two antiarrhythmic drugs, encainide and flecainide, has resulted in about 6,200 excess, unnecessary, and preventable deaths for every 100,000 near-normal postmyocardial infarction patients treated with these agents on a long-term prophylactic basis. Almost certainly, more than 100,000 of such patients have been treated, so that the absolute number of deaths is probably 7,000 or more. The term *excess death* refers to the difference in mortality between placebo (untreated) patients and those treated with these agents. An accurate estimate of excess mortality and excess morbidity usually requires a PRCCT.

The entire sequence of events involving the two drugs is a mass disaster and therefore an iatroepidemic. By comparison with the encainide-flecainide disaster, about 3,300 people died as a result of accidental poisoning at Bhopal, India. The latter disaster appropriately evoked universal horror and indignation. The encainide-flecainide disaster by contrast, was reported in seven paragraphs on page 9 of *The New York Times*.[78]

The excess mortality in patients not falling in the category of near-normal postmyocardial infarction receiving either of the drugs short term for tachyarrhythmias is unknown. It is probable that the excess mortality is even higher in such patients. An accurate estimate of the risk in that group of patients would require an independent prospective randomized, controlled clinical trial.

Contemporary Critical Medical History

The problem of arrhythmia following myocardial infarction in patients with increased ventricular irritability has troubled cardiologists for a number of years. Ventricular premature depolarizations are considered a risk factor for sudden or delayed cardiac death following myocardial infarction[49] and are commonly treated with antiarrhythmic drugs.[10] This problem is a component of an even larger problem, sudden death in patients with coronary artery disease, especially those with previous myocardial infarctions.[57–59]

A variety of different oral agents have been administered prophylactically to diminish the risk of sudden death, including quinidine, procainamide, lidocaine, tocainamide, phenytoin, mexiletine, disopyramide, amioderone, apresoline, and moricizene.

The use of oral long-term prophylactic encainide and flecainide was based on a series of extrapolations.

1. postmyocardial infarction ventricular premature beats (VPBs) are a risk factor for sudden death following acute myocardial infarction. Although such an extrapolation is logical, it is not based on a careful comparison of the rate of sudden death in a series of postmyocardial infarction patients without VPBs versus those with persistent VPBs. Without such data, the natural life history of untreated postmyocardial infarction VPBs cannot be accurately assessed. A number of studies that reported such an association are flawed and can hardly be considered as providing rigorous evidence that such an association exists.[57,60,61] None of those studies was adequately controlled, and the causes of death were not rigorously established. However, the "existence" of such a relationship became incorporated into clinical practice.

2. prevention of postmyocardial VPBs by antiarrhythmic drugs would decrease postmyocardial infarction mortality. A large number of studies cast great doubt on this hypothesis.

   Furberg surveyed from the literature a series of randomized, controlled clinical trials conducted during the early hospital phase after an acute myocardial infarction as well as after discharge.[62] All the surveyed trials failed to show improved patient survival with treatment. Included in his analysis were studies of quinidine, procainamide, disopyramide, lidocaine, phenytoin, tocainamide, mexiletine, and amioderone. Given the lack of benefit, he speculated on the causes of lack of efficacy: (1) antiarrhythmic treatment of ventricular arrhythmias does not improve prognosis; (2) treatment of ventricular arrhythmias does prolong life, but benefit has not been observed in the trials; and (3) control of ventricular arrhythmias helps some patients but harms others. His analysis did not include the possibility that the various agents resulted in net harm without corresponding benefit.

   A number of the trials showed that various agents were capable of suppressing ventricular ectopy, but this suppression did not lead to improved survival.[63,64] In a number of the studies the placebo group showed a lower mortality than the treatment group but the number of patients studied were too small to draw firm conclusions.

Given this vast amount of data, several facts are surprising.

1. The failure to show efficacy did not deter most clinicians and experts from the use of antiarrhythmic drugs in postmyocardial infarction patients. Perhaps most clinicians and experts were unaware of the evidence indicating lack of efficacy.
2. No emphasis was given to the possibility that the risk of the drugs was greater than the potential benefit. As a result the experts developed a two-alternative system, either the drug helped or did not help. The third alternative of a highly unfavorable risk-benefit ratio—because of increased risks specifically—was not considered.
3. A number of rigorous clinical trials indicated that one class of drugs, β-adrenergic blockers, did improve mortality after myocardial infarction.[58] β-Adrenergic blockers are not strictly speaking primary antiarrhythmic drugs. Perhaps the efficacy of these led to some confusion.
4. It is possible that adequate clinical trials would have shown (and might now show) excess mortality with the use of most or all antiarrhythmic drugs in addition to encainide and flecainide. Most previous trials were conducted on relatively small groups of patients. It is possible that the true excess mortality associated with the use of antiarrhythmic drugs generally is far larger than the 6,000/100,000 excess deaths associated with encainide-flecainide.
5. The final extrapolation from inadequate data was that prophylactic, long-term treatment with encainide-flecainide in near-normal patients with ventricular ectopy following myocardial infarction improved prognosis.

This hypothesis was a logical extension of hypotheses 1 and 2. Experts were convinced of the beneficial effects of antiarrhythmic therapy in reducing sudden death, and it seemed clear that an ideal agent had not been found. The selection of these two drugs was then a common approach in medicine, the search for the "magic bullet," even though the size or even existence of the target was (is) not known.

Encainide reached the pages of appropriate medical journals in 1979, and became incorporated into medical practice shortly after.[66] Flecainide was introduced into medical practice somewhat later.[67] Both drugs were originally used for short-term treatment of threatening ventricular arrhythmias often during hospitalization for acute myocardial infarction. Their long-term prophylactic use to "prevent" sudden death emerged somewhat later.

The details of Food and Drug Administration (FDA) approval of both drugs are not available (to us), but they undoubtedly included the usual three phases of human testing. Given the ultimate lethal effects of the two drugs it may be concluded that current FDA screening methods were (are) incapable of detecting the risks of such treatment. It is certain that as almost invariably occurs, no prospective randomized controlled clinical trials were performed prior to the introduction and widespread use of both drugs. This suggests that drugs with an excess mortality as high as 6% (or greater) cannot be detected by the current FDA drug-approval system.

Between 1983 and 1990, a series of poorly designed, inadequate studies were published claiming both efficacy and safety either for antiarrhythmic drugs generally or for encainide and flecainide specifically. Graboys et al.[68] treated 123 patients with malignant ventricular arrhythmias with antiarrhythmic drugs for an average of 30 months. Comparison of those treated with encainide showed that survival in this group was similar to that of patients considered drug responsive who were treated with other agents.

Swerdlow et al.[69] studied 239 patients with sustained ventricular tachycardia or acute ventricular fibrillation. Encainide-treated patients seemed to show a lower mortality than did other patients with sustained ventricular tachycardia.

Groups of postmyocardial infarction patients with VPBs, including some with congestive heart failure or coronary artery disease, showed moderate improvement in survival of encainide-treated patients compared with some other groups.[70] Such studies lacked adequate controls. A survey paper written by an employee of the pharmaceutical company marketing encainide could find no subgroup of encainide-treated patients with a mortality greater than published for comparable not-so-treated groups.[71] This same paper was also notable for retrospectively examining 1,245 patients with serious heart disease treated with encainide. The author concludes "The excellent hemodynamic and safety profile of encainide should provide a major advantage over currently available antiarrhythmic drugs."

The same paper also displayed the use of surrogate or indirect criteria to estimate safety. Surrogate criteria are those that do not directly involve quantity of life (mortality) or quality of life. In the case of encainide, the surrogate criteria included estimates that the drug did not accentuate hemodynamic abnormalities, precipitate or accentuate congestive heart failure, or result in proarrhythmic events. Ergo encainide must be safe. Outside consultants were employed by the pharmaceutical company and used retrospective, inadequate methods to "confirm" the efficacy and safety of encainide.[72]

Similar nonrigorous studies concluded that flecainide was both safe and effective. For example, in 15 patients with frequent VPBs "Flecainide was found to be highly effective and well tolerated." Side effects were described as "mild and tolerable."[73]

Another extrapolation crept undetected into clinical practice. This was the use of these agents for prophylactic long-term treatment of post myocardial infarction patients with ventricular ectopy. There is no record that it was considered that there might be a difference in safety and efficacy between the short-term and long-term use of these two drugs.

How widespread is the treatment of ventricular arrhythmia with antiarrhythmic drugs? An interesting study indicated that under some circumstances 80 to 100% of American cardiologists used these agents.[10] A shocking finding of this study is summarized by the investigators as follows:

"At the time of the survey (1990), most cardiologists treated patients with asymptomatic and symptomatic potentially malignant ventricular arrhythmia, although the interim results of the Cardiac Arrhythmias Suppression Trial (CAST) indicate reconsideration for therapy in such patients."

This is a most striking example of cultural lag. Now that the final results of the CAST studies are available with a demonstration of an excess mortality of 6%, it would be interesting to determine the impact of these results on practice habits. One would guess that many cardiologists have not changed their practice habits, a striking example of cultural arrest.

It should be pointed out in this historical survey that one study did appear in 1981, indicating the development of malignant ventricular tachyarrhythmias associated with the use of encainide. Eleven patients showed "toxic" arrhythmias following the use of encainide, two of whom died.[74] This paper did not anticipate the major problems that were to be uncovered and suggested rather that toxicity was found only in seriously compromised patients.

The study that preceded the ultimate CAST study appeared in 1988; this pilot study investigated the feasibility of large-scale clinical trials to evaluate the effect of ventricular arrhythmia suppression with antiarrhythmic drugs on mortality.[75] Four drugs were studied: encainide, flecainide, imipramine, and moricizene. It was recognized that the design of the study provided too few patients to detect differences in mortality or major arrhythmic events. Encainide and flecainide were found to be "effective for treating ventricular arrhythmia after acute myocardial infarction but also were [found to be] safe and well tolerated." The pilot study indicated that an adequate, full blown pro-

spective randomized controlled drug trial was feasible. The study now stands as a warning indicating the dangers of coming to firm conclusions about the results of prospective randomized controlled clinical trials in the absence of adequate numbers of patients studied. The paper committed what has been labeled as a type 3A error, given the small number of patients studied. Five patients would have died in the encainide-flecainide group versus two deaths in the placebo group. Such small numbers could not have permitted firm conclusions. This problem was recognized by the investigators.

This brief and by no means exhaustive review of the contemporary history of the use of encainide-flecainide provides an estimate of how much excess mortality of a drug can be present without detection by the usual approaches to clinical drug evaluation and use. A drug is fatal to 6% or more of the patients to whom it is administered without knowledge of lethality, using methods based on patient surveys, uncontrolled clinical trials, case comparison controls, mega- or mini-anecdotal evidence, clinical evaluations, and expert evaluations. Thus, neither current FDA procedures nor the commonly used clinical evaluative methods by which medical interventions are "validated" are adequate for patient protection.

Turning now to the CAST clinical trial of encainide and flecainide and its results, the study involved 1,498 patients.[76] Of the total, 755 patients received encainide or flecainide and 743 patients received placebo. After a mean follow-up period of 10 months, 69 patients receiving drug died, for a mortality of 8.3%. In the placebo group, 27 of 743 patients died, for a mortality of 2.1%. Excess mortality associated with drug treatment was 6.2% with $p < 0.01$.

The excess mortality associated with the use of the two drugs was not the only surprise. A substantial number of deaths were caused not by arrhythmia but by acute myocardial infarction with shock. Previous investigations of potential drug toxicity of the two agents focusing on proarrhythmias or abnormal hemodynamics would have overlooked approximately 27% of drug-related mortality. Of great interest was the relatively low annual death rate of 2.5% per year in the placebo group. A similar low annual death rate has been demonstrated in a placebo group of patients acting as controls for the effect of partial ileal bypass on mortality in postmyocardial infarction patients.[24]

It is not only certain that the treatment was worse than the disease, but that the untreated disease was less-bad/less-lethal than assumed by the cardiovascular community. The pressure to treat VPBs in postmyocardial infarction patients was badly misplaced despite numerous papers in the literature arguing the reverse. Thus, arguments to test other antiarrhythmic drugs or to persuade other patients to participate in controlled clinical trials of various antiarrhythmic drugs before the prognosis of untreated patients is established do not appear to be valid.

The results of the CAST study revealed other surprises. It has been maintained on the basis of uncontrolled studies that patients with no previous history of sustained ventricular arrhythmias were at very low risk of ventricular arrhythmias or mortality induced by such drugs as encainide and flecainide.[77] The CAST study has shown this to be false. The study also demonstrates that patients are susceptible to death during their entire period of drug exposure and not only during the early period after the drug is started. It appears that the longer the time of treatment, the higher the mortality. This finding has important consequences for all patients that continue to be treated with either drug.

The FDA's reaction was not surprising. An official was quoted in the press as follows[78]: "The drugs are useful for those people who are in a fairly desperate situation. There are a lot of drugs [to treat heart disease] and none of them work all the time. You need a full complement of drugs in that situation."

It should be noted that this statement is defensive. How can one fault the FDA for overlooking one minor aberrant behavior of two drugs that are generally useful and safe? It is hardly necessary to point out that the official has no acceptable data base from which to conclude that encainide and flecainide are safe for the treatment of other subgroups of patients with severe or life-threatening ventricular arrhythmias.

This brings up a subtle but important aspect of risk-benefit analysis. The risk-benefit ratio depends not on the value of the risk and not on the value of the benefit but on the ratio of the two. Critically ill patients with malignant ventricular tachycardia might show a favorable risk-benefit ratio from the use of the two drugs because the risk the disease is greater than the risk of the treatment. The value of permissible complications from various interventions depends on the value of the risks of untreated disease. To paraphrase Hippocrates, "desperate diseases require desperate treatment."[49] However, without appropriate rigorous data, patient welfare is not served by guesses. Too often, nondesperate diseases are treated with desperate measures.

The CAST investigators are to be congratulated for performing what should turn out to be a life-saving study. In particular, the fact that an independent monitoring group surveyed the data on an ongoing basis is highly commendable. Termination of the study when it was established that the drugs were unsafe saved lives. But there are also serious questions about the conduct of the study. As data accumulated suggesting excess mortality, were the patient volunteers who were still in the study notified that they might be taking a lethal drug? The CAST study continues investigating the risk-benefit ratio of another antiarrhythmic drug, moricizine. Have the patients in the experimental group taking moricizine been clearly notified that some of them might die as a result of their participation in that study? Have the families of the individual patients that died during the encainide-flecainide trial been notified that their death might have been caused by the drugs given during the trial? To what extent has an attempt been made to notify families of all post-myocardial infarction patients treated with the drugs and now deceased that their deaths may have been iatrogenic? How certain is it that all physicians (i.e., cardiologists) are sufficiently informed of the risks of these agents to ensure that no additional patients will die needlessly? Would not a moratorium in the use of these drugs be a better approach to prevent additional needless deaths than the routine way of notifying doctors with no assurance that the message has been received and heeded?

This brings up the issue of legal liability for the preventable deaths caused by encainide and flecainide. Do the two pharmaceutical houses that manufacture and market the drugs have any legal responsibility? Surely after August 10, 1989, the date of publication of the preliminary report of the CAST study, the legal system might question whether pharmaceutical houses, organized cardiology, and individual physicians reacted suitably to prevent further needless deaths. If there is excess mortality with the use of moricizine who, if anyone, should be held legally responsible? Will trial lawyers representing victims even learn that these important questions of tort law are involved in the encainide-flecainide disaster?

The above caveat on the use of moricizine was written before the data obtained by the CAST trial on this drug was made public. DuPont Pharmaceuticals[79] reported that the NHLBI discontinued its PRCCT of moricizine "due to unfavorable trends (i.e., translation: excess mortality) having evolved and to the remote likelihood of showing net benefit in reducing sudden cardiac death with continued therapy. Further evaluation of the data is being conducted by the CAST II investigation" (i.e., more near-normal patients will die preventable deaths from the use of moricizine).

The communication continues "moricizine is indicated for the treatment of documented ventricular arrhythmias, such as sustained ventricular tachycardia, that in the judgment of the physician are life-threatening. . . ." (i.e., we'll not give up our investment in this drug until a PRCCT is completed on such patients in 3 to 5 years—or more—unless the legal system catches up with us before then).

Benefits of the Prospective Randomized Controlled Clinical Trial

It may be useful to list formally the benefits of having organized such a trial and having implemented it:

1. It appears from the study that there are no net benefits from the two drugs in patients who have asymptomatic premature beats.
2. The study determined that the net risks of the use of these drugs in that patient group are very high. It is doubtful that without the trial, the risks of sudden death would have ever been detected; and thus it is probable that treated patients would have continued to die needlessly.
3. The results of the trial should and probably will save the lives of thousands of future patients.
4. The CAST study uncovered a new and unsuspected cause of death in patients treated with antiarrhythmic drugs, the development of shock and myocardial infarction.
5. The results of the trial raise the issue as to the accurate degree of risk of VPBs in patients who are postmyocardial infarction. It is our contention that the risks of ventricular ectopy in this setting have been grossly overestimated. This exaggeration has lead in turn to extensive overtreatment and excess mortality in treated cohorts. This opinion is largely based on the low rate of death in the placebo group.
6. If there has been an extensive overestimate of the true risks of VPBs in these patients, it is probable that no long-term treatment for VPBs in postmyocardial patients is warranted (with the exception of beta blockers and aspirin, since the use of both have been validated in postmyocardial infarction patients with or without VPBs).
7. The results of the CAST study suggest that excess mortality may be associated with the prophylactic long-term use of other antiarrhythmic drugs. (This has now been documented in the case of moricizine.)

Lessons of the Encainide-Flecainide Disaster

A number of important lessons emerge from the disaster:

1. A carefully controlled study of untreated patients with and without VPBs should have been (and still should be) performed to determine accurately and quantitatively the risks of VPBs in postmyocardial infarction patients. The failure to obtain such data prior to any treatment has cost numerous lives.
2. The present nonsystem for estimating efficacy and patient risk using mega or mini anecdotal data, using uncontrolled studies, using case control methods, using clinical consensus is simply inadequate to establish efficacy and to estimate risks. Even warning physicians that widely used, current approaches to drug evaluation are inadequate could, and would, still decrease the mortality from the use of the drugs. In this respect peer review, journal editorials, editorial boards, scientific meetings, and professional societies appear to offer little in terms of patient protection.
3. The present FDA system is not adequate for maximal public and patient protection. It is not only the physical plant of the FDA that is antiquated. Given the pace that new drugs, tests, and equipment are being introduced, the present system is clearly not adequate. Had the CAST study been performed before and not after the mass use of encainide and flecainide, thousands of lives would have been saved.

   It should be recognized that altering the FDA system and making it more complex has risks as well as benefits. By so doing, the introduction of truly effective and safe medical modalities may be delayed causing unnecessary mortality and morbidity. However, with the current rate of introduction of new modalities, there is little question that accurate determinations of safety and efficacy require new approaches.

   In this respect, recent proposals to modify the FDA procedure for new drug approval represents a form of cultural regression. In the present system, PRCCTs are not required. As a result, drugs with an unfavorable risk-benefit ratio are approved and widely used. The new proposal suggests that the present unsatisfactory system be made even less rigorous. As a result innumerable additional patients will be exposed to inadequately and nonrigorously tested drugs.
4. Medical school teaching, resident training, and cardiovascular training programs are deficient in teaching the elements of rigorous risk-benefit evaluation and thus gross errors, even once recognized, tend to have long lag periods before the practice is abandoned. These programs often fail to emphasize the major goal of medical care, improved patient outcome.
5. The occurrence of the encainide-flecainide disaster is only one of many similar disasters that have both specific and general features. Prevention of such disasters in cardiology will require more emphasis on risk benefit analysis than is currently provided.

One of the most remarkable aspects of the entire disaster is that no individual health care providers, no group connected with promulgating the disaster, no member of the CAST group, none of the pharmaceutical houses selling the drugs, and none of the professional cardiology organizations seems to have officially expressed grief at the needless death of thousands of patients in the general group administered the drugs or the patients who gave their lives during the CAST study. This does not reflect well on the humanistic basis of medicine. After all, the Union Carbide Company expressed remorse following the Bhopal disaster.

Pulmonary Artery Catheter Controversy

A recent ironic jest expresses one of the most fundamental problems in modern medicine: "The Hubble space telescope is perfect. It's the universe that is out of focus."[80]

Despite an ever-increasing influx of new technology and science into medicine, the relevance of many of these advances toward improving patient outcome is not at all clear. This dilemma is graphically illustrated by the controversy surrounding the clinical use of the pulmonary artery catheter (PAC). Improved patient outcome from its use has not been established. The mortality associated with its use is all too obvious.

Estimates of the total direct mortality associated with the use of PAC using very conservative estimates of risk[81] give rise to mortalities of 100,000 patients since the introduction of the catheter. Despite the large assumption errors involved in such an estimate, this figure is probably low.

A risk-benefit analysis would suggest that the catheter would have been required to save more than 100,000 lives to have an acceptable statistical risk-benefit ratio. As it has not been rigorously demonstrated that the use of the catheter has saved any lives, a rational system would require appropriate studies to demonstrate the accurate value of the risk-benefit ratio. Such studies have not been performed and in fact are actively resisted. A recent study reveals the problem facing adherents of its use.[40] An evaluation of the study can best be understood in terms of medical anthropology and medical archeology. The study was conducted under the sponsorship of a group called the Pulmonary Artery Catheter Study Group. The design of the study was to administer a 31-question multiple-choice examination regarding the use of the catheter to 496 physicians practicing in 13 medical facilities in the United States and Canada. In general, the physicians taking the test were in leading medical centers and represented the "best and the brightest" users (adherents).

The results were appalling and frightening. The mean score of accurate answers was 67% (approximately 21 of 31 correct answers). Sixty-one percent of the respondents were unable to recognize or respond appropriately to a blood-gas analysis consistent with arterial blood and 44% could not identify the determinants of oxygen delivery (not that the ability to do so

would guarantee efficacy of the use of the catheter). Furthermore, almost one-half (47%) the respondents were unable to calculate the pulmonary capillary wedge pressure from a clear tracing. The results of this quiz force an important conclusion:

For those who believe in the general efficacy of the use of the PAC, it must come from factors other than the objective interpretation of the data obtained from its use and the application of this data to patient care. That is, adherents of the use of the catheter are using the catheter as a form of primitive belief known as positive magic.[51] Merely inserting the catheter helps the patient.

Compare that approach with previous examples of positive magic in medicine.

Hippocrates advocated the following treatment for empyema:

> Having cut some bulbs or squill, boil in water, and when well boiled, throw this away, and having poured in more water, boil until it appears to the touch soft and well boiled; then triturate finely and mix roasted cumin, white sesames, young almonds pounded in honey, form into an electuary and give; and afterward sweet wine in draughts. Having pounded about a small acetabulum of white poppy, moisten it with water in which the summer wheat has been washed, add honey, and boil. Let him take this frequently during the day. And taking into account what happens give him supper.

And Galen, in claiming efficacy for a certain remedy, said as follows[82]: "All who drink of this remedy recover in a short time, except those whom it does not help, who all die. Therefore, it is obvious that it fails only in incurable cases."

We will return to an analysis of this study after but, lest the reader believe that we have furnished an extensively overdrawn picture, judge for yourself:

From a recent textbook on critical care medicine,[83] "The pulmonary artery flotation catheter changed the face of cardiovascular assessment at the bedside and gave an identity to the practice of critical care. It is more than an important development in critical care, it is critical care."

In the same textbook, 18 pages are devoted to what can only be classified as a catechism regarding calculations and interpretations of wedge pressures.[83] No acceptable data are provided to validate the use of this catechism in patient care, or indeed any purpose. The rules are provided "ex cathedra."

Contemporary Critical Medical History

The idea of a flotation catheter for insertion into the pulmonary artery apparently was conceived by one of the inventors after watching sailboats one sunny afternoon in Los Angeles. A balloon was substituted for a sail, and the catheter was originally tested in dogs.[84] To the best of our knowledge, the application to human use did not involve any careful consideration of possible risks either in dogs or in man. It must been assumed that the catheter at worse was harmless. For example, we do not know whether the dogs were sacrificed after several days of an indwelling catheter and examined pathologically for evidence of endocardial damage. That is a curious oversight. The catheter is anchored at one end to a transducer; the other end is more or less fixed in the pulmonary circulation. The intracavitary position of the catheter whips the endocardium during each cardiac cycle. If dogs are like humans in this respect, about 50% of them would have shown sufficient endocardial and/or valvular damage to be detected at postmortem.[25] Even if risks had been detected by the animal studies, it is doubtful that this would have slowed the use of the catheter in humans significantly.

It may be asked, for example, whether the FDA would have interfered with the catheter's introduction in the 1970s had the agency known about the potential risks associated with its use. The answer is almost certainly "no." FDA policy on approving medical tests and medical equipment was surprisingly lax during the 1970s and is surprisingly lax now.

Not only was the risk side of the use of the catheter completely ignored when the catheter was first described in the medical literature in 1970, it was assumed that the benefits of the catheter were obvious and required no documentation. This oversight stemmed from several factors. One of the most important of these was the widespread view that medical tests (and the use of the catheter is a form of medical test) did not have to be validated (justified). What criteria should be used in evaluating a test? From the standpoint of patient outcome, tests with acceptable benefits must meet the following standard. The results of the test statistically improves decision-making and, furthermore, improved decision-making significantly improves patient outcome. This standard also provides the mechanism for evaluating medical tests, namely that they are demonstrated (by rigorous trial) to increase the quantity of life (reduced mortality) or to improve the quality of life.

This simple concept can be supported by some abstract and poorly understood allusion to the fundamental role of the physician as a healer. Perhaps it can be more easily understood by many physicians in a different context: the economics of patient-physician relationships. Should it be acceptable to society that a patient pay, say, $1,000, for a test that does not improve patient outcome? If the answer to the question is "yes," it is difficult to find a social, legal, or philosophical justification for such an answer. Obviously,

the more risks associated with the test, the more clear cut should be the evidence that the benefits to be gained by the test justify the risks.

Despite the obvious objective of improved patient outcome as the criterion by which to judge the use of the pulmonary artery catheter (PAC), this concept has met with sharp opposition from numerous catheter users.

> One catheter acolyte states, "The lack of improved survival with PA catheters is not surprising because these catheters are meant to be a monitoring device and not a therapy."[83]

Furthermore,

> "Remember that the PA catheter is only a device for monitoring cardiovascular function and is not a therapy or panacea for hemodynamic problems."[83] Another opinion states that "pulmonary artery catheters are diagnostic devices that, in and of themselves, cannot be expected to provide improvement in a clinical condition, but only to monitor therapeutic interventions."[85]

Or a striking statement by one of the inventors of the catheter[86]:

> Although no carefully defined studies have established on a scientific basis the particular benefit of hemodynamic monitoring to the individual patient, it is reasonable to assume that a more precise and continuous knowledge of fundamental cardiovascular parameters would allow for more optimal decisions as to therapy, if not today then certainly in the future.

As stated in a rebuttal[86]:

> The first premise is debatable (it is not an issue that can be settled by pristine reason), and the second premise is chilling. Patients are being subjected to catheterization now so that future patients may benefit. This suggests that current patients are being used in experimental studies and subjected to risks, without their explicit understanding and informed consent, while being required to pay for the privilege of being studied in order to benefit future generations of patients.

Given the almost universally agreed-upon facts that (1) net patient benefit from the use of the catheter has not been documented, and (2) there are clear-cut patient risks from its use, what can one deduce from a review of the literature that accounts for the mass and perhaps escalating use of the catheter? Such deductions are always subject to reviewer bias, but the deductions are worth considering:

1. The catheter is user friendly, even though it may be usee unfriendly. The user almost always gains money, prestige, approval from peers, and acceptance into a select group.
2. Many physicians use the catheter without careful,

individual, explicit analysis. Having learned to use the catheter and having been influenced by the poorly documented opinions of various experts, physicians may go ahead with its use. This form of behavior by physicians has been called the lemming syndrome[87] and is very common not only among physicians but is found in many groups within different societies.

3. Many physicians believe that the use of the catheter provides a more scientific and accurate basis for evaluating patients than more simple clinical modalities such as physical examination and various laboratory studies. They derive a sense of security from its use even though the sense of security may be misplaced.

4. Some physicians believe that the use of the catheter can be justified by its research and educational value independent of its value to specific patients being studied.

5. The use of the catheter acts as a status symbol distinguishing users from nonusers, the latter being considered nonexperts.

6. Paramedical personnel such as ICU nurses are commonly but uncritically impressed with the value of the catheter and thus pressure physician nonusers to insert the catheter in specific patients who are not doing well.

7. The extensive nature of the risks associated with the use of the catheter is not appreciated by many physicians (see below).

8. Money.

9. Money.

10. Money: a gadget that brings about $2 billion/year into the medical system tends to be highly regarded.

Risks Associated with the Use of the Catheter

The qualitative nature of the risks associated with the use of the catheter have become increasingly clear with the passage of time. *Complications related to use of the pulmonary artery catheter* include the following[88]:

I. Local complications often recognized clinically
   A. Venous inflow
      1. Florid thrombosis
      2. Infection
   B. Cardiac
      Myocardial
      1. Insertion arrhythmias and heart block
      2. Right ventricular perforation
      Valvular
      1. Florid valve injury
      2. Bacterial endocarditis
   C. Pulmonary arterial
      1. Rupture
      2. Perforation
      3. Thrombosis
      4. Pulmonary embolism
      5. Pulmonary infarction
      6. Infection
   D. Miscellaneous
      1. Pneumothorax
      2. Arterial puncture
      3. Hemothorax
      4. Systemic sepsis

II. Local complications often or usually overlooked
   A. Venous inflow
      1. Subclinical thrombosis
      2. Infection
   B. Cardiac
      1. Late arrhythmias or heart block
      2. Direct myocardial injury, right ventricular hemorrhage, contusion, infarction, infection (battered myocardium syndrome)
      3. Valvular tricuspid/pulmonary injury, subclinical
   C. Pulmonary arterial
      1. Thrombosis in situ
      2. Infarction
      3. Late pulmonary embolism
      4. Infection

III. Technical problems
   A. Balloon rupture
   B. Sheath thrombosis/embolism
   C. Catheter knotting
   D. Catheter looping
   E. Failure to deflate balloon
   F. Failures of zeroing (obtaining proper baseline)
   G. Catheter misplacements

IV. Misinterpretation complications
   A. Iatrogenic overhydration related to increased myocardial compliance and/or increased ventricular volume
   B. Iatrogenic dehydration related to decreased myocardial compliance and/or decreased ventricular volume
   C. Miscellaneous

Several points require emphasis regarding this extensive list. One is that the frequency of the various complications is not known. Estimates derived from the literature based on inadequate, unrepresentative, uncontrolled experience vary widely. Arrhythmias are reported to occur in 35 to 70% of catheterized patients.[89,90] Catheter-related sepsis has been reported to occur at frequencies of 0 to 8%.[91,92] An accurate quantitative estimate would require a PRCCT.

It should be emphasized that a number of the complications occur covertly and are difficult or impossible to detect. Systemic sepsis may occur after the catheter is removed, and the development of sepsis may not be attributed to the use of the catheter. Late arrhythmias or heart block may be attributed to underlying independent heart disease. The battered endocardium syndrome usually requires a postmortem examination for detection and, with so few being performed, this diagnosis commonly escapes detection. Patients dying of the battered endocardium syndrome would usually be considered as having died of their underlying disease. Pulmonary embolism is a disease that has great intrinsic diagnostic difficulties and, even when accurately diagnosed, may not be attributed to complications caused by the PAC. Pulmonary artery thrombosis in situ is also difficult to diagnose and can mistakenly be attributed to the underlying disease. Pulmonary edema caused by overhydration may be attributed to the underlying disease rather than to a misinterpreted fluid challenge. This is likewise true of iatrogenic dehydration resulting in renal failure.

Given the apparent lack of basic knowledge concerning cardiac and pulmonary physiology among large numbers of catheter users, a variety of interpretive errors may be made that usually escape detection. It therefore seems probable that the mortality and morbidity associated with the use of the catheter are greatly underestimated by the experts and by individual physicians.

One important study concerned with the risks of the catheter was published in 1987, the so-called Worcester study. The Worcester study compared deaths in acute myocardial infarction with or without the use of a PAC. The data showed a 100% increase in mortality in those patients who were catheterized (no catheter: mortality 20%; catheter: mortality 40%, p <0.001).[91]

The first hypothesis to explain the results was the problem of selection bias. Seriously ill patients tend to be catheterized more frequently than are less seriously ill patients. However, subgroup analysis of patients with pulmonary edema, hypotension, and cardiogenic shock showed a dramatically higher mortality in patients with catheterization than in similar patients without catheterization. Multivariate analysis was performed to consider the impact of infarct size and severity. When these factors were taken in account, the excess mortality of 100% of those catheterized persisted. There were a number of (self-acknowledged) weaknesses of this study: retrospective chart analyses are not a precise way of determining excess risk, and multivariate analysis is not a precise tool for detecting differences between groups. The study concluded that a doubling of the mortality in patients in whom the PAC was used demonstrated a lack of benefit with the use of PAC in acute myocardial infarction (AMI). Indeed it did!

Based on the results of the study, one commentator called for a moratorium on the use of the catheter until a PRCCT was performed. This was based on the fact that, if the data were relevant, the catheter was causing 15,000 excess deaths per year in patients with acute myocardial infarction alone.[86] This modest proposal was thoroughly attacked even by one of the senior authors of the original Worcester paper.[85]

Since the original paper, three other epidemiologic studies have looked at the relationship between mortality and the use of the PAC in AMI. Two of these originated in studies from Israel. Both used the same data base made up of identical patients (5,841 patients having been reported in one paper and 5,839 patients reported in the second). Moreover, there was substantial overlap in the list of authors. One paper is a model of conservative analysis recognizing, no doubt, the limitations of retrospective studies and statistical analysis.[92] The paper demonstrated that females have a worse prognosis and have more serious disease than do men following an AMI. Despite the worse prognosis for women, the excess mortality associated with the use of the PAC is 1.61/1 as compared with the noncatheterized patients. Males, despite having less serious disease, show a higher relative excess mortality of 3.88/1 as compared with noncatheterized males. The authors correctly abstain from claiming that the data establish that selection bias has been eliminated as a less gravely ill group (males) have a significantly higher excess mortality associated with the use of the PAC than do more gravely ill females.

The resolution of retrospective statistical studies (however large a group of patients are studied) is not significantly high to permit such a conclusion. The second paper from the same group using the same data had as its objective to prove that the excess mortality in patients receiving PAC is related to "differences in the severity of CHF [congestive heart failure] which have not been assessed in every individual. It is unlikely that PAC increases mortality."[93]

There are at least two major problems with statistical analysis of uncontrolled data. One problem might be called the problem of *lumping*, and the other might be called the problem of *splitting*. Lumping increases the heterogeneity of groups being analyzed and ultimately may lead to comparing apples with oranges. Splitting (analyzing smaller and smaller subgroups of patients) may lead to the establishment of statistical significance merely based on random chance and having no etiologic relationship in real life.

To support its conclusions, the paper manages both to lump and to split. Lumping is accomplished by inventing a new category of patients with acute myocardial infarction called "pump failure." The heterogeneity of this group can be appreciated by the definition of pump failure as "the presence of symptoms or signs or radiologic features of CHF on admission, or their development during the patients' stay in the hospital, or the presence of cardiogenic shock, or the presence of systolic hypotension (systolic blood pressure below 90 mmHg) persisting 48 hours or more, or any combination of the foregoing."

What was done was to use a statistical construct to lump unlike patients together. A patient with radiologic evidence of pulmonary congestion (that might reflect anything from true pulmonary congestion, a radiologic error or interstitial lung disease unrelated to the acute myocardial infarction) differs fundamentally from a patient with cardiogenic shock. Their construct was such that they succeeded in eliminating the evaluation of clinicians who had cared for the patients in real life. The words of the authors are as follows: "related to difference in severity of CHF, which had not been assessed in every individual...." (translation: the clinicians caring for the patients often did not realize that their patients had pump failure). The implied message was that in such matters "The computer is mightier than the clinician."

Not only was there banning of the clinician from the bedside but apparently the pathologist was likewise banned. No histologic evidence or pathologic evidence was provided to validate the concept of "pump failure."

The failure to provide pathologic support may partially stem from an interesting cultural difference between Israel and the United States. A strict interpretation of Talmudic law pertaining to postmortem examination holds that an autopsy shall not be performed unless it is of direct benefit to the family of the decedent or to mankind. We presume (without accurate data) that the percent of autopsies in Israel is much smaller than even in the United States, where the percentage is quite small. In 1985 the autopsy rate in the United States was less than 15%, including autopsies done by statute for medical-legal purposes.[94] It is possible that some autopsies were performed on Palestinians and reformed Jews from whose families permission for an autopsy is more easily obtained.

Now having lumped the paper splits by dividing the pump failure group semiquantitatively into mild, moderate, and severe. By so doing the paper avoids the necessity for analyzing publicly the patients in terms of those with pulmonary edema, systemic hypotension, and cardiogenic shock. This avoids the necessity of comparing their results with the results previously obtained in the Worcester study (described earlier). The comparison would prove embarrassing because the results are so different. In the Worcester study, excess mortality was dramatically higher in patients receiving PAC compared with those not receiving PAC. Patients whose AMI was complicated by hypotension had an inhospital mortality of 48.3% when their management included PAC, compared with 32.2% if they were managed without a catheter (p

<0.001). In the Israeli study, there was no statistical difference between the two groups. What could explain such a striking difference in results? Could it be that Israeli patients with hypotension following an AMI are more hardy than patients in Massachusetts? Or is it possible that having artifactually set up groups of mild, moderate, and severe pump failure, now verbally synonymous with congestive heart failure, critically important quantitative relationships were obscured in a blur by using the term, congestive heart failure, to embrace virtually any complication related to AMI?

This was not the only potentially embarrassing result of the study. Comparison of mortality in patients not experiencing pump failure (presumably less ill patients) showed that those who had received PAC had a higher mortality than did those without the PAC. In the words of the paper, "this might arouse further suspicion that the use of PAC independently contributes to mortality." If this were the fact, the entire thesis of the paper would be invalidated, namely that it is CHF that kills patients with a PAC and not the PAC. The explanation raised more suspicions than did the higher mortality in the PAC group without pump failure. Five of the eight patients who died had the catheter introduced because of suspicion of a ruptured interventricular septum, a suspicion that proved to be well founded. The prevalence of ruptured interventricular septum in acute myocardial infarction is usually estimated at about 2%.[95] In the non-pump failure catheterized patients the prevalence was 9.4%. Why such a high value in this group? What was the corresponding prevalence in the pump failure group with and without a PAC? And what was the prevalence in the non-pump failure group without a PAC? These figures are not provided. What explains the 100% mortality in the five patients who died with a ruptured interventricular septum? With current surgical management, a mortality of 100% seems unusually high. How long was the PAC in place before frank rupture occurred? And was the catheter free floating, or was it anchored in the pulmonary circulation? What total length of time was the PAC in place? Was the site of rupture examined at autopsy to determine whether there was gross or microscopic evidence of the battered endocardium syndrome? Could the high rate of death be related to the use of the catheter itself? None of these obvious questions is answered in the paper.

Two of the non-pump failure patients died of "electromechanical disassociation following further blood pressure drop." What role, if any, did the PAC play in these two deaths? In particular, were these patients suffering from the battered endocardium syndrome? The eighth death occurred in a patient with brain death following resuscitation. Was a catheter complication the *coup de grace*? And why was a PAC placed in a patient with brain death? How long was the PAC in place?

The authors provide the gratuitous statement that "thus all the eight deaths in this group are explainable on the basis of the patients 'clinical conditions,' and there is no reason to believe that the introduction in any way contributed to their mortality." There are also no data presented that rule out catheter-related complications as the cause of some or all of the deaths.

There is another noteworthy aspect of the paper. Ex cathedra, the authors state "no randomized trials have been performed, nor would the development of such trials in the future be feasible." To document this sweeping assertion, the authors turn to a Higher Authority, one of the inventors of the PAC who actually stated in 1983 "elaborate randomized trials to prove effectiveness are impractical and would probably fail to provide the desired guidelines even if brought to completion."[96] Apparently in Israel as well as in the United States, the words of Higher Authorities are commonly misinterpreted.

The take-home message of this paper is that the mortality of patients with AMI subjected to the PAC was 53.1% compared with a mortality of those not receiving the catheter of 15.2%. The data as presented do not permit conclusions as to how much of the difference to attribute to the severity of AMI and how much to attribute to the intrinsic mortality of the PAC itself.

In an accompanying editorial, the editorialist is somehow content to accept the conclusions of the paper that differences in mortality do not arise from the use of the catheter in AMI.[97] He does believe that the benefits of the catheter have never been established. "What is not clear is whether the therapy that results from this procedure benefits patients. Given the potential complications of the procedure and its costs, I believe that we must determine if this procedure is of benefit to patients with acute myocardial infarction. As with other procedures and therapies, we need to assess efficacy by performing appropriately designed controlled clinical trials. Swan and Ganz are correct: Such clinical trials will be very difficult, but I believe they must be done."

Another retrospective study comparing mortality in patients with AMI with or without PAC is comprehensive, based on the records of almost 300,000 Medicare patients (Blumberg MS: personal communication, 1991). In summary, there appears to be about 20% excess mortality in AMI associated with the use of the catheter whether analyzed on an individual basis or analyzed on the basis of individual hospitals. The paper wisely indicates that its nature is exploratory. To what extent the excess mortality is based on complications of the PAC and to what extent the excess mortality is caused by the use of the PAC in sicker

patients cannot be extracted from the data. Determination of the factors involved in the increased mortality associated with the PAC use will require a PRCCT, and even such a trial may not answer all questions.

The paper is noteworthy for the number of patients studied. It presumably makes unnecessary any further retrospective medical record analyses on the use of PAC. It is also noteworthy for its honesty and provides an interhospital comparison of PAC usage and mortality.

A number of studies have looked at the patient benefits of PAC. To the best of our knowledge, only two of these have attempted some form of PRCCT and reported net benefit. Shultz et al.[98] examined the role of hemodynamic monitoring in patients with fracture of the hip. The monitored group of 35 patients demonstrated a 10-fold decrease in mortality relative to a nonmonitored group of 35 patients (3.9% versus 39%). Unfortunately, the control group had their surgery delayed a week or so as compared with the experimental group, while the investigators tried to convince the controls to undergo catheterization. It is well established in the orthopaedic surgical literature that early as compared with late surgery dramatically decreases mortality. A common design error in clinical trials is to treat the experimental group differently from the control group.

This episode is notable in several respects. The difference between the treatment of the two groups was not highlighted in the paper but had to be abstracted from the published paper. The justification for delaying surgery in 35 patients to obtain permission for insertion of a PAC, while knowing that delay added to the risks of the underlying disease, is not clear to us. Finally, the study demonstrated the spread of a technology to disciplines such as orthopedic surgery and obstetrics that usually would not use such methods.

The second modified PRCCT was performed by Shoemaker and Appel[99] in surgical patients. They used the data obtained from the catheter to calculate oxygen delivery and alter therapy accordingly. Unfortunately, the design was what might be called a coupled or catechism or smorgasboard design. To demonstrate benefit, it was necessary not only to use the PAC but to go through a precisely prescribed series of therapeutic measures. As a result, the efficacy of the catheter could not be separated from the efficacy of all the other steps, leaving the individual efficacy of the PAC open to question. It is clear that despite the use of 20 million to 30 million catheters in the United States alone, there is no rigorous demonstration of its efficacy in improving patient outcome in any disease state.

The world of PAC users has apparently been shaken by the publication of a study conducted in December 1990 and previously mentioned.[40] The study summarized the results of a 31-question quiz administered to 496 physicians from the United States and Canada affiliated with departments of medicine, surgery, and anesthesiology. Those taking the examination were considered to be among the best and brightest ("a select subset of Canadian and American physicians"). The results presumably provide an overestimate of the mean competence of all physicians using the PAC who, it may be inferred, would not do as well as the elite. As with the Vietnam War, the brightest and the best did not do well. The results were embarrassing. The mean test score was 67% (20.7 ± 5.4 SD). The examinees were more or less uniformly deficient in all subject areas covered, including insertion, complications, cardiac physiology, and interpretation of data covering interpretation of waveforms, PAC data, and pressure-volume relations.

A major and obvious implication of the study is that previous numerous claims of efficacy for the use of the catheter must be judged as grossly in error. If a substantial percentage of users do not know the basic rudiments of data interpretation derived from the use of a gadget, how can the gadget result in better care for patients? For example, if 47% or more of those using the PAC were unable "to determine the pulmonary capillary wedge pressure from a clear tracing," how can they possibly apply their fallacious estimate to improve patient outcome? (Incidentally, it would be of some interest to determine what percentage of experts, including those who prepared the quiz, know what wedge pressure measures and under what conditions the wedge provides inaccurate and potentially harmful estimates of pulmonary capillary pressure.)

The results indirectly but profoundly underestimate the risks of the catheter. An assumption is made that most risks derive from incompetent users. Many complications occur in the hands of the most skilled and experienced catheter users. For example, the battered endocardium syndrome results from the physical presence of the catheter inside of the heart and occurs despite the skill, knowledge, training, and good intentions of the user.

The tone of the article implies that the fault lies not in the catheter but in the catheterizers. That implication is simply not accurate. The priorities of the article are consistent with the ultimate suggestion for meeting the problems inherent in the use of the PAC. "Any such evaluation [PRCCT] must address questions of safety, efficacy [the instrument's ability to measure what is intended under ideal conditions], effectiveness [its ability to do what it is intended to do when deployed in the field], and effects on patients outcome."

It is no accident that the effects on patient outcome occupy the last place (have the lowest priority) on this list. This position goes to the core of a fundamental difference. To those who believe that the purpose of

medical care is to improve patient outcome, efficacy is defined as an improvement in the quantity or quality of patients' lives. To those like the authors of the quiz, efficacy is the ability of an instrument to measure what it is intended to measure. This form of medical ideology might be called "technophilia" (love of technology for its own sake) and its devotees called "technophiliacs." Technophilia is rampant in modern medicine. In this case, the technophiliacs propose that credentialing policies be established, thus restricting the use of the PAC to individuals with documented competence. Once most catheterizers have achieved a more exalted level of knowledge, a PRCCT could be considered.

For those who are primarily concerned with improved patient outcome, another sequence would be appropriate. The first step in determining the status of the PAC should be to determine whether, under conditions of an adequate clinical trial, there is clear evidence of net improvement of patient outcome. If, as appears probable, there is none, the use of the catheter should be interdicted. No training in its use would be required. If net benefit for the use of the catheter can be established, more intensive training and credentialing could be undertaken. It is hoped that no one is advocating additional training in the use of arsenic for anemia or oil of primrose for multiple sclerosis. Why advocate additional training in the use of a modality whose efficacy and safety remain to be determined and whose use thus is presumably moot at best?

One of the most interesting results of the publication of the study is the flood of criticisms of the incompetent use of the catheter in the hands of physicians other than the criticizer. The dogma appears to be, "I know how to use the gadget safely and effectively. No one else does." To the best of our knowledge, this art form has so far been confined to the United States and Canada. It can be safely predicted that soon colleagues in the United Kingdom, Holland, Australia, and New Zealand will be pointing a finger and indicating that it is only in the United States that such numbers of incompetent users are found. Such basic ignorance, they will say, is not found in the United Kingdom, Holland, or Australia, or wherever the home base of the criticizer happens to be.

It is instructive to take a closer look at the generators of the study, the Pulmonary Artery Catheter Study Group. Judging from a list of members, they include numerous physicians of various medical centers throughout the United States and Canada. Given the nature of the patient problems inherent in the PAC, they face two polar choices: (1) to act as technophiliacs whose mission is to defend the PAC, and (2) to act as defenders of patients. To date it appears that they have opted to act as defenders of the catheter. Among the 20 or so listed members of the group, it should be easy to find the nucleus for organizing an appropriate PRCCT. It is not difficult to predict what the choice will be or is.

Not that this group is alone responsible for failure to determine the risk-benefit ratio for the use of the PAC. For example, a recent survey was conducted by the American College of Physicians. Of the Directors of Internal Medicine Residency programs, 88% stated that their residents should learn the procedure.[100] They indicated that 10 separate insertions of the catheter would be required to master the procedure. What data base did these directors use to reach their conclusion? You have already seen that estimates of the risk of PAC are qualitative. There is almost universal agreement that there are no rigorous data that establish any net patient benefit from the use of the PAC. It thus seems clear that the opinion of the directors merely reflects current bias. In turn, such opinions led to a proliferation of a risky procedure of unknown benefit. This is a capsulized example of some of the major problems in medicine. For example, apparently none of the directors expressed concern about the welfare of the 10 patients during "the learning procedure." One of the major characteristics of technophiliacs is a relative indifference to patient welfare.

A highly instructive example of expert misinformation comes from a report issued recently by the American College of Cardiology/American Heart Association Task Force on Assessment of Diagnostic and Therapeutic Cardiovascular Procedures.[101] It was prepared by a subcommittee to develop guidelines for the early management of patients with acute myocardial infarction. The subcommittee includes 21 of the most illustrious cardiologists in the United States. Unfortunately, the report was completed and published about 10 months before it was established that about 50% of elite catheter users do not know how to use the catheter to calculate or interpret the data obtained from its use or how to apply these data to decision-making for patients.[40]

For the various interventions analyzed, patients were divided into three classes:

Class 1: usually indicated, always acceptable, and considered useful and effective
Class 2:
  a. a weight of evidence in favor of usefulness/efficacy
  b. not well established and probably not harmful
Class 3: not indicated; may be harmful

After a general paean of praise for the PAC, the classification in the various subgroups of patients with acute myocardial infarction goes as follows:

Class 1: Usually indicated, always acceptable, and considered useful and effective; severe and progressive congestive heart failure; cardiogenic shock or progressive hypotension; mechanical complications of acute infarction—the same groups of patients in whom the highest excess mortality has been demonstrated when compared with patients with the same complications of acute myocardial infarction, but without the use of the catheter
Class 2a:
  1. hypotension not responding to fluid administration without evidence of pulmonary congestion
  2. before giving a fluid challenge in a patient with circulatory insufficiency and suspected pulmonary congestion
  3. as a diagnostic tool

The first question that arises is the nature and quality of the data base that the 21 experts used to arrive at their conclusions. To the best of anyone's knowledge there is no such data base. Experts without adequate data are expressing mere opinions. No such disclaimer is provided. Being experts, of course, means that an acceptable data base is not required.

It is surprising that a group of expert cardiologists appear to be quite ignorant of Starling's law, failing to acknowledge the difficulties of interpreting pressure measurement during a fluid challenge without estimates of left ventricular volume and compliance.

The mention of risks in the statement refers only to the possibility of bleeding at the site of catheter insertion with thrombolytic therapy or the risk of infection. Not even the risks of malignant ventricular arrhythmias associated with a foreign body in the right ventricle are noted. Comparison of this discussion of risks with the tabulation on page 19 makes the paucity of emphasis on risks obvious.

This, then, is a body of experts without an acceptable data base who currently are faced with a fact that was previously unknown to them. The fact is that many cardiologists (including perhaps some of the above experts) lack knowledge of the bare fundamentals involved in the use of the PAC. Would knowledge of this fact have modified the certainty with which the guidelines were formulated? Probably not. And even a PRCCT that showed no net benefit and high risk might not change these opinions.

If approximately 50% of catheter users have been and are incompetent, since its first mass use in 1972, there may have been 100,000 deaths and 500,000 patients with complications related to their activities. Calculations of this type are subject to large assumption errors, but there is no doubt that the use of the catheter has been associated with mass morbidity and mortality.[81] No one in the Pulmonary Artery Catheter Study Group has expressed any contrition for the harm that has been done because of incompetence. Add to that the harm caused by *competent* catheterizers and the patient harm became astronomical—still, no one has expressed regrets.

In the issue of the *JAMA* that contains the study by the Pulmonary Artery Catheter Study Group there is an accompanying editorial of great interest.[37] The editorialist, while emphasizing the importance of PRCCT for high-tech medicine generally, somehow inexplicably omits a recommendation for such a trial in the case of the PAC. The editorial also opts for more formal credentialing of PAC users.

It is not difficult to determine the basis of these opinions. Physicians heavily involved in the use of a given technology have nothing to gain and much to lose by rigorous PRCCTs. If the technology is found valuable, it merely confirms their a priori feelings. If the technology is found useless or harmful, the devotees have much to lose in terms of prestige, power, and money.

In the case of the PAC there are approximately 2 billion reasons ($) per year to oppose actively or passively the development of such an adequate clinical trial. In 1986 there was a direct cost of catheters of $2 billion plus an additional $1 billion spent in treating its complications.[5] Everyone in medicine except patients and the public stands to lose if these vast sums are removed from the health care providers. It is not uncommon in medicine or other professions for the rationalizations for a given course of action to operate in such a way that the conclusions serve the perceived self-interests of the affected rationalizers. So much then for contemporary history.

Specific Elements of the PAC Controversy

Various proposals to grapple with the problems posed by the use of the PAC have been debated. One highly unpopular proposal has been to declare a moratorium on the use of the catheter pending a PRCCT that establishes an acceptable risk-benefit ratio.[86]

This proposal for a moratorium was made 3 years before it became apparent that a high percentage of catheter users are grossly deficient in their knowledge of such minutiae as insertion, cardiac physiology, interpretations, complications, and indications for the use of the catheter. How much more reasonable a proposal for a moratorium might appear now. There are, of course, medical and societal precedents for limited moratoriums on potentially dangerous drugs, appliances, manufactured products, and so forth. Thalidomide affords an excellent example. In 1961, the possibility of a relationship between the drug and phocomelia was raised. It required 7 years before the drug was withdrawn.[102]

Other dramatic examples include the use of clioquinol for diarrhea, resulting in several regional epidemics of subacute myeloopticoneuropathy particularly in Japan[103]; and the use of the β-blocker practolol that was shown to cause oculomucocutaneous syndrome, after which the oral form was withdrawn.[104] With each of these drugs, there was a substantial period of time during which physicians continued to administer the drugs and argued that the drugs were safe and that PRCCTs were not necessary.

The media makes frequent allusions to the withdrawal from the market of various automobiles and airplanes until safety can be guaranteed or remedial measures to improve safety can be undertaken. Why a medical technology should be exempt, especially one whose benefits have not been rigorously demonstrated, is not clear.

A typical and "convincing" argument against a moratorium is as follows:

> The editorial proposing a moratorium is 'distinctly wrong headed.'[85] [The readers should recognize that the senior author of this chapter (E.D.R.) first proposed a moratorium pending an appropriate PRCCT and thus may be biased.] It is difficult to find a cogent, reasonable argument against a moratorium. In the interest of fairness, we will supply one. Should the PAC turn out to have a strikingly favorable risk-benefit ratio, then large numbers of patient will have been deprived of a useful diagnostic tool. [The withdrawal of thalidomide deprived patients of a useful soporific.]

As we discussed above, the implementation of a PRCCT is considered controversial by some for a variety of reasons. Such a trial would be unethical, is impractical, is impossible to conduct, is not needed, and would not provide adequate answers. None of these arguments is accompanied by convincing evidence that the assertion is accurate. The format for such a trial could be easily generated. To quantitate risks using a population of patients with acute myocardial infarction might be optimal. To quantitate benefits, if any, a population of patients with adult respiratory distress syndrome (ARDS) might be optimal. When and if such a trial is implemented, the interpretation of the data should be under the direction of noncombatants. The trial format should include a neutral monitoring committee that would halt the trial as soon as either clear-cut benefits of the catheter or disappropriate risks were demonstrated.

Retrospective History of the Future

In the final analysis, the use of the PAC is a medical test. What will medical historians say of a health care system that used a gadget associated with thousands of deaths in patients without ever demonstrating that the gadget produced benefits that justified such a loss of life or perhaps was not associated with any benefits to patients?

Cardiac Deaths in Bronchial Asthma

It may seem unusual to analyze a disease, bronchial asthma, in a discussion devoted to risk-benefit analysis in cardiovascular disease. This seeming anomaly by itself illustrates an important limitation of current medical approaches. As medicine has become increasingly specialized, the focus of various experts in numerous areas of medicine has become more and more narrow. The benefit has been to provide experts with extensive knowledge about given small areas in medicine. In fact, an expert can be viewed as one who has learned more and more about less and less. In a reductio ad absurdum, the expert would be someone who knows everything about nothing.

One disadvantage of extensive specialization is that areas that subtend more than one discipline may be subject to substantial errors that could be avoided by participation of experts from "foreign" areas. This appears to be true of the field of bronchial asthma. It is clear that the lungs and heart are anatomically connected through one pulmonary circulation. It is also clear that bronchial asthma has important effects on the pulmonary circulation and thus the right heart. Finally, it is well known that a number of commonly used drugs in the treatment of bronchial asthma, such as the β-adrenergic agonists and xanthine derivatives (theophylline), have important adverse cardiovascular effects.[105] Despite this, the literature on bronchial asthma during the past 24 years has been pulmonologist dominated and has been scarcely participated in by cardiovascular-oriented experts.

One of the key problems in the area of bronchial asthma is a striking paradox. During the past 15 years, there have been a series of major advances in the knowledge base concerning asthma possessed by physicians. Some of the advances include knowledge about the immunologic basis of the asthmatic paroxysm, identification of some of the early mediators of airway obstruction, knowledge of late mediators released by the immunologic cascade of asthma, the potential cardiovascular effects of both early and late mediators, the cardiovascular effects of some forms of treatment, the existence of exercise-induced asthma and hyperreactive airway, the value of pulmonary function measurements in quantifying increased airway resistance, the development of potent new pharmacologic agents for treating asthmatics, and a number of other advances in knowledge and the application of this knowledge to the treatment of the disease. One might guess that, with such rapid scientific and medical progress, the prognosis of bronchial asthma must have improved substantially.

The paradox is that the reverse is happening. Population-specific deaths associated with bronchial asthma in the United States reached a nadir in 1977, when there were approximately 2,500 deaths per year, and has climbed progressively to approximately 6,000 deaths in 1990.[105] As a generalization, the increased mortality is not confined to the United States but is also found in the United Kingdom, New Zealand (where the increase is dramatic), Canada, Denmark, and Sweden.[106]

One of the major issues in the field of asthma is why mortality continues to climb despite substantial advances in the management of bronchial asthma. It appears certain that the upward shift is not an artifact related to a change in classification of the disease. It seems unlikely that the prevalence of the disease is increasing from some unknown cause. Nor does it appear likely that the increased mortality is related to better diagnostic methods, resulting in a higher rate of detection. There is no evidence to support the possibility that asthma is becoming a more virulent disease.[105]

It is of interest that the mechanism responsible for the rising mortality has, until recently, generally been judged to be ventilatory in origin. This assumption stems both from the obvious fact that bronchial asthma is a lung disease and from the fact that the experts involved in studies of the disease have been lung oriented. Until recently, scant attention has been focused on the possibility that some asthmatics die "with bronchial asthma" and not because of bronchial asthma. More specifically, the possibility that patients may die primarily of cardiac abnormalities rather than respiratory abnormalities has not received major attention.

Contemporary Critical Medical History

Between 1961 and 1967, a miniepidemic of deaths associated with bronchial asthma occurred in the United Kingdom. At peak the excess mortality was about 25 patients per year. In a remarkable paper in 1969, Inman and Adelstein[107] not only quantitated the excess mortality but also identified the proximate cause of the epidemic and set into operation corrective action that resulted in eradication of the excess mortality 2 years later.

The study established that the rising limb of mortality correlated with increasing use of β-agonists delivered by metered dose inhalers (MDI). The total use of β-agonists by the population of asthmatics was calculated from total sales and prescriptions issued per year for β-agonists in cannisters.

As β-agonist usage increased, so did mortality. A concerted educational effort was mounted among physicians to discourage the use of β-agonists delivered by MDI. The campaign succeeded and, as the use of aerosolized β-agonists decreased, there was a parallel decrease in mortality.

The effects of this epidemiologic study, on a very small scale, indicate the value of activist epidemiology. The British seem to have a genius for this form of medical investigation.

Edward Jenner became aware of a folk suspicion in Gloucestershire that dairy maids who had contracted cowpox through milking were immune to smallpox. Jenner conceived of the idea of applying the principle and, on May 14, 1796, performed an experiment on an innocent, healthy country boy, James Phipps. Jenner innoculated Phipps with cowpox matter from a milk maid and then with smallpox matter. When the boy did not die or become ill with smallpox he vaccinated 23 additional patients.[108] This entirely uncontrolled experiment led to the saving of millions of lives. That Jenner put the young lad and 23 patients at obvious jeopardy has not been (to our knowledge) specifically considered.[5]

John Snow correlated the development of cholera and the use of water obtained from a single well in London, the Broad Street Well. By removing the pump-handles from that well, he prevented additional cases of cholera during the epidemic of 1855.[108] Snow opposed the use of water from that well long before the germ theory of disease and long before *Vibrio* cholera had been described as the causative agent.

Snow may have been the first activist epidemiologist. His view that cholera was spread by water was hotly contested by William Farr, who is still revered as the father of vital statistics. Farr contended that cholera was caused by elevated atmospheric pressure. History does not record a consensus conference held to resolve the controversy.

It is not generally recognized that Inman and Adelstein used a powerful epidemiologic tool. Demonstrating both an ascending limb to the mortality-use curves as well as a descending limb, the thesis for a causal relationship between the two variables was enormously strengthened.

However, these results and others supporting a relationship evoked a controversy that is still waged today. Much of this controversy is based on misinterpretations, distortions, lack of accurate analysis, and simple misunderstanding.

The results of the study stimulated a continuing argument as to whether the excess mortality during the epidemic was caused by "overtreatment" or "undertreatment" of bronchial asthma. The fact that mortality increased as β-agonist use increased and that it decreased as β-agonist use decreased is, of course, quite inconsistent with an "undertreatment" theory.

The data in the original paper are badly misinterpreted by some of the controversialists. The study looked at two doses of the most commonly used β-agonist at that time. Isoprenaline MDI was available in two doses per inhalation, weak 0.2 mg and forte 0.4 mg. Weak isoprenaline was sold at almost twice the rate as forte. This was interpreted by some to indicate that the mortality dose curve was highest in the low treatment group. In fact, the slope of either weak or forte sales against total deaths is essentially indistinguishable, meaning that neither the weak nor the forte MDI preferentially was associated with excess mortality. In the words of Inman and Adelstein, "Both strong (forte) and weak preparations of isoprenaline show a similar pattern of rise and decline of their use. . . ."

A number of other distortions of the data developed with the passage of time. It has been stated that excess mortality was (almost) exclusively found in children. Actually, children over the age of 9 showed a steeper increase in mortality than did other age groups, but excess mortality was found in all age groups. It has been stated that excess mortality was related to essentially one β-agonist, isoprenaline. Actually there was increased mortality involving the use of metaproterenol (Alupent), isoetharine, and possibly norepinephrine. The fact that isoprenaline weak and forte accounted for the majority of sales strongly suggests that those drugs contributed to the increased mortality in asthmatics. It has been claimed that decreasing or eliminating the use of isoprenaline forte resulted in a cessation of the epidemic. Actually there was a global decrease in the use of β-agonists in general. Thus, no single β-agonist could be implicated.

One of the most important developments that occurred between 1962 and 1969 was the occasional suspicion that not every asthmatic who died with serious asthma died a ventilatory death. Lockett found that doses of isoprenaline 15 times smaller than those tolerated by a healthy heart-lung preparation were sufficient to stop a heart experimentally embarrassed by excessive pulmonary ventilation.[109] Greenberg and Pines[110] described eight patients with bronchial asthma who died suddenly following the long-term use of pressurized aerosols.

Usually, of course, ventilatory arrest in asthma does not occur suddenly (see below). Speizer et al.[111] investigated the death of 184 asthmatics; death had been sudden and unexpected in 80%. Among those deaths, 84% were known to have used MDIs, and in several cases, the use was excessive. However, most investigators did not use the "C (cardiac) word."

Inman and Adelstein were quietly and appropriately conservative. They recognized that epidemiologic studies frequently cannot by themselves provide mechanistic explanations. By 1970, the first epidemic had passed. It left a series of controversies focusing primarily on undertreatment versus overtreatment.

Even highly sophisticated and knowledgeable epidemiologists apparently not having performed a critical contemporary analysis of the relevant studies believed that most of the issues were satisfactorily addressed.[8]

A major compendium of adverse effects of drugs misstates and misinterprets the data emerging from the U.K. epidemic.[103]

The senior author of this chapter (E.D.R.) misinterpreted the events of the U.K. epidemic as follows[105]:

> Although absolute proof is not available, the epidemic subsided roughly concurrent with the time employment of high-dose cannisters was abandoned. There is no absolute certainty as to the cause of that epidemic of excess death because some of the facts are inconsistent with a simple one-medication overdose theory. Independent of the question of cause, investigation of the phenomenon benefited all asthmatics by reducing the potential dose to many patients, and focusing on the potential risks of therapy with isoprenaline.

To turn to anthropology, the events surrounding the first epidemic of deaths became transformed into a myth defined as "an imaginary fictitious story or unscientific account." The myth in turn became one of the causes of the present-day (new) epidemic of deaths in bronchial asthma.

Beginning in about 1977 and still gaining momentum, a new epidemic has appeared with excess deaths in the United Kingdom, New Zealand, and Australia, as well as the United States.[112] This recrudescence of fatal asthma is almost certainly associated temporally with increasing use of β-adrenergic agonists. An analysis from New Zealand showed that increased use of the β-adrenergic agonist, fenoterol, is associated with increased fatal asthma.[113] Asthmatics on this drug had an odds ratio of death of approximately 2, as compared with nonusers. In patients with severe asthma the odds ratio of death was approximately 10:1. In 1989, similar results were reported from New Zealand, but with minor shifts in the degree of increased risk.[114]

There were at least three problems with these studies: (1) they relied on case control methods; (2) they focused largely on a single β-adrenergic agonist, fenoteral; and (3) unlike the original study of Inman and Adelstein, there was no declining limb of utilization to study. Similar trends have been found in Australia, the United States, and Canada. With a sharply increasing use of β-adrenergic agonists, there has been no declining limb of the mortality-β-agonist relationship. It is to be hoped that, as evidence mounts, there will be an attempt to curtail usage of these drugs and that the seminal study of Inman and Adelstein will be brought up to date. Such a process is under way in the United Kingdom.[106]

Modes of Death in Bronchial Asthma

Two basic patterns may be extracted from the literature. One pattern is death from primary ventilatory failure and respiratory arrest. The second pattern is cardiac arrest. Primary ventilatory death in bronchial asthma occurs as a result of overwhelming increases in airway resistance under conditions in which cardiovascular effects are secondary to the abnormal ventilatory dynamics and subsequent changes in lung and tissue gas exchange.

Ventilatory failure with or without respiratory arrest occurs in several forms. The most common cause of death appears to be progressive increases in airway resistance often preceeded by increasing refractoriness to conventional asthmatic therapy (status asthmaticus). Death is usually not unexpected or unexplained and is usually not sudden. This mode of death is the common paradigm envisioned by most experts as fatal bronchial asthma. This group of patients have been characterized in a recent study showing marked hypercapnia ($PaCO_2$ more than 90) and respiratory acidosis (pH less than 7.23). Occasionally the hypercapnia is precipitated by too vigorous oxygen inhalation so that PaO_2 values can be relatively high.[115]

There is a small group of patients who quickly develop overwhelming ventilatory failure, followed by ventilatory arrest, in whom airway resistance appears to be normal or near-normal before ventilatory arrest. O'Hollaren et al., emphasized airborne pollutants in such patients.[116] Sensitivity to aspirin and nonsteroidal anti-inflammatory drugs (NSAIDs) has been described as a cause of rapid death due to ventilatory arrest.[117] Paradoxical reactions to β-agonists characterized by diffuse bronchial constriction have been reported.[118] In some patients of this group, no putative precipitating cause has been found.

Patients dying or near dead of ventilatory arrest may demonstrate an interesting physical sign during either resuscitative efforts or during the use of mechanical ventilation. This sign may be called "the supratight airway sign." The high airway resistance requires the use of high inspiratory pressures to inflate the lungs. The sign is elicited by the marked resistance to inflation using an Ambu bag attached to an endotracheal tube or peak ventilator inflation pressures at the mouth of more than 60 cm of H_2O to force adequate tidal volumes into the chest may be required.[119]

To our knowledge, the supratight airway sign is one of the first described physical sign associated with modern medicine and, as is true of most physical signs, its sensitivity, specificity, positive predictive value and negative predictive value are entirely unknown.

There are also several findings at postmortem examination consistent with high airway resistance. Under usual conditions, the isolated lungs, when removed from the chest, collapse. With ventilatory arrest in bronchial asthma, the lungs do not collapse because of major air trapping. The airways are filled with extensive, thick mucus, and there is diffuse mucus plugging. On microscopic examination, the usual findings of eosinophilic infiltration and hypertrophied bronchial smooth muscle are present. These microscopic changes are nonspecific and may be found in patients with chronic asthma who die of cardiac mechanisms.

Primary Cardiac Death

Primary cardiac death in bronchial asthma occurs as a result of alterations in cardiac function under conditions in which airway resistance is normal, moderately elevated or in some cases not sufficiently elevated to result in ventilatory arrest. Although primary cardiac death associated with bronchial asthma has not been emphasized, that there is such an association is by no means a new idea.

Greenberg and Pines[110] reported eight patients who had died suddenly, each of whom had used pressurized aerosols excessively. During the first English epidemic of the 1960s, attention was focused on the possibility that Freon or other fluorocarbon propellants affected the myocardium in such a way as to produce excess deaths. A substantial number of animal studies and clinical reports examined this possibility with no definite resolution.[120] These efforts distracted attention not only from possible adverse myocardial effects of β-adrenergic agonists but also from the probability that many of the deaths were related to cardiac and not airway mechanisms.

Kurland et al. reported fatal myocardial toxicity during continuous intravenous infusion of isoproterenol.[121] The development of myocardial ischemia during intravenous β-adrenergic agonist treatment has been reported.[122] A significant incidence of cardiac arrhythmia was reported in patients receiving slow-release salbutanol and slow-release terbutaline for asthma.[123] There is a case report of a 39-year-old woman who inhaled a megadose of isoproterenol and showed an ECG pattern consistent with acute myocardial infarction.[124]

Since at least 1982, the Physician's Desk Reference (PDR) reports that "Fatalities have been reported using excessive use of Alupent [metaproteranol sulfate] as with other sympathicomimetic inhalation preparations and the exact cause is unknown. Cardiac arrest was noted in several cases."[125] This warning turns out to be prophetic, as it mentions asystole rather than arrhythmia as the cause of death. Thus, the anecdotal clinical evidence is quite strong that primary cardiac deaths occur and that such deaths can be associated with the use of β-adrenergic agonists.

One of the major lines of emerging evidence that cardiac deaths occur with inhaled β-adrenergic agonists comes from the occurrence of ultrarapid, unexpected, unexplained death in patients with bronchial asthma—sudden asthmatic death syndrome (SADS). This occurs under circumstances that are simply too rapid for ventilatory arrest. Postmortem examinations

are not consistent with overwhelming airway disease. We have previously reported four such cases[126] and have now accumulated seven more examples. Postmortem findings in a number of these patients were inconsistent with ventilatory arrest related to overwhelming asthma. All patients were being treated with inhaled β-adrenergic agonists at the time of death.

Several mechanisms for cardiac toxicity are found in patients with bronchial asthma. Myocardial contraction band necrosis (MCBN) was originally described in animals infused with large doses of β-adrenergic agonists.[127] The cardiac lesion is quite different from the changes of coagulation necrosis and ischemic change in the heart associated with acute myocardial infarction. In MCBN myocardial cells die in tetanic contraction with intracellular calcium overload.[128] MCBN was found in 4 of 13 children who died with acute asthma.[128] Although MCBN can be induced by cathechol administration, MCBN was found in the hearts of children who died without receiving β-agonists suggesting that other mechanisms might be operative. The possible arrhythmogenic effects of β-agonists has been emphasized.

It is highly probable that severe asthma is usually accompanied by pulmonary hypertension.[123] Increased alveolar pressure and the existence of hypoxemia and hypercapnia in many patients and a direct effect of some of mediators released on pulmonary vascular smooth muscle are all mechanistic explanations for the not uncommon right ventricular hypertrophy seen in some asthmatic patients.[129] Moreover, during inhalation of β-adrenergic agonists, relatively large doses must diffuse directly across the alveolar-pulmonary capillary membranes, resulting in a first-pass exposure of the left ventricle without preliminary metabolic degradation. It should also be emphasized that increased cardiac toxicity results from the combined effects of β-adrenergic agonists and xanthine derivatives, two agents commonly used in bronchial asthma.[130]

A recent key study in this area leaves no doubt that inhaled β-adrenergic agonists are capable of producing abnormal cardiac function even in the usual dose range.[131] Eight subjects with bronchial asthma were studied while subjected to fenoterol, salbutanol, terbutaline, or placebo, all by MDI. The design was a double-blind crossover study. All three β-agonists caused abnormal changes in three cardiac or paracardiac functions. With increasing dose, there was of course an increase in heart rate. Serum K^+ fell in a dose-dependent fashion. The fall in plasma K^+ was presumably caused by a shift of extracellular K^+ into cells. As a result, the Nernst ratio, $[K^+]e/[K^+]i$, must have changed resulting in an alteration of resting transmembrane potential.

Finally, there was an increase in QTc (rate corrected QT) interval on the ECG. The QT interval measures the time of ventricular depolarization and repolarization and reflects key events in bioelectric events in cardiac function. All three β-agonists studied produced these effects, although the degree of effect depended on the specific agent used.

These results are important not only in indicating mechanisms for cardiac toxicity over the usual dose range of inhaled β-agonists. The results provide a method for monitoring potential cardiac toxicity of β-agonists by measurements of QTc before and after inhaled doses of β-agonists. They supply a new dimension for controlling some of the excess mortality associated with bronchial asthma. Bronchial asthma is now a disease in which the cardiologist as well as the pulmonologist should interact for maximum patient safety. It is of interest that these results, which have caused significant changes in current thinking about the doses and the use of β-agonists in the United Kingdom and New Zealand, seem to have largely escaped the scrutiny of the American medical community.[131] The importance of these observations is underscored by recent studies of the role of a prolonged QT interval in the pathogenesis of sudden death in nonasthmatics.

For the past 20 years, it has been known that the autonomic nervous system is involved in the pathogenesis of malignant ventricular arrhythmias.[132] During the past decade, an idiopathic long QT interval syndrome has emerged associated with sudden death particularly in subjects with coronary artery disease.[133] This syndrome presents itself as recurrent episodes of syncope or cardiac arrest associated with torsades de pointes, sometimes precipitated by mental or physical stress demonstrating QT prolongation on the surface ECG.

Of great interest is the uncovering of a DNA marker of the syndrome at the Harvey ras-1-gene locus.[134] This suggests that analysis of leukocyte might serve as a marker to identify patients at high risk from sudden death associated with a prolonged QT interval. Surgical denervation of the left cardiac sympathetic supply is being employed in patients with idiopathic long QT interval with arrhythmias.[135]

A noncongenital form of sudden death associated with prolonged QT interval has been described in young males in Southeast Asia and Japan.[136] Sudden and unexplained death during sleep has been documented in substantial numbers of young males. In a group of young males considered at high risk of sudden death, it was noted that there is both a prolonged QT interval as well as hypokalemia. In the young Asian males, this association represents an acquired disorder since it is not found in young Asians that no longer live in the area. Thus, in young Asians and asthmatics treated with β-agonists, there is an acquired defect that can lead to sudden death. There have been no studies of the frequency of Harvey ras-1 gene in the population at risk of sudden death either in Southeast Asian young males or in asthmatics treated with β-agonists.

Given the present state of knowledge, it is possible to classify the sudden death prolonged QT interval association as follows:

I. Endogenous
   A. Abnormal ras-1 gene locus
   B. Others
II. Exogenous
   A. Asthmatics treated with β-agonists
   B. Acquired prolonged QT interval in young males in Southeast Asia
   C. Others

While considering risks, it is always important to consider benefits. A careful human double-blind placebo-controlled randomized crossover study of the effects of regular versus on-demand inhaled bronchodilator therapy in mild asthmatics was conducted.[137] Regular inhalation of β-agonists was associated with deterioration of asthma control in most subjects. Thus, patients appear to be subjected to enhanced risks and decreased benefits by a treatment regimen that essentially all pulmonologists have believed to be both safe and effective.

Often when confronted with a plea for PRCCT, the response is that these are not needed because so much effective therapy in medicine is used without going through the crucible of adequate clinical trials. Until recently, no such trials were conducted to test the safety of β-adrenergic agonists in bronchial asthma. The climbing mortality in bronchial asthma is a stark reminder that not having the data from such trials courts disaster for our patients.

Partial Ileal Bypass to Lower Serum Cholesterol: A Mini-iatroepidemic

Assume that a pharmaceutical company develops a (mythical) drug, Cholesterol Fighter (ChF) said to be promising with respect to lowering serum cholesterol. Assume that ChF is chemically similar to a previous drug, Obesity Fighter (ObF), formerly used to treat obesity. The use of ObF was abandoned because of a grossly unfavorable risk-benefit ratio and multiple undesirable side effects, including death.

Assume further that a long-term PRCCT is organized in 1975 and terminated in 1990. The purpose of the trial was to determine the efficacy of ChF in decreasing total mortality and mortality related to myocardial infarction: the subjects selected for study range in age from 30 to 64 years and have survived previous myocardial infarction. In general, aside from a previous myocardial infarct, the health status of the group is excellent. No subject has arterial hypertension, obesity, or diabetes. They are also free of overt congestive failure and have normal ejection fractions.

As the PRCCT is pursued, the administration of ChF results in the following complications. Two of the 399 patients in the experimental group die within 30 days of starting the drug. The relative risk of the development of gallstones in the experimental group increases fourfold. The development of renal stones in the experimental group increases sixfold. The administration of the drug increases the requirement for abdominal surgery eightfold or more to treat drug complications; in 100% of the experimental group, chronic and persistent diarrhea develops, and in 6 to 8%, the diarrhea is associated with watery or frothy stools. Suppose that 14% of the experimental group developed at least one episode of bowel obstruction and that in 4% of patients bowel surgery was required to treat the intestinal obstruction. Assume that the patients in the experimental group (none of whom were obese to begin with) lost 5.3 kg of body weight and could not regain their initial body weight because of malabsorption produced by the drug.

At the conclusion of this 15-year study, it is confirmed that the treatment did result in a dramatic and sustained decrease in serum cholesterol, a dramatic decrease in LDL, and a modest increase in HDL, but did not reduce significantly the total mortality or the mortality from coronary artery disease.

It also turns out, on examination of the placebo group, that the risks of AMI were less than had been anticipated by the investigators. In fact, in untreated patients, the total mortality per year was 1.57%. As the mortality from coronary artery disease was 1.0%/year, the treatment could have at best resulted in a slightly improved patient prognosis, while patients in the experimental group had suffered the complications resulting from the administration of ChF.

Even if the prognosis of the control group did not become apparent until the 15 years of the study had been completed, similar data were already available in the literature. In the Coronary Artery Surgery Study (CASS), the medically treated group (when compared with patients treated with coronary bypass surgery) showed an annual mortality of 1.6%.[138]

A similar relatively low mortality in untreated post-myocardial infarction patients with ventricular premature beats is reported, the annual mortality being 2.1%.[76] There is little question that the threat to life is less than generally believed. As a result, any acceptable rate of complications is also relatively small. Otherwise, the treatment of a disease may be substantially more perilous to the patient than the disease itself.

Imagine what a furor these results would create. The media would be up in arms. Congressional committees would rush to investigate the flow of events, especially when it became apparent that the PRCCT had consumed more than $50 million of state and federal taxpayers' money.

You may imagine what would happen in the courts as the injured parties brought a class action suit against the government and against the investigators and their institutions. Given these facts, what jurors would decide that those in the experimental group had not suffered needless harm?

Now, substitute a nonmythical surgical procedure, partial ileal bypass, for the drug ChF, a form of intestinal bypass that was studied for its possible efficacy in reducing both total mortality and specific mortality related to CAD. Add to the list of complications the pain, suffering, and infections secondary to the performance of surgery and reoperation in some subjects. Add the deaths and disability caused by serial diagnostic studies, and the deterioration of quality of life caused by chronic diarrhea and malabsorption syndrome during the past 15 years and an accurate picture emerges of a recently described miniepidemic.[24]

Perhaps the most amazing fact is that the results of the study were enthusiastically perceived by a number of surgeons and investigators. To determine the pathogenesis of this miniepidemic of partial ileal bypass, two separate historical trends should be analyzed: (1) the general efficacy of cholesterol-lowering regimens in reducing CAD mortality; and (2) the misuse of human volunteers in clinical investigations.

Cholesterol and Paracholesterol Hypotheses

Space does not permit an adequate review of the current status of the various hypotheses and controversies surrounding the use of lipid manipulation to lower the prevalence of CAD and cardiovascular deaths.

Despite widespread acceptance of the virtues of low plasma cholesterol or high HDL or low LDL in reducing deaths from CAD there is considerable evidence to the contrary. In overall terms, there is firm evidence that deaths from CAD began to decrease long before the current medical and societal emphasis on modifying cholesterol by drugs or diet became a national obsession.[139] During the past 5 years, while millions of Americans have religiously adhered to diets based on cholesterol or lipid restriction, the rate of decline in mortality from CAD (the decline began in 1972) remains unchanged. This lack of effect on mortality rate during years of emphasizing lipid lowering is at least curious for this reason: we have seen a significant decrease in the in-hospital mortality of acute myocardial infarction related to the increased use of thrombolytic agents (see below). This benefit, coupled with any measurable benefits from lipid lowering, would be expected to appear in recent mortality rate tables, but such has not been the case. This sequence does not prove that such diets or cholesterol-lowering medicine do not affect the prevalence of coronary artery disease. But it is a rather surprising finding, occurring as it does during a period when in-hospital CAD fatality rates from AMI have dropped dramatically because of the use of thrombolytic agents. Individual readers will decide for themselves as to the validity of the claims made for aggressive management of cholesterol.

Several references dating back to the 1960s provide excellent summaries of the scientific evidence raising substantial question about the validity of speculations about cholesterol. Interestingly, some of the most cogent sources are provided by nonphysicians.[141,142]

Inadvertently, the investigators involved in the partial ileal bypass study provide a relatively accurate, if biased, summary of current data as follows[24]:

> The findings of the National Heart, Lung, and Blood Institute Type II Coronary Intervention Study implied that a reduction in the total plasma cholesterol level by cholestyramine slowed the progression of atherosclerotic coronary heart disease as assessed by serial coronary arteriograms. This finding, however, lacked statistical significance, and no differences were observed between the intervention group and the control group in the rate of atherosclerotic events. A more definite conclusion was reached in the Cholesterol-Lowering Atherosclerosis Study. There was significantly less progression of coronary atherosclerosis in the native circulation and the coronary-artery bypass grafts on the arteriograms of patients treated with colestipol and nicotinic acid (P = 0.001). That trial was not designed to measure overall or cardiovascular mortality or to evaluate the validity of the use of sequential changes on coronary arteriograms as surrogate end points of clinical atherosclerotic events. In the Helsinki Heart Study, the rate for the combined end point of three clinical events—fatal myocardial infarction, confirmed nonfatal myocardial infarction, and sudden cardiac death—was significantly lower in patients treated with gemfibrozil (P = 0.02). However, no statistically significant difference in overall mortality was noted. The cholesterol-lowering trial that has been most widely cited is the Lipid Research Clinics-Coronary Primary Prevention Trial (LRC-CPPT), in which patients were treated with cholestyramine or placebo. The difference between the study groups in overall mortality was negligible; there was evidence of benefit with respect to the combined end points of death due to atherosclerotic coronary heart disease and confirmed nonfatal myocardial infarction, but only by a one-sided test of significance.
>
> With the failure of individual trials to validate conclusively the benefit of cholesterol lowering, the pooling of results from independent trials, conducted in vastly different populations, has been suggested. Meta-analysis, when applied to trials of diet and drug therapy for the reduction of plasma cholesterol, has demonstrated a decrease in deaths due to atherosclerotic coronary heart disease and an increase in deaths due to noncardiovascular diseases, with no net effect on overall mortality.
>
> And further, like the LRC-CPPT, the Helsinki Heart Study was unable to show significant decreases in overall mortality, in cause-specific mortality, or in individual coronary heart disease end-points after lipid modification. Only by combining numerous coronary heart disease end-points could a statistically significant result be obtained. This trial also provides evidence for, but does not prove, the lipid-atherosclerosis theory.

In other words, statistical subgroup analysis is fraught with difficulties. Keep this quotation in mind during the analysis of the partial ileal bypass study (below).

The authors of this ileal bypass study also offer us a chilling statement contrasting compliance with surgery as compared with medical therapy: "Partial ileal bypass therapy is obligatory as long as the operation is not reversed." It is now established that partial ileal bypass does not improve significantly either total mortality or mortality from CAD. The patients who underwent partial ileal bypass face what even for a Hobson's choice is grim. Should they undergo a second surgery to escape the consequences of the original surgery? Or should they hope that the so-called "reduction of atherosclerosis progression" will somehow ultimately be translated into increased longevity or improved quality of life for themselves? The hope seems tenuous because after 15 years the "inhibition of atherosclerotic progression" has not improved mortality significantly.

Another interesting issue is raised by the authors of the study and has become increasingly apparent. An increase in noncardiac mortality appears to accompany most previous attempts to reduce hypercholesterolemia.[143] This includes the Lipid Research Clinics Trial,[144] The Helsinki Heart Study,[145] The Los Angeles Veteran's Administration dietary trial,[146] the Helsinki Mental Hospitals trial,[147] and with some modification the Oslo Heart Study.[148]

At first, increased noncardiac mortality associated with aggressive cholesterol intervention was thought to be some statistical aberration. This opinion is no longer tenable, although the precise mechanism(s) for increased noncardiac death is not known. Increased noncardiac mortality selectively affects younger subjects.[149] The reality of increased noncardiac death is even more troubling, as aggressive cholesterol manipulation is now being recommended in young children.[150] Given the present data, it must be asked, What shall it avail a man to lower his cholesterol, if he thereby suffers an increased rate of noncardiac death?

So much for excess noncardiac deaths related to cholesterol manipulation. Until recently, the long-term impact of cholesterol manipulation had not been studied. The results are most disturbing.[151] A 15-year follow-up was provided of a PRCCT performed on two groups of middle-aged men. One group of subjects were seen by physicians every 4 months, subjected to intensive-hygiene measures and treated actively with hypolipemic and antihypertensive drugs as judged necessary. The control group was not seen by the investigators.

At the end of the 15 years, not only was there a significant increase in total deaths in the manipulated group, but there was a highly significant increase in cardiac deaths in the experimental group (p = 0.002).

The long-term effect of active medical intervention was to increase and not decrease cardiac mortality! The investigators who have been active in picking aggressive intervention were obviously shocked, stating, "These unexpected results may not question multifactorial intervention as such [the validity of this statement is not clear] but do support the need for research for the selection of methods used in the primary prevention of cardiovascular diseases." This presumably is a plea for perhaps another $50 to 100 billion of research funds.

In a defensive editorial,[152] it is commented, "We believe that the issue of an excess number of deaths not attributable to physical illness in individuals subject to current preventive measures against coronary artery disease cannot be brushed under the rug." This statement is made as the editorialists attempt assiduously to brush under the rug the fact of excess cardiac mortality in the subjects treated according to current dogma.

Finally, it will turn out that the data provided by the partial ileal bypass experiment provide a shattering blow against easy acceptance of aggressive cholesterol management. Believers in that practice have stated that more beneficial outcome from such management could be demonstrated if only it would be possible to produce more dramatic decreases in cholesterol or LDL and to maintain these decreases for a longer time. Readers will be able to judge for themselves what happened to mortality from coronary artery disease and total mortality when such reductions were accomplished over an average of 9 years by partial ileal bypass.

It is useful to consider the societal roots of beliefs such as cholesterol lowering as a form of management. We believe that the medically trained reader can gain more perspective in evaluating the cholesterol approach to coronary artery disease by reading the classic *The Golden Bough* by Frazer[51] than by reading conventional medical literature. Here is a synopsis of some of the pertinent portions.

In primitive societies, there were (and are) two forms of magical practices, as discussed above: negative magic or taboos that involve avoidance of specific measures, and positive magic that involves taking specific measures. To repeat, the hoped-for benefit of negative magic is to avoid unfavorable circumstances or outcomes for individuals, or for society as a whole; for example, to avoid death or disease or to avoid certain undesirable characteristics or outcomes. Positive magic consists of active acts designed to achieve the same objectives.

Left to themselves, human societies usually select diets that reflect the food available and other factors. It is this propensity that is altered by positive and negative magic. Here is an example. The Fans of West Africa would never eat tortoises because this would slow them down. However, old men could eat tortoises freely because the seniors had already lost the ability to run quickly.

The Namaquas abstained from eating rabbit meat because they believed it would make them as fainthearted as a hare. Bushmen will not give their children jackel heart to eat because it might make the children timid like a jackel. Among the Dyaks of Borneo, young men and warriors may not eat deer meat because it will make them timid as deer. So do the Kayans of the same region.

Jewish people traditionally do not eat pork. It has been claimed that this originally represented a way of avoiding the parasitic disease trichinosis. This claim is hardly tenable as the religion also interdicts eating clams, mussels, oysters, lobster, and crab, forms of food not readily available on the Sinai Desert when the pork taboo first developed. No one has claimed that those taboos were attempts to avoid hepatitis or salmonella infection.

In old Madagascar, soldiers were prohibited from eating hedgehog lest the soldiers acquire the propensity of those animals to curl up when in danger. No soldier could eat an ox's knee lest the soldier (like the ox) become weak in the knees.

The Zaparo Indians of Ecuador would not (unless from necessity) eat heavy meats such as tapir and peccary because ingesting slow animals would make the ingestor slow. Brazilian Indians would eat no beast, bird, or fish that ran, flew, or swam slowly lest, by partaking of such flesh, they would lose their ability to escape from enemies.

Caribs abstained from eating pig lest it cause them to have small eyes (like pigs).

The cholesterol taboo began as a North American belief and then spread through the medical world. It is of some interest to describe some early native American forms of negative food magic.[153]

Some North American Plains Indians favored eating venison over the clumsy bear, the dunghill fowls, the slow-footed cattle, or heavy wallowing swine. As a result, the abstainers became swifter and smarter.

Among the Alequas (Wood Indians of California), pork and fat bear flesh (negwitsch) were forbidden and permitted only to old women. Among most tribes, except for the Yokuts, eating dog was an absolute taboo and dog meat was considered a deadly poison. Among the Yokuts the flesh of birds of prey and carrion were forbidden.

The Chukchansi were highly selective in their food taboos. The gopher snake, water snakes and frogs were rejected but lizards, turtles, and rattlesnake meat were acceptable. Oddly enough, the neighboring Miwok and Salinores ate snake, lizard, and frog. The resemblance of these practices, to eggs-no eggs; saturated-unsaturated fats; 37% to 30%-less-than-30% dietary fat negative magic practices should be obvious to the reader.

Another issue has recently brought perspective to the cholesterol control issue. Suppose that all the assumptions underlying active manipulation of cholesterol were true. How much additional time would, on the average, be added to life expectancy?

Two recent studies using models provide interesting estimates. In one study, the impact of a reduction of fat in the diet from 37% to 30% was evaluated.[149] It was calculated that the benefit "equivalent to an increase in average life expectancy of 3 to 4 *months* would accrue chiefly to people over the age of 65 years." The investigators went on to state "if recent concerns about the possibly harmful effects of cholesterol lowering on noncardiovascular mortality are valid . . . these relatively modest benefits would be overestimates of the actual effect."

In an independent study using a different model, it was concluded that (somehow) decreasing serum cholesterol in men with cholesterol levels exceeding 200 mg/dl would gain 0.5 to 4.2 years in life expectancy and women would gain 0.4 to 6.3 years.[154]

Analyses based on models are, of course, quite sensitive to the assumptions underlying the models. However, whatever the assumptions, the implicit conclusions from two different models is that dietary control of fat results in a barely significant increase in life span.

The relevance of these studies bears on an evaluation of the risk-benefit ratio of cholesterol manipulation. Even granting the claims that have been made for the general efficacy of cholesterol interventions, if the ultimate increase in life expectancy is trivial, the basis for cholesterol intervention no longer exists. To achieve these putative (and now recognized) trivial improvements in life span, the use of invasive surgery such as partial ileal bypass is impossible to justify.

As is generally the case, attacks on orthodoxy usu-

ally evoke strong counterassaults; soon after the media reported the two studies, an epidemiologist rushed to the fray. He trotted out the old chestnut[155]: "surveys of Japanese and Greek populations show that their diets contain far less animal fat than Americans consume and that their death rate from heart disease is barely a tenth of the American death rate." This constitutes a remarkable non sequitur that can best be appreciated by reviewing similar false reasoning in the 1950s and 1960s. A strong proponent of the fat-cholesterol heart disease thesis summarized his impression of current data (1964) as follows[141]:

> There is a remarkable relationship between the death rate from degenerative heart disease and the proportion of fat calories in the national diet. A regular progression exists from Japan through Italy, Sweden, England and Wales, Canada and Australia to the United States. No other variable in the mode of life besides the fat calories in the diet is known which shows . . . such a constant relationship to the mortality rate from coronary or degenerative heart disease.

Two creative epidemiologists, Yerushalmy and Hilleboe, wondered why the statistics were based on only seven countries.[141] They decided to examine data from 22 countries, whereupon the relationship fell apart. They found that Israel consumed as much fat per capita as Mexico but the Israeli death rate from cardiovascular disease was eight times that of Mexico. Italy had more heart disease than the Netherlands on less fat per capita. The United States consumed only a small amount of fat more than Norway but the U.S. death rate per capita from cardiovascular disease was three times that of Norway.

It became clear why only seven countries had been cited in the original report. These countries provided data that fitted the bias of the proponent of the fat-cholesterol-heart disease theory. When the number of countries analyzed was increased, the theory was demolished.

We hesitate to add to the literature the next step taken by Yerushalmy and Hilleboe lest it be seized upon by certain meatpacking industry executives or some voluntary health organizations. Tongue in cheek they examined the statistical relationship between dietary protein and heart disease. They found that "the association between dietary protein and heart disease is at least as strong as that between dietary fat and heart disease. This clearly suggests that the dietary fat-heart disease association is not unique or specific since the association between fat and heart disease mortality is not as strong as that between animal protein and heart disease."

In primitive societies, there were (and are) two forms of magical practices, as discussed above: negative magic or taboos that involve avoidance of specific measures, and positive magic that involves taking specific measures. To repeat, the hoped-for benefit of negative magic is to avoid unfavorable circumstances or outcomes for individuals, or for society as a whole; for example, to avoid death or disease or to avoid certain undesirable characteristics or outcomes. Positive magic consists of active acts designed to achieve the same objectives.

The cholesterol, lipid, unsaturated fat, egg, what-have-you taboos, are different in three respects from those examples. First, a scientific or statistical veneer is used to justify the taboos. The validity of the veneer in terms of increasing either the quantity of life or the quality of life is moot. Nor is it likely that further studies will add much shine to that veneer. Second, with the development of methods of mass communication the taboos have been thoroughly dispensed throughout society so that there are very few nonbelievers. Our children will grow up believing in the cholesterol taboo. Finally, the taboo has become a huge source of money, prestige, and position for some members of society and some professionals. Given those vested interests, any questioning of the belief provokes a sharp attack. To oppose the taboo is to oppose the "truth."

Treatment of Human Volunteers in Clinical Trials

There is a long and precontemporary history that involves the use and often the abuse of human "volunteers" in medical research. We will begin arbitrarily in 1966 in the United States, relying heavily on a recent account of the events as summarized by Rothman.[156] In essence, Henry K. Beecher, an anesthesiologist, summarized 22 examples of what he considered breaches of medical ethics in the conduct of human research. All the studies were conducted in the United States, and most of them at leading medical centers. Some of the most distinguished physicians and medical scientists committed some of the worst aggressions against innocent people. The results of these experiments were published in the best medical journals. Some of the worst examples include thymectomy in children to study the effect on skin-homograft survival; the deliberate precipitation of hepatic coma in cirrhotics given certain nitrogenous substances; ammonium tolerance in liver disease studied by catheterization of the hepatic vein; the deliberate exposure of mentally defective institutionalized children to hepatitis virus; the injection of cancer cells into innocent victims and the homotransplantation of a melanoma resulting in death from the tumor.

Cardiology is overrepresented in the list of examples. In two studies, antibiotic therapy was deliberately withheld from subjects documented to have streptococcal infection; cerebral ischemia was deliberately induced by hypotension; the relationship between end diastolic pressure and ventricular contraction was studied in patients with mitral stenosis and atrial fibrillation; the sequence of ventricular contraction was studied by simultaneous catheterization of both ventricles; hepatic blood flow was measured in volunteers; left atrial pressure was measured by direct insertion of a needle through a bronchoscope; in a similar study, left heart catheterization was performed by the transbronchial route; and a study of the effect of exercise on cardiac output and pulmonary arterial pressure was studied in patients with cardiovascular disease and pulmonary emphysema.

It can be seen that none of the studies dealt directly with the welfare of the individuals being studied. Rather, the subjects were used as experimental preparations. It should also be emphasized that the experts who engaged in the studies were among the "best and the brightest." Their involvement in these studies, in a number of examples, advanced the careers of those performing the studies.

Rothman contends that the publication by Beecher resulted in a revolutionary change for the better and that the evaluation of institutional human protection committees has resulted in enormous changes for the better. That contention is open to great question.

Two key areas are involved in the issue of patient protection against unacceptable experimental practices. One area is the adequacy of research ethics committees in truly protecting subjects from unacceptable experimental processes. The second area involves the process of informed consent. This issue explores the two questions of insuring that subjects truly understand the risks of the study and that investigators insure that the subjects be provided with sufficient and ongoing information so that they are in a position to accept or decline participation in the study.

Four recent examples are quite revealing. In one study performed in Naples, Italy, two experimental groups were investigated to determine the effects of intracoronary injection of the neurotransmitter, serotonin. The rate of serotonin release in coronary vasospastic disease (Prinzmetal's variant angina) is a topic of substantial research interest at this time.[157] Seven of the 14 patients were free of obvious coronary artery disease. Each had mild to moderate mitral stenosis and had been referred to the laboratory for routine (almost certainly) right-sided catheterization. They were persuaded to undergo bilateral ventricular catheterization as well as coronary artery catheterization. Serial 2-minute intracoronary infusions of vasoactive agents were delivered into a branch of the coronary artery, including graded concentrations of serotonin. Finally nitroglycerin was administered directly into the coronaries as a control.

At the end of each infusion, coronary arteriograms were performed. It appears that seven sets of coronary arteriograms were performed in each subject. Please note that seven subjects with known CAD were subjected to the same protocol. Several questions come immediately to mind. What was the approval of the institutional review board of the University of Naples based upon? Did they realize that routine coronary arteriography has an intrinsic mortality per se even without other injections into the coronary arterial bed? Did the review board distinguish between approval of the study in patients with established coronary artery disease and those with mild to moderate mitral stenosis? Did the board realize that a PRCCT in 1984 had shown that ketanserin was without therapeutic value in Prinzmetal's angina?[158] And most important, did the board review the proposed informed consent process and monitor the process to guarantee that the subjects had provided truly informed consent?

Did the subjects give their consent to the studies based on an honest, thorough process so that each subject understood the risks of the study and the lack of personal benefit to themselves, especially the group with mild to moderate mitral stenosis? To answer this question, the reader has only to consider whether any even moderately knowledgeable cardiologist with mild to moderate mitral stenosis would agree to submit personally to the specific protocol or whether a moderately knowledgeable cardiologist would agree to have a member of his family participate in the study.

A second, similar, study was performed in Hammersmith Hospital in London, England.[159] In this study, 22 patients were admitted for routine cardiac catheterization. It is not made clear whether routine refers to standard cardiac catheterization or to left ventricular catheterization for performing coronary arteriograms. There were three groups of patients. The first group had atypical chest pain but proved not to have coronary artery disease. Group 2 suffered from chronic stable effort-induced angina and were positive on exercise testing. Group 3 had a history of spontaneous early morning angina. Ergonovine testing produced angina and ST depression. All patients had shown discreet coronary artery stenosis on coronary arteriography.

Patients were tested by an infusion of various concentrations of serotonin directly into the coronary arterial bed. Following the completion of serotonin injections, each patient received intracoronary isosorbide dinatrate.

In all patients in group 2, angina developed at the highest infused dose of serotonin accompanied by ST-segment depression in most patients. All patients in group 3 showed angina with focal occlusion of epicardial vessels and a shift in ST segments (elevation in three and depression in two). It is stated that no subjects died during the study nor was transmural infarction reported. The study protocol had been approved by the Research Ethics Committee of Hammersmith Hospital.

The basis on which the Research Ethics Committee approved the study is, of course, not provided. Nor are the details of the process by which consent was obtained. We do not know whether group 3 patients entering the study late in its development were informed that potentially dangerous complications had been observed in previously studied patients.

Given the fact that ketanserin had already been shown to be ineffective in the treatment of variant angina,[158] it is difficult to reconcile the performance of both studies with a concern for the outcome of the subjects studied.

In fact, the mind-set of both investigative teams seem close to that of Dr. Pangloss in Voltaire's Candide.[160] You may recall that Dr. Pangloss believed that noses were made to wear spectacles, legs were visibly instituted to be breeched, stones were formed to be quarried and built into castles, and pigs were invented so that we could eat pork. Apparently there is a school of cardiologists who believe that Prinzmetal's angina was invented so that various agents could be injected directly into the coronary circulation.

Careful analysis of both studies reveals that the subjects were viewed as physiologic preparations for inclusion in hazardous studies designed to advance knowledge in a field that, while important, was not directly relevant to their own status.

Overall these studies were quite similar to previously criticized studies, such as the measurement of cerebral hemodynamics during cerebral ischemia deliberately induced by acute hypotension[161] performed 37 years before, or measurements of the effects of exercise in normal subjects and patients with emphysema on cardiac output and pulmonary artery pressure performed 43 years before.[162]

The main differences are the absence of ethical committees and less strict (perhaps) requirements for informed consent in those earlier, less enlightened times. There is no clear-cut public information on the quality of the ethical committees approval either in Naples or Hammersmith or clear evaluation of the quality of the informed consent process in the subjects; it can only be speculated that both processes were quite deficient. The basis for this speculation is the near-certain rejection of both studies by knowledgeable cardiologists or their families if they were asked to participate as subjects. There is, of course, no record that any member of the institutional review board of the University of Naples or the Research Ethics Committee of Hammersmith Hospital volunteered to serve as normal controls. There is no mention of the risks inherent in producing angina, ST segment changes, and epicardial vascular occlusion.

The two papers evoked an editorial comment in the journal publishing the original paper.[163] The editorialists likewise refrained from commenting on the risks that the subjects were exposed to during the study. They developed an elegant physiologic theory to explain the results thereby strengthening the impression that the subjects, in reality, served as physiologic preparations rather than as human beings. They evoked an indirect, somewhat far fetched benefit for the studies involving the use of aspirin or thrombolytic agents in non-Q wave infarction, neither of which therapies has any clear relevance to the studies that were performed.

A third study was performed in the United States. This study involved a multicenter prospective randomized controlled trial to determine whether comprehensive life-style changes affected coronary artery atherosclerosis after one year.[164] The effect that was studied was the degree of coronary vessel stenosis. To examine that issue 28 subjects (the experimental group) were assigned to a low-fat vegetarian diet. They stopped smoking, pursued stress management and performed moderate exercise. Twenty subjects (controls) were assigned to a usual-care control group. Overall, 82% of experimental group patients had an average change toward regression of coronary lesions and progressed minimally compared to the control group. None of the patients at the end of 1 year showed significant differences in the frequency of chest pain, or chest pain duration, but the experimental group reported a significant subjective decrease in the severity of chest pain.

To obtain data, a minimum of 56 coronary arteriograms were performed on both groups in which 28 angiograms were performed for purpose of the study. However, prior to admission to the study, a total of 193 patients underwent quantitative coronary arteriography so that the exact number of arteriograms performed solely for the study is difficult to determine.

The study was a multicenter study and the usual approval was forthcoming from the relevant ethical committees.

The design of the study was flawed in several respects. The research question asked: would this evidence of (moderate) regression of atherosclerotic lesions of the coronary arteries by life-style changes be deemed desirable by numerous physicians? The only question of interest to the subjects was: does a "more healthy lifestyle" result in a decreased morbidity or mortality from coronary artery disease? The subjects were asked to risk their lives undergoing quantitative coronary arteriography (again, exact mortality not known, perhaps 1/1,000 or 5/1,000) to examine a surrogate criterion, partial or nonregression of coronary lesions.

The use of surrogate criteria to assess subject outcome is very common in this field. Blankenhorn et al.[7] noted a reduction in about 14% of lesions after using combined colestipol-niacin treatment for about 2 years. It is not claimed at present that this combination has been shown to demonstrate a favorable risk-benefit ratio in prevention or treatment of coronary artery disease. Whether partial regression, even if maintained, improves outcome requires a PRCCT that looks at mortality and morbidity. Whether prospective subjects were so informed is not at all clear.

A second flaw is that the study involved lumped or linked or smorgasbord criteria. A more healthy lifestyle includes a low fat vegetarian diet without animal products except egg white and one cup of nonfat milk or yogurt per day. Coffee was eliminated. The diet was supplemented with vitamin B_{12}. Stress management included stretching exercises, breathing techniques, meditation, progressive relaxation and imagery. Patients were asked to practice these stress management techniques for at least 1 h/d. Only one patient in the experimental group was smoking at baseline and she agreed to stop on entry. How many smokers there were in the control group is not stated, nor is it recorded how many of the controls continued to smoke.

Which, if any, of the numerous aspects of a more healthy life contributed to the modest regression of coronary lesions cannot be extracted from the data. It is unfortunate that the control group of patients was not asked to chant mantras each day. It might have established that the chanting of mantras accelerates atherogenesis. In summary, subjects were asked to undergo a study with imprecise and fuzzy boundaries when the measuring modality had as its ultimate risk death. None of the ethical committees in various institutions failed to approve of the study.

The fourth example is very interesting as it comes from Japan.[165] It cites no approval by ethics committees or signatures affirming informed consent. The Japanese health care system apparently lacks (lacked) these refinements in patient protection. In fact, there is a growing movement within Japan to affirm the fact that "patients are human, also."[166] A formal requirement for informed consent was not inaugurated until October 1, 1990 in Japan. The failure to protect individual patient rights in Japan stems from an important cultural difference between that society and our own. Traditionally Japan regards a person as a collective and not an individual reality. This view is, for example, incompatible with the notion of individual brain death (complicating organ transplantation in Japan).[167]

Given the lack of patient safeguards and cultural differences between Japan and Western society, the

Japanese study may be regarded as a control for the three studies cited above. How well or poorly protected are patients without ethics committees or efforts to obtain informed consent? The disconcerting answer is, judging by these unrepresentative and limited examples, there is little fundamental difference.

The Japanese study[166] involved the use of a new angioscope to perform percutaneous transluminal angioscopy. One hundred consecutive patients deemed *anatomically* suitable for the procedure were studied. The quality of angioscopic image was deemed good enough for analysis in 84 patients. The patient mix included 14 with acute myocardial infarction (within 8 hours of onset), 16 with recent myocardial infarction (3 days to 2 months since onset), 24 with old myocardial infarction, 10 with stable angina, and 20 with unstable angina. Coronary arteriography was performed in many of the patients.

The findings appear somewhat less than world-shaking. Occlusive thrombi were more common in patients with acute myocardial infarction than in those with unstable angina. Xanthomatous plaques were more common in patients with acute coronary disorders than in those with stable angina or old myocardial infarcts. Angioscopy was thought to display the intracoronary lumen better than coronary arteriography.

During angioscopy transient rises in the ST segment occurred in nine patients, with chest pain in seven. Coronary spasm was seen in 1 patient alleviated by withdrawal of the angioscope and/or intracoronary injection of glyceryl trinitrate. No major complications such as acute myocardial infarction or death occurred during the procedure. No follow-up data are provided. As the study was uncontrolled, excess mortality or morbidity could not be determined.

The major objective of the study appeared to be the trial of a new gadget. The results were cast in a pathogenetic frame of reference. One suspects that without that bow to medical science, the study would not have been publishable (*in a Western medical journal*).

The assertion that this final study is not fundamentally different from the first three studies described above in terms of attitude towards patients is supported by the acceptance of the Japanese paper by peer reviewers and editorial board of a prestigious medical journal without any questions about ethics committees, informed patient consent, or any protest against using patients to test out a new and dangerous gadget.

Contemporary Critical Medical History

Having been employed in rabbits, dogs, pigs, and later in primates, the first partial ileal bypass was performed in a human on May 29, 1963. We can be certain of the exact date because the authors of the report must have felt that the day should live in history and managed to publish the exact date in medical articles.[168-170] To set this surgical procedure in a proper historical perspective, it is useful to review two other surgical trends.

Ineffective surgical treatment of patients with coronary artery disease using a number of different approaches is not all that rare. Ablation of the thyroid left patients not only with their intrinsic CAD but with induced hypothyroidism as well.[171] Thoracic sympathectomy, epicardial abrasion, and internal mammary ligation came and went,[138] leaving behind a large number of patients injured or dead from useless surgery.

It is interesting that the precise number of patients so injured and so dying is unknown. It is not conventional to keep track of either the total number of patients undergoing useless (or useful) surgery or the morbidity and mortality of such surgery.

Nor do we know the rate at which these discredited forms of surgery were abandoned by surgeons and no longer used. Our general impression is that this form of cultural lag is a prominent aspect of surgical management.

The surgical history of partial ileal bypass provides some important lessons. Surgical procedures designed to lower cholesterol were exported from the primary site of partial ileal bypass in two forms.

One form involved the use of partial ileal bypass by a number of surgeons in the United States and abroad.[172-174] What could the surgeons have known about the results of the bypass? They could have only known that the procedure was effective in lowering cholesterol and altering lipid metabolism. When they applied the surgery to patients, they could not have known whether the surgery was efficacious in terms of improving patient outcome. They could not have had adequate information on the number and nature of the risks. These elementary requirements did not deter them.

In fact, one Finnish group used the procedure in 27 patients with heterozygous familial hypercholesterolemia.[174] The results were dismal for these patients but were excellent for one of the investigators who used the experiment for his dissertation at the University of Helsinki.[175]

In fact, one British surgeon did attempt to provide some sense of perspective for evaluating partial ileal bypass in 1990[176]: "whether the authors [Buchwald et al.] can give us any comfort that patients have had benefits from the primary prevention point of view because we rather regret that from the secondary prevention point of view, lipid lowering at a rather late stage of disease may have limited value." This same physician was not totally clear in his analysis. "This historical work that we have heard . . . is most courageous." Whose courage was he saluting, the surgeon's or the patient's? This peculiar custom of saluting the courage of surgeons rather than the courage of their experimental subjects seems to be a recurrent practice.

Here is a comment provided by a surgeon commenting on the apparently ill-fated performance of partial ileal bypass on children.[177]

"I would like to congratulate Dr. Buchwald and his associates on . . . also on their wisdom and daring, if you will, in applying these principles to the pediatric age group particularly in patients with the terrible problem of familial hypercholesterolemia." Unlike adults, these children did not even have the option of informed choice.

The second form of surgical attack consisted of various procedures different from partial ileal bypass but designed to lower serum cholesterol. Starzl and associates described end-to-side portacaval anastomosis for management of a hyperlipidemic patient.[178] This procedure metastasized to South Africa[179] and elsewhere. We assume that this form of surgery for hypercholesterolemia has now been abandoned, leaving behind its quota of the dead and the disabled. Young children did not escape. Starzl and colleagues performed cardiac and liver transplantation in a young girl, age 6 years 9 months, with severe homozygous type 2 hyperlipidemia.[180] Shaw and colleagues also combined liver transplant with cardiac transplant in several patients with end-stage coronary artery disease and type 2 hyperlipidemia.[181] All of this suggests that the use of experimental surgical procedures on humans urgently requires tighter regulation in the interests of patient safety.

The second historical antecedent of partial ileal bypass was the use of jejunal-ileal bypass for the treatment of morbid obesity. This procedure was introduced into clinical medicine during the 1960s in the same institution and by some of the same surgeons who later introduced partial ileal bypass.[182] This discredited and (largely) abandoned form of surgery was associated with extensive problems. By 1977, the list of recognized complications was very large including a surgical mortality of 4%.[183]

One list of complications published in 1979[183] (and modified by us) is as follows:

1. Early
   a. Perioperative mortality
   b. Thromboembolic disease
   c. Wound infection
   d. Renal failure
   e. Severe nausea and vomiting
   f. Wound dehiscence
2. Late
   a. Urinary calculi
   b. Severe electrolyte imbalance
   c. Acute cholecystitis
   d. Progressive liver disease
   e. Intestinal obstruction
   f. Peptic ulcer
   g. Osteoporosis
3. Minor
   a. Diarrhea
   b. Weakness
   c. Hypokalemia
   d. Hypoproteinemia
   e. Vomiting
   f. Thirst
   g. Hypocalcemia
   h. Arthralgias
   i. Incisional hernias
   j. Hyperuricemia
   k. Anemias (Fe, B_{12}, folate)
4. General complications
   a. Malnutrition
   b. Syndrome of bacterial overgrowth
   c. Bypass enteropathy
   d. Increased incidence of tuberculosis
   e. Enteropathic non-vitamin B_{12} ataxia
   f. Hypoglycemia
   g. Pseudo-obstructive megacolon
5. Required reanastomosis and bowel continuity restoration with second wave mortality and morbidity.

The same investigator after reviewing the risks and the benefits concludes that "It is, therefore, the opinion of this commentator that intestinal bypass surgery is justified for some of the grossly obese individuals who are severely impaired in their social or medical functions." In fact, in 1978 a National Institute of Health Consensus Conference endorsed bypass surgery, and only in 1991 was intestinal bypass frowned upon.[184] Sometime after 1979 the surgery was largely abandoned.[183] The basis of this abandonment is not entirely clear. It may be that there was almost universal recognition that the surgical procedure was more morbid than the obesity. It may have been that a new and equally unvalidated surgical procedure, gastric banding, became available.[185] Current favorites include vertical banded gastroplasty and Roux-en-Y gastric bypass.[186] Surgical styles may have simply changed. The rise and fall of jejunal-ileal bypass provides several lessons:

1. Dangerous and discredited surgical procedures usually do not die. They either fade away or, occasionally, they are replaced by new, equally ineffective, procedures.
2. Cultural lag is common in surgery as well as in other branches of medicine.
3. The use of procedures without data derived from a

PRCCT is at least as dangerous in surgery as in other branches of medicine.

4. Surgical procedures are not abandoned until there is a new surgical procedure waiting in the wings to replace the surgery.

5. Jejunal-ileal bypass was even more complication-associated than partial ileal bypass. As a result, the investigators involved in the latter procedure may have underestimated the impact of partial ileal bypass on the quality of life.

Given the surgical mileau at the home of jejunal-ileal bypass, it is not surprising that partial ileal bypass on human subjects arose at the same instution.

In an early summary publication it was reported that a total of four patients underwent partial ileal bypass.[169] The indication in each was elevated serum cholesterol with values of 300 to 600 mg. The ages of the patients are not provided. They were all said to have a family history of and exhibit signs of atherosclerotic vascular disease.

It is certain that *informed* consent could not have been obtained from these four patients. What could the subjects have been told to be truly informed? A new surgical procedure with risks unknown to the investigators was being tried for a chemical abnormality, hypercholesterolemia, whose risks to individual patients were even more uncertain then than now? An uninformed investigator cannot possibly inform a prospective experimental subject. The risks of the procedure were unknown. Institutional approval was not the norm in 1963. After all, this was the decade during which thymectomy was studied with respect to skin homograft survival in children,[187] melanoma was being transplanted into human "volunteers,"[189] and the newborn subjected to large doses of x-ray to outline the ureterovesical junction.[190]

Whether it is reasonable to criticize the use of the first four patients as largely unprotected experimental animals requires a discussion that is too extensive for this chapter. We do know that the three common errors that plague experimental surgery on human subjects were made by these investigators: too few subjects, too short a period in postoperative follow-up and an optimism about the results of one's own experiments.

"To date there have been no untoward after effects of the operation: There is no evidence of malnutrition or inadequate carbohydrate and protein absorption in any of the patients, the thin patients have all gained weight without difficulty."[187]

In 1970, there was the extension of the experimental group to include children.[191] The rationale was to arrest atherogenesis in its earliest phase during childhood. Seven pubertal or prepubertal youngsters, the youngest aged 7, each with a presumed diagnosis of familial hypercholesterolemia underwent partial ileal bypass. The degree of civilization of a society is often reflected in its treatment of young children. Performing surgery on these children in this poorly conceived experiment is reminiscent of the administration of infectious hepatitis virus to mentally deficient children to determine the incubation period of the virus.[192] The enthusiasm for performing partial ileal bypass on children with familial hypercholesterolemia persisted until at least 1974.[187]

These seven children (any survivors are now adults) disappeared from the medical literature until 1990 when a passing reference is made as follows[193]:

"This may have been due to the inclusion of several younger patients afflicted with homozygous (actually 6 or more were heterozygous), familial hypercholesterolemia in this analysis (20-26 year post surgery follow-up)." Then follows a Delphian statement, "These patients with severely elevated total cholesterol values responded poorly to partial ileal bypass." Does this mean that the changes in cholesterol metabolism were limited, or does this mean that the youngsters did poorly?

We believe that society has a right to know. Did the bypass with its obligatory malabsorption interfere with normal growth and development of the young children? In how many of the seven patients did bowel obstruction and/or diarrhea develop? How many are still alive? How many require long-term medical care because of partial ileal bypass? How many of them died as a result of short-term or long-term complications of the procedure? What were their parents told? What do their parents know now?

We believe that the fate of the missing seven children is an integral, legitimate and critical concern for those seeking to evaluate partial ileal bypass. The fate of the missing seven children urgently requires clarification.

In this respect, what responsibility was taken by the various granting agencies supporting the studies such as the Helen Hay Whitney Foundation, the Heart, Lung, and Blood Institute, the Life Insurance Research Fund? Did the Expert Panel Report of the National Cholesterol Education Program consider at all the fate of the missing seven?

A chronology of the various complications with the surgery (partial ileal bypass) is as follows: The material are largely extracted from the numerous publications of Buchwald and collaborators. When other sources are used, an asterisk followed by a reference is provided.

Chronic diarrhea
    1963: Not mentioned.
    1966: Diarrhea mentioned.
    1969: Outside group reports that postoperative diarrhea is troublesome and persists for months to years.* [194]

1974: "Only" 18% of patients had 6 to 10 stools a day; one patient required restored bowel continuity because of intractable diarrhea.

1981: 50% of patients had frequent bouts; in two patients, diarrhea controlled with cholestyramine.* [174]

1990: Frequent bowel movements are the rule; however, not one surviving patient believed that this required any life-style modification.

1990: Less than 2% of patients have had operative restoration of intestinal continuity because of intractable diarrhea.

1990: Diarrhea is 100%. 6 to 8 percent of patients had watery to frothy stools.

Bowel obstruction

1963: Not mentioned.

1964: Three patients with small bowel obstruction caused by adhesive bands requiring surgery in all three.

1981: Not mentioned.

1990: Not mentioned.

1990: The incidence of late bowel obstruction secondary to adhesions (2%) and late development of incisional hernia are identical to those observed after any surgical procedure (perhaps, but these patients had their surgical procedure to influence lipid metabolism).

1990: 57/399 (14%) patients had at least one episode of bowel obstruction of which 15/399 (4%) required surgical intervention.

Weight loss

1963: Not mentioned.

1974: Not mentioned.

1981: Patients did not lose weight "but in contrast to controls did not gain weight either."

1990: Not mentioned.

1990: "No long term loss of weight has been reported."

1990: This non obese group of 399 patients lost a mean of 5.3 kg.

Gallstones and renal stones

1963: Not mentioned.

1974: "We have not been able to demonstrate the formation of gallstones in our material. In our entire postoperative series only one patient has developed cholelithiasis. Another individual has, on the basis of x-ray evidence, shown conversion of a "strawberry gallbladder to a normal appearing structure" (no suggestion fortunately that partial ileal bypass be used to dissolve gallstones).

1981: The incidence . . . viz. biliary and renal stones known to be increased in ileal dysfunction tended to be higher in our ileal bypass patients than the control patients but the differences were not statistically significant.

1980: "Cholelithiasis appears to develop at an increased rate after partial ileal bypass." "Nephrolithiasis develops at an increased rate."

1990: "An increased incidence of calcium oxalate renal stones has been observed after partial ileal bypass." No mention of gallstones. However, "excessive foul-smelling flatus and the gas-bloat syndrome" encountered after partial ileal bypass.

1990: A higher incidence of kidney stones and gallstones was observed among the patients who had undergone partial ileal bypass. The incidence rate of kidney stone was approximately 4% per year in the surgery group . . . 14 partial ileal bypass patients underwent cholecystectomy during the first 5 years of follow-up . . . 40 of these patients had gallstones detected by oral cholecystography or ultrasonography.

Malabsorption and Other Complications

Malabsorption of vitamin B_{12} has been documented in patients undergoing partial ileal bypass and this vitamin is generally administered parenterally after surgery.[195] The absorption of vitamin A appears to be reduced possibly related to steatorrhea.[196] The absorption of dietary calcium is reduced by about 15% although usually there are no signs of calcium deficiency.[197] One case of asymptomatic hypocalcemia has been reported and treated with calcium supplementation and vitamin A.[198]

One case of potassium deficiency has been reported that responded to potassium supplementation.[199]

In two patients partial ileal bypass caused an increase in serum alkaline phosphatase. With the restoration of bowel continuity in one patient, alkaline phosphatase values returned to normal.[173]

Partial ileal bypass may impair the absorption of monosaccharides as shown by a reduction in d-xylose absorption.[198]

Modest rises in serum alanine amino transferase, aspartate amino transferase, alkaline phosphatase, and other liver enzymes have been reported.[197] In one patient restoration of bowel continuity induced a fall toward normal in amino transferase and aspartate aminotransferase. The effects of partial ileal bypass on liver function and histology have not been systematically studied.

Many of these data were assembled in a review of partial ileal bypass in 1986.[173]

It is not possible to extract the rate of surgery to

restore intestinal continuity from the data in the literature. It is not clear whether there was operative mortality associated with surgery to restore intestinal continuity, with gallbladder surgery with renal stone removal or with surgery for intestinal obstruction. Three serious complications of jejunal-ileal bypass are specifically denied; electrolyte depletion secondary to diarrhea although no data are provided; the arthropathy associated with jejuno-ileal bypass and the liver disease associated with jejuno-ileal bypass.[193] Sequential liver function studies are not reported in the literature. Finally, it appears that the perioperative mortality was relatively low with partial ileal bypass as compared with jejuno-ileal bypass. Mortality is listed as less than 1% in the former surgical procedure and as about 3% in the latter.[183]

The statements made in the medical literature about the kinds and frequency of risks were often contradictory. In general, the more time that elapsed, the higher the rate of complications. In a general way, some concern about the rate of complications has paralleled accumulating data. It seems clear that many studies in the survey have consistently tended to underestimate the rate of complications. Some potential complications have not been adequately investigated. Finally, it should be emphasized that without accurate information about risks it is impossible for physicians to provide adequate information to potential subjects for a clinical trial so that they can make an informed choice.

The POSCH Experiment

We turn now to the results of the prospective randomized controlled trial of partial ileal bypass conducted over a 15-year period (1975 to 1990) in an attempt to determine the value of partial ileal bypass in reducing mortality from coronary artery disease in patients with one prior myocardial infarction by lowering serum cholesterol or altering some of the associated biochemical variables said to be pathogenetic in the development of CAD.[24] As stated above (p. 31), the multiinstitutional, multiinvestigator, multiauthored study population consisted of 838 patients, 417 in the control group and 421 in the surgery group.

In the assembly and interpretation of the data a very peculiar decision was made. Peculiar, because epidemiologic expertise abounded. To repeat, 22 patients refused surgery. For unclear reasons, during statistical analysis the results of this group was included with patients undergoing surgery. One of the results of this maneuver was to lower erroneously the rate of complications. Only 399 patients were subjected to partial ileal bypass, and this number was the valid denominator to use in calculations. Whether this error affected the calculated rates of total deaths or of deaths from myocardial infarction cannot be extracted from the data. On the one hand, if none of the 22 died then this error would lower the calculated mortality in the control group. On the other hand, if all 22 lived it would decrease the mortality in the experimental group.

As other data were calculated, such as the percentage of patients with a low ejection fraction, the exact effect of (erroneously) including the 22 unoperated patients in the experimental group is unknown.

The results in the experimental group with respect to decreases in plasma cholesterol and related variables were dramatic and similar to the changes previously noted in rabbits, dogs, pigs, monkies, and about 200 patients who had undergone partial ileal bypass prior to the POSCH study.

From the standpoint of patient outcome, the results showed no significant difference in total mortality and mortality from coronary artery disease between those having partial ileal bypass and the controls.

The failure to show a significant decrease in general or specific mortality despite a 23% decrease in serum cholesterol, a decrease of 38% in LDL and an increase of 4.3% in HDL, as pointed out by Moore[200] challenges proponents of aggressive management of cholesterol metabolism. Moreover, these changes were maintained for an average of 8.9 years. It is therefore evident that not only partial ileal bypass but other modes of treatment would be ineffective in improving total mortality or specific mortality of CAD by virtue of cholesterol manipulation.

Faced with these unpleasant facts, the investigators appeared to redefine the study so as to declare victory.

They evaluated a series of surrogate values. They combined (1) death due to coronary artery disease and confirmed nonfatal myocardial infarction or changes in arteriograms of the coronary arteries or outcome in patients with (2) patients with normal ejection fractions to show significance. Despite having previously criticized subgroup analysis performed for the same purpose to establish statistical significance in the Helsinki Heart Study, the investigators now engaged in the same practice. In so doing, there appeared to be a subtle but definite shift in the fundamental objectives of partial ileal bypass.

The surgery could not be demonstrated to improve patient outcome significantly. Now it was claimed that the surgery halted atherosclerotic progression. This attempt is a two-edged sword. The results of the study show that despite "improvement" of atherosclerotic involvement of coronary and peripheral arteries but not cerebral vessels, there is no significant improvement in total mortality. However, the watchwords of cholesterol manipulators may become atherosclerotic regression or halting atherosclerotic progress rather than reducing CAD mortality.

It is important to raise other issues. For a study that extended over 15 years, one must ask not only what the investigators knew and when did they know it, but also what were the patients in the trial told and when were they told? These questions are pertinent not only for the period of recruitment into the trial (1975 to 1982) but also for the entire period when knowledge of the rate of and nature of complications became known to the investigative team.

Informed consent must involve not only what is known in the way of hazards when a PRCCT is started but what information is accumulated during the trial that has important relevance to the welfare of the participants. We doubt that many knowledgeable cardiologists would have volunteered to participate in the experiment knowing what was at stake in partial ileal bypass. And even fewer would have remained in the trial had timely information been provided.

There is one more pertinent issue. Who paid for the treatment of surgical complications of partial ileal bypass? Hopefully not the subjects in the experiment. Who will pay for the treatment of surgical complications as these continue to accumulate? Who will pay for reversal of the bypass as this becomes increasingly frequent with the passage of time?

It is worth emphasizing that an independent monitoring group is essential to reduce the risks of experimental medical studies in human subjects. The experiment could have and would have been terminated in less than 15 years had a suitable monitoring group supervised the study.

The paper appears to contain no statement that the experiment was approved by ethics committees at the four sponsoring medical institutions. Is it possible that this extensive 15-year study was conducted without formal local review?

It is known that the experiment was approved by various granting agencies, by various peer review committees, by peer reviewers and editorial boards for various medical journals, and by a large number of experts that participated in the experiment. Could a 15-year human experiment be performed without any criticism of the basic safety of the experiment?

Another lesson involves the importance of independent, external monitoring committees whose function is to insure patient protection and to insure that patients are fully informed as data about risks is accumulated and as it becomes known that the risk-benefit ratio is favorable or unfavorable for the subjects being studied.

The study was rich in committees and boards. There was an 11-member data monitoring committee, a 4-member mortality review committee, and so forth.[201] Did the fact of universal diarrhea in the experimental patients somehow escape attention? What about the 14% incidence of intestinal obstruction? This did not become suddenly obvious in 1990. An incidence of kidney stones of 4% per year could have been detected

long before 1990. The finding that 40 (10%) experimental patients developed gallstones suggests that this complication could have been detected or that 14 surgery group patients required cholecystectomies during 5 years of follow-up should have come as no surprise in 1990. Many lives were saved in the encainide-flecainide study by an independent monitoring overview committee. This mechanism should certainly be mandatory for all invasive experimental studies.

IATROBOONS AND THROMBOLYTIC THERAPY FOR ACUTE MYOCARDIAL INFARCTION

Readers having completed the previous sections outlining iatroepidemics may consider that our discussion lacks adequate balance. This is accurate although in a chapter dealing with medical risks, such lack of balance is perhaps unavoidable.

However, it is obvious that medicine, including cardiology, offers much that is life-saving and welfare enhancing. It is probably not necessary to introduce a new term for the benefits provided by medicine. It is probably gratuitous to coin a term, iatroboon, which is defined as the development and widespread use of a management modality with a strongly favorable risk/benefit ratio resulting in an increase in the quantity of life or an improvement in the quality of life for masses of patients. The general (but mistaken) perception is that most of medical practice operates in that fashion. However, it may be worth closing this chapter with one example out of many of an iatroboon (*iatros:* Greek "physician," *boon:* Archaic "welcome benefit").

The widespread use of thrombolytic agents in patients with acute myocardial infarction has reduced in-hospital mortality from about 20 to 5%.[202] This means an annual saving of about 60,000 lives in the United States alone. The use of these agents also permits earlier hospital discharge improving the quality of life. In all probability, thrombolytic therapy is myocardium-sparing and provides an improved lifestyle.

Moreover, this giant contribution has been rigorously evaluated by a series of PRCCTs so that the magnitude of neither the benefits nor the risks require guess work. This is an enormous contribution to patients throughout the world. ISIS III is a remarkable testimony to cooperative studies in medicine.[203]

Not that the process of introducing and applying available agents has been entirely altruistic. For example, the early approval and favorable handling of the use of recombinant TPA involved a sharp conflict of interest by two members of the approving board. But no part of our society can be entirely free of politics and economics.

There are still important uncertainties. The addition of heparin to thrombolytic therapy improves survival but increases the incidence of brain hemorrhage.[202] Whether to use heparin or not is a difficult decision in which the final decision should be left to the patient if he or she is able to make it, understanding the risks and benefits. Many patients might wish to have their brain spared at the expense of small additional protection of the myocardium.

There are also important problems in logistics to be solved. Thrombolytic therapy becomes less effective with the passage of time after an acute myocardial infarction.[202] Should we not develop a system for administration of this therapy in the field, possibly by paramedics? And finally, we must learn what the impact of thrombolytic therapy is on long-term prognosis. Just as the net impact of the encainide-flecainide disaster causes us shame, the net impact of thrombolytic therapy on patient outcome should give cardiologists pride.

REFERENCES

1. Blendon RJ: The public's view of the future of health care. JAMA 259:3587, 1988
2. Eddy DM: The quality of medical evidence: implications for quality of care. Health Affairs 7:19, 1988
3. Wennberg JE: Dealing with medical practice variations: a proposal for action. Health Affairs 3:7, 1984
4. Landenson PW: Editorial. Treatment for Grave's disease. N Engl J Med 324:989, 1991
5. Califano JA: American's Health Care Revolution: Who Lives? Who Dies? Who Pays? p. 105. Random House, New York, 1986
6. Robin ED: Saltem plus boni quam mali efficere conare: At least try to do more good than harm. Pharos 50:40, 1987
7. Blankenhorn DH, Nassin SA, San Marino ME et al: Beneficial effects of combined colestipol-niacin therapy on coronary arteriosclerosis and coronary venous bypass grafts. JAMA 257:3233, 1987
8. Feinstein AR: Clinical Epidemiology: The Architecture of Clinical Research. WB Saunders, Philadelphia, 1985
9. Robin ED, Lewiston NS: Type 3 and type 4 errors in the statistical evaluations of clinical trials. Chest 98:463, 1990
10. Morganroth J, Bigger JT, Jr, Anderson JL: Treatment of ventricular arrhythmias by United States cardiologists: a survey before the cardiac arrhythmia suppression trial results were available. Am J Cardiol 65:40, 1990
11. Registry for Research on Hormonal Transplacental Carcinogenesis: 1977 Newsletter, Chicago.
12. Gofman JW, O'Conner E: X-rays Health, Effects of Common Exams. Sierra Club, San Francisco, 1985
13. Robin ED, Theodore J: Iatroepidemics and iatroepidemiology. West J Med 133:131, 1980
14. Robin ED: A critical look at critical care. Crit Care Med 2:144, 1983
15. Robin ED: Matters of Life and Death. WH Freeman, New York, 1984
16. Robin ED: Iatroepidemics: a probe to examine systematic, preventable errors in medicine. Am Rev Respir Dis 135:1152, 1987
17. Robin ED: Overdiagnosis and overtreatment of pulmonary embolism. Ann Intern Med 87:775, 1977
18. Moertel CG, Fleming TR, Creagen ET: High-dose Vitamin C versus placebo in the treatment of patients with advanced cancer who have had no prior chemotherapy. N Engl J Med 312:137, 1985
19. Grossman W: Cardiac Catheterization and Angiography. Lea & Febiger, Philadelphia, 1986, p. 30
20. Robin ED: Iatroepidemics: a probe to examine systematic preventable errors in (chest) medicine. Am Rev Respir Dis 135:1152, 1987
21. Rossouw JB, Rifkin LB: The value of lowering cholesterol after acute myocardial infarction. N Engl J Med 16:1112, 1990
22. Weinstein PR, Rodriguezy Baena R, Chater NL: Results of extracranial-intracranial arterial bypass for intracranial internal carotid artery stenosis: review of 105 cases. Neurosurg 15:787, 1984
23. The EC/IC Bypass Study Group: Failure of extracranial-intracranial arterial bypass to reduce the risk of ischemic stroke. Results of an international randomized trial. N Engl J Med 313:1191, 1985
23A. Haynes RB, Mukherjee J, Sackett DL et al: Functional status changes following medical or surgical treatment for cerebral ischemia. JAMA 257:2043, 1987
24. Buchwald H, Varco RL, Matts, JP, and the POSCH Group: Effect of partial ileal bypass on mortality and morbidity from coronary heart disease in patients with hypercholesterolemia. N Engl J Med 323:946, 1990
25. Rowley KM, Clabb KS, SMith GI et al: Right sided infective endocarditis as a consequence of flow-directed pulmonary artery catheterization: a clinicopathological study of 55 autopsied patients. N Engl J Med 311:1152, 1985
26. Robin ED: Death by pulmonary artery flow-directed catheter: time for a moratorium? (Editorial.) Chest 92:727, 1987
27. Ziporyn T: Scoliosis management now subject to question. JAMA 254:3009, 1985
28. Hoffman DA, Lonstein JE, Morin MM et al: Breast cancer in women with scoliosis exposed to multiple diagnostic x-rays. JNCI 81:1307, 1989
29. Goodwin JS, Goodwin JM: The tomato effect: rejection of highly efficacious therapy. JAMA 251:2387, 1984
30. Fuster V, Cohen M, Halperin J: Aspirin in the prevention of coronary disease. N Engl J Med 321:183, 1989
31. Steering Committee: Physicians Health Study Research Group. Final report on the aspirin component of the ongoing physicians health study. N Engl J Med 321:129, 1989
32. Pocock SJ, Hughes MD, Lee RJ: Statistical problems in the reporting of clinical trials. N Engl J Med 317:426, 1987
33. Spector TD, Thompson SG: The potential and limitations of meta-analysis. J Epidemiol Community Health 45:89, 1991

34. Thompson SG, Pocock S: Can meta-analysis be trusted. Lancet 2:1127, 1991
35. Robin LJ: Primary pulmonary hypertension. (Letter.) Chest 93:894, 1988
36. Blom JJ: Descartes: His Moral Philosophy and Psychology. New York University Press, New York, 1978
37. Hill RKH, Jr: Gray matters. Pressure 20:7, 1991
38. Raphael JC, Elkharrit P, Jars-Guincoestre MC et al: Trial of normobaric and hyperbaric oxygen for acute carbon monoxide intoxication. Lancet 2:414, 1989
39. Dedhia HV, Schiebel F, Teba L: Letter re Robin ED: Risk-benefit analysis in chest medicine—Defenders of the pulmonary artery catheter. Chest 93:1059, 1988
40. Iberti TJ, Fischer EP, Andrew B et al, and the Pulmonary Artery Catheter Study Group: A multicenter study of physicians knowledge of the pulmonary artery catheter. JAMA 264:2928, 1990
41. Bone RC: High-tech predicament: pulmonary artery catheter. (Editorial.) JAMA 264:2933, 1990
42. Sollman TH: A Manual of Pharmacology and Its Applications to Therapeutics and Toxicology. WB Saunders, Philadelphia, 1942, p. 1024
43. Oakley A: The history of ultrasonography in obstetrics. Birth 13:1, 1986
44. Joyce J: Ulysses. Modern Library, New York, 1940
45. Carlyle T: On Heroes and Hero-Worship. Oxford University Press, Oxford, 1928
46. Gibbon E: Decline and Fall of the Roman Empire. Modern Library, New York, 1940
47. Ford H: Statement made during Chicago Tribune lawsuit trial, July 1919
48. Hegel GWF, cited in Shaw GB: The Revolutionist's Handbook. Bancroft, New York, 1962
49. Hippocrates: Aphroisms. François Rabelais (ed). Lyon, 1532
50. Robin ED: Death from bronchial asthma. Chest 91:616, 1988
51. Frazer JG: The Golden Bough. Macmillan, New York, 1922
52. Robin ED: Overdiagnosis and overtreatment of pulmonary embolism: the Emperor may have no clothes. Ann Intern Med 88:775, 1977
53. Hull RD, Hirsh J, Carter C et al: Diagnostic value of ventilation-perfusion scanning in patients with suspected pulmonary embolism. Chest 88:819, 1985
54. PIOPED Investigators: Value of the ventilation/perfusion scan in acute pulmonary embolism: results of the Prospective Investigation of Pulmonary Embolism Diagnosis (PIOPED). JAMA 263:2753, 1990
55. Fyke FE, III: Transesophageal echocardiography and cardiac masses. (Editorial.) Mayo Clin Proc 66:1171, 1991
56. Lowen B: Sudden cardiac death: the major challenge confronting contemporary cardiology. Am J Cardiol 43:313, 1979
57. Ruberman W, Weinblatt E, Goldberg JD et al: Ventricular premature beats and mortality after myocardial infarction. N Engl J Med 297:750, 1977
58. Hinkle LE, Jr, Carver ST, Stevens M: The frequency of asymptomatic disturbances of cardiac rhythm and conduction in middle aged man. Am J Cardiol 24:629, 1969
59. Moss AJ, De Camilla J, Mietiowski W et al: Prognostic grading and significance of ventricular premature beats after recovery from myocardial infarction. Circulation, suppl III. 52:111, 1975
60. Kitlier MN, Tabatznik B, Mower MN, Tominaga S: Prognostic significance of ventricular ectopic beats with respect to sudden death in the late post infarction period. Circulation 47:959, 1973
61. Mukharji J, Rude RE, Poole WK et al: Risk factors for sudden death after myocardial infarction: two years follow up. Am J Cardiol 54:31, 1984
62. Furberg CD: Effect of antiarrhythmic drugs on mortality after myocardial infarction. Am J Cardiol 52:32C–36C, 1983
63. Ryden L, Arnman K, Conradson TB et al: Prophylaxis of ventricular tachyarrhythmias with intravenous and oral tocainide in patients with and recovery from acute myocardial infarction. Am Heart J 100:1006, 1980
64. Hockings BEF, George T, Mahrous F et al: Effectiveness of amiodarone on ventricular arrhythmias during and after acute myocardial infarction. Am J Cardiol 60:967, 1987
65. Yusuf S, Petro R, Lewis J et al: Beta-blockade during and after myocardial infarction: an overview of the randomized studies. Prog Cardiovasc Dis 27:335, 1985
66. Kesteloot H, Stroobandt R: Clinical experience of encainide (MJ 9067): A new antiarrhythmic drug. Eur J Clin Pharmacol 16:323, 1979
67. Duff HS, Roden DM, Mattuci RJ et al: Suppression of resistant ventricular arrhythmias by twice daily dosing with flecainide. Am J Cardiol 48:1133, 1981
68. Graboys TB, Lowen B, Podrid P, DeSilva R: Long-term survival of patients with malignant ventricular arrhythmias treated with antiarrhythmic drugs. Am J Cardiol 50:437, 1982
69. Swerdlow CD, Winkle RA, Mason JW: Determinants of survival in patients with ventricular tachyarrhythmias. N Engl J Med 308:1436, 1983
70. DiBianco R, Fletcher RD, Cohen A et al: B. Treatment of frequent ventricular arrhythmias with encainide assessment using serial ambulatory electrocardiograms, intracardiac electrophysiologic studies, treadmill exercise tests and radionuclide cineangiographic studies. Circulation 65:1135, 1982
71. Soyka LF: Safety of encainide for the treatment of ventricular arrhythmias. Am J Cardiol 58:96C, 1986
72. Harrison DC, Winkle R, Somi M, Mason J: Encainide: a new and potent antiarrhythmic agent. Am Heart J 100:1134, 1980
73. Meinertz T, Zehender MK, Geibel A et al: Long-term antiarrhythmic therapy with flecainide. Am J Cardiol 54:91, 1984
74. Winkle RA, Mason JW, Griffin JC, Ross D: Malignant ventricular arrhythmias associated with the use of encainide. Am Heart J 102:857, 1981
75. Cardiac Arrhythmia Pilot Study (CAPS) Investigators: Effects of encainide, flecainide, imipramine and moricizine on ventricular arrhythmias during the year after myocardial infarction: the CAPS. Am J Cardiol 61:501, 1988
76. Cardiac Arrhythmia Suppression Trial, Echt D, Liebson

PR, Mitchell LB et al: Mortality and morbidity in patients receiving encainide, flecainide or placebo. N Engl J Med 324:781, 1991

77. Ruskin JN: The cardiac arrhythmia suppression trial (CAST). (Editorial.) 321:386, 1989

78. Temple R: Quoted in: Two heart drugs called useful though cropped from study. The New York Times. July 29, 1989: p. 9

79. STAT/GRAM: DuPont Pharmaceutical, Aug 9, 1991

80. Attributed to William Geoge at the 101st meeting American Pediatric Society 1991 quoted in Lancet, 837:1215

81. Robin ED: Pulmonary artery catheters. (Letter.) JAMA 265:2339, 1991

82. Hippocrates quoted in Silverman WH: Human Experimentation. Oxford Medical Publications, Oxford, 1985

83. Marino PL: The I.C.U. Lea & Febiger, Philadelphia, 1991

84. Swan HJC: In Sprung CL (ed): The Pulmonary Artery Catheter Methodology and Clinical Applications. Aspen Systems, Rockville, MD, 1983

85. Boucek CO: Published in Robin ED. Defenders of the pulmonary artery catheter. Chest 93:1059, 1988

86. Robin ED: Death by pulmonary artery flow-directed catheter. Time for a moratorium? (Editorial.) Chest 92:727, 1987

87. Robin ED: Hydras, lemmings, and diagnostic tests. Arch Int Med 147:1704, 1987

88. Robin ED, Morin M: The unvalidated mass use and lethal risk of the pulmonary artery flow-direction (Swan-Ganz) catheter. pp. 178–190. In Winterbaner RH (ed): Debate in Medicine. Vol. 2. Year Book Medical Publishers, Chicago, 1989

89. McGrath RB: Invasive bedside hemodynamic monitoring. Prog Cardiovasc Dis 29:129, 1986

90. Damean J, Bolton D: A prospective analysis of 1400 pulmonary artery catheterizations in patients undergoing cardiac surgery. Acta Anaesthesiol Scand 30:386, 1986

91. Gore JM, Goldberg RJ, Spodich DH et al: A community-wide assessment of the use of pulmonary artery catheters in patients with acute myocardial infarction. Chest 92:721, 1987

92. Greenland P, Reicher-Reiss H, Goldboert U et al, and the Israeli Spring Investigators: In-hospital and 1 year mortality in 1,524 women after myocardial infarction, comparison with 4,315 men. Circulation 83:484, 1991

93. Zion MM, Balkin J, Rosenmann D et al: Use of pulmonary artery catheters in patients with acute myocardial infarction. Analysis of experience in 5,841 patients in the SPRINT Registry. Chest 98:1331, 1990

94. Council on Scientific Affairs: Autopsy. A comprehensive review of current issues. JAMA 258:364, 1987

95. Honan MB, Harrell FE, Jr, Reimer KA et al: Cardiac rupture, mortality and the timing of thrombolytic therapy: a meta-analysis. J Am Coll Cardiol 16:359, 1990

96. Swan HJC, Ganz W: Hemodynamic measurements in clinical practice. J Am Coll Cardiol 1:103, 1983

97. Dalen JE: Does pulmonary artery catheterization benefit patients with acute myocardial infarction? (Editorial.) Chest 98:1313, 1990

98. Schultz RS, Whitfield JF, La Murra JJ et al: The role of physiologic monitoring in patients with fracture of the hip. J Trauma 25:309, 1985

99. Shoemaker WC, Appel PL: Use of physiologic monitoring to predict outcome and assist in clinical decisions in critically ill postoperative patients. Am J Surg 146:43, 1983

100. Wigton RS, Nicolos BA, Blank LL: Procedural skills training in internal medicine residencies: a survey of program directors. Ann Intern Med 111:932, 1989

101. ACC/AHA Guidelines for the early management of patients with acute myocardial infarction. Office of Scientific Affairs. American Heart Association, 7320 Greenville Ave. Dallas, TX 75321. Circulation 67:664, 1990

102. Robinson K: Parlimentary debates. House of Commons Official Report 677. Log 439:109, 1963

103. Mann RD: Drug-induced disorders of central nervous system function. p. 113. In Iatrogenic Diseases. D'Arcy IF, Guffen SP (eds): Oxford University Press, New York, 1986

104. Felix RH, Ives FA, Dahl MGC: Cutaneous and ocular reactions to practalol. Br Med J 4:321, 1974

105. Robin ED: Death from bronchial asthma. Chest 93:614, 1988

106. Editorial: Beta agonists in asthma: relief, prevention, morbidity. Lancet 2:1411, 1990

107. Inman WHW, Adelstein AM: Rise and fall of asthma mortality in England and Wales in relation to pressurized aerosols. Lancet 2:279, 1969

108. Fielding H, Garrison A: An Introduction to the History of Medicine. WB Saunders, Philadelphia, 1914

109. Locke HMF: Dangerous effects of isoprenaline in myocardial failure. Lancet 2:104, 1963

110. Greenberg MS, Pines A: Pressurized aerosols in asthma. Br Med J 1:563, 1967

111. Speizer FE, Doll R, Neaf P: Observations on recent increases in mortality from asthma. Br Med J 3:245, 1968

112. Sly RM: Increases in death from asthma. Ann Allergy 53:20, 1984

113. Pearce N, Grainger J, Atkinson M et al: Case control study of prescribed fenoterol and death from asthma in New Zealand 1981–83: case-control study. Lancet 1:917, 1989

114. Crane J, Flatt A, Jackson R et al: Prescribed fenoterol and death from asthma in New Zealand 1981–1983: case-control study. Lancet 1:917, 1989

115. Molfino NA, Nannini LS, Martelli AN, Slutsky AS: Respiratory arrest in near fatal asthma. N Engl J Med 324:285, 1991

116. O'Hollaren MT, Yunginger JW, Oxford KP et al: Exposure to an aerosol as a possible precipitating factor in respiratory arrest in young patients with asthma. N Engl J Med 324:359, 1991

117. Guidelines for the diagnosis and management of asthma: Pediat Asthma Allergy Immunol. 5:183, 1991

118. D'Arcy PF, Guffen JP (eds): Iatrogenic Diseases. Oxford University Press, Oxford, 1986, p. 204

119. Eason J, Cottan S, Beard C et al: Manual chest compression for total bronchospasm. (Letter.) Lancet 337:366, 1991

120. Taylor GJ, Harres WS: Cardiac toxicity of aerosol propellants. JAMA 214:81, 1970

121. Kurland G, William SJ, Lewiston N: Fatal myocardial

toxicity during continuous infusion isoproteranol. J Allergy Clin Immunol 63:407, 1979

122. Shovlin CK, Tam FWK: Salbutamol nebulizer and precipitation of critical cardiac ischemia. Lancet 336:1258, 1990

123. Rolf SS, Ryder C, Kendall MS, Holder R: Cardiovascular and biochemical responses to nebulized salbutamol in normal subjects. Br J Clin Pharmacol 18:641, 1984

124. Alenoy Y, Laks MN, Beall G: An electrocardiographic pattern of acute myocardial infarction associated with excessive use of aerosolized isoproteranol. Chest 68:107, 1975

125. Nicklas RA: Paradoxical bronchospasm associated with the use of beta agonists. J Allergy Clin Immunol 85:959, 1990

126. Robin ED, Lewiston N: Unexpected, unexplained sudden death in young asthmatic subjects. Chest 98:790, 1989

127. Schoen F: Cardiac pathology in asthma. J Allergy Clin Immunol 80:419, 1987

128. Drislane F, Samuels M, Kozakewich H et al: Myocardial contraction band lesions in patients with fatal asthma: possible neurocardiologic mechanisms. Am Rev Respir Dis 135:498, 1987

129. Calverly PMA, Cattarall JR, Shapiro C, Douglas NS: Cor pulmonale in asthma. Br J Dis Chest 77:303, 1983

130. Nicklas RA, Balazs T: Adverse effects of theophylline-beta agonist interactions. J Allergy Clin Immunol 78:806, 1986

131. Wong CS, Pavord ID, Williams J et al: Bronchodilator, cardiovascular and hypokalemic effects of fenoterol, salbutamol, and terbutaline in asthma. Lancet 2:1396, 1990

132. Verrier RL, Haggard EL: Role of the autoimmune nervous system in sudden death. p. 41. In Josephensen ME (ed): Sudden Cardiac Death. FA Davis, Philadelphia, 1985

133. Editorial. Neural mechanisms in sudden cardiac death: insights from long QT interval. Lancet 2:1181, 1991

134. Keating M, Atkinson D, Dunn C et al: Linkage of a cardiac arrhythmia, the long QT interval and the Harvey ras-1 gene. Science 252:704, 1991

135. Swartz PJ, Locati EH, Moss AJ et al: Left cardiac sympathetic denervation in the therapy of the congenital long QT syndrome. Circulation 84:503, 1991

136. Munger RG, Prineas RJ, Crow RS et al: Prolonged QT interval and risk of sudden death in South-East Asian males. Lancet 2:280, 1991

137. Sears MR, Taylor DR, Print CG et al: Regular inhaled beta-agonist treatment in bronchial asthma. Lancet 2:1391, 1990

138. Cass Principal Investigators and their Associates. Coronary Artery Surgery Study (CASS): A randomized trial of coronary artery surgery (CASS) bypass surgery survival data. Circulation 68:939, 1983

139. Pell S, Fayerweather WE. Trends in the incidence of myocardial infarction and in associated mortality and morbidity in a large employed population 1957–83. N Engl J Med 312:1005, 1985

140. White HD, Norris RM, Brown MA: Effect of intravenous streptokinase on left ventricular function and early survival after acute myocardial infarction. N Engl J Med 317:850, 1987

141. Carter RC: Your Food and Your Health. New York, 1964

142. Moore TJ: The cholesterol myth. Atlantic Monthly 266:37, 1989

143. Oliver MF: Might treatment of hypercholesterolemia increase noncardiac mortality. Lancet 2:1529, 1991

144. Lipid Research Clinics Coronary Prevention Trial: I. Reduction in incidence of coronary heart disease. II. The relation of reduction in incidence of coronary heart disease to cholesterol lowering. JAMA 251:351, 1984

145. Frick MH, Elo O, Haaps K et al: Helsinki Heart Study: primary prevention trial with gemfibrozil in middle aged men with dyslipidemia. N Engl J Med 317:1227, 1987

146. Dayton S, Pearce ML, Hashimoto S et al: A controlled trial of a diet high in unsaturated fat in preventing complications of atherosclerosis. Circulation 39/40:1, 1969

147. Turpeinen O, Karvonen MJ, Pekkarinen M et al: Dietary prevention of coronary heart disease. The Finnish Mental Hospital Study. Int Epidemiol 8:99, 1979

148. Hypermann J, Byre KV, Holme I, Leren P: Effect of diet and smoking intervention on the incidence of coronary heart disease. Lancet 2:1303, 1981

149. Browner WS, Westenhouse J, Tice JA: What if Americans ate less fat? A quantitative estimate of the effect on mortality. JAMA 265:3285, 1991

150. Committee on Nutrition: Indications for cholesterol testing in children. Pediatrics 83.141, 1989

151. Strandberg TE, Soloman VV, Neukkarinen VA et al: Long term mortality after 5 year multifactorial primary prevention of cardiovascular diseases in middle aged men. JAMA 266:1225, 1991

152. Paul O, Hennekens CH: The latest report from Finland. (Editorial.) JAMA 266:1267, 1991

153. Heizer RF, Whipple MA: The California Indians. University of California Press, Berkeley, 1971

154. Tsevat J, Weinstein MC, Williams LW et al: Expected gains in life expectancy from various coronary heart disease risk factor modifications. Circulation 83:1194, 1991

155. Luepker R quoted by Perlman D in San Francisco Chronicle 1991

156. Rothman DJ: Strangers at the Bedside. Basic Books, New York, 1991

157. Golino P, Piscone F, Willerson JT et al: Divergent effects of serotonin on coronary artery dimensions and blood flow in patients with coronary atherosclerosis and control patients. N Engl J Med 324:641, 1991

158. DeCaterina R, Carpeggione C, L'Abbate AA: A double blind placebo controlled study of kentonserin in patients with Prinzmetal's angina. evidence against a role for serotonin in the genesis of coronary vasospasm. Circulation 69:889, 1984

159. McFadden EP, Clarke JG, Davies GJ et al: Effect of intracoronary serotonin on coronary vessels in patients with stable angina and patients with variant angina. N Engl J Med 324:648, 1991

160. Voltaire FMA: Candide. New York Hartsdale House 1930

161. Finnerty FA, Jr, Witkin L, Fazegos JF: Cerebral hemodynamics during cerebral ischemia induced by acute hypotension. J Clin Invest 33:1227, 1954

162. Hickam JB, Cargill WH: Effect of exercise on cardiac output and pulmonary arterial pressure in normal persons and in patients with cardiovascular disease and pulmonary emphysema. J Clin Invest 27:10, 1948

163. Hillis LD, Lange RA: Serotonin and ischemic heart disease. (Editorial.) N Engl J Med 324:688, 1991

164. Ornish D, Brown SE, Scherwitz LW et al: Can lifestyle changes reverse coronary heart disease? The lifestyle heart trial. Lancet 2:336:129, 1990

165. Mizuno K, Miyamoto A, Satomura K: Angioscopic coronary macromorphology in patients with acute coronary disorders. Lancet 2:809, 1991

166. Masonori F: Quoted in Kansai Time Out. Oct 1990, 8–9

167. Nudeshima J: Obstacles to brain death and organ transplantation in Japan. Lancet 2:1063, 1991

168. Buchwald H: A surgical operation to lower circulating cholesterol. Circulation 28:649, 1963

169. Buchwald H: Lowering of cholesterol absorption and blood levels by ileal exclusion: experimental basis and preliminary clinical report. Circulation 29:713, 1964

170. Buchwald H, Moore RB, Varco RL: Surgical treatment of hyperlipidemia III. Clinical studies of the partial ileal bypass operation. Circulation 50:1008, 1974

171. Fishberg AM: Heart Failure. Lea & Febiger, Philadelphia 1940

172. Chalstrey LS, Winder AF, Galton DJ: Partial ileal bypass in treatment of familial hypercholesterolemia. J R Soc Med 75:851, 1982

173. Schouten JA, Beynen AC: Partial ileal bypass in the treatment of heterozygous familial hypercholesterolemia. Artery 13:240, 1986

174. Koivisto PA, Mittinen TA: Long term effects of ileal bypass on lipoproteins in patients with familial hypercholesterolemia. Circulation 70:290, 1984

175. Koivisto P: Partial ileal bypass in the treatment of familial hypercholesterolemia. Dissertation. University of Helsinki, Helsinki, 1982

176. Greenholgh R: Discussion 20–26 year partial ileal bypass results. Ann Surg 212:318, 1990

177. Scott HW, Jr: Comments in Buchwold H, Moore RB, Frantz ID Jr, Varco RL. Cholesterol reduction by partial ileal bypass in pediatric population. Surgery 68:1101, 1970

178. Starzl TE, Chase HP, Ahrens EH et al: Portacaval Shunt in patients with familial hypercholesterolemia. Ann Surg 198:273, 1983

179. Stein EA, Mieny C, Spitz L et al: Portacaval shunt in four patients with homozygous hypercholesterolemia. Lancet 1:832, 1975

180. Starzl TE, Bahnson HT, Hardesty RL et al: Heart liver transplantation in a patient with familial hypercholesterolemia. Lancet 2:1382, 1984

181. Shaw BW, Bahnson HT, Hardesty RL et al: Combined transplantation of the heart and liver. Ann Surg 202:667, 1985

182. Mason EE: Surgical Treatment of Obesity. WB Saunders, Philadelphia, 1981

183. Bray GA: Current status of intestinal bypass surgery in the treatment of obesity. Diabetes 26:1072, 1977

184. Gastrointestinal Surgery for Severe Obesity. p. 1. National Institutes of Health Consensus Development Conference Consensus Statement. Vol 9. March 1991

185. Brolin RE, Kenler HA, Gorman RC, Cody RP: The dilemma of outcome assessment after operations for morbid obesity. Surgery 105:337, 1989

186. Benotti PN: Vertical banded gastroplasty in the treatment of severe obesity. (Editorial.) Mayo Clin Proc 66:662, 1991

187. Buchwald H, Moore RB, Varco RL: Surgical treatment of hyperlipidemia. Circulation, Suppl I. 49:1–22–I37, 1974

188. Zollinger RM, Jr, Lindern MC, Filler RM et al: Effect of thymectomy on skin-homograft survival in children. N Engl J Med 270:707, 1964

189. Scanlon EP, Hawkins RA, Fox WW, Smith WS: Fatal homotransplanted melanoma. A case report. Cancer 18:782, 1965

190. Lich RJ, Jr, Howerton LW, Jr, Goode LS, Davis LA: The ureterovesical junction in the newborn. J Urol 92:436, 1964

191. Buchwald H, Moore RB, Frantz ID, Jr, Varco RL: Cholesterol reduction by partial ileal bypass in a pediatric population. Surgery 68:1101, 1970

192. Krugman S, Ward R, Giles JP et al: Infectious hepatitis: detection of virus during the incubation period and in clinically inapparent infection. N Engl J Med 261:729, 1959

193. Buchwald H, Stoller DK, Campos CT et al: Partial ileal bypass for hypercholesterolemia 20–26 year follow-up of the first 57 consecutive cases. Ann Surg 212:318, 1990

194. Van Niekerk JLM, Hendriks T, de Boer HHM: The treatment of familial hypercholesterolemia by partial ileal bypass surgery. A review of the literature. Neth J Med 27:18, 1984

195. Buchwald H: Vitamin B12 absorption deficiency following bypass of the ileum. Am J Dig Dis 9:755, 1964

196. Helsinger N, Rootwelt K: Partial ileal bypass. Nord Med 45:1409, 1415, 1969

197. Faergeman O, Heinertz H, Hylander E et al: Effects of side-effects of partial ileal bypass surgery for familial hypercholesterolemia. Gut 23:558, 1982

198. Chalstrey LJ, Winder AF, Galton DJ: Partial ileal bypass in treatment of familial hypercholesterolemia. J R Soc Med 75:851, 1982

199. Russell D, Fritz V, Miery CJ et al: Treatment of familial hypercholesterolemia by partial ileal bypass. S Afr Med J 55:237, 1979

200. Moore TJ: Letter. N Engl J Med 324:563, 1991

201. Buchwald H, Matts JP, Fitch LL et al: Program on the surgical control of the hyperlipidemia (POSCH) design and methodology. J Clin Epidemiol 42:1111, 1989

202. Julian DG: Time as a factor in thrombolytic therapy. Eur Heart J, suppl F. 53:5, 1990

203. ISIS-3 (Third International Study of Infarct Survival) Collaborative Group. ISIS-3: a randomised comparison of streptokinase vs tissue plasminogen activator vs anistreplase and of aspirin plus heparin vs aspirin alone among 41,299 cases of suspected acute myocardial infarction. Lancet 1:(339):753, 1992

2

Cardiovascular Disease in the United States: Mortality, Prevalence, and Incidence*

Richard F. Gillum
Manning Feinleib

Diseases of the heart remain the leading cause of death and cerebrovascular diseases, the third leading cause of death in the United States.[1] Of the 2,123,323 total deaths in 1987, diseases of the heart accounted for 760,353 (35.8%) and cerebrovascular diseases for 149,835 (7.1%). Patterns of mortality, prevalence, and incidence for these and other cardiovascular diseases are generally characterized by strong associations with age, sex, and race. Using data from the National Center for Health Statistics (NCHS), this chapter highlights some important aspects of the epidemiology of cardiovascular disease.

HEART DISEASE

Mortality

In 1987, diseases of the heart accounted for the following percentages (number of deaths) of total deaths by sex and race: white males 35.8% (342,063), white females 37.5% (333,669), black males 27.9% (38,934), and black females 33.7% (38,813).[1] Table 2-1 shows age-adjusted death rates for diseases of the heart for

selected years, 1950 to 1987.[1] This category is defined since 1979 by the following codes of the International Classification of Diseases, Ninth Revision (ICD-9), for the underlying cause of death: 390 to 398, 402, 404 to 429. Age adjusted death rates for all causes in 1987 were 73% higher in males than in females and 52% higher in blacks than in whites; for diseases of the heart, rates were 89% higher in males than in females and 38% higher in blacks than in whites.[2] The ratio of rates in blacks to those in whites was much higher in younger compared with older persons. Diseases of the heart were the third leading cause of years of potential life lost (YPLL) before age 65 and the leading cause of YPLL before age 85.[3]

Morbidity

Hospital Discharges

Data from the 1987 National Hospital Discharge Survey (NHDS) indicate an estimated 3.0 million discharges among whites, 381,000 among nonwhites, and 357,000 among persons of unknown race with a first-listed diagnosis of heart disease (ICD-9-Clinical Modification (cm) 391–392.0, 393–398, 402, 404, 410–416, 420–429).[4] The rate of discharges was 1,546 per 100,000 for all ages, 3.5 for under 15 years, 212 for 15

TABLE 2-1. Age-Adjusted Death Rates for Diseases of Heart by Race and Sex: United States, 1950 to 1987

Year	White Male	White Female	Black Male	Black Female	Race Ratio Male	Race Ratio Female
1950	381.1	223.6	415.5	349.5	1.09	1.56
1960	375.4	197.1	381.2	292.6	1.02	1.48
1970	347.6	167.8	375.9	251.7	1.08	1.50
1980	277.5	134.6	327.3	201.1	1.18	1.49
1983	257.8	126.7	308.2	191.5	1.20	1.51
1984	249.5	124.0	300.1	186.6	1.20	1.50
1985	244.5	121.7	301.0	186.8	1.23	1.53
1986	234.8	119.0	294.3	185.1	1.25	1.56
1987	225.9	116.3	287.1	180.8	1.27	1.55

(From the National Center for Health Statistics.[2])

to 44 years, 2,731 for 45 to 64 years, and 7,507 for 65 years and over. It should be noted that NHDS samples discharges, not individual patients.

Prevalence

Prevalence of self-reported heart disease was obtained from the National Health Interview Survey (NHIS).[5] During 1983 to 1985, an estimated annual average of 19.3 million persons reported having heart disease in the civilian, noninstitutionalized population. The rate per 1,000 rose from 21.4 under 18 years to 339.2 at 75 years and over.

Coronary Heart Disease

Mortality

More than one-half of deaths due to diseases of the heart in 1987 were attributed to ischemic heart disease (IHD) (ICD-9 410-414), the percentage being lower for blacks than for whites: white males, 71.5% (244,461); white females, 66.6% (222,229); black males, 52.7% (20,521); and black females, 52.9% (20,549). Table 2-2 shows death rates for ischemic heart disease (IHD) by age, sex, and race.[6] Also shown are rates for IHD subgroups, acute myocardial infarction (ICD-9 410), and chronic IHD (ICD-9 412, 414). At younger ages, rates were higher in black men than in white men (Fig. 2-1). At all ages below 75, rates were higher in black women than in white women. Black-to-white ratios were higher for chronic IHD than for acute myocardial infarction (AMI).

Recent analyses of data from 40 states revealed that death due to IHD was more likely to occur out of hospi-

TABLE 2-2. Death Rates for Ischemic Heart Disease by Age, Sex, and Race: United States, 1987

Age (y)	Rate per 100,000 Men White	Men Black	Women White	Women Black	Race Ratio[a] Men	Women
	Ischemic heart disease					
35–44	33.0	51.1	6.6	16.1	1.5	2.4
45–54	146.0	182.5	35.4	76.8	1.3	2.2
55–64	425.8	431.2	142.8	246.8	1.0	1.7
65–74	1,005.2	920.1	463.1	595.5	0.9	1.3
75–84	2,375.6	1,875.4	1,450.2	1,410.6	0.8	1.0
0–85 +[b]	161.7	150.8	76.9	93.6	0.9	1.2
	Acute myocardial infarction					
35–44	19.9	27.4	4.0	8.8	1.4	2.2
45–54	91.1	98.7	22.6	44.7	1.1	2.0
55–64	253.3	230.5	87.4	135.7	0.9	1.6
65–74	564.9	483.9	266.7	320.7	0.9	1.2
75–84	1,198.9	887.7	719.9	692.5	0.7	1.0
0–85 +[b]	88.2	77.3	40.0	48.5	0.9	1.2
	Chronic ischemic heart disease					
35–44	12.7	22.9	2.5	6.8	1.8	2.7
45–54	52.9	79.8	12.2	31.0	1.5	2.5
55–64	167.6	192.5	53.9	106.8	1.1	2.0
65–74	432.1	422.6	192.6	266.7	1.0	1.4
75–84	1,158.4	963.1	719.0	704.8	0.8	1.0
0–85 +[b]	72.0	71.0	36.2	43.7	1.0	1.2

[a] For blacks and whites.
[b] Age adjusted by the direct method, standard: 1940 U.S. population.

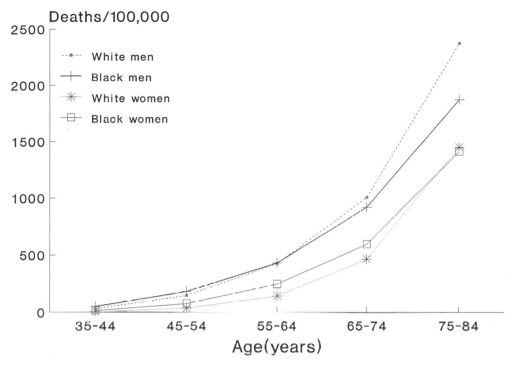

Fig. 2-1. Death rates for ischemic heart disease by age, sex, and race: United States, 1987.

tal or emergency departments among blacks than among whites, in men than in women, and in younger than in older persons.[7] Figure 2-2 shows the percentage of men dying of IHD whose death was coded as occurring out of hospital or in the emergency department in 1985. IHD death rates declined between 1968 and 1985 in all race and sex groups. However, during 1968 to 1975, rates declined faster for blacks than for whites, while during 1976 to 1985, rates for white males declined faster than for blacks or for white women.[8] Substantial geographic variation has been documented for levels and trends not only in coronary

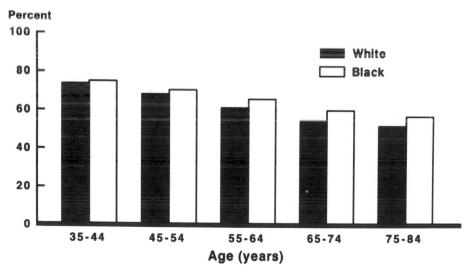

Fig. 2-2. Percentage of men dying of ischemic heart disease whose place of death was coded as out of hospital or in the emergency department by race and age: 40 states, 1985. (From Gillum,[7] with permission; data from National Center for Health Statistics, National Vital Statistics System, 1985.)

heart disease (CHD) mortality rates but also in percentages of CHD deaths occurring out of hospital.[9,10]

Morbidity

Hospital Discharges

Numbers, rates, and trends in hospital discharges for AMI and IHD in the United States were obtained from the NHDS.[11-13] In contrast to death rates, no decline was seen since 1970 in hospitalization rates for first-listed or all-listed AMI or ischemic heart disease. Since 1982, a marked increase was noted in rate of discharges for unstable angina pectoris. There was also a decrease in the rate of discharges for chronic IHD.

In 1987, there were 760,000 hospital discharges with a first-listed diagnosis of AMI.[4] There were 5.9 deaths per 100 discharges for persons under 65 years of age and 19.8 for persons aged 65 and over. For all ages, the rate of discharges for AMI was 314 per 100,000 but was 615 at ages 45 to 64 and 1,458 at ages 65 and over. Average length of stay was 8.5 days resulting in more than 6.4 million days of care. Table 2-3 shows numbers and rates of discharges for AMI and other categories of CHD. Using imputation of missing data and case-control techniques, several analyses of NHDS data have concluded that AMI discharge rates were lower, and in hospital AMI mortality rates were higher for blacks than for whites in the United States during the 1980s.[11,14]

In 1987, there were 332,000 coronary artery bypass procedures, 152,000 in persons aged 65 and over. There were 184,000 other procedures for removal of coronary artery obstruction, most of which were percutaneous transluminal angioplasties. The rapid increases in procedure rates since 1979 contrasts with the minimal changes in AMI discharge rates.[12] Coronary artery bypass surgery rates were lower among blacks than among whites.[15,16]

Prevalence

The prevalence of CHD was estimated in the Health Examination Survey of 1960 to 1962 using all available clinical data.[17,18] At ages 55 to 64, percentages with definite CHD were as follows: white males, 10.3%; black males, 5.7%; white females, 4.7%; and black females, 5.5%. Percentages with definite or suspect CHD were as follows: white males, 14.4%; black males, 13.4%; white females, 10.0%; and black females, 9.8%. However, more recent estimates have been based on self-reported history of diagnosis or on symptom questionnaires.[5,19,20] During 1983 to 1985, an estimated annual average of 6.97 million persons reported having IHD in the NHIS. Average annual

TABLE 2-3. Number and Rate of First-Listed Diagnoses of Ischemic Heart Disease for Inpatients Discharged from Short-Stay Nonfederal Hospitals by Discharge Diagnosis, Sex, and Age of Patient: United States, 1987

Diagnosis	Age			
	45–64		≥65	
	N[a]	Rate[b]	N[a]	Rate[b]
Both sexes				
Acute myocardial infarction	279	615.4	435	1,458.0
Other acute and subacute IHD	182	402.8	306	1,025.7
Angina pectoris	132	292.1	163	547.0
Coronary atherosclerosis	178	393.5	174	584.3
Other chronic IHD	100	221.4	93	310.6
Males				
Acute myocardial infarction	207	956.3	232	1,914.6
Other acute and subacute IHD	108	497.1	124	1,025.6
Angina pectoris	79	367.0	70	579.5
Coronary atherosclerosis	127	585.1	102	841.1
Other chronic IHD	71	327.4	54	445.9
Females				
Acute myocardial infarction	72	303.1	203	1,145.7
Other acute and subacute IHD	75	316.4	182	1,025.7
Angina pectoris	53	223.5	93	524.8
Coronary atherosclerosis	51	217.9	72	408.7
Other chronic IHD	29	124.3	39	218.0

[a] Number in thousands.
[b] Rate per 100,000 civilian population.
Abbreviations: ICD-9-CM, International Classification of Diseases, Ninth Revision, Clinical Modification; IHD, ischemic heart disease.
ICD-9-CM codes: acute myocardial infarction, 410; other acute and subacute IHD, 411; angina pectoris, 413; coronary atherosclerosis, 414.0; other chronic ischemic heart disease, 412, 414.1–414.9.

prevalence rates per 1,000 of reported IHD by sex and race at ages 55 to 64 during 1982 to 1984 were as follows: white males, 141.7; black males, 59.7; white females, 59.7; and black females, 38.0.[20] The London School of Hygiene Chest Pain Questionnaire was administered in the Second National Health and Nutrition Examination Survey (NHANESII), yielding the following age-adjusted prevalence rates of angina pectoris at ages 25 to 74 years: black males, 6.2%, black females, 6.8%; white males, 3.9%, and white females, 6.3%.[21] Thus, no firm conclusions were possible about the prevalence of CHD for the United States because of varying results of surveys, which depended on the methods used and the years covered.

Incidence

The NHANESI Epidemiologic Follow-up Study (NHEFS) provided national estimates of the incidence of CHD.[22-24] Case ascertainment was based on death certificate and hospital discharge diagnoses, with data limitations as described elsewhere.[25,26] After 10 years of follow-up, the incidence of CHD events (percentage of group) by baseline ages was as follows: age 55 to 64 years: white males, 17.4%; white females, 8.0%; black males, to 11.6%; black females, 10.1%; age 65 to 74 years: white males, 28.1%; white females, 22.7%; black males, 23.4%; and black females, 21.7%. Multiple logistic analyses confirmed the importance of systolic blood pressure, diabetes, and cigarette smoking as risk factors for CHD at ages 55 to 74 in whites. Lower educational attainment also was a predictor of CHD in this cohort.[23] When persons aged 40 to 74 years were included, serum cholesterol was a significant predictor of CHD mortality in whites.[24] The risk model for CHD mortality based on the Framingham Heart Study was very similar to a corresponding model based on NHEFS white adults.[24] Systolic blood pressure in men and diabetes in women were significant predictors of CHD in blacks. However, follow-up evaluation of larger cohorts of blacks would be desirable. Useful analyses of total mortality have appeared for both blacks and whites.[23–27]

Correlations Among the Measures of CHD

Feinleib et al.[28] presented data on CHD mortality, AMI hospital discharges, AMI hospital case fatality, and prevalence of CHD obtained from data systems of NCHS to examine possible causal relationships between trends in medical care and the decline in CHD mortality. When displayed by region, a pattern was seen of declining mortality and declining AMI case fatality and of increasing prevalence of CHD in each region in men aged 55 to 64 years, between 1970 and 1984. Trends in mortality and morbidity were examined within each of the regions. In the Northeast, a pattern of slight declines in AMI hospital discharge rate and case fatality rate, a marked decline in mortality rates, and an increase in prevalence was considered consistent with an increase in CHD survival rates and a slight decline in incidence. In the Midwest, a considerable decline in AMI case fatality and CHD mortality rates, little change in AMI hospital discharge rates, and an increase in CHD prevalence was consistent with an improvement in survival from CHD. In the South, declining CHD mortality and AMI case fatality, stable or increasing AMI discharge rates, and increasing CHD prevalence were consistent with improving effectiveness of medical care. In the West, marked declines in AMI discharge rates, AMI case fatality rates, and CHD mortality rates, with a relatively small increase in prevalence, were consistent with declining CHD incidence. Although not conclusive, owing to methodologic limitations, these data were believed to indicate a significant role for improved medical care in the decline in CHD mortality rates between 1970 and 1984 in middle-aged men in the United States.[28]

National levels and trends in the major risk factors—elevated blood pressure, cigarette smoking, and elevated serum cholesterol—are published regularly.[2] The need persists for longitudinal studies to establish the relative importance of these and other coronary risk factors in blacks, women, and the elderly.[22,29]

Other Heart Diseases

National data from the NCHS have been reported for several other heart diseases. Age-adjusted death rates for acute rheumatic fever and rheumatic heart disease combined (ICD-9 390–398) were higher in women than in men and slightly lower in blacks than in whites.[30] Death rates for congestive heart failure (ICD-9 428) were higher in older than in younger, in male than in female, and in black than in white persons.[31] A similar pattern was seen for hospital discharge rates.[31,32] Cardiomyopathy (ICD-9 425) death rates were higher in older than in younger, in male than in female, and in nonwhite or black than in white persons.[33,34] The age-adjusted hospital discharge rates for blacks were 2.2 times higher than those in whites aged 35 to 74. Pulmonary embolism (ICD-9 415) death and hospital discharge rates were also higher in blacks than in whites.[35]

Summary

Diseases of the heart were the leading cause of death in the United States in 1987. Most of these deaths were attributed to IHD. More than one-half of IHD deaths occurred out of hospital or in emergency departments in persons aged 35 to 74. National data for prevalence and incidence provide useful information on heart disease epidemiology, despite limitations. Continued monitoring and analysis of patterns and trends in mortality and morbidity are needed to monitor progress in primary and secondary prevention of heart disease.

CEREBROVASCULAR DISEASE

Mortality

In 1987, cerebrovascular diseases (ICD-9 430–438) were the third leading cause of death overall, as well as the third leading cause in black females and white females and the fourth leading cause in black males and white males (accidents and adverse effects were

TABLE 2-4. Age-Adjusted Death Rates for Cerebrovascular Disease by Sex and Race: United States, 1950 to 1987

Year	White Male	White Female	Black Male	Black Female	Race Ratio Male	Race Ratio Female
1950	87.0	79.7	146.2	155.6	1.68	1.95
1960	80.3	68.7	141.2	139.5	1.76	2.03
1970	68.8	56.2	124.2	107.9	1.81	1.92
1980	41.9	35.2	77.5	61.7	1.85	1.75
1983	35.2	29.6	64.2	53.8	1.82	1.82
1984	33.9	28.9	62.8	51.8	1.85	1.79
1985	32.8	27.9	60.8	50.3	1.85	1.80
1986	31.1	27.1	58.9	47.6	1.89	1.76
1987	30.3	26.3	57.1	46.7	1.88	1.78

(From the National Center for Health Statistics.[2])

the third leading cause in males).[1] Table 2-4 shows the death rates for selected years by age, sex, and race.[2] In 1987, age-adjusted death rates were 16% higher in males than in females and 82% higher in blacks than in whites. The relative excess mortality among blacks rose sharply with decreasing age. Stroke mortality rates were much higher in the Southeast than in other U.S. regions among blacks but not among whites in 1980.[36] The long-term decline in stroke mortality rates accelerated after 1973 for each race-sex group.[37,38] Recent analysis shows that a deceleration in the decline during 1979 to 1986 compared with 1973 to 1978 occurred for stroke for each race and sex group, as previously reported for CHD mortality among major segments of the population.[8,38,39] Cerebrovascular disease

was the tenth leading cause of YPLL before age 65 and the fifth leading cause of YPLL before age 85.[3]

A recent report suggested that, since the late 1970s, improved diagnostic accuracy of death certificate diagnoses permitted examination of death rates for stroke subgroups.[40] Between 1979 and 1985, the relative decline in rates was greater for nonhemorrhagic stroke (NHS) (ICD-9 433–438) than for intracranial hemorrhage (IH) (ICD-9 431–432) in both nonwhites and whites (Figs. 2-3 and 2-4). Further studies of the validity of death certificate diagnoses of stroke subgroups are needed to confirm these findings.

Morbidity

Hospital Discharges

Epidemiologic patterns of stroke hospitalization, prevalence, incidence, and risk factors, all generally higher in blacks than in whites, were also treated in a recent article and review.[39,41] In 1987, there were 895,000 hospital discharges with a first-listed diagnosis of cerebrovascular disease, 684,000 of whites, 108,000 of nonwhites, and 103,000 of persons for whom race was not stated.[4] The rate of discharges was 370 per 100,000 overall, rising from 423 at ages 45 to 64 to 2,230 at ages 65 and over. These rates decreased between 1985 and 1987, reversing the upward trend observed between 1979 and 1985.[39,42] The average length of stay was 10.1 days, resulting in more than 9 million days of short-stay hospital care. One analysis found aged-adjusted hospital discharge rates for first-

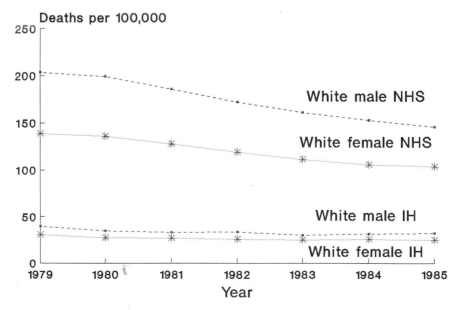

Fig. 2-3. Death rates for nonhemorrhagic stroke (NHS) and intracranial hemorrhage (IH) in whites aged 65 to 74 by sex: United States, 1979 to 1985.

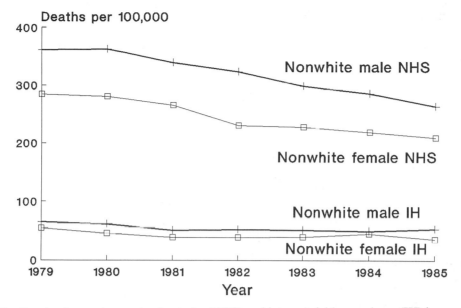

Deaths per 100,000

Nonwhite male NHS

Nonwhite female NHS

Nonwhite male IH

Nonwhite female IH

Year

Fig. 2-4. Death rates for nonhemorrhagic stroke (NHS) and intracranial hemorrhage (IH) in nonwhites aged 65 to 74 by sex: United States, 1979 to 1985.

listed cerebrovascular disease to be 30% higher in blacks than in whites at ages 35 to 74 years.[11] Numbers and rates of first-listed cerebrovascular disease are shown by diagnostic subgroup in Table 2-5.

Prevalence

In the 1982 to 1984 NHIS, the average rates for stroke prevalence by history per 1,000 persons aged 65 and over were as follows: white males, 62.9; black males, 108.0; white females, 50.4; and black females, 75.8.[20] These rates are for the civilian noninstitutionalized population.

Incidence

National estimates of stroke incidence have been produced from the NHANESI Epidemiologic Follow-up Study.[43] The 10-year incidence of cerebrovascular disease for persons aged 65 to 74 years at baseline was about 21%, and about 7.5% for those aged 55 to 64. Most common were events categorized as ill-defined (probably a mixture of hemorrhagic and thromboembolic events), followed by thromboembolic and hemorrhagic. Survival following a cerebrovascular event was markedly compromised, with poorer survival for hemorrhagic than for thromboembolic events, ill-defined being intermediate. Approximately one-half the survivors of cerebrovascular events were disabled at follow-up. Multivariate analyses confirmed older age, male sex, black race (among men), elevated blood pressure, diabetes, heart disease, and elevated hemoglobin

TABLE 2-5. Number and Rate of First-Listed Diagnoses of Cerebrovascular Disease for Inpatients Discharged from Short-Stay Nonfederal Hospitals by Discharge Diagnosis, Sex, and Age of Patient: United States, 1987

	Age			
	45–64		≥65	
Diagnosis	N[a]	Rate[b]	N[a]	Rate[b]
Both sexes				
Intracranial hemorrhage	24	53.5	43	144.6
Cerebral artery occlusion	42	93.6	188	629.7
Transient cerebral ischemia	42	92.3	162	542.4
Acute, ill-defined CVD	38	83.7	159	532.4
Other CVD	45	99.8	114	381.5
Males				
Intracranial hemorrhage	10	46.1	17	142.7
Cerebral artery occlusion	24	111.3	66	548.7
Transient cerebral ischemia	22	100.0	70	579.6
Acute, ill-defined CVD	22	100.8	67	552.1
Other CVD	25	115.1	52	431.3
Females				
Intracranial hemorrhage	14	60.4	26	145.9
Cerebral artery occlusion	18	77.4	121	685.1
Transient cerebral ischemia	20	85.2	92	516.9
Acute, ill-defined CVD	16	68.1	92	518.9
Other	20	85.9	62	347.4

[a] Number in thousands.
[b] Rate per 100,000 civilian population.
Abbreviations: ICD-9-CM, International Classification of Diseases, Ninth Revision, Clinical Modification; CVD, cerebrovascular disease.
ICD-9-CM codes: intracranial hemorrhage, 430–432; cerebral artery occlusion, 434; transient cerebral ischemia, 435; acute, ill-defined CVD, 436; other CVD, 433, 437, 438.

levels as risk factors for thromboembolic stroke. Older age, elevated blood pressure, elevated hemoglobin level, diabetes, and black race were independent risk factors for hemorrhagic stroke. Thirty to 37% of risk of all types combined could be attributed to four risk factors: diabetes, systolic blood pressure above 149 mmHg, hemoglobin above 15.7 g/dl, or evidence of prior heart disease.

Summary

Cerebrovascular disease was the third leading cause of death in 1987, with age-adjusted death rates 82% higher in blacks. Between 1979 and 1985, death rates declined more for NHS than for IH. Recent surveys showed prevalence, incidence, and hospitalization rates for stroke to be higher in blacks than in whites. Continued monitoring of mortality, prevalence, incidence, and survivorship trends for stroke and stroke subgroups is needed.

HYPERTENSIVE DISEASE

Mortality

In 1987 there were 31,338 deaths, with the underlying cause coded as hypertensive disease (ICD-9 401–404, HD), 24.7% of which were of blacks. Of

20,678 hypertensive heart disease (ICD-9 402, HHD) deaths, 25.5% were of blacks. Data on underlying cause of death underestimate the impact of hypertension. Analyses of multiple causes of death have attempted to assess the broader impact of hypertension on mortality of blacks and whites in the United States.[44,45]

Death rates were higher in males than in females and in blacks than in whites. Rates declined for HD and HHD in each sex-race group between 1979 and 1987. Death rates for HD and HHD varied considerably among geographic divisions of the United States for each sex and race group (Fig. 2-5). The variation in rates among divisions points to major variations in hypertension prevalence, treatment, control and possibly other factors including death certification for sequelae of hypertension.

Morbidity

Hypertension

Documented in a number of NCHS publications are epidemiologic patterns and trends in hypertension and blood pressure distributions in the United States.[5,19,46–49] Possible explanations for the well-doc-

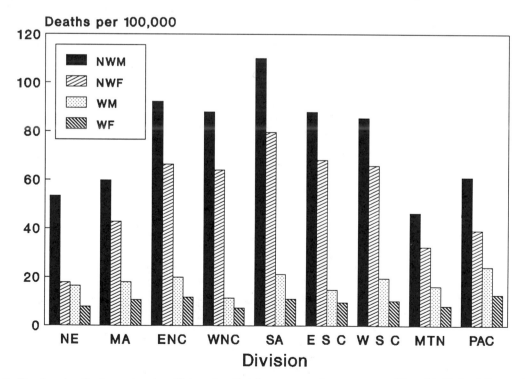

Fig. 2-5. Death rates for hypertensive disease by division, sex, and race at ages 55 to 64: United States 1979 to 1985 combined. WM, white male; WF, white female; NWM, nonwhite male; NWF, nonwhite female. NE, New England; MA, Middle Atlantic; ENC, East North Central; WNC, West North Central; SA, South Atlantic; ESC, East South Central; WSC, West South Central; MTN, Mountain; PAC, Pacific.

umented higher prevalence and incidence of hypertension in blacks than in whites have been reviewed.[50] Comparison of data from NCHS surveys conducted during 1960 to 1962, 1971 to 1974, and 1976 to 1980 revealed decreases in mean systolic blood pressure (SBP), the proportion with SBP above 139 mmHg, and increases in the proportions of hypertensives who where treated and controlled among all race and sex groups.[49] However, among men, only 20% of blacks and 25% of whites who had definite hypertension had their blood pressure controlled to less than 160/95 mmHg in 1976 to 1980.[47] Data from the NHEFS suggested that for most age-sex-race subgroups, the frequency of medication use for hypertension increased further between 1976 to 1980 and 1982 to 1984.[51] Changes were most evident for men.

Among black females, rates of uncontrolled hypertension and severe blood pressure elevations were higher in the Southeast than in other regions, corresponding to higher stroke mortality rates.[36] Higher rates of severe hypertension in black males in the Southeast were also consistent with higher stroke mortality.

Hospital Discharges

In 1987, there were 201,000 hospital discharges with a first-listed diagnosis of essential hypertension, 24,000 specifically coded as malignant essential hypertension. Only 5,000 discharges were coded as secondary hypertension. HHD was the first-listed diagnosis for 57,000. However, essential hypertension was mentioned more than 3 million and HHD over 345,000 times among all listed diagnoses. Further hypertension may have played a role in some of the nearly 1.8 million discharges with a diagnosis of heart failure mentioned, even though hypertension was not mentioned.

Prevalence

National data on the prevalence of HHD are more limited. In the National Health Examination Survey of 1960 to 1962, the prevalence of HHD derived from physical examination, electrocardiogram (ECG), and chest radiography of a national sample aged 18 to 79 years.[52] Among men, rates were 33.1% in blacks and 11.7% in whites aged 55 to 64. Among women of the same age, rates were 46.4% in blacks and 19.5% in whites. Recent analyses of data from the NHANESI Epidemiologic Follow-up Study demonstrated higher prevalences of left ventricular hypertrophy by several ECG criteria in blacks than in whites and documented its prognostic significance.[53–55]

Summary

Substantial numbers of deaths are attributed to HD, including HHD. In addition, hypertension contributes to mortality and morbidity from IHD and cerebrovascular disease. Despite the improvements in hypertension control of the past two decades, vigorous efforts are still needed, particularly among blacks in the South Atlantic states.

PERIPHERAL ARTERIAL OCCLUSIVE DISEASE

Chronic peripheral arterial disease of the extremities (ICD-9CM 440.2, 443.9, or 447.1) was listed as the underlying cause for fewer than 4,000 deaths in 1985.[56] However, during 1985 to 1987, an average of 55,000 males and 44,000 females were discharged from U.S. hospitals with such a first-listed diagnosis. Average annual discharge rates at ages 65 and over were 278 per 100,000 for males and 171.2 for females. The average annual number of coded procedures during 1985 to 1987 was 88,000 for arteriography of the femoral and other leg arteries, 31,000 for aorta-iliac-femoral bypass, 74,000 for other peripheral shunt or bypass, and 17,000 for endarterectomy of leg arteries. An average of 110,000 discharges per year had any diagnosis of acute peripheral arterial occlusive disease (ICD 9 444.21, 444.22, 444.81) among up to seven diagnoses coded in the NHDS. Embolectomy or thrombectomy of leg arteries was listed for 28,000 discharges per year.

In the first National Health and Nutrition Examination Survey (NHANES I), the prevalence of intermittent claudication by questionnaire at age 65 to 74 was 2.0% in males and 0.4% in females for definite diagnoses and 3.1% and 2.5%, respectively, for definite and possible diagnoses. Among whites aged 40 to 74, 13.1% of men and 9.2% of women had at least one diminished or absent dorsalis pedis pulse in preliminary analyses (Harris T: personal communication).

CONCLUSIONS

In 1987 heart disease was the leading cause of death and cerebrovascular disease the third leading cause of death for both blacks and whites in the United States. Of the estimated $32.5 billion in personal health care expenditures for diseases of the circulatory system in 1980, $14.3 billion was spent for heart disease, $5.0 billion for cerebrovascular disease, $4.4 billion for hypertension, and $8.8 billion for other circulatory diseases.[57,58] Despite improvements in control of hypertension and declines in mortality rates for all groups, cardiovascular disease remains a major public health problem. Epidemiologic monitoring of several indicators of disease over time can assist in guiding research and prevention efforts. Data from longitudinal studies including sizable numbers of women and blacks are needed to enhance understanding of the factors influencing cardiovascular risk.

REFERENCES

1. Advance Report of Final Mortality Statistics, 1987. National Center for Health Statistics. Monthly Vital Stat Rep, Suppl 38:5, 1989
2. Health, United States, 1989. DHHS Publ No. (PHS)90-1232. Public Health Service. National Center for Health Statistics, Washington, DC, 1990
3. Centers for Disease Control: Years of potential life lost before ages 65 and 85—United States, 1987 and 1988. MMWR 39:20, 1990
4. Graves EJ: National Hospital Discharge Survey: annual summary, 1987. National Center for Health Statistics. Vital Health Stat 13(99):1, 1989
5. Collins JC: Prevalence of Selected Chronic Conditions, United States, 1983–85. Advance Data from Vital and Health Statistics. No. 155. DHHS Publ No. (PHS) 88-1250. National Center for Health Statistics. US Public Health Service, Hyattsville, MD, 1988
6. Vital Statistics of the United States, 1987. Vol. II. Mortality, Part A. DHHS Publ No. (PHS) 90-1101. US Public Health Service. National Center for Health Statistics, Washington, DC, 1990
7. Gillum RF: Sudden coronary death in the United States: 1980–1985. Circulation 79:756, 1989
8. Sempos C, Cooper R, Kovar MG, McMillen M: Divergence of the recent trends in coronary mortality for the four major race-sex groups in the United States. Am J Public Health 78:1422, 1988
9. Ingram D, Gillum R: Regional and urbanization differentials in coronary heart disease mortality in the United States, 1968–85. J Clin Epidemiol 42:857, 1989
10. Gillum R: Geographic variation in sudden coronary death. Am Heart J 119:380, 1990
11. Gillum RF: Acute myocardial infarction in the United States, 1970–1983. Am Heart J 113:804, 1987
12. Feinleib M, Havlik RJ, Gillum RF et al: Coronary heart disease and related procedures: National Hospital Discharge Survey Data. Circulation, suppl I. 79:I–13, 1989
13. Centers for Disease Control: Hospitalization rates for ischemic heart disease—United States, 1970–1986. MMWR 38:275, 281, 1989
14. Roig E, Castaner A, Simmons B, Patel R et al: In-hospital mortality rates from acute myocardial infarction by race in U.S. hospitals: findings from the National Hospital Discharge Survey. Circulation 76:280, 1987
15. Ford E, Cooper R, Castaner A et al: Coronary arteriography and coronary bypass surgery among whites and other racial groups relative to hospital-based incidence rates for coronary artery disease: findings from NHDS. Am J Public Health 79:437, 1989
16. Gillum RF: Coronary artery bypass surgery and coronary angiography in the United States, 1979–1983. Am Heart J 113:1255, 1987
17. Gordon T, Garst CC: Coronary Heart Disease in Adults, United States, 1960–62. Vital and Health Statistics. Series 11, No. 10, PHS Publ No. 1000. US Public Health Service. National Center for Health Statistics, Washington, DC, 1965
18. Gillum RF: Coronary heart disease in black populations. I. Mortality and morbidity. Am Heart J 104:839, 1982
19. Collins JC: Prevalence of selected chronic conditions, United States, 1979–81. Vital and Health Statistics. Series 10, No. 155, DHHS Publ No. (PHS) 86-1583. US Public Health Service. National Center for Health Statistics, Washington, DC, 1986
20. Havlik RJ, Liu BM, Kovar MG et al: Health Statistics on Older Persons, United States, 1986. Vital and Health Statistics. Series 3, No. 25 DHHS Publ No. (PHS) 87-1409. US Public Health Service. National Center for Health Statistics, Washington, DC, 1987
21. LaCroix AZ, Haynes SG, Savage DD, Havlik RJ: Rose Questionnaire angina among United States black, white, and Mexican-American women and men. Prevalence and correlates from the Second National and Hispanic Health and Nutrition Examination Surveys. Am J Epidemiol 129:669, 1989
22. Leaverton PE, Havlik RJ, Ingster-Moore LM, et al: Coronary heart disease and hypertension, p. 53. In Cornoni-Huntley JC, Huntley RR, Feldman JJ (eds): Health Status and Well-being of the Elderly. Oxford University Press, New York, 1990
23. Makuc DM, Feldman JJ, Gillum RF: Educational differentials in heart disease incidence and case-fatality rates in a national sample. Am J Epidemiol 128:892, 1988
24. Leaverton PE, Sorlie PD, Kleinman JC et al: Representativeness of the Framingham risk model for coronary heart disease mortality: a comparison with a national cohort study. J Chron Dis 40:775, 1987
25. Madans JH, Kleinman JC, Cox CS et al: Ten years after NHANES I: report of initial follow-up, 1982–84. Public Health Rep 101:465, 1986
26. Madans JH, Cox CS, Kleinman JC et al: Ten years after NHANES I: mortality experience at initial follow-up, 1982–84. Public Health Rep 101:474, 1986
27. Cornoni-Huntley J, LaCroix AZ, Havlik RJ: Race and sex differentials in the impact of hypertension in the United States. The National Health and Nutrition Examination Survey I Epidemiologic Follow-up Study. Arch Intern Med 149:780, 1989
28. Feinleib M, Lentzner H, Collins J et al: Regional variation in coronary heart disease mortality and morbidity. p. 31. In Higgins M, Leupker R (eds): Trends in Coronary Heart Disease Mortality. Oxford University Press, New York, 1988
29. Eaker ED, Packard B, Thom TJ: Epidemiology and risk factors for coronary heart disease in women. Cardiovasc Clin 19:129, 1989
30. Gillum RF: Trends in acute rheumatoic fever and chronic rheumatic heart disease—a national perspective. Am Heart J 111:430, 1986
31. Gillum RF: Heart failure in the United States 1970–1985. Am Heart J 113:1043, 1987

32. Ghali JK, Cooper R, Ford E: Trends in hospitalization rates for heart failure in the United States, 1973–1986. Arch Intern Med 150:769, 1990

33. Gillum RF: Idiopathic cardiomyopathy in the United States, 1970–1982. Am Heart J 111:752, 1986

34. Gillum RF: The epidemiology of cardiomyopathy in the United States. Prog Cardiol 2:11, 1989

35. Gillum RF: Pulmonary embolism and thrombophlebitis in the United States, 1970–1983. Am Heart J 114:1262, 1987

36. Rocella EF, Lenfant C: Regional and racial differences among stroke victims in the United States. Clin Cardiol 12:IV18, 1989

37. Klag MJ, Whelton PK, Seidler AJ: Decline in US stroke mortality: demographic trends and antihypertensive treatment. Stroke 20:14, 1989

38. Cooper R, Sempos C, Hsieh SC, Kovar MG: The slowdown in the decline of stroke mortality in the United States, 1978–1986. Stroke, 21:1274, 1990

39. Gillum RF: Stroke in blacks. Stroke 19:1, 1988

40. Iso H, Jacobs DR, Wentworth D et al: Serum cholesterol levels and six-year mortality from stroke in 350,977 men screened for the Multiple Risk Factor Intervention Trial. N Engl J Med 320:904, 1989

41. Gillum RF: Cerebrovascular disease morbidity in the United States, 1970–1983. Age, sex, region, and vascular surgery. Stroke 17:656, 1986

42. Centers for Disease Control: Hospital discharge rates for cerebrovascular disease—United States, 1970–1986. MMWR 38:194, 1989

43. White LR, Losonczy KG, Wolf PA: Cerebrovascular disease. p. 115. In Cornoni-Huntley JC, Huntley RR, Feldman JJ (eds): Health Status and Well-being of the Elderly. Oxford University Press, New York, 1990

44. Wing S, Manton KG: The contribution of hypertension to mortality in the US: 1968, 1977. Am J Public Health 73:140, 1983

45. Tu EJ: Multiple cause-of-death analysis of hypertension-related mortality in New York state. Public Health Rep 102:329, 1987

46. Persky V, Pan WH, Stamler J et al: Time trends in the US racial difference in hypertension. Am J Epidemiol 124:724, 1986

47. Drizd T, Dannenberg AL, Engel A: Blood pressure levels in persons 18–74 years of age in 1976–80, and trends in blood pressure from 1960 to 1980 in the United States. Vital Health Stat [11] (234):1–68, 1986

48. Roberts J, Maurer K: Blood pressure levels of persons 6–74 years, United States, 1971–74. Vital and Health Statistics. Series 11, No. 203. DHEW Pub. No. (HRA) 78-1648. Health Resources Administration. National Center for Health Statistics, Washington, DC, 1977

49. Dannenberg AL, Drizd T, Horan MJ et al: Progress in the battle against hypertension. Changes in blood pressure levels in the United States from 1960 to 1980. Hypertension 10:226, 1987

50. Gillum RF: Pathophysiology of hypertension in blacks and whites. A review of the basis of racial blood pressure differences. Hypertension 1:468, 1979

51. Havlik RJ, LaCroix AZ, Kleinman JC et al: Antihypertensive drug therapy and survival by treatment status in a national survey. Hypertension, suppl I. 13:I-28, 1989

52. Gordon T, Devine B: Hypertension and Hypertensive Heart Disease in Adults, United States, 1960–62. Vital and Health Statistics. Series 11, No. 13. PHS Publ No. 1000. US Public Health Service. National Center for Health Statistics, Washington, DC, 1966

53. Rautaharju PM, LaCroix AZ, Savage DD et al: Electrocardiographic estimate of left ventricular mass versus radiographic cardiac size and the risk of cardiovascular disease mortality in the epidemiologic follow-up study of the First National Health and Nutrition Examination Survey. Am J Cardiol 62:59, 1988

54. Rautaharharju PM, Lacroix AZ, Savage DD et al: Heart size estimates indexed optimally to body and chest size. I. The effect of age and hypertensive status. Am J Noninvas Cardiol 4:104, 1990

55. Rautaharju PM, Cox CS, Madams JH et al: Heart size estimates indexed optimally to body and chest size. II. Prognostic value for cardiovascular disease mortality. Am J Noninvas Cardiol 4:187, 1990

56. Gillum RF: Peripheral arterial occlusive disease of the extremities in the United States: hospitalization and mortality. Am Heart J 120:1414, 1990

57. Hodgson TA, Kopstein AN: Health care expenditures for major diseases in 1980. Health Care Financ Rev 5:1–12, 1984

58. Hodgson TA: Health care expenditures for major diseases in 1980. Health Care Financ Rev 6:128, 1984

3
Epidemiology of Established Major Cardiovascular Disease Risk Factors

Gregory L. Burke
Teri A. Manolio

Cardiovascular disease (CVD) mortality rates have declined by approximately 50% from the mid-1960s to the early 1990s. However, CVD still remains the leading cause of morbidity and mortality among U.S. adults. A substantial amount of previous work has documented specific cardiovascular disease risk and protective factors. This has been accomplished by (1) assessing disease patterns and risk factors in different populations; (2) observing risk factors within populations; and (3) intervening on these major risk factors to document the efficacy of risk reduction on subsequent CVD morbidity and mortality. This chapter focuses primarily on the epidemiology of major cardiovascular disease risk factors, including blood pressure, lipids, smoking, diabetes, obesity, and left ventricular hypertrophy (LVH). In numerous studies, similar relationships for these CVD risk factors have been observed, but for purposes of clarity, this chapter presents data from three studies: the Framingham Heart Study, the Second National Health and Nutritional Examination Survey (NHANES II), and the Minnesota Heart Survey (MHS). Framingham data are used to document known cardiovascular disease risk factors; NHANES II data are used to describe the distribution of known risk factors across age, race, and gender groups; and Minnesota data are used to describe re-

cent trends in cardiovascular disease risk factors in U.S. adults.

RISK FACTORS FOR CARDIOVASCULAR DISEASE

This section describes the relationship between risk factors and CVD. These include blood pressure, lipids, cigarette smoking, diabetes, coagulation factors, obesity, and LVH. Figures presented are based on Framingham data documenting the relationship between baseline risk factors and 8-year risk of CVD events in participants free of CVD at baseline. For purposes of clarity, other risk factors were set to normal levels in these gender-specific multiple logistic function analyses.

Elevated Blood Pressure

Figure 3-1 presents 8-year risk of CVD (fatal and nonfatal CHD) by baseline diastolic blood pressure level in 60-year-old nonsmokers with no LVH, diabetes, or hypercholesterolemia. Elevated levels of diastolic blood pressure were related to an increased risk of incident CVD morbidity and mortality.[1] Risk of CVD

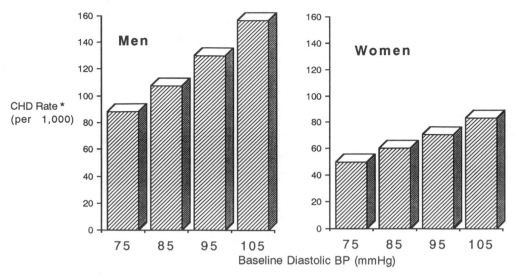

Fig. 3-1. Eight-year CHD incidence by baseline diastolic blood pressure level. *, no other major risk factors at baseline (smoking, LVH, diabetes, hypercholesterolemia). (Data from Abbott and McGee.[1])

was continuous across the blood pressure distribution, with increasing risk of heart disease sequelae observed even in those patients with only borderline elevated levels of blood pressure.[2–4] Elevated systolic and diastolic blood pressure appear to be associated with increased risk, both independently and in combination. Prospective clinical trials,[5,6] have shown that reduction of hypertension has resulted in reduced risk from CVD in the treated versus the placebo/usual care group. Data from the Systolic Hypertension in the Elderly Program (SHEP) have shown that treatment of isolated systolic hypertension resulted in a significant reduction of CVD risk in older adults.[7] This increased risk from systolic blood pressure includes both risk of cerebrovascular disease where hypertension is the primary risk factor, as well as increased risk of coronary heart disease (CHD). Thus blood pressure is an important risk factor for cardiovascular disease and reduction of blood pressure levels results in a significant decrease in both cardiovascular and cerebrovascular disease.

Lipids and Lipoproteins

Figure 3-2 presents 8-year-risk of CVD (fatal and nonfatal CHD) by baseline blood cholesterol level in 60-year-old nonsmokers with no LVH, diabetes, or hypertension.[1] Increased risk of CVD was observed with increasing levels of baseline cholesterol in both men and women. Ecologic studies such as the Seven-Country Study have shown that countries with the highest levels of CHD also had the highest blood cholesterol levels.[8] Dyslipidemia has been shown to be associated with increased risk of CHD in many other studies.[9–13]

These prospective studies within populations have shown that blood cholesterol, low-density lipoprotein cholesterol (LDL-C), and triglycerides have all been associated with an increased risk of subsequent morbidity and mortality of CVD, while high-density lipoprotein cholesterol (HDL-C) has been shown to be a protective factor. The Lipid Research Clinic Primary Prevention Trial was a double-blind, placebo-controlled study of the effects of reduction of hypercholesterolemia on subsequent CHD risk.[14] This study showed a significant decline in fatal and nonfatal events in participants followed over a 5-year period. Data from the Lipid Research Clinic study suggested that every 1% decline in the level of serum cholesterol resulted in a 2% decline in CHD mortality. These data document the importance of blood lipids as a risk factor for cardiovascular disease and that improvement of lipid profile results in an improvement in risk of CVD.

Cigarette Smoking and Cardiovascular Disease

The public perception has been that cigarette smoking is more strongly linked to risk from cancer than to CVD mortality. In actuality, given the higher prevalence of heart disease in the U.S. population, cigarette smoking causes more morbidity and mortality from heart disease than from cancer. Figure 3-3 shows 8-year CVD incidence in smokers compared with nonsmokers.[1] Within each age and gender group, smokers have higher CVD rates. Cigarette smokers are at increased risk of both myocardial infarction (MI) and sudden death.[15] The increased risk between smoking

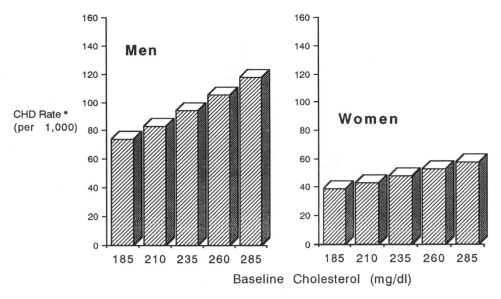

Fig. 3-2. Eight-year CHD incidence by baseline serum cholesterol level. *, major risk factors normal at baseline (smoking, diabetes, hypertension). (Data from Abbott and McGee.[1])

and MI is even greater in the presence of other risk factors, such as hyperlipidemia. The likely mechanism for the association observed between cigarette smoking and CHD is related to the increased thrombogenesis and decreased oxygen carrying capacity in cigarette smokers. Longitudinal studies have shown that the risk of MI decreases after smoking cessation and that the improvement in risk occurs very rapidly after cessation of cigarette smoking.[16,17] In the MRFIT study, men who quit smoking reduced their CHD mortality rates by about 50% over those who did not quit smoking.[18] Thus, there are compelling data documenting the reversible adverse relationship between smoking and CVD.

Diabetes and Cardiovascular Disease

Patients with diabetes mellitus are at increased risk of CVD. Most studies assessing diabetes and CVD were done in type II diabetics, as reflected by the relation-

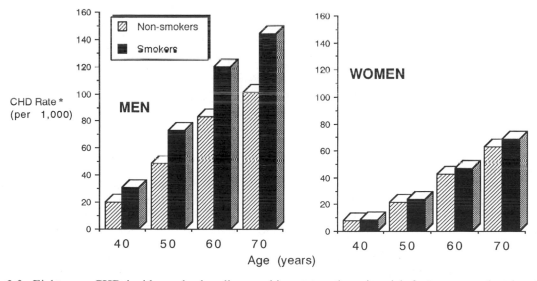

Fig. 3-3. Eight-year CHD incidence by baseline smoking status. *, major risk factors normal at baseline (diabetes, LVH, hypertension, hypercholesterolemia). (Data from Abbott and McGee.[1])

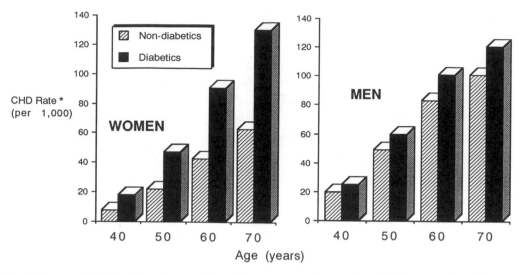

Fig. 3-4. Eight-year CHD incidence by baseline diabetes status. *, no major risk factors at baseline (smoking, LVH, hypertension, hypercholesterolemia). (Data from Abbott and McGee.[1])

ships presented. The increased risk in diabetics appears to be mediated in part by the increased prevalence of hypertension and dyslipidemia. Even after consideration of these risk factors, however, diabetics are still at increased risk of the morbidity and mortality associated with CVD. Figure 3-4 presents 8-year-risk of CVD (fatal and nonfatal CHD) by baseline diabetes status (1). Increased risk of CVD was observed for diabetics in all age and gender categories. It is of particular interest that the differences in CVD between diabetics and nondiabetics were greater in women than in men, suggesting that the gender difference in CVD susceptibility is substantially less or virtually eliminated in diabetics. Recent data suggest that increased insulin resistance and hyperinsulinemia in diabetics may be associated both with their abnormal CVD risk profile and with their increased risk of CHD.[19–21] Less well known is the issue of how control of glycemic status impacts on risk of CHD; it is beyond the scope of this book to provide an in-depth appraisal of this issue. Thus, diabetics are at increased risk of morbidity and mortality associated with CVD, which may be explained in part by their CVD risk profile.

Coagulation Factors in Cardiovascular Disease

Given that CVD events likely represent both an atherosclerosis phase as well as a thrombosis/occlusion phase, a pathophysiologic mechanism for the association between hemostatic factors and CVD is quite plausible. Levels of fibrinogen and Factor VII activity have been associated with increased risk of CHD events.[22,23] Alterations in hemostatic factors may me-

diate in part the relationship between smoking and cardiovascular morbidity and mortality, emphasizing the importance of chronic factors associated with atherosclerosis and acute factors associated with risk of a thromboembolic episode precipitating the acute CHD event.

Left Ventricular Hypertrophy and Cardiovascular Disease

LVH has been linked to increased risk of CVD. This is shown in Figure 3-5, which presents 8-year CVD risk in participants with and in participants without baseline LVH.[1] In participants with no CVD risk factors at baseline, the rates of CVD events were greater in those with LVH than in those without LVH. This was true in all age and gender groups. Framingham data have suggested that LVH not only is independently related to CVD, but also that it is one of the strongest CVD risk factors in their study.[24] Thus, interventions based on reducing the prevalence of LVH seem appropriate to reduce the risk of CVD sequelae in high-risk groups.

Obesity and Cardiovascular Disease

Evidence exists documenting the presence of an independent relationship between obesity and CHD.[25] In addition, obesity has been associated with a more adverse CVD risk profile. Obesity has been linked to a greater prevalence of hypertension, dyslipidemia, and abnormalities in glycemic status.[26–28] The association between obesity and hypertension has been observed in numerous studies; even a modest weight loss results in significant decline in risk factors.[29–31] Obesity has

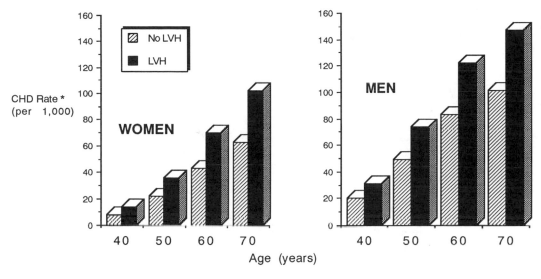

Fig. 3-5. Eight-year CHD incidence by baseline left ventricular hypertrophy (LVH). *, no major risk factors at baseline (smoking, diabetes, hypertension, hypercholesterolemia). (Data from Abbott and McGee.[1])

also been shown to be related to increased levels of serum cholesterol, triglycerides, VLDL cholesterol, and LDL cholesterol. HDL cholesterol levels are lower in obese than in nonobese patients. Obesity has been associated with a higher prevalence of glucose intolerance, and obesity may result in increased hyperinsulinemia and increased peripheral insulin resistance. Thus, obesity is both an independent CHD risk factor and a marker for higher levels of established CHD risk factors.

Physical Activity and Coronary Heart Disease

The observed inverse relationship between physical activity and CHD likely manifests itself through known cardiovascular disease risk factors. Cohort studies have shown that persons who are more physically active have a lower risk of subsequent CHD than do those who are not physically active. This finding has been observed both in occupational cohorts and in nonoccupational cohorts.[32–36] Specifically, the Harvard Alumni Study has shown that those college students who reported higher levels of leisure time physical activities had lower rates of subsequent CHD events.[35] Given the difficulty in self-selection of healthier persons in more vigorous occupational activities and the high degree of concordance between life-style factors such as cigarette smoking and diet with leisure time physical activity, it is difficult to separate out potential confounding factors in the relationship between physical activity and CHD. Despite this concern, it should be noted that at least part of the direct association between exercise and CHD is mediated by a lower prevalence of cigarette smoking, lower levels of blood pressure, and an improved lipid profile.

Diet and Coronary Heart Disease

Numerous studies have shown an ecologic relationship between dietary intake and prevalence of CHD in different countries.[8] Populations that consume a high percentage of their calories from fat are at increased risk of heart disease. Likewise, increased consumption of dietary sodium has been linked to an increased prevalence of hypertension in studies across populations.[37] While these differences have been observed across populations, the relationship between diet and cardiovascular disease within populations are less clearly observed. This stems from both the relative homogeneity of dietary factors within populations and the difficulties in accurate quantification of a patient's dietary intake. The association between dietary fat consumption and serum cholesterol levels has been established in a number of settings. In addition, more recent data suggest that dietary cholesterol intake in independently associated with CHD events.[9] Thus, dietary factors play a key role in the genesis of CVD risk factors and, hence, risk of CVD.

DISTRIBUTION OF CARDIOVASCULAR DISEASE RISK FACTORS IN U.S. POPULATIONS

NHANES II data are used to present the distribution of known cardiovascular disease risk factors in U.S. adults across age, ethnicity, and gender groups. Given

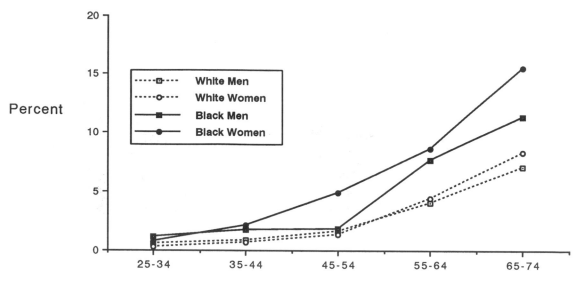

Fig. 3-6. Hypertension prevalence in U.S. adults by age, race, and gender. *, BP 160/95 or taking antihypertensive medications. (Data from Drizd et al.[38])

the importance of the above CVD risk factors, the distribution of these factors among and within populations are likely associated with differential CVD risk. Age-, race-, and gender-specific differences in CVD risk, for example, may be mediated in large part by risk factor differences between the groups.

Blood Pressure

Blood pressure levels increase with age in U.S. populations from young adulthood through middle age. The prevalence of hypertension (BP > 160/95 or on medication) by age, race, and gender is presented in Figure 3-6.[38] The prevalence of hypertension increased with age, with higher rates observed in black than in white adults. Similar age and racial differences in blood pressure level have been observed in other studies of U.S. populations.[39–42] In addition, these studies have noted that blood pressure levels are higher in men than in women. These observed differences have been linked to differences in cerebrovascular disease morbidity and mortality (i.e., higher stroke rates in U.S. blacks than in U.S. whites).

Lipids and Lipoproteins

Blood cholesterol levels increase from young adulthood to middle and older age groups. In men, population total cholesterol levels peak approximately in their 50s and are lower in older age groups, while in women's levels peak in their early 60s with a rapid rise observed following menopause[43] (Fig. 3-7). Serum cholesterol levels tend to be lower in black adults than in white adults, while HDL cholesterol levels are sig-

nificantly higher in black populations.[39,44,45] Thus, the prevalence of dyslipidemia is higher in U.S. whites. The lower levels of cholesterol observed in older age groups is likely a result of early mortality from CHD in patients with the highest levels of cholesterol. Recent data suggest that of patients with hypercholesterolemia, more than two-thirds were unaware of their increased cholesterol and only approximately 5% reported being on any current treatment.[46] These data suggest that, although improvements in the prevalence of dyslipidemia have occurred in the United States, substantial numbers of U.S. adults remain at high risk based on their lipid profile.

Smoking

The prevalence of smoking in the United States varies across age cohorts, with the highest prevalence of smoking observed in middle-aged adults and the lowest prevalence of smoking observed in older adults (in part because of a survivorship effect). Smoking prevalence rates are significantly higher in black Americans than in white Americans.[47,48] In addition, smoking has been shown to be inversely associated with education, with higher smoking rates observed in patients with lower education versus higher education.[48] U.S. smoking rates are higher in men than in women, with the exception of younger cohorts in which a similar prevalence of smoking has been observed across gender.

Diabetes

Figure 3-8 shows the prevalence of self-reported diabetes by age, race, and gender group in participants in the NHANES II Study.[49] The prevalence of diabetes

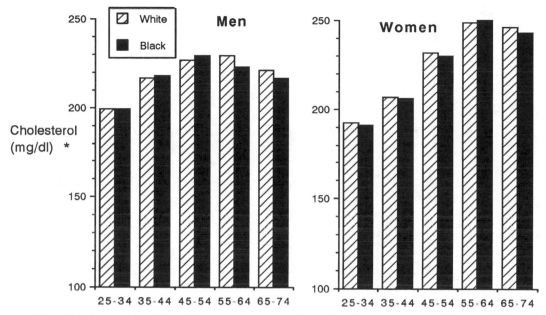

Fig. 3-7. Blood cholesterol in U.S. adults by age, race, and gender. *, mean serum cholesterol. (Data from Fulwood et al.[43])

increased with age in all race and gender groups. In addition, the prevalence of diabetes was significantly higher in U.S. blacks than in U.S. whites. The importance of this risk factor is emphasized by the fact that by age 65 to 74 years, at least 10% of all race and gender groups reported having diabetes.

Obesity

Figure 3-9 shows the prevalence of obesity (greater than the 85th percentile for body mass index [BMI], using the gender-specific means at ages 20 to 29 as the standard) by age, race, and gender group.[27] The prevalence of obesity in U.S. adults increased from young adulthood to middle age groups. In men no consistent racial differences were observed, with a higher prevalence of obesity observed in middle-aged black men only. In women a substantially greater prevalence of obesity has been observed in U.S. blacks compared with U.S. whites. Similar findings have been observed in other studies and document the high prevalence of obesity in U.S. adults.[50,51]

TRENDS IN CARDIOVASCULAR DISEASE RISK FACTORS

Significant time trends in CVD mortality have been observed in the United States. CVD mortality rates increased after World War II and peaked in the mid-1960s.[52] Subsequent to that period, a consistent decline has been observed from the mid-1960s through

the early 1990s. Given these dramatic changes in CVD mortality, there have also been substantial and dramatic changes in heart disease risk factors during the same time.[53] This section describes trends in cardiovascular risk factors during the 1970s and 1980s. Data from the community-based surveys of CVD risk factors done in Twin Cities of Minneapolis-St. Paul are presented. Data from the Lipid Research Clinics population survey conducted during 1973 to 1974 are compared with subsequent Minnesota Heart Survey examinations conducted during 1980 to 1982 and 1985 to 1987.[53]

Blood Pressure Trends

Blood pressure levels have consistently declined from the 1970s through the mid-1980s. Diastolic blood pressure declined by 2.6 mmHg in men and 1.5 mmHg in women from 1973 to 1987 (Fig. 3-10). Similar findings were observed for systolic blood pressure levels. The National High Blood Pressure Education Program was initiated in 1973, coinciding with a period of very marked improvement in hypertension status in U.S. adults. Other studies have noted that this decline in blood pressure levels has occurred in men, women, different ethnic groups, and in middle and older ages.[54]

Blood Lipids

Figure 3-11 presents blood cholesterol trends from 1973 to 1987 in Twin Cities adults. Blood cholesterol levels have declined consistently from the early 1970s

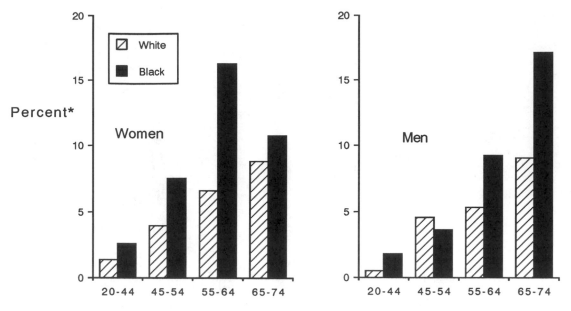

Fig. 3-8. Prevalence of diabetes in U.S. adults by age, race, and gender. *, self-reported diabetes. (Data from Hadden and Harris.[49])

through the 1980s (8 mg/dl in men and 11 mg/dl in women). The prevalence of hypercholesterolemia (>240 mg/dl) has also declined during this same period.[46] These improvements in population cholesterol levels can be attributed in part to marketplace changes in the foods (e.g., more choices, less saturated fatty acids) and also to an increasing awareness and treat-

ment of hypercholesterolemia in high risk populations. Surveys have shown that during this period both physician and patient have become more knowledgeable and motivated toward the reduction of cholesterol levels.[46,55,56] In addition, the number of available cholesterol-lowering medications has also increased dramatically during this period.

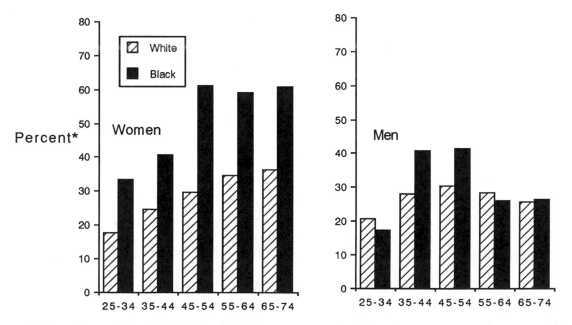

Fig. 3-9. Prevalence of obesity in U.S. adults by age, race, and gender. *, percent exceeding sex-specific 85th percentile of body mass index (BMI) for ages 20 to 29. (Data from Najjar and Rowland.[27])

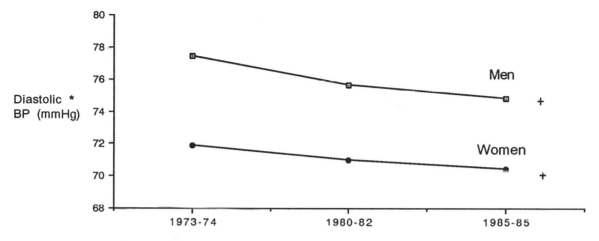

Fig. 3-10. Diastolic blood pressure trends in Twin Cities adults from 1973 to 1987. *, age-adjusted, adults aged 25 to 59; +, significant trend from 1973 to 1987 (p <0.05). (Data from Burke et al.[40])

Cigarette Smoking Trends

The prevalence of cigarette smoking has decreased by approximately 10% from the 1970s into the 1980s[53] (Fig. 3-12). Over the past 30 years, there has been a shift in the profile of the "typical smoker" from the higher socioeconomic status groups to the lower socioeconomic status groups in large part because the most rapid declines in smoking occurred in the higher socioeconomic status groups. In addition, while smoking rates have decreased among black Americans, their prevalence of smoking still remains significantly higher than white Americans.

Obesity

Figure 3-13 shows time trends in body mass index in Minnesota adults.[53] Body mass index increased consistently from 1973 to 1987 in both men (a 1-unit increase) and women (a 2.7-unit increase). Similar trends in obesity have been observed in national data[57] and in younger age groups.[58] Therefore, this secular trend of increasing obesity has been observed in virtually all ages and also across different ethnic and gender groups. Of interest, this increasing prevalence of obesity is likely at least part of the reason for the increases observed in diabetes prevalence.

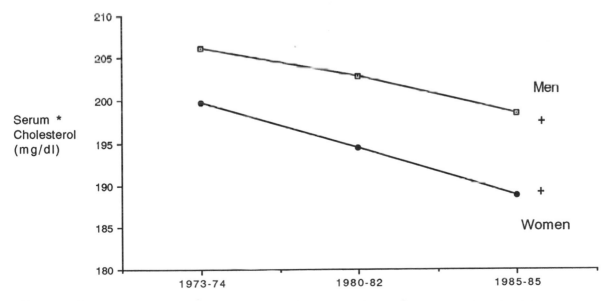

Fig. 3-11. Blood cholesterol trends in Twin Cities adults from 1973 to 1987. *, age-adjusted, adults 25 to 59; +, significant trend from 1973 to 1987. (p <0.05). (Data from Burke et al.[40])

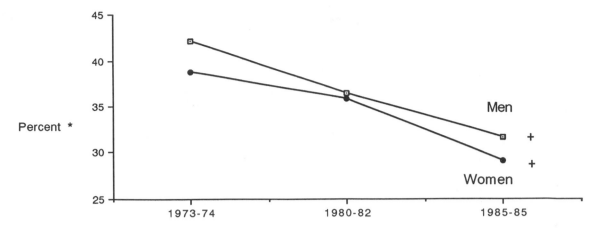

Fig. 3-12. Cigarette smoking trends in Twin Cities adults from 1973 to 1987. *, age-adjusted, adults aged 25 to 59; +, significant trend from 1973 to 1987 (p <0.05). (Data from Burke et al.[40])

Life-style Factors

A number of time trends in life-style factors have been observed. The prevalence of physical activity has increased from the 1960s into the 1970s, with only very minor changes after that.[59] Intake of dietary fat and cholesterol decreased during the 1980s.[60] Although it is difficult to assess long-term trends in dietary factors accurately, significant marketplace changes have occurred in food composition, with lower fat and sodium, and a higher polyunsaturated to saturated fatty acid ratio. It is likely that the dietary changes in the United States occurred both by increased individual choice of heart-healthy foods, as well as by marketplace changes (which do not require individual choices). In summary, major changes have occurred in CVD risk factors, which are concurrent with decreasing cardiovascular disease mortality rates.

SUMMARY

Major CVD risk factors have been well defined in both prospective cohort studies and clinical trials. These risk factors include blood pressure, lipids and lipoproteins, cigarette smoking, diabetes, LVH, and obesity. In addition, these factors are directly influenced by diet and physical activity. Major differences were observed in the CVD risk profile across age, race, and gender groups. The heterogeneity of risk factors between these groups mediates the observed differ-

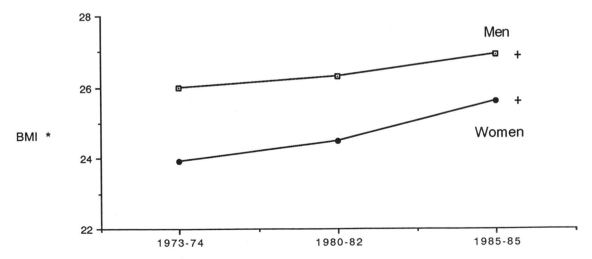

Fig. 3-13. Body mass index trends in Twin Cities adults from 1973 to 1987. *, age-adjusted, adults aged 25 to 59; +, significant trend from 1973 to 1987 (p < 0.05). (Data from Burke et al.[40])

ences in CVD morbidity and mortality. The overall decline in CHD mortality in the United States from the 1960s to the 1990s can be explained by the improvements seen in CVD risk factors. It should be noted that, although substantial improvements have been seen in the risk profile of U.S. adults during this time frame, there remain a large number of adults with treatable/modifiable CVD risk factors.

REFERENCES

1. Abbott RD, McGee D: The Framingham Study, Section 37: The probability of developing certain cardiovascular diseases in eight years at specified values of some characteristics. NIH Publ No. 87-2284. NIH, Washington, DC, 1987
2. Hypertension Detection and Follow-Up Program Cooperative Group: The effect of treatment on mortality in "mild" hypertension—results of the hypertension detection and follow-up program. N Engl J Med 307:976, 1982
3. Pooling Project Research Group: Relationships of blood pressure, serum cholesterol, smoking habit, relative weight and ECG abnormalities to incidence of major coronary events. Final report of the Pooling Project. J Chronic Dis 31:201, 1978
4. Veterans Administration Cooperative Study Group on Antihypertensive Agents: Effects of treatment on morbidity in hypertension: results in patients with diastolic blood pressure averaging 90 through 114 mmHg. JAMA 213:1143, 1970
5. Veterans Administration Cooperative Study Group on Antihypertensive Agents: Effects of treatment on morbidity in hypertension: results in patients with diastolic blood pressure averaging 115 through 129 mmHg. JAMA 202:1028, 1967
6. Hypertension Detection and Follow-Up Program Cooperative Group: Five-year findings of the Hypertension Detection and Follow-Up Program. I. Reduction in mortality of persons with high blood pressure, including mild hypertension. JAMA 242:2562, 1979
7. SHEP Cooperative Research Group: Prevention of stroke by antihypertensive drug treatment in older persons with isolated systolic hypertension: final results of the Systolic Hypertension in the Elderly Program (SHEP). JAMA 265:3255, 1991
8. Keys A, Aravanis C, Blackburn HW et al: Epidemiological studies related to coronary heart disease: characteristics of men aged 40-59 in seven countries. Acta Med Scand 460:1, 1967
9. Shekelle RB, Shryock AM, Paul O et al: Diet, serum cholesterol, and death from coronary heart disease: the Western Electric Study. N Engl J Med 304:65, 1981
10. Reed D, Yano K, Kagan A: Lipids and lipoproteins as predictors of coronary heart disease, stroke, and cancer in the Honolulu Heart Program. Am J Med 80:871, 1986
11. Stamler J, Wentworth D, Neaton JD: Is relationship between serum cholesterol and risk of premature death from coronary heart disease continuous and graded? Findings in 356,222 primary screenees of the Multiple Risk Factor Intervention Trial (MRFIT). JAMA 256:2823, 1986
12. Castelli WP: Epidemiology of coronary heart disease: the Framingham Study. Am J Med 76:4, 1984
13. Rose G, Shipley M: Plasma cholesterol concentration and death from coronary heart disease: 10 year results of the Whitehall Study. Br Med J 293:306, 1986
14. Lipid Research Clinics Program: The Lipid Research Clinic Coronary Primary Prevention Trial Results. II. The relationship of reduction in incidence of coronary heart disease to cholesterol lowering. JAMA 251:365, 1984
15. Doll R, Hill AB: Mortality in relation to smoking: ten years observations of British doctors. Br Med J 1399, 1964
16. Salonen J: Stopping smoking and long-term mortality after acute myocardial infarction. Br Heart J 43:463, 1980
17. Wilhelmsson E, Vedin JA, Elmfeldt D et al: Smoking and myocardial infarction. Lancet 1:415, 1975
18. Multiple Risk Factor Intervention Trial Research Group: Multiple Risk Factor Intervention Trial. Risk factor changes and mortality results. JAMA 248:1465, 1982
19. Reaven GM: Insulin resistance and compensatory hyperinsulinemia: role in hypertension, dyslipidemia, and coronary heart disease. Am Heart J 121:1283, 1991
20. Manolio TA, Savage PJ, Burke GL, et al: Correlates of fasting insulin levels in young adults: the CARDIA study. J Clin Epidemiol 44:571, 1991
21. Stout RW: Hyperinsulinemia as an independent risk factor for atherosclerosis. Int J Obes 6:111, 1982
22. Kannel WB, D'Agostino RB, Belanger AJ: Fibrinogen and risk of cardiovascular disease. JAMA 258:1183, 1987
23. Meade TW, Mellows S, Brozovic M et al: Haemostatic function and ischemic heart disease: principal results of the Northwick Park Heart Study. Lancet 2:533, 1986
24. Levy D, Garrison RJ, Savage DD: Prognostic implications of left ventricular mass. N Engl J Med 322:1561, 1990
25. Hubert HB, Feinlieb M, McNamara PM, Castelli WP: Obesity as an independent risk factor for cardiovascular disease: a 25 year follow-up of participants in the Framingham Heart Study. Circulation 7:968, 1983
26. Smoak CG, Burke GL, Webber LS et al: Relation of obesity to clustering of cardiovascular disease risk factors in children and young adults: the Bogalusa Heart Study. Am J Epidemiol 125:364, 1987
27. Najjar MF, Rowland M: Anthropometric reference data and prevalence of overweight, United States 1976-1980. Vital and Health Statistics, Series 11-No. 238. DHHS Publ No. 87-1688, 1-73. NCHS, Hyattsville, MD, 1987
28. Gillum RF: The association of body fat distribution with hypertension, hypertensive heart disease, coronary heart disease, diabetes and cardiovascular risk factors in men and women aged 18-79 years. J Chronic Dis 40:419, 1987
29. Berkowitz D: Metabolic changes associated with obesity before and after weight reduction. JAMA 187:399, 1964
30. Fletcher AP: The effect of weight reduction on the blood pressure of obese hypertensive women. J MED 47:331, 1954
31. Newburgh LH: Control of hyperglycemia of obese diabetics by weight reduction. Ann Intern Med 17:935, 1942

32. Morris JN, Kagan A, Pattison DC et al: Incidence and prediction of ischaemic heart disease in London busmen. Lancet 2:552, 1966

33. Breslow L, Buell P: Mortality from coronary heart disease and physical activity of work in California. J Chronic Dis 11:421, 1960

34. Cassel J, Heyden S, Bartel AC et al: Occupation and physical activity and coronary heart disease. Arch Intern Med 128:920, 1971

35. Paffenbarger RS, Jr, Brand RJ, Sholtz RI et al: Energy expenditure, cigarette smoking and blood pressure level as related to death from specific diseases. Am J Epidemiol 108:12, 1978

36. Pomrehn PR, Wallace RB, Burmeister LF: Ischemic heart disease mortality in Iowa farmers: the influence of lifestyle. JAMA 248:1073, 1982

37. Stamler J, Rose G, Stamler R et al: INTERSALT study findings: public health and medical implications. Hypertension 14:570, 1989

38. Drizd T, Dannenberg AL, Engel A: Blood pressure levels in persons 18-74 years of age in 1978-80 and trends in blood pressure from 1960 to 1980 in the United States. Vital and Health Statistics Series II, No. 234. DHHS Publ. No. 86-1684. USPHS, Washington, DC, 1986

39. Sprafka JM, Burke GL, Folsom AR, Hahn LP: Hypercholesterolemia prevalence, awareness and treatment in blacks and whites: the Minnesota Heart Survey. Prev Med 18:423, 1989

40. Burke GL, Voors AW, Shear CL et al: Cardiovascular disease risk factors from birth to seven years of age: the Bogalusa Heart Study. Part III. Blood Pressure. Pediatrics 80:784, 1987

41. Hypertension Detection and Follow-Up Program Cooperative Group: Race, education and prevalence of hypertension. Am J Epidemiol 106:351, 1977

42. Stamler R, Stamler J, Riedlinger WF et al: Weight and blood pressure: findings in hypertension screening of 1 million Americans. JAMA 240:1607, 1978

43. Fulwood R, Kalsbeck W, Rifkind B et al: Total serum cholesterol levels of adults 20-74 years of age: United States, 1976-80. Vital Statistics Series II, No. 236. DHHS Publ. No. (PHS) 86-1686. DHHS, Washington, DC, 1976

44. Tyroler HA, Heyden S, Bartel A et al: Blood pressure and cholesterol as coronary heart disease risk factors. Arch Intern Med 128:907, 1971

45. National Institutes of Health: The Lipid Research Clinics Population Studies Data Book. Vol I. The prevalence study. NIH Publ. No. 80-1527. NIH, Washington, DC, 1980

46. Burke GL, Sprafka JM, Hahn LP et al: Trends in cholesterol levels, treatment and control from 1980 to 1987: the Minnesota Heart Survey. N Engl J Med 324:941, 1991

47. National Center for Health Statistics: Health, United States, 1986. DHHS Publ. No. (PHS) 87-1232. USPHS, Washington, DC, 1986

48. Wagenknecht LE, Perkins LL, Cutter GR et al: Cigarette smoking is strongly related to education level: the CARDIA study. Prev Med 19:158, 1990

49. Hadden WC, Harris MI: Prevalence of diagnosed diabetes, undiagnosed diabetes and impaired glucose tolerance in adults 20-74 years of age, United States, 1976-80. Vital and Health Statistics, Series II. No. 237 DHHS Publ. No. (PHS) 87-1687. DHHS, Washington, DC, 1987

50. Burke GL, Jacobs DR, Sprafka JM et al: Obesity and overweight in young adults: The CARDIA Study. Prev Med 19:476, 1990

51. Harsha DW, Voors AW, Berenson GS: Racial differences in subcutaneous fat patterns in children aged 7-15 years. Am J Phys Anthropol 53:333, 1980

52. Thom TJ, Kannel WB: Downward trend in cardiovascular mortality. Annu Rev Med 32:427, 1981

53. Burke GL, Sprafka JM, Folsom AR et al: Trends in coronary heart disease mortality, morbidity and risk factors from 1960 to 1986: the Minnesota Heart Survey. Int J Epidemiol suppl 1. 18:S73, 1989

54. Rowland ML, Fulwood R: Coronary heart disease risk factor trends between the first and second National Health and Nutrition Examination Surveys, United States 1971-80. Am Heart J 108:771, 1984

55. Schucker B, Bailey K, Heimbach JT et al: Change in public perspective on cholesterol and heart disease. JAMA 258:3527, 1987

56. Schucker B, Wittes JT, Cutler JA: Change in physician perspective on cholesterol and heart disease. JAMA 258:3521, 1987

57. Burton BT, Foster WR, Hirsch J, Van Itallie TB: Health implications of obesity: an NIH Consensus Development Conference. Int J Obes 9:155, 1985

58. Shear CL, Freedman DS, Burke GL et al: Prevalence of secular trends of obesity in early life: the Bogalusa Heart Study, (abstracted). Circulation 74:426, 1986

59. Jacobs DR, Hahn LP, Folsom AR et al: Time trends in leisure-time physical activity in the upper midwest 1957-1987: University of Minnesota Studies. Epidemiology 2:8, 1991

60. Graves KL, McGovern PG, Sprafka JM, Folsom AR: Trends in serum cholesterol levels and dietary intake in a Metropolitan area between 1980-1982 and 1985-1987: the Minnesota Heart Survey, abstracted. Circulation 82(4):III-347, 1990

4

Lipoprotein Abnormalities and Atherosclerosis Risk

H. Robert Superko

The link between lipoprotein abnormalities and atherosclerosis has become well established during the past two decades. Epidemiologic and clinical trials have validated the cholesterol hypothesis, namely, elevated plasma cholesterol increases the risk of coronary artery disease (CAD) and reduction in plasma cholesterol results in reduction of this risk. Recent clinical trials employing arteriography as an risk end point have established that aggressive manipulation of plasma lipoproteins can result in decreased lumen obstruction and decreased clinical events. The future of atherosclerosis treatment is bright, and advances in molecular biology and genetics may substantially improve our ability to manipulate atherosclerotic plaques metabolically.

This chapter highlights three topics: (1) epidemiologic and clinical trial evidence that indicate CAD patients deserve aggressive lipoprotein management; (2) current topics in lipidology that help explain the lack of precision in risk prediction when only measures of lipoprotein cholesterol are used; and (3) the future of lipoprotein treatment and atherosclerosis that will substantially improve risk prediction and treatment.

EPIDEMIOLOGY AND CLINICAL TRIALS

Epidemiology

The risk of the development of clinically significant CAD is correlated with plasma total cholesterol and low-density lipoprotein cholesterol (LDL-C) concentration. However, as many as 80% of persons who suffer a myocardial infarction have total cholesterol concentrations within the same range as do those who do not suffer a myocardial infarction.[1] A portion of these persons with "normal" LDL-cholesterol and excess CAD risk can be identified by measurement of high-density lipoprotein (HDL)-cholesterol, triglycerides, or other lipoprotein measurements that include LDL and HDL subclass distribution, apoproteins, Lp(a), apoprotein isoforms, and perhaps oxidation potential. Because of the important role of detailed measures of lipoproteins that are not routinely determined in epidemiologic investigations, epidemiologic studies are useful guides to risk assessment but lack the detail necessary to be of substantial clinical use on a 1:1 patient basis unless well-defined lipoprotein abnormalities are present.

Several epidemiologic investigations have contributed to our knowledge regarding blood cholesterol concentrations and CAD risk. These studies are useful in developing general guidelines and have taught us valuable lessons. The Seven Country Study was a 10-year investigation in more than 12,000 middle-aged men that revealed a significant (r = 0.80) correlation between serum cholesterol and CAD death.[2] This was one of the first large investigations that supported a link between abnormally elevated blood cholesterol and CAD. Blood cholesterol is not the only lipid risk factor. In the Stockholm Prospective Study more than 3,400 subjects were studied for 14 years, and the investigators determined that both total cholesterol and triglycerides are independent risk factors for CAD and that triglycerides are the more important of the two.[3]

One of the largest and most-cited studies, the Framingham Study, is an ongoing surveillance study of more than 5,000 men and women that is more than 30 years old.[1] This study confirmed the stepwise CAD risk increase as total serum cholesterol and LDL-cholesterol increased and revealed several additional findings. The cholesterol relationship was particularly powerful for men under 50 years of age, and low HDL-cholesterol (less than 25 mg/dl) was reported to have the strongest correlation to CAD. This investigation has resulted in substantial information relating risk of the development of CAD to several medical and lifestyle factors. Tables of risk prediction developed from this investigation are useful as general guides and reflect group risk. They illustrate the powerful effect of increasing the number of risk factors and increased risk.

The interaction of multiple risk factors may involve persons genetically predisposed to developing hypertension and lipoprotein abnormalities. Hypertensive dyslipidemia is a term used to describe families with the combination of hypertension, dyslipidemia, and increased CAD risk.[4] A similar spectrum of abnormalities and CAD risk that includes insulin resistance has been termed "Syndrome X."[5] These syndromes may indeed overlap, but they consistently illustrate the significantly increased CAD risk associated with these multiple risk factors.

Important differences in lipoprotein subclass distribution can be obscured by simple measures of lipoprotein cholesterol. Information on lipoprotein subspecies and CAD risk was initially revealed in the landmark study performed by Dr. John Gofman 30 years ago. The Livermore Study was a 10-year follow-up study of more than 1,900 men that employed the analytic ultracentrifuge to determine lipoprotein subclass distribution in great detail. During the late 1960s, this study determined that both HDL2 and HDL3 (mass) were inversely related to CAD events.[6] This was the first investigation that addressed the fact that VLDL, LDL, and HDL classes are made up of numerous subclasses and the differences in subclass distribution is associated with CAD.

The relative importance of LDL subclass distribution, or "type," was revealed in the Boston Area Health Study and helps explain how a patient with "normal" cholesterol concentration may still be at significant CAD risk.[7] In this case-control investigation of 789 subjects, a significant association of small-dense LDL (LDL phenotype B) with post-myocardial infarction (MI) patients, compared with LDL-cholesterol matched "healthy" subjects was revealed. This difference between cases and controls was not apparent from measurement of total or LDL-cholesterol and contributed to our understanding of the role of lipoprotein heterogeneity in CAD.

Two large observational follow-up investigations have revealed associations that tend to conflict with previous dogma. In the Multiple Risk Factor Intervention Trial, more than 360,000 men were screened and followed for 6 years.[8] This study indicated that CAD risk increases progressively above a value of 180 mg/dl and strongly suggests that the concept of a "safe" cholesterol level may be erroneous. The Lipid Research Clinics Prevalence Study followed more than 7,500 men and women for 8 years and found that in women HDL-cholesterol was more closely related to CAD than LDL-cholesterol and that HDL-cholesterol increments of 10 mg/dl were similar in regard to CAD mortality as LDL-cholesterol decrements of 30 mg/dl.[9] This study indicated that gender differences in lipoprotein levels and their relative association with CAD risk are clinically relevant.

Clinical Trials

In order to test the hypothesis that actively altering plasma lipoprotein concentrations will have a beneficial impact on CAD, clinical trials have monitored clinical CAD events following a specific intervention. Clinical CAD events are often defined as the appearance of angina pectoris, fatal or nonfatal MI, coronary bypass surgery, or a positive graded exercise test. It is helpful to have a control (nonintervention) group in order to accurately assess change since these studies are often many years long. Nonpharmacologic and pharmacologic trials that illustrate this approach are listed in Table 4-1.

Nonpharmacologic Trials

Nonpharmacologic treatment has primarily employed diet and smoking manipulation. One of the earlier studies involved 846 men, aged 55 to 89 years, in the Los Angeles Veterans Administration Study.[10] In this 8-year investigation, subjects were randomized to

TABLE 4-1. Clinical Trials That Have Reported Change in Cardiovascular Endpoints with Lipoprotein Modification

Investigation	Number	Treatment	Outcome
L.A. Veterans Study	846	Diet	13% reduction in total cholesterol; nonsignificant reduction in coronary events
Oslo Trial	1232	Diet Stop smoking	13% reduction in total cholesterol 47% reduction in MI (p < 0.03)
Leiden Trial	39	Diet	46% no new CAD lesions
Stockholm Study	555	Diet, niacin, clofibrate	Significant reduction in CAD mortality
WHO	15,745	Clofibrate	Significant reduction in nonfatal MI; 25% more deaths in the clofibrate group
CDP	8,341	Niacin Estrogen Clofibrate Dextrothyroxine	Significant reduction in nonfatal MI (niacin) Significant medication side effects
CPPT	3,806	Cholestyramine	Significant reduction in CAD events
Helsinki	4081	Gemfibrozil	Significant reduction in CAD events

Abbreviations: CAD, coronary artery disease; MI, myocardial infarction.

a control diet (40% fat), or the study diet (50% less cholesterol, P:S − 2:1), which resulted in a 13% reduction in serum cholesterol. A trend toward fewer coronary events in the treatment group was noted, but this was not statistically significant.

The effect of combining diet and smoking cessation advice was tested in the Oslo Study Diet and Antismoking Trial.[11] In this investigation, 1,232 healthy, middle-aged hypercholesterolemic (TC = 290-380 mg/dl) men were randomized to a control group or to receive diet and antismoking advice. The intervention resulted in a 13% reduction in serum cholesterol (p < 0.01), a 20% reduction in triglycerides (p < 0.01), a 20% increase in HDL-C (p < 0.01) and a 45% reduction in smoking, compared with the control group. At the end of the study, the incidence of myocardial infarction (fatal and nonfatal) and sudden death was 47% lower (p = 0.03) in the intervention group. The difference in CHD incidence was due mainly to the reduction in serum cholesterol and, at most, 25% of the difference was attributed to smoking cessation.

Pharmacologic Trials

A number of investigations have tested the cholesterol hypothesis by achieving blood cholesterol reduction with medications and by observing differences in clinical signs of CAD. These trials generally require large numbers of participants and 4 to 10 years of active participation.

The effectiveness of this approach in preventing a second coronary event in patients who have survived at least one event (secondary prevention) has been tested, and is beneficial in the proper situation. The effect of combining diet, clofibrate (1 g bid) and nicotinic acid (1 g tid) was investigated in 555 MI survivors in the Stockholm Ischemic Heart Disease Secondary Prevention Study.[12] In addition, hypertension treatment and advice to stop smoking was given. 50% of the patients had elevated triglyceride concentrations and 13% were hypercholesterolemic. Compliance to the medications was variable, 40% took ≥2.5 g of nicotinic acid and ≥1.5 g of clofibrate, 12% took <1.5 g nicotinic acid and <1 g clofibrate. Overall, serum cholesterol was reduced 13% and triglycerides 19% more in the treatment group compared with the control group. Total mortality and CAD mortality were significantly (p < 0.05) reduced in the treatment group.[13] An interesting result that has clinical significance was that the clinical benefit of this combination treatment appeared to be mainly in patients with elevated plasma triglyceride concentration (baseline triglyceride >133 mg/dl). In the 44% of the treatment group that achieved greater than 30% reduction in triglycerides, CAD mortality was reduced by 60% (p < 0.01). There was no such relationship for serum cholesterol concentration.

Another secondary prevention trial was the Coronary Drug Project. This double-blind, randomized, placebo-controlled clinical trial used five medication groups to reduce elevated blood cholesterol in patients who had previously survived a myocardial infarction.[14] Three medication groups were discontinued prematurely due to an excess of drug-related morbidity and mortality. Subjects who completed the trial and who were treated with niacin had an approximate 10% mean reduction in serum cholesterol. In the niacin group, the incidence of nonfatal MI was 27% (p < 0.01) lower (8.9%) than in the placebo group (12.2%). Niacin was also associated with a higher incidence of atrial fibrillation. Fifteen years after the start of the program, all cause mortality was similar in all groups except for the group treated with niacin. In the niacin-treated group, mortality was 11% lower (p < 0.002) than in the placebo-treated group.[15]

Primary prevention trials are conducted in subjects without documented disease with the intent of delaying the clinical expression of the disease in the treatment group. Three large, well-designed prospective trials have provided overwhelming evidence that subjects with elevated blood cholesterol can benefit from pharmacologic blood cholesterol reduction. One of the earlier studies, the World Health Organization (WHO) Cooperative Trial, was a double-blind trial that used the medication clofibrate and illustrates a potential hazard associated with pharmacologic cholesterol reduction and cardiovascular benefit.[16] One-half of the 15,745 men who were enrolled, had elevated serum cholesterol. Serum cholesterol was reduced approximately 9% by the medication and resulted in a significant reduction in nonfatal MI's (p < 0.05). Unfortunately, 25% more deaths from all causes were noted in the clofibrate group as compared with the control group (p < 0.01) and a greater number of cholecystectomies were reported in the clofibrate treated group (p < 0.001). This study has cast doubt on the safety of long-term treatment with fibrates, but the data are currently being reviewed and the Helsinki trial used the fibric acid derivative gemfibrozil and did not reveal similar adverse effects.

The longest and most meticulously conducted trial of this kind was the Lipid Research Clinics, Coronary Primary Prevention Trial (CPPT). This double-blind, randomized trial treated hypercholesterolemic male subjects (total cholesterol >265 mg/dl) with cholestyramine or placebo for 10 years.[17] The treatment group revealed an 8.5% and 12.6% greater reduction in total cholesterol and LDL-C, respectively, than the placebo group. This difference resulted in a 24% reduction in definite CAD death and a 19% reduction in nonfatal myocardial infarction. Using the proportional hazards model it was predicted that a 25% reduction in TC would result in a 49% reduction in CAD risk. Significant reductions in other clinical signs of CAD were also seen including the need for bypass surgery, new angina, and ischemic treadmill tests.

The effect of a fibrate (gemfibrozil) was tested in the Helsinki Trial. This 5-year double-blind randomized trial was conducted in healthy middle-aged men with elevated LDL-C and/or VLDL-C.[15] 63% of the group was classified as Fredrickson type IIa, 28% IIb, and 9% IV. The total number of CAD events was significantly lower (p < 0.02, two-tailed test) in the gemfibrozil-treated group compared to the placebo group. The greatest reduction was in nonfatal MI (37%, p < 0.05), consistent with the Coronary Drug Project results. The greatest benefit was in subjects with elevations in triglycerides and/or low HDL-C.

These trials indicate a reduction in blood cholesterol achieved with drugs is associated with a significant reduction in cardiovascular events. The major event in two of the trials was nonfatal MI while the other two included all MIs and CHD death. The amount of cholesterol reduction achieved in these trials can be considered quite moderate and averaged around 10%.

Arteriographic Trials

Studies employing the amount of change of coronary obstruction, assessed by arteriography, have indicated progression, delayed progression, and regression associated with alterations in lipoproteins and lipoprotein subclass distribution. Studies lacking a control group date back to 1967 and have been reviewed.[18] In these studies, the initial plasma cholesterol value is often elevated and the degree of plasma cholesterol reduction substantial. For example, over a period of 7 years, Kuo and associates demonstrated a plasma total cholesterol reduction from 413 ± 24 mg/dl to 270 ± 11 mg/dl with the use of diet and a bile acid binding resin. Twenty-one of these 25 men demonstrated a lack of progression of their disease as assessed by arteriography.[19]

To be convincing and clinically relevant, trials of this nature must have control groups since knowledge regarding change in coronary artery diameter due to natural progression or other medical intervention, is incomplete. Coronary arteries initially respond to the atherosclerotic process by enlarging their diameter, and functionally important lumen stenosis may be delayed until the lesion occupies 40% or more of the internal elastic lamina area.[20] Thus, substantial disease can be present that is not reflected by coronary arteriography, which measures only lumen obstruction.

Measurements of coronary artery maximum diameter reduction obtained with quantitative coronary arteriography in the Coronary Artery Surgery Study (CASS) indicates that in a CAD population, a mean reduction in maximum diameter of approximately 6% per year can be expected.[21] However, change in CASS was highly variable. Arteriographic CAD progression has been related significantly to the number of diseased vessels, age, smoking status, and blood cholesterol.[22] Patients who showed progression had a mean total cholesterol of 250 ± 42 mg/dl compared with patients with no progression who had a mean total cholesterol of 216 ± 48 mg/dl. With multivariate logistic regression, the number of segments (p = 0.001), smoking status (p < 0.05), and cholesterol level (p < 0.05) remained significant predictors of progression. This issue takes on added importance in the coronary artery bypass population were progression is 3 to 6 times greater in grafted versus ungrafted arteries, and 45% of all grafts have significant occlusive disease 5 years following surgery.[23]

Therapies not designed to manipulate plasma lipoproteins may affect arteriographically assessed CAD progression. The effective of calcium antagonists have been reported in two such trials.[24,25] While some reduction in the rate of disease progression was reported, the results did not suggest a powerful role for calcium antagonists in the metabolic manipulation of atherosclerosis at this time.

Nonpharmacologic Trials

The effectiveness of vegetarian diets on treating arteriographically defined CAD has been explored. In the Leiden Intervention Trial (Leiden, the Netherlands), 39 CAD patients with documented disease of greater than 50% obstruction of at least one vessel were treated for 2 years with a vegetarian diet having a P:S > 2 and <100 mg dietary cholesterol per day.[26] Unfortunately, there was no control group. In 18 of the 39 patients (46%) who completed the trial, no new lesion growth was documented on coronary arteriography Lesion growth correlated with TC/HDL-C ($r = 0.50$, $p < 0.001$) and in patients with TC/HDL-C <6.9, no new lesion growth was seen. The Lifestyle Heart Study involved a specially designed and administered diet along with mild exercise and stress reduction for 1 year.[26a] Unfortunately, 58% of the subjects randomized to the control group, and 47% of the subjects randomized to the treatment group, refused to accept randomization. In the 78% in the experimental group who completed the trial, reductions in LDL-C (38%) and HDL-C (3%), and increases in TG (22%), were reported and coronary arteriograms suggest less luminal obstruction. This study is difficult to interpret due to the high drop-out rate and significant differences ($p < 0.03$) in baseline HDL-C (52.3 mg/dl control, 38.7 mg/dl treatment).

Pharmacologic and Diet Trials

Six well-designed trials offer important information regarding altering rates of progression of coronary atherosclerosis following intervention with diet and lipid-lowering medications. These studies and primary outcomes are listed in Table 4-2.

The first double-blind trial of the effect of lipid-lowering medication on coronary artery diameter was reported by Cohn in 1975.[27] Forty CAD patients were treated with clofibrate (n = 16) or a placebo (n = 24) for 1 year, at which time repeat coronary arteriograms were obtained. Total serum cholesterol was reduced 6% and triglycerides 16%. Out of 64 coronary arteries, 19 (30%) revealed progression in the clofibrate group compared to 24 out of 96 (25%) in the placebo group. The difference was not statistically significant. In this early study, the treatment duration was relatively brief and the amount of cholesterol reduction relatively small.

More aggressive lipoprotein manipulation was reported by Duffield et al.,[28] when they assessed change in femoral artery atherosclerosis using the medications cholestyramine, nicotinic acid, and clofibrate. In his investigation 24 patients with peripheral vascular disease were randomly assigned to a usual-care group, or treatment with diet and medications. Patients were treated for an average of 19 months, and LDL-C was reduced 28%, triglycerides 45%, and HDL-C increased 41%. Significantly fewer ($p < 0.01$) segments showed progression in the treatment group (10 versus 27). He concluded that the rate of progression was reduced 60% by hypolipidemic treatment.

The first randomized coronary arteriographic investigation was the NHLBI Type II study and involved 116 type 2 hyperlipidemia subjects who were treated with diet therapy and either placebo or cholestyramine for 5 years.[29,30] Change in the placebo and cholestyramine groups, respectively, were triglyceride (+26%, +28%), LDL-C (−5%, −26%), HDL-C (+2%, +8%). Compared with baseline, triglycerides increased significantly in the placebo and cholestyramine groups (+30 mg/dl, $p < 0.001$; +37 mg/dl, $p <$

TABLE 4-2. Triglyceride and Lipoprotein Cholesterol Change Difference Between Control and Intervention Groups in Controlled Investigations Using Arteriography to Assess Change in Artery Lumen Obstruction

Study	Years	No. of Subjects	Medication	Change Triglyceride	LDL-C	HDL-C	Outcome
Cohn	1		Clofibrate	−16%	NA	NA	No difference
Duffield	1.5		Cholestyramine Clofibrate Niacin	−38%	−27%	+43%	Reduction in rate of progression
NHLBI-II	5		Cholestyramine	+1%	−22%	+8%	Reduction in rate of progression
CLAS	2		Colestipol + Niacin	−19%	−38%	+35%	14% CAD regression
FATS	2.5		Colestipol + Niacin	−45%	−25%	+34%	28% CAD regression
			Colestipol + Locastatin	−24%	−38%	+10%	21% CAD regression
SCOR	2		Colestipol + Niacin + Lovastatin	−25%	−27%	+25%	20% CAD regression
SCAMP	4	300	Colestipol, niacin, Lovastatin, gemfibrozil	−20%	−20%	+7%	11% CAD regression

NA = data currently not available.

0.001), LDL-C decreased significantly (-10 mg/dl, p < 0.001, -64 mg/dl, p < 0.001), and HDL-C increased significantly only in the cholestyramine group (0 mg/dl, p = NS; $+3$ mg/dl, p < 0.001) Between-group differences were significant only for LDL-C (p < 0.001).

This study revealed that in lesions causing 50% or greater stenosis at baseline, 33% of placebo and 12% of cholestyramine treated patients revealed lesion progression (p < 0.05). When the patient's arteriograms were examined independent of treatment group, a significant (p < 0.05) association was seen with LDL-C reduction, HDL-C increase, and the extent of coronary atherosclerosis progression. In the group with the smaller change in HDL-C, 47% demonstrated progression and in the group with the greater HDLC change, 15% demonstrated progression. Unfortunately, this investigation met with some difficulty due to adherence problems. It did demonstrate that lack of disease progression was significantly correlated with the change in LDL-C and HDL-C values and in particular, the HDL subspecies HDL_{2A} and HDL_{2B}. This investigation also revealed a significantly greater decrease in progression in the group that achieved greater reduction in small LDL ($S_f 0-7$) and IDL (Sf12-20).[31] This is clinically relevant since it highlights the benefit of reduction in triglyceride rich lipoproteins and aspects of CAD risk that are not apparent from routine measurements of total cholesterol, LDL-C and HDL-C.

Important lessons regarding treatment of bypass patients and patients with total cholesterol of 185 to 240 mg/dl were learned in the Cholesterol Lowering and Atherosclerosis Study.[32] This trial involved 162 post-coronary bypass patients randomly assigned to placebo or treatment with colestipol and niacin. Following 2 years of treatment, the average number of lesions that progressed was significantly less (p < 0.03) in the drug treatment group. The number of subjects with new atheroma formation in native coronary arteries (p < 0.03) and changes in bypass grafts (p < 0.04) was also significantly less. Atherosclerosis regression was reported to have occurred in 16.2% of the drug treated patients (p < 0.002). Lipoprotein management was aggressive and drug treatment resulted in a mean 43% reduction in LDL-C, 22% reduction in triglycerides, and a 37% increase in HDL-C.

The role of lipid modification in patients following coronary artery bypass surgery (CABS) has been unclear. It is commonly accepted that a patient with an established diagnosis of hyperlipidemia clearly requires aggressive plasma lipid therapy. However, the risk-benefit issue of pharmacologically altering plasma lipids not in the classic (>95th percentile) hyperlipidemia range has been debated.[33] CLAS indicates benefit from pharmacologic lipid reduction at virtually all levels of plasma cholesterol. Additionally, a retrospective analysis of 82 CABS patients 10 years

following surgery indicates that in those patients that did not develop new or progressive disease, plasma cholesterol and triglyceride values were significantly lower (p < 0.01) than in those who demonstrated disease progression.[34] Furthermore, the levels of HDL-C and LDL-apoprotein B best distinguished the group that revealed progression from the group that did not.

CLAS-II was a 2-year extension to the CLAS-I investigation and revealed similar results.[35] Nonprogression of coronary disease was seen on a third arteriogram significantly more (p < 0.0001) in the treatment group (52%) compared with the placebo group (15%), as was regression, 18% versus 6%, respectively. New lesions appeared less (p < 0.001) in the treatment group in native arteries, 14% versus 40%, and bypass grafts (p < 0.006), 16% versus 38%. There was no difference in clinical cardiovascular events between the treatment and placebo groups. One case of cystoid macular edema that reversed with cessation of niacin therapy was reported.

Patients with specific lipoprotein abnormalities may be more resistant to treatment. This possibility was investigated in the Familial Atherosclerosis Treatment Study (FATS), which was a randomized 2.5-year trial of drug therapy in patients with coronary disease documented with quantitative coronary arteriography.[36] It is the first arteriographic investigation reported that used quantitative coronary arteriography. Quantitative arteriography allows greatly enhance precision of arterial lumen measurements.[37,38] Subjects (n = 146) were recruited on the basis of apolipoprotein B > 125 mg/dl (total cholesterol > 270 mg/dl). There were three treatment groups, lovastatin (40 mg/d) + colestipol (n = 38), niacin (4 g/d) + colestipol (n = 36), and the control group was treated with placebo + colestipol (n = 46) The goal of therapy was to achieve an LDL-C <120 mg/dl. Substantial change in LDL-C, Apo B, and HDL-C concentration was achieved, which was significantly (p < 0.001) related to coronary artery obstruction change. Results were as follows:

	% Change				
	LDL-C	HDL-C	ApoB	Progression	Regression
Placebo + colestipol	-9	$+3$	$+5$	46	11
Lovastatin + colestipol	-48	$+14$	-36	21	32
Niacin + colestipol	-34	$+41$	-28	25	39

The most recent of the regression trials to be published is the University of California, San Francisco, Familial Hyperlipidemia Study (SCOR).[39] Seventy-two patients with familial heterozygous hyperlipidemia were randomized to a control group (n = 32) or treatment group (n = 40). The control group was treated with colestipol and the treatment group received colestipol, niacin, and lovastatin. Quantitative coronary arteriography was performed and evaluated in a manner similar to the FATS trial. This study is unique in that it included both men and women, and the patients did not suffer from obvious coronary heart disease.

The subjects were approximately 42 years old, 41 female and 31 male, with the following mean values: total cholesterol = 370 mg/dl, triglycerides = 120 mg/dl, LDL-C = 280 mg/dl, HDL-C = 49 mg/dl. In these asymptomatic but hypercholesterolemic subjects, the mean coronary artery percent stenosis was 52%. An important clinical lesson is that only 15% had less than a 10% obstruction on the first arteriogram and provides clinically useful arteriographic information on asymptomatic young hypercholesterolemic men and women. Following 2 years of treatment results were as follows:

	% Change				
	TG	LDL-C	HDL-C	Progression	Regression
Control	+5	−12	−0.5	41	12.5
Treatment	−22	−39	+26	20	32.5

There was a strong trend (p = 0.06) toward regression and away from progression in the treatment group compared with the placebo group. The change in percentage area stenosis was better correlated with on-trial LDL-C levels than with change from baseline, which suggests absolute LDL-C values may be a better goal than percentage change from baseline. Women and men had similar changes in LDL-C and HDL-C but women had slightly greater reductions in TG than men (25% versus 11%, p = 0.10). Within the gender groups, the change in mean percent area stenosis was significant in women (p = 0.05) but not in men.

These arteriographic studies employed a strict pharmacologic treatment plan for approximately 2 years. A more flexible treatment approach for 4 years was tested in the Stanford Coronary Risk Intervention Project (SCRIP). SCRIP was designed to employ a practical low fat diet, smoking cessation, exercise, and multiple drug lipoprotein management[40,41]; 300 male and female subjects with coronary artery disease documented by quantitative coronary arteriography were randomized to a usual care or special intervention group. The usual care group was returned to their personal physicians for usual care. The special intervention group was seen approximately every 2 months

for 4 years and underwent diet, weight loss, smoking cessation, exercise, and pharmacologic management designed to optimize all known CAD risk factors. The change in lipoprotein values were as follows:

	Usual Care (%)	Special Intervention (%)
Triglycerides (mg/dl)	−1	−20
Total cholesterol	−1	−16
LDL-C	−4	−23
HDL-C	5	+12

Quantitative coronary arteriography indicated that progression occurred in 49.6% of the Usual Care versus 50.4% of the Special Intervention group while regression was reported in 10% of the Usual Care versus 21% of the Special Intervention group. There was a significantly greater (p < 0.01) annualized rate of minimum diameter change for diseased vessels in the Usual Care group compared to the Special Intervention group.

CURRENT TOPICS OF CLINICAL IMPORTANCE

Recent advances in lipidology help clarify the lack of precision in individual risk prediction based on the classic measures of blood cholesterol and triglycerides. These topics will be of clinical importance during the 1990s. At the present time, many of these tests are available only in lipid research laboratories, but they will soon be available to practicing clinicians.

LDL Phenotype B

Hypertriglyceridemia as a CAD risk factor is a subject that has received much debate and a National Institutes of Health consensus on this topic has been published.[42,43] Associated with mild to moderate elevations in plasma triglycerides is the dense LDL subclass pattern (LDL phenotype B), which is a heritable trait determined by a single major dominant gene (the *alp* locus).[44,45] This trait has been linked to a locus on chromosome 19, at or near the LDL receptor gene.[46] The full expression of this trait occurs following puberty in men and after menopause in women. Based on Hardy-Weinberg equilibrium, 35% of people are heterozygous for *alp* and another 5% are homozygous. The dense LDL subspecies is a marker for a common genetic trait that effects lipoprotein metabolism and increases CAD risk. The LDL pattern B trait is associated with a tendency toward elevated levels of triglyceride, VLDL, and IDL, and reduced levels of HDL, however, the LDL phenotype B persists, even when levels of triglyceride, VLDL, and HDL are normal. Subjects classified as phenotype B appear to have an enhanced response to nicotinic acid compared to phenotype A subjects.[47] This common trait may account for at least a portion of the heart disease risk associated with mild elevations of triglyceride and reductions in HDL in the general population.

The Boston Area Health Study was a case-control study that shed some light on the triglyceride controversy.[7] In this study, 366 individuals with a recent documented myocardial infarction were compared to 423 individuals selected randomly and controlled for gender, age, and place of residence. Gradient gel electrophoresis was used to identify LDL subclasses in 109 MI cases, and 121 control subjects.[45] Mean lipid and lipoprotein cholesterol differences in MI cases and controls were as follows:

	MI Cases	Controls	p
Total cholesterol (mg/dl)	226	215	NS
LDL-C (mg/dl)	144	138	NS
HDL-C (mg/dl)	33	40	<0.01
Triglycerides (mg/dl)	214	157	<0.01

There were significantly more (p < 0.01) LDL pattern Bs in the male MI subjects (54%) compared with the control group (31%). While 29% of the women MI cases were LDL phenotype B compared to 4% of the control group. LDL phenotype B carried a three fold greater risk of CAD despite no difference in LDL-C. A clinical clue to the presence of LDL phenotype B can be obtained from routine tests of triglyceride and lipoprotein cholesterol. Triglycerides, and intermediate density lipoprotein were significant in predicting LDL phenotype B (p < 0.05), and HDL-C was inversely significant (p < 0.05) in predicting LDL phenotype B.

The atherogenicity of small LDL particles may relate to the increased uptake of small LDL into the arterial wall.[48] In an animal model, a 16% reduction in LDL diameter is related to a 40% increase in the rate of LDL uptake into the arterial wall. Once in the arterial wall, oxidation of the LDL particle, recruitment of macrophages, and foam cell generation could occur.[49]

Hyperapobetalipoproteinemia

Unfortunately, few large clinical trials involving triglycerides and CHD report apoprotein B values. This is of importance since approximately 50% of CAD is not explained by the conventional risk factors, including elevated plasma cholesterol, and due to the high incidence of hyperapobetalipoproteinemia (81%) in the post-MI population that exhibit relatively "normal" LDL-C, elevated plasma triglycerides (>200 mg/

dl, mean = 350 mg/dl), and elevated LDL apoB (>120 mg/dl).[1,50] Seventy percent of normotriglyceridemic (<200 mg/dl, mean = 143 mg/dl) post-MI patients with relatively normal LDL-C have been reported to have abnormal elevations in LDL apoB.[51] Individuals with this condition have an overabundance of small, dense LDL particles that are similar to those noted in patients with familial combined hyperlipidemia and patients shown to have more progression of CAD demonstrated on arteriography.[32] This condition appears to be due to increased apoprotein B-100 synthesis and transmitted as a dominant trait. Incorporation of fatty acids into lipid esters appears to be decreased and results in abnormal processing of dietary fat and postprandial increases in free fatty acids. HDL and apoA-I are reduced and in the postprandial state, a sharp decrease in HDL₂-cholesterol has been reported.[52] Thus, in this relatively common condition, several abnormalities in lipoprotein metabolism that are not reflected in the LDL-C measurement, could contribute to CAD.

Lp(a)

[a] is a large protein composed of multiple protein conformations quite similar to kringle 4 in plasminogen.[53] Cross-sectional studies and in vitro work indicate this is a powerful CAD risk factor that may be more important than LDL-C and HDL-C. Lp(a) is an independent risk factor for myocardial infarction in young men and is independently associated with arteriographically defined coronary disease.[54,55] While as yet not well defined, a differential genetic distribution is suggested by the report that Lp(a) levels are significantly higher (p = 0.007) in post-MI black patients (31.7 mg/dl) compared to white patients (20.4 mg/dl).[56] Furthermore, opposite correlations were observed with HDL-C so that in blacks, Lp(a) correlated positively (r = 0.31, p − 0.03) and whites negatively (r = −0.16, p = 0.02). Similar differences are suggested from the Bogalusa Heart Study in which Lp(a) levels were 1.7 fold higher (p < 0.0001) in black than white children and females were slightly greater than males (p < 0.05).[57] Lp(a) has been consistently detected in 30 hypertriglyceridemic patients, but not in hypercholesterolemic patients who were normotriglyceridemic.[58] This suggests an interaction of fasting triglyceride levels and Lp(a).

The incidence of clinical events may be associated with Lp(a) concentration. In FATS, cardiovascular events were fewer in the group with less Lp(a).[37] The effect of lipid-lowering medications on Lp(a) has not been investigated in a systematic manner. Some investigations report the effect through post hoc analysis but the studies have not been designed to address the hypothesis that medications may alter Lp(a) or [a] isoforms. In 16 subjects treated with resin, Lp(a) values varied between <2mg% to >180 and there was no consistent effect on Lp(a).[59] Niacin alone or used in combination with neomycin has been reported to reduce Lp(a) levels.[60,61] Lp(a) *isoforms* track by a simple Mendelian pattern of inheritance.[62] The relative atherogenicity of [a] isoforms has yet to be determined.

Apo E Polymorphism

One of the most common genes affecting LDL levels is the gene for apoE, which has three major isoforms, E2, E3, and E4.[63] The most common allele, E3, has a frequency of approximately 0.78, while E4 has a frequency of 0.15, and E2 a frequency of 0.07.[64] Several studies have established that the E4 allele is associated with higher and the E2 with lower levels of LDL cholesterol and apo B than is the E3 allele. It has been found that the fractional catabolic rate of LDL is greater in individuals with the apo E2 genotype than in those with apo E3.[65,66] This is consistent with the suggestion that hepatic LDL receptor activity is relatively higher in individuals with the apoE2 genotype because of decreased uptake of apoE2-containing triglyceride-rich lipoproteins, resulting in less suppression of LDL receptors.[67–70] Conversely, fractional catabolic rate of LDL is reduced in individuals with the apoE4 genotype,[64] and this may be related to enhanced clearance of apoE4-containing remnants and suppression of LDL receptors. The disease, type III hyperlipoproteinemia, is an example of an interaction of the apoE2 homozygous state with other genetic or environmental factors leading to accumulation of triglyceride-rich lipoprotein remnants and atherosclerosis.[71] It is useful in analyzing potential differences in response to a therapeutic intervention, since one group may respond more favorably but the response diluted due to the inclusion of a nonresponsive E isoform group in the analysis.

Familial Defective apoB-100 (FDB)

FDB results from a single nucleotide mutation in the apoB gene and results in approximately 32% of the receptor-binding activity of the normal LDL apoB-100.[72] Approximately 1 in 500 individuals may be affected and 3% of the hypercholesterolemic population may suffer from FDB.[73] Average total plasma cholesterol concentrations have been reported to vary between 269 mg/dl and 369 mg/dl.[74] The association of CAD with this recently described condition is not well established, although a similar plasma cholesterol associated risk is anticipated.

LDL Modification

Oxidation of apoprotein B has been shown to result in a modified LDL particle that is taken up rapidly by tissue macrophages resulting in atherogenic foam cell formation.[75] Incubation of LDL with cultured endothelial cells also results in a modified LDL (m-LDL) that is taken up by macrophages 3 to 10 times more rapidly than native LDL resulting in foam cell formation.[76,77] An alternative, non apoB, high-affinity receptor for LDL exists in arterial endothelial cells and macrophages that avidly takes up the m-LDL and a specific macrophage receptor that recognizes oxidized LDL but not acetylated LDL has been described.[78,79] This m-LDL undergoes many structural changes most of which depend on peroxidation of polyunsaturated fatty acids in the LDL lipids, which can be inhibited by vitamin E.[80,81] In plasma, aldehydes (i.e., malondialdehyde or 4-hydroxynonenal) are generated by peroxidation of polyunsaturated fatty acids, which are part of LDL phospholipids. These aldehydes may alter lysine residues of apoprotein B and result in m-LDL.[82,83]

The human pathologic effects of m-LDL are thought to occur in the arterial wall since addition of plasma to the in vitro system results in inhibition of cell-induced oxidation in part due to naturally circulating antioxidants. Once the LDL contains fatty acid lipid peroxides, there follows a propagation that amplifies the number of free radicals and leads to extensive fragmentation of the fatty acid chains.[84] HDL and the associated apoproteins, A-I and A-II, may play a protective role in inhibiting oxidation of apoprotein B on the LDL particle. Apoprotein A-I, A-I/A-II, and HDL itself have a protective effect on Cu^{2+} catalyzed oxidation of human LDL.[85]

Postprandial Lipemia

Lipoprotein metabolism during the hours following a typical American meal is quite dynamic and with the exception of total plasma cholesterol, the lipoprotein values can be dramatically altered. A relation between postprandial lipemia and coronary heart disease was reported by Harlan in 1964 but the precise relationship between changes in postprandial lipemia and atherosclerosis remain elusive and are under active investigation.[86] A pathophysiologic link is quite reasonable, and lipoprotein disorders associated with a higher incidence of CAD have been demonstrated to have abnormalities in postprandial lipemia.[51,87–89]

GENETICS AND THE FUTURE

During the 1990s, aggressive manipulation of plasma lipoproteins by dietary and pharmacologic intervention will provide the physician with a powerful tool to manipulate atherosclerosis metabolically.[90] Combining therapies involved with platelet action, prostaglandins, thromboxins, growth factors, and immunology will provide extremely powerful therapies.[91] However, the underlying defect in patients with

CAD is frequently being associated with defined genetic abnormalities. Elucidation of these conditions, development of clinically available diagnostic tools, and, eventually, gene therapy will provide physicians in the not-too-distant future the possibility of eradicating atherosclerosis from our society.

Plasma concentrations of lipoproteins, lipoprotein subclass distribution, and apoproteins are powerful predictors of CAD risk. However, every clinician has a group of patients who exhibit many CAD risk factors yet live into their ninth decade, and other patients who lead exemplary life-styles yet surcum to premature CAD. This variation in clinical experience and in individual variation in response in clinical trials has long been thought to be in large part due to genetic variation. Until recently it was technically impossible to obtain enough genetic material to investigate this issue at the DNA level. Five technologic advances have allowed an explosion in understanding of the genetic aspects of CAD.[92] Restriction endonucleases are enzymes that allow specific DNA segments to be made available for study by clipping them out of the human genome. Molecular cloning allows the restriction fragments to be inserted into foreign DNA and replicated many fold in organisms such as *Escherichia coli*. The construction of DNA libraries provide cloned DNA fragments that represent all of the source DNA sequences. The ability to select the clone with the DNA sequence of interest has been refined, and finally, DNA sequencing has been established that permits determination of the sequence of the foreign DNA of interest.

These technological advances have provided the opportunity to investigate the etiology of atherosclerosis at the DNA level. This has tremendous diagnostic and therapeutic implications. The human genome is complex and estimated to have at least 10^6 genes. Thus, selecting a specific gene that contributes to CAD appears to be an overwhelming task. One approach has been described as the "candidate gene approach."[93,94] This approach involves selecting genes in which an allelic variation might produce a lipoprotein abnormality contributing to CAD. Genes that code for apoproteins, enzymes, receptors, vessel wall proteins, growth factors, and coagulation factors are obvious candidates. Since CAD appears to be a polygenic disease, multiple genetic and environmental conditions probably contribute to the cumulative atherogenic potential.

Genetic causes for variation in plasma lipoproteins is common. Studies indicate that approximately 50% of interindividual variability of LDL-C and HDL-C can be attributed to genetic factors.[95,96] Nineteen rare genetic variations affecting lipid transport in humans have been identified and at least fifteen common gene polymorphisms associated with plasma lipid phenotypes or CAD have been reported.[93,97] The chromosomal organization of these genes have been organized into "fat maps" that will eventually enable us to pinpoint the DNA location of lipoprotein and atherosclerosis abnormalities.[97] Twenty such locations have been mapped in the human Chromosome and are in Table 4-3. In the future, DNA markers may be used to more accurately predict genetic susceptibility to atherosclerosis and provide the clinician with invaluable

TABLE 4-3. Chromosomal Location of Genes Affecting Plasma Lipoproteins

Gene	Chromosome	Function
APOA2	1	Structural gene for apoprotein AII
CR39-1	1	Prenyltransferase
Ath-1	1	HDL levels and susceptibility to diet-induced atherosclerosis
APOB	2	Structural gene for apoprotein B100
LFABP	2	Fatty acid binding protein
APOD	3	Structural gene for apoprotein D
CRBP and CRBP-II	3	Proteins that bind vitamin A
IFABP	4	Intestinal fatty acid binding protein
HMCGS	5	Structural gene for 3-hydroxy-3-methylglutaryl coenzyme A synthase
HMGCR	5	Structural gene for 3-hydroxy-3-methylglutaryl coenzyme A reductase
APOA	6	Structural gene for [a]
LPL	8	Encodes lipoprotein lipase
APOAI, APOC3 APOA4	11	Gene cluster encoding apoproteins, AI, CIII, and AIV
CR39-15	15	Hybridized with CR 39
HL	15	Structural gene for hepatic lipase
CETP	16	Encodes cholesteryl ester transfer protein
LCAT	16	Encodes lecithin-cholesterol acyltransferase
LDLR	19	Encodes the LDL receptor
APOC1, APOC2 APOE	19	Encodes apoproteins CI, CII, and E
CR39-X	21	Hybridizes to CR39 cDNA

(From Lusis and Sparkes,[97] with permission.)

information regarding which patient requires aggressive manipulation of environmental and physiologic parameters to prevent or cure CAD.[98]

CONCLUSION

By incorporating measurement of apoproteins and lipoprotein subclass distribution the clinician can enhance the precision and accuracy of CAD risk prediction and identify subjects with a "normal lipid profile" that is in fact at high CAD risk. The effectiveness of diet and pharmacologic interventions is in part dependent on specific lipoprotein and apoprotein abnormalities. Clinically available measurement of these abnormalities will be available during the 1990s that will help guide diagnosis and treatment. The future of lipoprotein and atherosclerosis diagnosis and treatment lies in the field of molecular genetics.

REFERENCES

1. Kannel WB, Castelli WP, Gordon T: Cholesterol in the prediction of atherosclerotic disease. Ann Intern Med 90:85, 1979
2. Keys A: Seven Countries. Harvard University Press, Cambridge, Massachusetts, 1980
3. Bottiger LE, Carlson LA: Risk factors for ischemic vascular death in men in the Stockholm Prospective study. Atherosclerosis 36:389, 1980
4. Williams RR, Hopkins PN, Hunt SC et al: Population-Based frequency of dyslipidemia syndromes in coronary-prone families in Utah. Arch Intern Med 150:582, 1990
5. Zavaroni I, Dall'Aglio E, Bonora E et al: Evidence that multiple risk factors for coronary artery disease exist in persons with abnormal glucose tolerance. Am J Med 83:609, 1987
6. Gofman JW, Young W, Tandy R: Ischemic heart disease, atherosclerosis and longevity. Circulation 34:679, 1966
7. Hennekens CH, Buring JE, O'Conner GT et al: Moderate alcohol consumption and risk of myocardial infarction. Circulation, suppl 4. 76:501, 1987
8. Martin MJ, Hulley SB, Browner WS et al: Serum cholesterol, blood pressure, and mortality: implications from a cohort of 361,662 men. Lancet 2:933, 1986
9. Lipid Research Clinics Program: The Lipid research clinics coronary primary prevention trial results. I. Reduction in incidence of coronary heart disease. JAMA 251:351, 1984
10. Dayton S, Pearce ML, Hashimoto S et al: A controlled clinical trial of a diet high in unsaturated fat in preventing complications of atherosclerosis. Circulation, suppl II. 39/40, 1969
11. Hjermann I, Holme I, Velve BK, Leren P: Effect of diet and smoking intervention on the incidence of coronary heart disease. Lancet 2:1303, 1981
12. Carlson LA, Danielson M, Ekberg I et al: Reduction of myocardial reinfarction by the combined treatment with clofibrate and nicotinic acid. Atherosclerosis 28:81, 1977
13. Carlson LA, Rosenhamer G: Reduction of mortality in the Stockholm ischaemic heart disease secondary prevention study by combined treatment with clofibrate and nicotinic acid. Acta Med Scand 223:405, 1988
14. Coronary Drug Project Research Group: Natural history of myocardial infarction in the coronary drug project: Long-term prognostic importance of serum lipid levels. Am J Cardiol 42:489, 1978
15. Frick MH, Elo O, Haapa K et al: Helsinki heart study: Primary-prevention trial with gemfibrozil in middle-aged men with dyslipidemia. N Engl J Med 317:1237, 1987
16. Oliver MF, Heady JA, Morris JN et al: A cooperative trial in the primary prevention of ischemic heart disease using clofibrate. Report from the Committee of Principal Investigators. Br Heart J 40:1069, 1978
17. Lipid Research Clinics Program: The lipid research clinics coronary primary prevention trial resutls. I. Reduction in incidence of coronary heart disease. II. The relationship of reduction in incidence of coronary heart disease to cholesterol lowering. JAMA 251:351, 1984
18. Superko HR, Wood PD, Haskell WL: Coronary heart disease and risk factor modification. Is there a threshold? Am J Med 78:826, 1985
19. Kuo PT, Hayase K, Moreyra AE: Use of combined diet and colestipol in long-term treatment of patients with type II hyperlipoproteinemia. Circulation 59:199, 1979
20. Glagov S, Weisenberg E, Zarins CK et al: Compensatory enlargement of human atherosclerotic coronary arteries. N Engl J Med 316:1371, 1987
21. Optimal detection of the progression of coronary artery disease: comparison of methods suitable for risk factor intervention trials. Circulation 74:1235, 1986
22. Moise A, Théroux P, Taeymans Y, Waters DD: Factors associated with progression of coronary artery disease in patients with normal or minimally narrowed coronary arteries. Am J Cardiol 56:30, 1985
23. Kroncke GM, Kosolcharoen P, Clayman JA et al: Five-year changes in coronary arteries of medical and surgical patients of the veterans administration randomized study of bypass surgery. Circulation, suppl I. 78:I–144, 1988
24. Lichtlen PR, Hugenholtz PG, Rafflenbeul W et al: Retardation of angiographic progression of coronary artery disease by nifedipine. Results of the International Nifedipine Trial on antiatherosclerotic therapy (INTAC) Lancet 2:1109, 1990
25. Waters D, Lesperance J, Francetich M et al: A controlled clinical trial to assess the effect of a calcium antagonist upon the progression of coronary atherosclerosis, abstracted. Circulation 80:II–266, 1989
26. Arntzenius AC, Kromhout D, Barth JD et al: Diet, lipoproteins, and the progression of coronary atherosclerosis. The Leiden intervention trial. N Engl J Med 312:805, 1985
26a. Ornish D, Brown SE, Scherwitz LW et al: Can lifestyle changes reverse coronary heart disease? Lancet 336:129, 1990
27. Cohn K, Saki FJ, Langston MF: Effect of clofibrate on progression of coronary disease—A prospective angiographic study in man. Am Heart J 89:591, 1975

28. Duffield RGM, Lewis B, Miller NE, et al: Treatment of hyperlipidaemia retards progression of symptomatic femoral atherosclerosis. Lancet 2:639, 1983

29. Levy RI, Brensike JF, Epstein SE et al: The influence of changes in lipid values induced by cholestyramine and diet on progression of coronary artery disease: results of the NHLBI type II coronary intervention study. Circulation 69:325, 1984

30. Brensike JF, Levy RI, Kelsey SF, et al: Effects of therapy with cholestyramine on progression of coronary atherosclerosis: results of the NHLBI type II coronary intervention study. Circulation 69:313, 1984

31. Krauss RM, Lindgren FT, Williams PT et al: Intermedicate-density lipoproteins and progression of coronary artery disease in hypercholesterolaemic men. Lancet 2:62, 1987

32. Blankenhorn DH, Nessim SA, Johnson RD et al: Beneficial effects of combined colestipol-niacin therapy on coronary atherosclerosis and coronary venous bypass grafts. JAMA 257:3233, 1987

33. AMA Scientific Council Report: Dietary and pharmacologic therapy for the lipid risk factors. JAMA 250:1873, 1983

34. Campeau L, Enjalbert M, Lesperance J et al: The relation of risk factors to the development of atherosclerosis in saphenous-vein bypass grafts and the progression of disease on the native circulation. N Engl J Med 311:1329, 1984

35. Cashin-Hemphill L, Mack WJ, Pogoda JM et al: Beneficial effects of colestipol-niacin on coronary atherosclerosis. JAMA 264:3013, 1990

36. Brown G, Albers JJ, Fisher LD et al: Regression of coronary artery disease as a result of intensive lipid-lowering therapy in men with high levels of apolipoprotein B. N Engl J Med 323:1289, 1990

37. Alderman EL, Hamilton KK, Silverman J et al: Anatomically flexible, computer-assisted reporting system for coronary angiography. Am J Cardiol 49:1208, 1982

38. Brown BG, Bolson EL, Dodge HT: Arteriographic assessment of coronary atherosclerosis. Review of current methods, their limitations, and clinical applications. Arteriosclerosis 2:2, 1982

39. Kane JP, Malloy MJ, Ports TA et al: Regression of coronary atherosclerosis during treatment of familial hypercholesterolemia with combined drug regimens. JAMA 264:3007, 1990

40. SCAMP AHA abstract

41. Alderman EL, Haskell WL, Fair JM et al: Beneficial angiographic and clinical response to multifactor modification in the Stanford Coronary Risk Project. Arteriosclerosis 11:1400a, 1991

42. Hulley SB, Rosenman RH, Bawol RD, Brand RJ: Epidemiology as a guide to clinical decisions: the association between triglyceride and coronary heart disease. N Engl J Med 302:1383, 1980

43. NIH Consensus Development Conference Summary: Treatment of Hypertriglyceridemia. 4(8): NIH PD5GR-2152-D-1, 1984

44. Austin MA, King MC, Vranizan KM, Krauss RM: Atherogenic lipoprotein phenotype. A proposed genetic marker for coronary heart disease risk. Circulation 82:495, 1990

45. Austin MA, Breslow JL, Hennekens CH et al: Low density lipoprotein subclass patterns and risk of myocardial infarction. JAMA 260:1917, 1988

46. Nishina PM, Johnson JP, Naggert JK et al: Linkage of atherogenic lipoprotein phenotype to the low-density lipoprotein receptor locus on the short arm of chromosome 19. Proc Natl Acad Sci USA 89:708, 1992

47. Superko HR, Krauss RM: Differential effects of nicotinic acid in subjects with different LDL subclass patterns. Atherosclerosis 1992 (in press)

48. Nordestgaard BG, Zilversmit DB: Comparison of arterial intimal clearances of LDL from diabetic and nondiabetic cholesterol-fed rabbits. Differences in intimal clearance explained by size differences. Arteriosclerosis 9:176, 1989

49. Tribble DL, Holl LG, Wood PD et al: Variations in oxidative susceptibility among six low density lipoprotein subfractions of differing density and particle size. Atherosclerosis 93:189, 1992

50. Kwiterovich PO: HyperapoB: a pleiotropic phenotype characterized by dense low-density lipoprotein and associated with coronary artery disease. Clin Chem 34:B71, 1988

51. Sniderman AD, Wolfson C, Teng B et al: Association of hyperapobetalipoproteinemia with endogenous hypertriglyceridemia and atherosclerosis. Ann Intern Med 97:833, 1982

52. Genest J, Sniderman A, Cianflone K: Hyperapobetalipoproteinemia. Arteriosclerosis 6:297, 1986

53. Scanu AM, Gless GM: Lipoprotein (a). Heterogeneity and biological relevance. J Clin Invest 85:1709, 1990

54. Sandkamp M, Funke H, Schelte H et al: Lipoprotein(a) is an independent risk factor for myocardial infarction at a young age. Clin Chem 36:20, 1990

55. Dahlen GH, Guyton JR, Attar M et al: Association of levels of lipoprotein Lp(a), plasma lipids, and other lipoproteins with coronary artery disease documented by angiography. Circulation 74:758, 1986

56. Pearson T, Davidson L, Jenkins P et al: Lipoprotein (a) levels in Blacks versus Whites: marked differences in levels and correlations with other lipids, abstracted. Circulation 82:III–120, 1990

57. Srinivasan SR, Dahlen GH, Jarpa RA et al: Black-White differences in serum Lp(a) levels and its relation to parental myocardial infarction among children. Bogalusa Heart Study, abstracted. Circulation 82:III–20, 1990

58. Selinger E, Dallongeville J, Davignon J: Lp(a) is presnet in plasma of density <1.006 g/ml in hypertriglyceridemia. Circulation, abstracted. 82:III–90, 1990

59. Vessby B, Kostner G, Lithell H, Thomis J: Diverging effects of cholestyramine on apolipoprotein B and lipoprotein Lp(a). Atherosclerosis 44:61, 1982

60. Carlson LA, Hamsten A, Asplund A: Pronounced lowering of serum levels of lipoprotein Lp(a) in hyperlipidaemic subjects treated with nicotinic acid. J Intern Med 226:271, 1989

61. Gurakar A, Hoeg JM, Kostner G, et al: Levels of lipoprotein Lp(a) decline with neomycin and niacin treatment. Atherosclerosis 57:293, 1985

62. Gaubatz JW, Ghanem KI, Guevara J et al: Polymorphic forms of human apolipoprotein[a]: inheritance and relationship of their molecular weights to plasma levels of lipoprotein[a]. J Lipid Res 31:603, 1990

63. Mahley RW: Apolipoprotein E: cholesterol transport protein with expanding role in cell biology. Science 240:622, 1988

64. Lusis AJ: Genetic factors affecting blood lipoproteins: the candidate gene approach. J Lipid Res 29:397, 1988

65. Gabelli C, Greff RE, Zech LA et al: Abnormal low density lipoprotein metabolism in apolipoprotein E deficiency. J Lipid Res 27:326, 1986

66. Utermann G: Apolipoprotein E polymorphism in health and disease. Am Heart J 113:433, 1987

67. Brown MS, Goldstein JL: Lipoprotein receptors in the liver. J Clin Invest 72:743, 1983

68. Gregg RE, Zech LA, Schaefer EJ, Brewer HB: Type III hyperlipoproteineima: defective metabolism of an abnormal apolipoprotein E. Science 211:584, 1981

69. Gregg RE, Zech LA, Schaefer EJ et al: abnormal in vivo metabolism of apolipoprotein E4 in humans. J Clin Invest 78:815, 1986

70. Weintraub MS, Eisenberg S, Breslow JL: Different patterns of postprandial lipoprotein metabolism in normal, type IIa, type III, and type IV hyperlipoproteinemic individuals. J Clin Invest 79:1110, 1987

71. Mahley RW: Atherogenic hyperlipoproteinemia. The cellular and molecular biology of plasma lipoproteins altered by dietary fat and cholesterol. Med Clin North Am 66:375, 1982

72. Innerarity TL, Weisgraber KH, Arnold KS et al: Familial defective apolipoprotein B-100: Low density lipoproteins with abnormal receptor binding. Proc Natl Acad Sci USA 84:6919, 1987

73. Innerarity TL: Familial hypobetalipoproteinemia and familial defective apolipoprotein B100: genetic disorders associated with apolipoprotein B. Current Opinion Lipidol 1:104, 1990

74. Tybjaerg-Hansen, Nordestgaard BG, Gerdes LU et al: Variation of Apo B gene is associated with myocardial infarction level and lipoprotein levels in Danos. Atherosclerosis 89.69, 1991

75. Steinberg D, Parthasarathy S, Carew TE et al: Beyond cholesterol. Modifications of low-density lipoprotein that increase its atherogenicity. N Engl J Med 320:915, 1989

76. Henriksen T, Mahoney EM, Steinberg D: Enhanced macrophage degradation of low density lipoprotein previously incubated with cultured endothelial cells: recognition by receptor for acetylated low density lipoproteins. Proc Natl Acad Sci USA 78:6499, 1981

77. Henriksen T, Mahoney EM, Steinberg D: Enhanced macrophage degradation of biologically modified low density lipoprotein. Arteriosclerosis 3:149, 1983

78. Sparrow CP, Parthasarathy S, Steinberg D: A macrophage receptor that recognizes oxidized low density lipoprotein but not acetylated low density lipoprotein. J Biol Chem 264:2599, 1989

79. Goldstein BD, Lodi C, Collinson C, Balchum OJ: Ozone and lipid peroxidation. Arch Environ Health 18:631, 1969

80. Morel DW, DiCorleto PE, Chisolm GM: Endothelial and smooth muscle cells alter low density lipoprotein in vitro by free radical oxidation. Arteriosclerosis 4:357, 1984

81. Steinbrecher UP, Parthasarathy S, Leake DS et al: Modification of low density lipoprotein by endothelial cells involves lipid peroxidation and degradation of low density lipoprotein phospholilids. Proc Natl Acad Sci USA 83:3883, 1984

82. Fogelman AM, Shechter I, Saeger J et al: Malondialdehyde alteration of low density lipoproteins leads to cholesterol ester accumulation in human monocyte-macrophages. Proc Natl Acad Sci USA 77:2214, 1980

83. Jurgens G, Lang J, Esterbauer H: Modification of human low-density lipoprotein by the lipid peroxidation product 4-hydroxynonenal. Biochim Biophys Acta 875:103, 1986

84. Esterbauer H, Jurgens G, Quehenberger O, Koller E: Autooxidation of human low density lipoprotein: loss of polyunsaturated fatty acids and vitamin E and generation of aldehydes. J Lipid Res 28:495, 1987

85. Ohta T, Takata K, Horiuchi S et al: Protective effect of lipoproteins containing apoprotein A-I on Cu^{2+} catalyzed oxidation of human low density lipoprotein. FEBS 257:435, 1989

86. Harlan WR, Beischer DE: Changes in serum lipoproteins after a large fat meal in normal individuals and in patients with ischemic heart disease. Am Heart J 61, 1963

87. Zilversmit DB: Atherogenesis: a post prandial phenomenon. Circulation 60:473, 1979

88. Superko HR, Wood PD, Laughton C, Krauss RM: Low Density Lipoprotein (LDL) Subclass patterns and postprandial lipemia. Arteriosclerosis 10:826a, 1990

89. Bersot TP, Innerarity TL, Pitas RE, Rall SC, Jr et al: Fat feeding in humans induces lipoproteins of density less than 1.006 that are enriched in apolipoprotein (a) and that cause lipid accumulation in macrophages. J Clin Invest 77:622, 1986

90. Superko HR: Drug therapy and the prevention of atherosclerosis in humans. Am J Cardiol 64.31G, 1989

91. Ross R: The pathogenesis of atherosclerosis-an update. N Engl J Med 314:488, 1986

92. Breslow JL: Molecular genetics of lipoprotein disorders. Circulation 69:1190, 1984

93. Lusis AJ: Genetic factors affecting blood lipoproteins: the candidate gene approach. J Lipid Res 29.397, 1988

94. Galton DJ, Ferns FAA: Candidate genes for atherosclerosis. p. 95. In Lusis AJ, Sparkes RS (eds): Genetic Factors in Atherosclerosis: Approaches and Model Systems. Vol. 12. Monographs in Human Genetics. S. Karger, New York, 1989

95. Moll PP, Powsner R, Sing CF: Analysis of genetic and environmental sources of variation in serum cholesterol in Techumseh, Michigan. V. Variance components estimeted from pedigrees. Ann Hum Genet 42:343, 1979

96. Rao DC, Morton NE, Gulbrandsen CL et al: Cultural and biological determinants of lipoprotein concentrations. Ann Hum Genet 42:467, 1979

97. Lusis AJ, Sparkes RS: Chromosomal organization of genes involved in plasma lipoprotein metabolism: Human and mouse "Fat Maps." p. 79. In Lusus AJ, Sparkes SR (eds): Genetic Factors in Atherosclerosis: Approaches and Model Systems. Monographs in Human Genetics, Vol 12. S. Karger, Basel, 1989

98. Frossard PM, Vinogradov S: Using DNA markers to predict genetic susceptibility to atherosclerosis. p. 110. In Lusis AJ, Sparkes SR (eds): Genetic Factors in Atherosclerosis: Approaches and Model Systems. Monographs in Human Genetics. Vol. 12. S. Karger, Basel, 1989

5

Risk Assessment and Prognosis of Patients With Diabetes and Heart Disease

Richard W. Nesto
Masoor Kamalesh

The association of heart disease and diabetes was recognized more than 100 years ago. Vergely[1] in 1883 recommended urine testing for glucose for all patients with angina. Over the years, there has been a substantial increase in the survival of diabetics, largely because of the discovery of insulin, which reduced the mortality related to ketoacidosis; the development of antibiotics for effective treatment of infections; and the availability of various modalities to manage renal failure. These developments have resulted in a relative increase in morbidity and mortality from cardiovascular disease, as indicated by the Joslin Clinic[2] and the Framingham Study[3,4] (Fig. 5-1). Mortality attributable to diabetes has decreased from the late 1960s throughout the 1970s and has since remained at a plateau, although age-adjusted death rates for diabetics increased by 3% between 1987 and 1988. As of 1988, however, diabetes ranks as the seventh leading cause of death in the United States. Since these statistics are based on underlying cause of death, the overall impact of diabetes on mortality is underestimated.[5] In actuality, diabetes contributes to a much larger number of deaths, as it is the thirteenth leading cause of years of potential life lost before the age of 65, accounting for

128,229 (1.1%) of all years of potential life lost. Although relatively uncommon compared with other major cardiovascular risk factors, diabetes has a tremendous impact on coronary artery disease (CAD) mortality. For a prevalence of only 2.8%, the nonadditive population-attributable risk (PAR) (i.e., percentage of mortality attributable to diabetes) is 5.1% compared with hypertension, the overall prevalence of which is 29.7%, with a population attributable risk of 32.9%.[6] In other words, mortality due to coronary artery disease in diabetes is expressly linked to the prevalence of diabetes in the population, while hypertension, although more prevalent, has less of an impact on CAD mortality (Table 5-1). Thus, any small change in the prevalence of diabetes will have a profound effect on mortality from CAD.

This chapter briefly reviews the major areas of cardiovascular involvement in diabetes and discusses factors that have an impact on overall prognosis and risk assessment. The principal clinical expressions of diabetes-related cardiac disease include (1) atherosclerotic CAD, (2) cardiomyopathy (including preclinical systolic and diastolic left ventricular dysfunction), and (3) autonomic nervous system dysfunction. In addi-

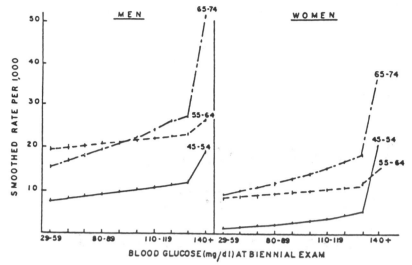

Fig. 5-1. Average annual incidence of coronary heart disease according to blood glucose level in patients aged 45 to 74. Framingham study, 16-year follow-up. (From Castelli,[131] with permission.)

tion, there are important derangements of hemostatic functions and lipid metabolism in diabetes that contribute both to the chronic development of atherosclerosis and to more acute manifestations of vascular disease, such as atherosclerotic plaque rupture or superimposed thrombosis, or both.

ATHEROSCLEROTIC CORONARY ARTERY DISEASE

A number of studies have shown that the incidence of atherosclerotic CAD is increased in diabetics as compared with the general population[7–13] (Table 5-

2). Autopsy studies reveal that the occurrence is even higher than clinical indications suggest.[14–23] The incidence of CAD rises with duration of diabetes, although some studies do not show a correlation between duration of disease and risk of CAD.[24] Furthermore, it has also been observed that diabetics treated with insulin have the highest risk of the development of CAD, while those controlled on diet have the least.[24] Angiographic and autopsy studies, which permit direct visualization of the arterial system, have further shown that, compared with nondiabetics, diabetics have a greater involvement of the coronary arteries, including a greater number of vessels involved, more distal vessel disease, and greater degree of stenosis.[25–27]. Whether diabetics

TABLE 5-1. Coronary Heart Disease Indices—United States

Risk Factor	Prevalence (%)	Crude Relative Risk	Population-attributable Risk (%; Nonadditive)	Estimated Preventable Deaths (Nonadditive)
Smoking (current)	26.5	1.7	15.6	92,525
Hypertension				
(>159 mmHg)	17.7	2.9	25.2	149,464
(140–159 mmHg)	12.0	1.7	7.7	45,670
Diabetes	2.8	2.9	5.1	30,249
Cholesterol				
(>240 mg/dL)	24.9	3.0	33.2	196,913
(200–239 mg/dL)	31.1	1.7	17.9	106,167
High-density lipoprotein				
(<35 mg/dL)	11.2	2.4	13.6	80,663
Inactivity	58.8	1.9	34.6	205,216
Overweight				
MRW > 130	26.6	2.0	21.0	124,553
MRW 110–129	41.4	1.5	17.1	101,422

(Adapted from U.S. Center for Disease Control.[6])

TABLE 5-2. Coronary Artery Disease in Living Diabetic Patients

Author	Year	Group	Pathology	Age	N	Percent
Liebow[14]	1955	Diabetic	CAD	10–90	383	42
			MI			7
			AP			10
Bryfogle[15]	1957	Diabetic	CAD	40	394	56
			AP			12
Anderson[16]	1961	Diabetic	CAD	23–88	100	55
Liebow[17]	1964	Diabetic	CAD	40–70	58	33
UGDP[18]	1970	Diabetic	CAD	20–79	1017	9.5
Kannel[19]	1961	Framingham	CAD	30–62	4469	1.6
Epstein[20]	1965	Tecumseh	CAD	16–70+	5129	4.1

Abbreviations: AP, angina pectoris; CAD, coronary artery disease.
(From Kannel,[45] with permission.)

have a greater incidence of diffuse disease, which makes them less amenable to corrective interventional or surgical therapy, remains debatable.[28–33]

The incidence of myocardial infarction (MI) is increased in diabetic patients. In addition, diabetics frequently have a more extensive and complicated infarction (see below). Another feature, noted by some clinicians, is the frequent occurrence of silent MI in diabetics.[34–49] This has been attributed inconsistently to the increased incidence of autonomic neuropathy in such patients.[39,40]

CARDIOMYOPATHY

During the 1970s, several reports documented the presence of intramyocardial "small vessel disease" in the absence of major epicardial CAD.[11,42] Pathologic examination of the heart in these studies demonstrated increased amounts of connective tissue in the myocardium. One of the earliest studies to report on the structure of small intramural arteries was conducted by Blumenthal et al.[44] in 1960, who identified proliferative lesions in the medium-sized vessels in the diabetic heart. Similar observations were made later by Hamby and colleagues,[41] who examined 73 patients with idiopathic cardiomyopathy and found a greater incidence of diabetes in these patients. Autopsy in three of four patients who died showed that the large coronary arteries were patent and free of atherosclerosis, while proliferative changes were seen in the small vessels in the myocardium. By contrast, in autopsies of 28 patients who had cardiomyopathy without diabetes, only one patient was found to have such small (70 to 150 μm) coronary vessel disease.[45] Capillary microaneurysms have also been demonstrated in diabetic hearts.[46] These data point to the presence of a characteristic microvascular disease in the diabetic heart.

In a subset of these diabetics with cardiomyopathy, myocardial dysfunction, in the absence of ischemic, valvular, or hypertensive heart disease, is frequently seen.[47] Prior to the development of systolic dysfunction these patients have subclinical impairment of diastolic function.[48,51] This abnormality has not been found to be related to duration of diabetes or the presence of microvascular complications, nephropathy, or neuropathy.[52]

Furthermore, many of these patients may have angina with normal coronary arteries.[49] The pathogenesis of impaired left ventricular (LV) function in the absence of significant CAD is unclear. Pathologic studies have demonstrated small vessel disease in some but not all such patients.[53]

Clinical implications of this microangiopathy are illustrated by the findings of 18-year follow-up study of 5,192 diabetic subjects in the Framingham study,[54] in which congestive heart failure (CHF) developed in 97 men and 86 women. Comparing the incidence of CHF in diabetics and nondiabetics, men were found to have a 2.4-fold increase and women had a 5.1-fold increase in the incidence of congestive heart failure (Fig. 5-2). Multivariate analysis showed diabetes to be independently associated with an increased incidence of CHF. A number of invasive and noninvasive studies have since demonstrated the presence of myocardial dysfunction in the absence of significant CAD.

HEMOSTATIC ABNORMALITIES

During the 1970s, a large number of reports documented the existence of various abnormalities of the hemostatic system in diabetics. Increased platelet aggregability,[55] decreased platelet count in peripheral blood,[56] reduced platelet survival,[57] increased platelet reactivity,[58] and increased platelet adhesion[56] have been demonstrated in such patients. Such platelet ab-

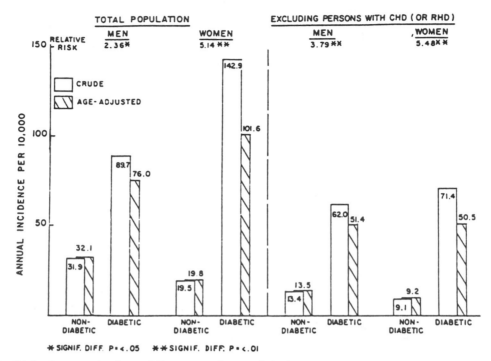

Fig. 5-2. Risk of congestive heart failure according to diabetic status each biennial examination of men and women aged 45 to 74 years. The Framingham Study, 18-year follow-up. (From Kannel,[45] with permission.)

normalities are also seen in nondiabetics with vascular disease. It is therefore not clear whether the platelet disorders are a cause or effect of vascular disease. Improved glycemic control reverses some of these hemostatic abnormalities.[58,59] Other changes in the coagulation and fibrinolytic system suggesting the existence of a 'hypercoagulable state' in diabetics include elevated levels of fibrinogen,[60] factor VIII,[61] and reduced levels of coagulation inhibitors, such as AT-III.[62] Rheologic changes in diabetes contributing to an increased tendency to thrombosis include increased blood viscosity,[63] increased hematocrit,[64] reduced erythrocyte deformability,[63] and increased erythrocyte aggregation.[65] This 'hypercoagulable' state in diabetics is important in the pathogenesis of unstable angina involving the formation of a thrombus on a ruptured atherosclerotic plaque.[66] Hemostatic abnormalities in diabetics would favor more rapid progression of thrombus formation, resulting in complete occlusion of the artery.

CARDIAC AUTONOMIC NEUROPATHY

Autonomic involvement of the heart occurs as a part of generalized autonomic neuropathy.[5,67] Abnormal heart rate response to Valsalva maneuver,[67] deep breathing,[68] and standing[69] are seen with parasympathetic involvement while exaggerated postural blood pressure responses to standing[70] and sustained handgrip[71] indicate sympathetic involvement.

In most large series, abnormal autonomic function is found in 17 to 40% of consecutively or randomly selected diabetics[71–73] and is even higher in patients with CAD. Resting tachycardia and fixed heart rates are common findings in these patients. Ewing et al.[74,75] found that diabetics without involvement of the autonomic nervous system (ANS) had the lowest resting heart rates, those with parasympathetic damage alone had the highest, and those with additional sympathetic damage had slightly lower rates (Fig. 5-3). Another important finding by the same group was that there was a loss of the usual diurnal variation of heart rate in diabetics compared with nondiabetics (Fig. 5-4). This persistently higher heart rate would increase oxygen demand, thus acting as a continuous stress. Other abnormalities include diminished heart rate variation with respiration,[68] loss of tachycardia with standing,[76] loss of relative bradycardia with lying down,[77] small heart rate responses to bicycle exercises,[78] and sustained handgrip[79] and flat response to tilt.[80]

Abnormalities of blood pressure control include postural hypotension,[67] and improper response (i.e., <10

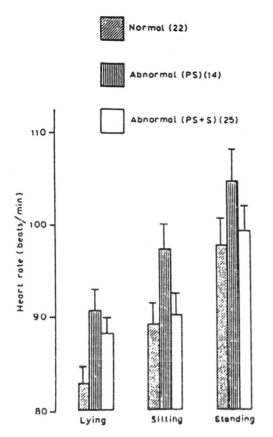

Fig. 5-3. Mean resting heart rates (+SEM) while lying, sitting, and standing, in 22 diabetics with normal cardiovascular reflexes, 14 with abnormal parasympathetic function and 25 with abnormal parasympathetic and sympathetic function. (From Ewing et al.,[74] with permission.)

mmHg rise in diastolic blood pressure following maximum voluntary contraction for as long as possible or up to 5 minutes) to sustained handgrip[81] and bicycle exercise.[82] Furthermore, it has been observed that in diabetics with autonomic damage, the fall in blood pressure after nitroglycerin administration was greater than in normal subjects or in diabetic patients without autonomic dysfunction.[83] Autonomic neuropathy has distinct effects on the overall management and prognosis of diabetics with heart disease.

LIPID AND LIPOPROTEIN ABNORMALITIES

Lipid and lipoprotein abnormalities in diabetics are a complex subject; only the important features are highlighted here. A detailed discussion can be found in a recent review article.[84] Lipid abnormalities represent an important cardiovascular risk factor.[85] In type 2 diabetes, there is an overproduction of very low-density lipoprotein (VLDL), decreased clearance of low-density lipoprotein (LDL), and decreased production of high-density lipoprotein (HDL). Obesity, which is frequently present in type 2 diabetics, modulates these lipoprotein abnormalities. Type 1 diabetics are rarely obese. In addition, their lipoprotein metabolism is influenced by the fact that they are insulin deficient. VLDL elevation in these patients correlates well with the degree of diabetic control. Extreme elevations in VLDL are commonly seen in diabetic ketoacidosis. Both LDL and VLDL levels decrease with improved glycemic control. Increased levels of LDL and VLDL

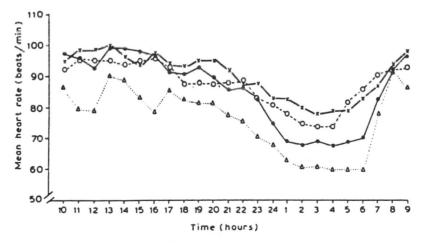

Fig. 5-4. Mean 24-hour heart rate pattern in normal subjects (*n* = 21) and in three diabetic groups: normal cardiovascular reflexes (*n* = 20); abnormal parasympathetic function (*n* = 10); and abnormal parasympathetic and sympathetic function (*n* = 24) (x--x). Group mean hourly heart rate values are shown. (From Ewing et al.,[75] with permission.)

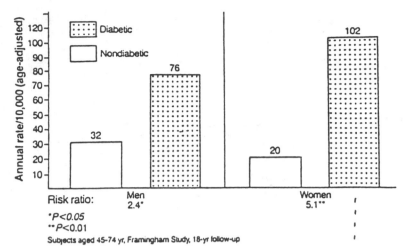

Fig. 5-5. Risk of coronary heart disease in high-risk and low-risk persons by serum cholesterol and diabetic status. (From Kannel,[85] with permission.)

are typically seen in poorly controlled diabetics. Insulin deficiency is associated with decreased HDL, and insulin administration increases HDL levels.

The Framingham study clearly shows the profound effects of lipoprotein abnormalities on the incidence of CHD[85] in diabetics compared with nondiabetics[85] (Fig. 5-5). Female but not male diabetic subjects had higher serum cholesterol levels as compared with the nondiabetics (Table 5-3). Even among males in whom atherosclerotic cardiovascular disease developed, total cholesterol was lower than in nondiabetic males. In this cohort HDL, however, was consistently lower in diabetic patients of both sexes than in those without diabetes. In the general population, and presumably in the diabetic individual as well, the risk of CAD at

any total serum cholesterol level is greatly influenced by the percentage of various lipoprotein fractions. Thus, at any atherogenic LDL cholesterol value, risk is inversely related to HDL cholesterol (Fig. 5-6). Multivariate regression coefficients, standardized for different units of measurements and range of values, suggest that the protective influence of HDL is twice that of the atherogenic influence of LDL cholesterol in the general population. In women, the triad of obesity, low HDL cholesterol, and diabetes carries an especially high risk of CAD. Among type 1 diabetics, it has been suggested that excess cardiovascular disease and lipoprotein abnormalities become clinically significant only after onset of proteinuria and decreased renal function.[84]

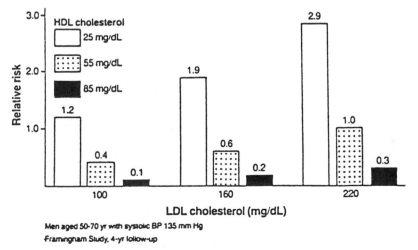

Fig. 5-6. Relative risk of coronary heart disease by high-density lipoprotein (HDL) and low-density lipoprotein (LDL) cholesterol. (From Kannel,[85] with permission.)

TABLE 5-3. Level of Risk Factors in Diabetics versus Non-diabetics: Framingham Study, 20-Year Follow-up

Cardiovascular Risk Factors	Men		Women	
	Diabetic	Nondiabetic	Diabetic	Nondiabetic
Serum cholesterol	230	233	259	250
HDL cholesterol	44	46	54[b]	58
LDL cholesterol	135	142	157	155
Triglycerides	138	135	141[c]	133
Systolic BP	148[c]	139	150[c]	139
Relative weight	126[c]	122	129[c]	121
Cigarettes	9	12	6	5

[a] $p < 0.005$.
[b] $p < 0.01$.
[c] $p < 0.001$.

Abbreviations: BP, blood pressure; HDL, high-density lipoprotein; LDL, low-density lipoprotein.

(From Kannel,[85] with permission.)

PROGNOSIS OF DIABETICS WITH CAD

Several long-term follow-up studies have demonstrated an increased risk of cardiovascular disease in diabetics. One of the largest studies was conducted in Framingham, Massachusetts, in 5,000 men and women aged 30 to 62 years, who were followed for 18 years.[85] Mortality and morbidity from all cardiovascular causes were increased in diabetics; this increase was present after accounting for other associated risk factors, such as smoking, hypertension, and high cholesterol. In particular, the relative risk of the development of heart failure was much higher in women (7.7) than in men (2.8) (Fig. 5-7). Other studies have shown that morbidity and mortality is higher in patients with insulin-dependent diabetes mellitus (IDDM) and that patients with nephropathy have the worst prognosis.[86,87] The Pittsburgh IDDM mortality study[88] demonstrated a correlation between cardiovascular mortality and duration of diabetes, which accounted for a substantial increase in cardiovascular morbidity and mortality seen in those patients whose diabetes exceeded 20 years in duration (Fig. 5-8).

The impact of asymptomatic hyperglycemia as a cardiovascular risk factor has been addressed by the Paris Prospective study,[89] the Tecumseh study,[90] and the Chicago Heart Association Detection Project.[91] These studies strongly suggest that asymptomatic hyperglycemia is an independent risk factor for CAD mortality. The Tecumseh study cohort consisted of 921 men and 937 women aged 40 and over who had no evident CAD at entry into study during 1959 to 1965. Their outcome was determined during 1977 to 1979. While diabetes was a statistically significant independent risk factor for CAD mortality in both sexes (17.8 deaths/1,000, as opposed to 5.9/1,000 in nondiabetics),

an elevated blood glucose (1 hour after oral glucose challenge) in nondiabetics was also independently associated with excess CAD mortality. The magnitude of this effect, however, was substantially below that of diabetics, with a relative rate of 1.21 compared with nondiabetics. Interestingly, this study showed no excess mortality in women over men. It was concluded that postchallenge hyperglycemia may identify or serve as a marker for patients who have other conditions that increase the risk of CAD, such as obesity, high blood pressure, hyperlipidemia, and hyperinsulinemia. Asymptomatic hyperglycemia was not believed to be an independent predictor of CAD. Similar findings were noted in the Chicago Heart Association Detection Project in which 9-year follow-up data were collected for 11,230 white men and 8,030 white women aged 35 to 64 years at entry into the study. Both diabetes and asymptomatic hyperglycemia were associated with increased mortality from CAD. The extent of association was greater in women than in men in regard to relative risk, while absolute excess risk of both diabetes and asymptomatic hyperglycemia was greater for men. For men, no independent effect of asymptomatic hyperglycemia was apparent, while it was of borderline significance in women. More recently, Wilson et al.[92] reported on the relationship of nonfasting blood glucose levels to CAD incidence. On a 10-year follow-up of this cohort from the Framingham Heart Study, age-adjusted CAD incidence was positively associated with blood glucose levels in nondiabetic females in whom diabetes did not develop during follow-up. No such association was seen in men. Multivariate analysis confirmed the independent association of blood glucose levels with subsequent CAD in nondiabetic women. This study suggests that hyperglycemia in the original Framingham cohort is an independent risk factor for CAD in women but not in men.

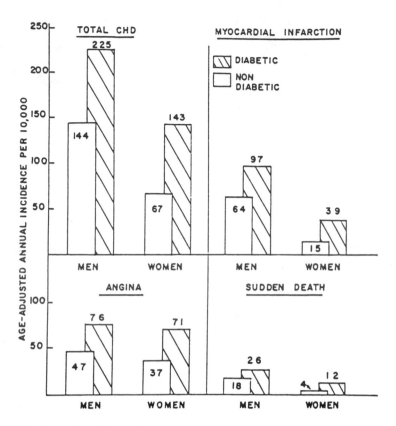

Fig. 5-7. Risk of clinical manifestations of coronary heart disease according to diabetic status each biennial examination of men and women aged 45 to 74 years. Framingham study, 18-year follow-up. (From Kannel,[45] with permission.)

MYOCARDIAL ISCHEMIA AND DIABETES

There are several important ways in which diabetes has an impact on the clinical presentation of myocardial ischemia. Clinical experience suggests that ischemia in diabetics presents either atypically or entirely free of recognizable angina pectoris. Because angina is frequently used as a barometer of the activity of CAD, diabetics may not only experience accelerated atherosclerosis but may also lack angina as a reliable warning signal that CAD may be progressing. Over the years, numerous studies have examined the relationship of symptoms to ischemia in diabetics.[34–40,93–95] Most, but not all, of these studies demonstrate a higher incidence of silent (asymptomatic) ischemia in diabetics. Some studies report a higher incidence of painless ischemic episodes in patients with autonomic neuropathy,[93] while others show no such difference.[94] The importance of bearing this in mind is borne out by

studies that show the patients with silent ischemia are at higher risk of the development of clinically apparent heart disease[39] and cardiac events. These considerations become pertinent when assessing cardiac risk for a patient before a surgical procedure.[96]

We studied 50 consecutive diabetics and 50 consecutive nondiabetics using exercise thallium 201 scintigraphy to examine the relationship of angina and ischemia.[97] The indications for testing were similar in each group and included chest pain typical of angina pectoris, stratification of risk postinfarction, evaluation of adequacy of coronary angioplasty and coronary bypass surgery, or atypical chest pain, or as a screening test in patients with multiple risk factors for coronary disease. In this study, angina was present in only 14 of 50 diabetics with ischemia compared with 34 of 50 nondiabetic patients with similar degree of ischemia on thallium scanning. There was no difference between the two groups with regard to the extent of infarction or ischemia, exercise capacity, submaximal or peak double products, time to ST-segment depres-

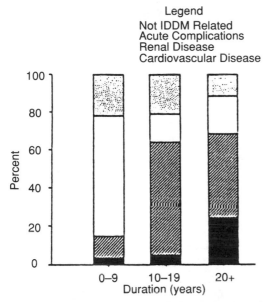

Fig. 5-8. Distribution of cause of death by duration of diabetes. The Pittsburgh IDDM Mortality Study. (From Barrett-Connor and Orchard,[88] with permission.)

sion, or maximal ST-segment depression. In assessing the magnitude of ischemia related to angina, thallium segment scoring showed no difference in the extent of ischemia or infarction between those patients who had diabetes and those who did not. These data indicate that angina is frequently absent in the diabetic patient despite myocardial ischemia and is not predicted by a clinical parameter. On the contrary, Chipkin et al.[40] reviewed 211 exercise tolerance tests that were positive for ischemia. Although there was a high incidence of silent ischemia, diabetic patients did not seem to experience a greater frequency of silent exertional ischemia (54 versus 47%; p − NS). The difference in results between these two studies could be due in part to inherent differences in the study population and the objective tests used to determine ischemia.

Using ambulatory ST-segment monitoring, Chiariello et al.[98] demonstrated that silent ischemia in Holter monitoring in the diabetic population was more frequently observed than in a similar nondiabetic group (35% versus 17%). In our experience, Holter monitoring of diabetics with documented CAD and angina during out-of-hospital activities reveals that only 3 to 5% of ischemic events are associated with chest pain. This absence of pain with ischemia adversely effects prognosis in multiple ways. Soler and associates[35] found that diabetic patients with AMI commonly had nonanginal symptoms; as a result, many of these patients were not admitted to the intensive care unit (ICU). The frequency and characteristics of angina are commonly used to assess treatment mo-

dalities or the need for diagnostic interventions. It is likely that clinical appreciation of ischemia is greatly underestimated when one relies on angina pectoris in evaluating diabetic patients with CHD. Ischemic episodes with and without pain are associated with similar degrees of left ventricular dysfunction. Such episodic LV dysfunction may be responsible for symptoms of dyspnea or fatigue that, in the absence of angina, might not be considered ischemic in origin. We and others in the past have shown that in patients in whom anginal frequency was stable, ambulatory ST-segment monitoring might demonstrate an alarming density of painless ischemic episodes prior to MI. In a large Veterans Administration (VA) study,[99] Hultgren and Peduzzi[99] found that severity of angina was not related to severity of CAD or long-term prognosis and that mild or infrequent angina might not indicate mild coronary disease. Weiner and associates[100] looked at 2,982 patients with angiographically proven CAD (greater than 70% narrowing of one or more major coronary arteries) from the Coronary Artery Surgery Study (CASS) Registry who underwent exercise testing and were followed up for 7 years. Survival rates were similar for patients with and without angina on exercise testing (76% compared with 77%). Thus, prognosis in CAD is related more directly to degree of inducible ischemia and not necessarily to the presence or absence of angina.

MYOCARDIAL INFARCTION AND DIABETES

Myocardial infarction is the cause of death in as many as 20% of diabetic patients.[101] The Framingham data showed that diabetics who survived MI appear to have a poorer short and long-term prognosis than do nondiabetic patients. One explanation for this observation is that diabetics experience a greater degree of LV dysfunction despite similar size and site of infarction. Factors that may account for this observation include (1) antecedent subclinical LV dysfunction as a result of prior remote silent infarction,[102] (2) a higher incidence of clinical or subclinical cardiomyopathy, and (3) hypertension that, to a variable extent, may cause systolic and diastolic dysfunction. Studies conducted at the Joslin Clinic during the 1960s revealed a nearly three times higher mortality during the first 2 months post-MI as well as at 5-year follow-up,[34] as compared with the nondiabetic population. One investigator[34] studied the course of 258 hospitalized diabetic patients after acute myocardial infarction (AMI). During the first 2 months, there were 78 deaths among the 205 patients who had experienced their initial infarction, for an immediate mortality of 38%. Of the 53 patients with their second infarction, 29 succumbed, for a mortality of 54.7%. On 5-year follow-up of the survivors, the results of mortality were 62% and 75%, respectively. This study also showed a high incidence of CAD among female diabetic patients (with women outnumbering men 144 to 114 in the total series), consistent with prior studies. Factors adversely affecting outcome were increased age at presentation, duration of diabetes, presence of microvascular and macrovascular diseases, and associated hypertension. Soler et al.[35] in 1975 reporting on 285 patients with MI found similar results. In a retrospective study of 21,447 diabetic patients over a 26-year period from the Joslin Clinic, Kessler[103] observed that the excess mortality of diabetic patients (as compared with the general population) disappeared when diabetes mellitus and coronary disease were eliminated as causes of death.

Greenland and associates[104] recently reported on the in-hospital and 1-year mortality in 1,524 women and 4,315 men after myocardial infarction. Age-adjusted in-hospital mortality and 1 year mortality in patients surviving hospitalization were significantly higher for women. In separate multivariate analyses for each gender, a major factor that emerged as a predictor of outcome in women but not in men was a reported history of diabetes.

AUTONOMIC NEUROPATHY AND DIABETIC HEART DISEASE

The development of ANS dysfunction may be a marker for shortened survival in diabetics. The mortality rate among patients with symptomatic autonomic neuropathy is greater than among those without symptoms (27% versus 10% after 10 years).[67] Although most of these deaths are due to renal failure, a significant number of the nonrenal deaths are cardiac in origin.

Whether a causal relationship exists between autonomic neuropathy and mortality from cardiac disease is not clear, but lack of recognition of the extent of CAD may be partially responsible. Diabetic patients may not experience typical anginal symptoms despite significant myocardial ischemia or infarction, presumably because of associated neuropathy. In a recent combined retrospective and prospective review of 1,653 exercise tests,[105] 247 were diagnostic of ischemia. Of the 29 diabetic patients with positive tests, 20 (69%) had painless ST depression compared with 77 (35%) of the 218 nondiabetic patients. Diabetics with silent ischemia were characterized by a longer duration of diabetes and a higher incidence of microvascular complications. In the prospective study, of 30 diabetics with positive exercise tests, 11 of 12 (92%) with

severe neuropathy had painless ST depression compared with 7 of 18 (39%) without severe neuropathy. This study underscores the importance of lack of symptoms with ischemia that might prevent the diabetic patient from being "warned" that progression of CHD may have occurred.

In addition, diabetics with autonomic neuropathy have a prolongation of the QT interval.[106,107] Prolongation of the QT interval has been reported in association with abnormalities of the sympathetic nervous system and is known to increase the risk of ventricular arrhythmia and sudden death.[108] A correlation between the presence of autonomic neuropathy and depressed ventricular function (assessed by radionuclide ventriculography) has also been shown.[51] Among 28 patients with IDDM, those with cardiac autonomic neuropathy had depressed LV diastolic filling compared with subjects free of autonomic neuropathy. The strongest correlate of impaired diastolic filling was orthostasis. CHD as a cause of abnormal diastolic function was excluded in all patients with a stress-thallium test. In addition, patients with diastolic dysfunction were noted to have low plasma catecholamine levels. Although this finding does not establish a causal relationship between autonomic dysfunction and diastolic filling abnormalities, it does suggest an association between the two. Since the strongest correlate was with orthostasis (which uses the sympathetic pathway predominantly), as opposed to beat-to-beat variability in heart rate (which uses the parasympathetic pathway), it was suggested that sympathetic pathway might be especially important for diastolic filling. Long-term studies will be needed to assess the clinical significance of this relationship between ANS dysfunction and intrinsic myocardial function.

METABOLIC CONTROL AND DIABETIC HEART DISEASE

Whether treatment for hyperglycemia affects cardiovascular morbidity and mortality has been debated for some time. The Framingham Study[85] shows that reduced risk of CAD in the diabetic patient depends more on the control of obesity, correction of hypertension, elimination of cigarette smoking, and improvement of LDL-to-HDL ratio than on the control of hyperglycemia. The risk of CAD in diabetic subjects is distinctly lower in those who have few other accompanying risk factors. Concerning control of hyperglycemia, Waller et al.[33] studied the extent of atherosclerosis in the coronary arteries of 229 diabetic patients and found that the type of treatment received by the patients (diet, insulin, or oral agents) or their adherence to the therapeutic regimen did not correlate with number of severe coronary narrowing. The results of three prospective studies[109–111] suggest a nonlinear relationship with a threshold phenomenon in the upper range of the distribution of blood glucose values after an oral glucose load. Multivariate analysis demonstrated that the association between blood glucose levels and cardiovascular disease was not independent from the other major risk variables. Hence it is not clear whether tight metabolic control of blood glucose directly reduces risk of the development of cardiovascular disease in diabetics.

Studies on the relationship between metabolic control and prognosis post-MI has also yielded mixed results. Recently, Yudkin and Oswald[112] studied the clinical features and hospital outcome of 83 diabetic patients admitted with AMI and found that neither incidence nor case fatality of AMI in diabetic patients was positively associated with cumulative glycemic exposure (as assessed by HbA1C measurements). Other studies with larger patient populations show a poorer short-term post-MI outcome in relationship to the blood glucose control (as measured by HbA1C or blood glucose directly).[113,114] Long-term prognosis in 73 male diabetics who survived a first MI showed a cumulative survival rate of 82%, 78%, and 58% at 1, 2, and 5 years post-MI, as compared with 94%, 92%, and 82% in nondiabetics.[115] There were no difference in mortality rate among patients with type 1 diabetes as compared with those with type 2, nor among patients treated with diet, insulin, or oral agents. Thus, difference in the type of treatment does not appear to influence outcome. In an uncontrolled small trial, Clark et al.[116] treated 29 diabetics who suffered an AMI and found a fall in the incidence of cardiac arrhythmias associated with a regimen of continuous insulin infusion.

CONGESTIVE HEART FAILURE AND DIABETIC HEART DISEASE

Compared with nondiabetics, the development of CHF in diabetics appears to confer a particularly unfavorable prognosis. In a recent review of the clinical course of 183 diabetics hospitalized with AMI at our institution,[117] death attributable to CHF occurred in 22% of diabetic women as compared with 6% of diabetic men. CHF accounted for 26 of the 52 total deaths. Thus, the development of CHF post-MI has a pernicious influence on prognosis in diabetics overall but particularly for female patients. Prior studies[34,113,114] show similar findings. The Multicenter Investigation for Limitation of Infarct Size (MILIS) study looked at the course of acute infarction in 85 diabetic patients with a mean follow-up of 34.9 months, all of whom had serial assessment of LV function.[118] The diabetic

patients experienced a more complicated in-hospital and postdischarge course than did the nondiabetic patients, including a higher incidence of postinfarct angina (42% versus 31%), infarct extension (14% versus 7.5%), heart failure (42% versus 24%), and death (7.1% versus 1.9%), despite the development of a smaller infarct size and similar levels of LV ejection fraction. Diabetic women started with a poorer baseline risk profile and experienced an almost twofold increase in cardiac mortality despite development of the smallest infarct size during the index event. The investigators concluded that this adverse outcome might be related to an acceleration of atherosclerosis, the presence of diastolic dysfunction associated with diabetic cardiomyopathy, or other as yet unidentified factors. Other features of MI that may be more common in diabetics than in nondiabetics include a greater incidence of myocardial rupture[34] and recurrent infarcts.[115]

INTERVENTIONAL/SURGICAL PROCEDURES AND DIABETIC HEART DISEASE

Percutaneous transluminal coronary angioplasty (PTCA) in diabetics is associated with a higher restenosis rate than in nondiabetics.[119] Prognosis after coronary artery bypass graft (CABG) surgery in diabetics has been the subject of several investigations. A study at our institution evaluated the results of CABG in 13 type 1 diabetic subjects with a mean follow-up of 4 years. At the end of 4 years, 12 of 13 patients were alive, with 8 of the 12 being either in New York Hospital Association (NYHA) class 1 or 2.[120] In this retrospective analysis of a small group of patients, CABG was safely performed with good long term results in some type 1 diabetics. Furthermore, follow studies of saphenous vein graft coronary artery surgery demonstrated high patency rates with recurrence of angina being related more commonly to progression of native CAD than to graft occlusion. In a more recent and larger study with longer follow-up,[121] preoperative angiographic findings revealed no significant difference in the number of vessels diseased or integrity of LV function between 212 diabetic and 1,222 nondiabetic subjects. Perioperative mortality was similar in diabetics and nondiabetics (7.1% versus 4.5%), as was improvement in anginal symptoms. However, on long-term follow-up, 15-year survival probability was worse for diabetics (36%) than for nondiabetics (53%). Within the diabetic group, type 1 diabetics fared the worst, with a 15-year survival of only 19% compared with 33% for those on oral agents, while diet-only-treated diabetics did the best (43%). Thus, although CABG was effective in all groups for relief of symptoms, survival rates were different among different diabetic subgroups. Another large, long-term study, by Salomon et al.[122] showed that 10-year survival post-CABG was lower in diabetics than in nondiabetics, but the type of treatment in the diabetic group did not influence survival rates. While proximal localized stenoses occurred with comparable frequency in diabetics and nondiabetics undergoing surgery, diffuse distal disease was more prevalent in the diabetics, as was the average number of grafts placed. Thus, although most studies indicate that the frequency and extent of CAD is higher in diabetics, it does not appear that there is any difference in the indications for CABG between diabetics and nondiabetics. CABG is an effective form of therapy for CAD in diabetics despite the nature of glycemic control, although overall survival rates are not as good when compared with nondiabetics.

Perioperative mortality and morbidity in diabetics undergoing CABG was not different from that in nondiabetics in the study by Lawrie et al.[122] This has been borne out by other large studies.[122,123] A more recent large retrospective study, done by Clement et al.[124] showed that the only difference between diabetics and nondiabetic population regarding complications of CABG was that the hospital stay tend to be longer for diabetics. The diabetic patients requiring intra-aortic balloon pump (IABP) support had a significantly higher incidence of all postoperative complications analyzed compared with diabetics without IABP, whereas the nondiabetic subset requiring IABP exhibited only a significantly higher incidence of renal failure and neurologic complications.

ASSOCIATED RISK FACTORS AND DIABETIC HEART DISEASE

Most studies indicate a peculiarly noxious effect of diabetes in women. In fact, the presence of diabetes negates the premenopausal cardioprotective effect associated with female gender.[125] Why does diabetes portend a poorer prognosis in women than in men? Favorable lipoproteins, especially HDL, have been shown to be lower in diabetic women than in diabetic men.[126]

Barrett-O'Connor and associates[127] suggest that the higher hazard associated with diabetes in women appears to be largely a function of their superior survival in the absence of diabetes, that is, the diabetes-by-sex interaction was not due to higher rates in females versus male diabetics but rather to lower rates in female versus male nondiabetics. Their conclusion is based on a report of 14-year sex-specific effect of non-IDDM on the risk of fatal ischemic heart disease in a geographically defined population of men and women—the Rancho Bernardo study. By 11 years, female survival approached male survival among diabetics, while the female survival advantage persisted among nondiabetics (Fig. 5-9).

Associated risk factors of smoking and hypertension substantially worsen the prognosis in diabetics. The incidence of high blood pressure as shown by the Framingham study is much higher in the diabetic than in the nondiabetic population. Hence, it is very important to monitor for presence of hypertension and achieve good control of the same. The recent prospective study from Pittsburgh,[129] whose data strongly suggest that cigarette smoking among diabetics should be avoided in order to improve longevity and decrease mortality from CAD, makes a compelling case for smoking cessation in diabetics.

STRESS TESTING FOR RISK ASSESSMENT IN DIABETICS

Noninvasive risk assessment for CAD involves the use of the treadmill test, stress echocardiography, and exercise thallium scintigraphy, in combination with certain clinical variables. Rubler and co-workers[129] performed exercise thallium tests in 68 men with diabetes who had no symptoms of cardiac disease. Fifty-two men were followed for 12 to 18 months. The only parameter that identified those who subsequently had a coronary event was the duration of exertion. The shorter the duration of exercise, the greater the risk of complications. Moreover, risk rates of a coronary event were raised 36-fold with a positive thallium finding and more than 7-fold with ST-segment changes on the treadmill. The predictive accuracy of a positive electrocardiographic (ECG) response was 30%, while the negative predictive value was 88%. For thallium scintigraphy, predictive value of a positive response was only 38%, but the ability of a negative test to exclude CAD was 96%. In fact, in patients with both negative ECG and thallium findings, no cardiac events occurred. Other clinical variables, such as blood pressure, cholesterol, family history, or maximal heart rate with exercise, were not predictive. Rubler and colleagues[130] concluded that diabetic men who can exercise for 440 seconds on a treadmill using a Bruce protocol are at a low risk of coronary event and that in those with negative thallium with no ECG changes on treadmill testing, overt disease was unlikely to develop. Furthermore, clinical variables added little to risk assessment once exercise duration and thallium scintigraphy are used for evaluation.

In a larger study, done by Felsher et al.[130] exercise thallium was performed in 123 patients (73 men and 46 women) with a follow-up of up to 36 months; 75% of

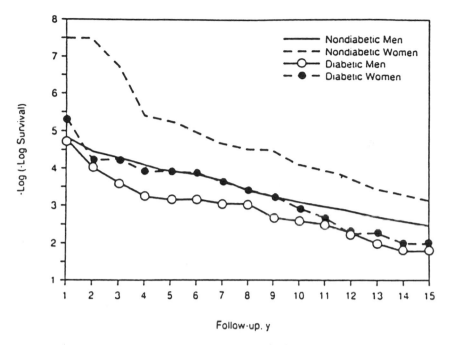

Fig. 5-9. Age-adjusted ischemic heart disease −log(−log survival) by sex and diabetes. Rancho Bernardo, CA, 1972 to 1988. Curves were estimated by Cox model blocked on both sex and diabetic status and adjusted for age. (From Barrett-Connor et al.,[127] with permission.)

these patients had symptoms of angina to begin with, unlike the previous study, which included only asymptomatic patients. Multivariate analysis of patients who had cardiac events showed that only two variables contributed independent information: the presence of abnormal exercise thallium images (p = 0.02) and exercise heart rate (p = 0.09). Unlike the study by Rubler and co-workers, duration of exercise did not predict events. Patients with normal thallium images and peak exercise heart rates of 120 beats/min had no events, patients with abnormal thallium images and exercise heart rate of 120 beats/min or less had a 22% event rate, and the remaining patients had an intermediate risk (Table 5-4). Actuarial life-table analysis showed a significant difference in survival in these

three groups (Fig. 5-10). To account for chronotropic incompetence in diabetes caused by autonomic neuropathy, they examined a group without diabetes and found that exercise heart rates and exercise duration were significantly lower in diabetic patients, whether the thallium images were normal or abnormal. Thus, as in the previous study, patients with abnormal thallium images are at a particularly high risk of future cardiac events, and a normal thallium study predicts freedom from subsequent events, particularly when exercise heart rates are high. The presence of diabetic autonomic neuropathy, however, reduces the predictive value of thallium imaging by producing an inadequate heart rate response.

CONCLUSION

From the data in this chapter, it is abundantly clear that diabetes adds substantially to morbidity and mortality from heart disease. As far as risk assessment is concerned, it appears that noninvasive modalities can be reliably used to predict future cardiac events in this population. Although control of diabetes itself is an attainable goal in most cases, our ability to affect the observed enhanced cardiovascular morbidity and mortality is limited in part by a lack of understanding of the underlying mechanisms that account for cardiac

TABLE 5-4. Incidence of Events in Relation to Exercise Heart Rate and Thallium Imaging

	Patients	Events (%)
Abnormal images and Ex HR ≤ 120 bpm	27	6 (22)
Abnormal images or Ex Hr ≤ 120 bpm	52	6 (11.5)
Normal images and Ex HR > 120 bpm	44	0 (0)

Abbreviations: HR, heart rate; Ex, exercise; bpm, beats per minute.
(From Felsher et al.,[131] with permission.)

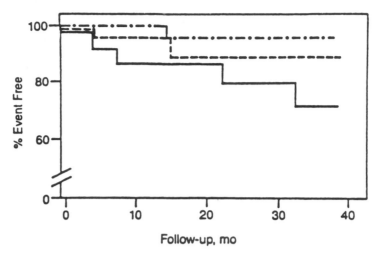

Fig. 5-10. Actuarial analysis showing event-free survival in relationship to results of exercise thallium 201 imaging and exercise heart rate. -··-, patients with normal images and exercise heart rate >120 beats/min; - - -, patients with either abnormal images or exercise heart rates of ≤120 beats/min; ---, patients with abnormal images and exercise heart rates of ≤120 beats/min. Mantel-Cox X^2 = 4.95; p = 0.08. (From Felsher et al.,[130] with permission.)

dysfunction in such patients; furthermore, heart disease in diabetics is usually advanced by the time it is clinically recognized.

REFERENCES

1. Vergely P: De l'angine de poitrine dans ses rapports avec le diabete. Gaz Hebd Med Paris, Ser 2. 20:364, 1883
2. Kessler II: Mortality experience of diabetic patients: a twenty six year follow up study. Am J Med 51:715, 1971
3. Garcia MJ, McNamara PM, Gordon T et al: Morbidity and mortality in diabetics in the Framingham population: sixteen year follow up study. Diabetes 23:105, 1974
4. Kannel WB, Hjortland M, Castelli WP: Role of diabetes in congestive heart failure: the Framingham study. Am J Cardiol 34:29, 1974
5. U.S. Center for Disease Control: Trends in diabetes mellitus mortality: MMWR 37:769, 1988
6. U.S. Center for Disease Control: Chronic disease reports: Coronary heart disease mortality—United States, 1986. MMWR 38:285, 1989
7. Liebow IM, Hellerstein HK, Miller M: Arteriosclerotic heart disease in diabetes mellitus. Am J Med 18:438, 1955
8. Bryfogle JW, Bradley RF: The vascular complications of diabetes mellitus: a clinical study. Diabetes 6:159, 1957
9. Anderson RS, Ellington A, Gunter LM et al: Incidence of atherosclerotic heart disease in negro diabetic patients. Diabetes 10:114, 1961
10. Liebow IM, Newill VA, Oseasohn R: Incidence of ischemic heart disease in a group of diabetic women. Am J Med Sci 248:403, 1964
11. Klimt CR, Knatterud GL, Meinert CI et al: A study of

the effects of hypoglycemic agents on vascular complications in patients with adult onset diabetes. Diabetes 19:747, 1970
12. Kannel WB, Dawber TR, Kagan A et al: Factors in the development of coronary heart disease—six year follow up experience. Ann Intern Med 55:33, 1961
13. Epstein FH, Ostrander LD, Jr, Johnson BC et al: Epidemiological studies of cardiovascular disease in a total community—Tecumseh, Michigan. Ann Intern Med 62:1170, 1965
14. Uusitupa M, Siitonen O, Aro A et al: Prevalence of coronary heart disease, left ventricular failure and hypertension in middle aged, newly diagnosed type 2(non-insulin dependent) diabetic subjects. Diabetologia 28:22, 1985
15. Uusitupa M, Siitonen O, Pyorala K et al: The relationship of cardiovascular risk factors to the prevalence of coronary heart disease in newly diagnosed type 2 (non-insulin dependent) diabetes. Diabetologia 28:653, 1985
16. Blotner H: Coronary disease in diabetes mellitus. N Engl J Med 203:709, 1930
17. Enklewitz M: Diabetes and coronary thrombosis: an analysis of cases which came to necropsy. Am Heart J 9:386, 1934
18. Nathanson MH: Coronary disease in 100 autopsied diabetics. Am J Med Sci 183:495, 1932
19. Root HF, Fland EF, Gordon WH et al: Coronary atherosclerosis in diabetes mellitus: a post-mortem study. JAMA 113:27, 1939
20. Hart JF, Lisa JR: Diabetes mellitus and atherosclerosis—effect of duration and severity on arterial change. NY State J Med 44:2479, 1944
21. Stearns S, Schlesinger MJ, Rudy A: Incidence and clinical significance of coronary artery disease in diabetes mellitus. Arch Intern Med 80:463, 1947
22. Clawson BJ, Bell ET: Incidence of fatal coronary disease

in non-diabetic and diabetic persons. Arch Pathol 48: 105, 1949

23. Goldberg S, Alex M, Blumenthal HT: Sequelae of atherosclerosis of aorta and coronary arteries. Diabetes 7: 98, 1958

24. Lemp GF, Vander Zwaag R, Hughes JP et al: Association between the severity of diabetes mellitus and coronary artery atherosclerosis. Am J Cardiol 60:1015, 1987

25. Robertson WB, Strong JP: Atherosclerosis in persons with hypertension and diabetes mellitus. Lab Invest 18: 538, 1968

26. Hamby RI, Sherman L, Mehta J et al: Reappraisal of role diabetic state in coronary artery disease. Chest 70: 251, 1976

27. Dortimer AC, Shenoy PN, Shiroff RA et al: Diffuse coronary artery disease in diabetic patients: fact or fiction? Circulation 57:133, 1978

28. Schlesinger MJ, Zoll PM: Incidence and localization of coronary artery occlusion. Arch Pathol 32:178, 1941

29. Pitt B, Zoll PM, Blumgart HL et al: Location of the coronary artery occlusion and their relation to the arterial pattern. Circulation 28:35, 1963

30. Montenegro MR, Eggen DA: Topography of atherosclerosis in the coronary artery. Lab Invest 18:586, 1968

31. Vlodaver Z, Edwards JE: Pathology of coronary atherosclerosis. Prog Cardiovasc Dis 14:256, 1971

32. Dash H, Johnson RA, Dinsmore RE et al: Cardiomyopathic sequelae due to coronary artery disease. Br Heart J 39:740, 1977

33. Waller BF, Palumbo RA, Lie JT et al: Status of coronary arteries at necropsy in diabetes mellitus with onset after age 30 years. Am J Med 69:498, 1980

34. Partamian JO, Bradley RF: Acute myocardial infarction in 258 cases of diabetes. N Engl J Med 273:455, 1965

35. Soler NG, Bennett MA, Pentecost BL et al: Myocardial infarction in diabetics. Q J Med 44:125, 1975

36. Bradley RF, Schonfeld A: Diminished pain in diabetic patients with acute myocardial infarction. Geriatrics 17:322, 1962

37. Margolis JR, Kannel WS, Feinleib M et al: Clinical features of unrecognized myocardial infarction—silent and symptomatic: Eighteen year follow up: the Framingham study. Am J Cardiol 32:1, 1973

38. Christensen PD, Kofoed PE, Seyer-Hansen K: Painless myocardial infarction in diabetes—a myth? Dan Med Bull 32:273, 1985

39. Hume L, Oakley GD, Boulton AJ et al: Asymptomatic myocardial ischemia in diabetes and its relation to diabetic neuropathy: an exercise electrocardiographic study in middle-aged diabetic men. Diabetes Care 9: 384, 1986

40. Chipkin SR, Frid D, Alpert JS et al: Frequency of painless myocardial ischemia during exercise tolerance testing in patients with and without diabetes mellitus. Am J Cardiol 59:61, 1987

41. Hamby RI, Zoneraich S, Sherman L: Diabetic cardiomyopathy: JAMA 229:1749, 1974

42. Rubler S, Dlugash J, Yuccoglu YZ et al: New type of cardiomyopathy associated with diabetic glomerulosclerosis. Am J Cardiol 30:595, 1972

43. Regan TJ, Lyons MM, Ahmed SS et al: Evidence for cardiomyopathy in familial diabetes mellitus. J Clin Invest 60:885, 1977

44. Blumenthal HT, Alex M, Goldenberg S: A study of lesions of the intramural coronary branches in diabetes mellitus. Arch Pathol 70:13, 1960

45. Kannel WB: Role of diabetes in cardiac disease. pp. 97–112. In Zoneraich S (ed): Diabetes and the Heart, Charles C Thomas, Springfield, IL, 1978

46. Factor SM, Minase T, Sonnenblick EH: Clinical and morphological features of human hypertensive-diabetic cardiomyopathy. Am Heart J 99:446, 1980

47. Fein FS, Sonnenblick EH: Diabetic cardiomyopathy. Prog Cardiovasc Dis 27:255, 1985

48. Rynkiewicz A, Semetkowska-Jurkiewicz E, Wyrzkowski B: Systolic and diastolic time intervals in young diabetics. Br Heart J 44:280, 1980

49. Midenbeger RR, Bar-Shlomi B, Druck MN et al: Clinically unrecognized ventricular dysfunction in young diabetic subjects. J Am Coll Cardiol 4:234, 1984

50. Airaksinen J, Ikaheimo M, Kaila J et al: Impaired left ventricular filling in young female diabetic. An echocardiographic study. Acta Med Scand 216:509, 1984

51. Kahn JK, Zola B, Juni JE et al: Radionuclide assessment of left ventricular diastolic filling in diabetes mellitus with and without cardiac autonomic neuropathy J Am Coll Cardiol 1303, 1986

52. Zarich SW, Arbuckle BE, Cohen LR et al: Diastolic abnormalities in young asymptomatic diabetic patients assessed by pulsed doppler echocardiography. J Am Coll Cardiol 12:114, 1988

53. Ledet T: Diabetic cardiopathy. Quantitative histological studies of the heart from young juvenile diabetics. Acta Pathol Microbiol Scand [A] 84:421, 1976

54. Kannel WB, Hjortland M, Castelli WP: Role of diabetes in congestive heart failure: the Framingham study. Am J Cardiol 34:29, 1974

55. Colwell JA, Halushka PV, Sarji KE et al: Platelet function and diabetes mellitus. Med Clin North Am 62:753, 1978

56. Fuller JH, Keen J, Jarrett et al: Hemostatic variables associated with diabetes mellitus and its complications. Br Med J 2:964, 1979

57. Abrahamson AF: Platelet survival studies in man with special reference to thrombosis and atherosclerosis. Scand J Haematol suppl. 3:1, 1968

58. Preston FE, Ward JD, Marcola BH et al: Elevate beta-thromboglobulin levels and circulating platelet aggregates in diabetic microangiopathy. Lancet 1:238, 1978

59. Juhan I, Vague P, Buonocore M et al: Abnormalities of erythrocyte deformability and platelet aggregation in insulin-dependent diabetics corrected by insulin in vivo and in vitro. Lancet 1:535, 1982

60. Banerjee RN, Kumar V, Sahni AL: Plasma thrombin clotting time and plasma fibrinogen in diabetes mellitus and atherosclerosis. Ind J Med Res 60:1432, 1972

61. Lufkin EG, Fass DN, O'Fallon et al: Increased von Willebrand factor in diabetes mellitus. Metabolism 28:63, 1979

62. Monnier L, Follea G, Mirouze J: Antithrombin III deficiency in diabetes: influence on vascular degenerative complications. Horm Metab Res 10:470, 1978

63. Barnes AJ: Blood viscosity in diabetes mellitus. p. 26. In Lowe, GDO, Barberel JC, Forbes CD (eds): Clinical Aspects of Blood Viscosity and Cell Deformability. Springer-Verlag, Berlin, 1981

64. Lowe GDO, Lowe JM, Drummond MM et al: Blood viscosity in young male diabetics with and without retinopathy: Diabetologia 18:359, 1980

65. Volger E: Effect of metabolic control and concomitant diseases upon the rheology of blood in different states of diabetic retinopathy. In Pathogenetic Concepts of Diabetic Microangiopathy. Thieme-Stratton, 1981

66. Fuster V, Stein B, Ambrose JA et al: Atherosclerotic plaque rupture and thrombosis; evolving concepts. Circulation, suppl. 82:47, 1990

67. Watkins PJ: Diabetic autonomic neuropathy. N Engl J Med 322:1078, 1990

68. Wheeler T, Watkins PJ: Cardiac denervation in diabetes. Br Med J 4:564, 1973

69. Ewing DJ, Hume L, Campbell IW et al: Autonomic mechanisms in the initial heart rate response to standing. J Appl Physiol 49:809, 1980

70. Hilsted J, Parving HH, Christensen NJ et al: Hemodynamics in diabetic orthostatic hypotension. J Appl Physiol 68:1427, 1981

71. Ewing DJ, Irving JB, Kerr F et al: Cardiovascular responses to sustained handgrip in normal subjects and in patients with diabetes mellitus: a test of autonomic function. Clin Sci Mol Med 46:295, 1974

72. Sharpey-Schafer EP, Taylor PJ. Absent circulatory reflexes in diabetic neuritis. Lancet 1:559, 1960

73. Hilsted J, Jensen SB: A simple test for autonomic neuropathy in juvenile diabetics. Acta Med Scand 205:385, 1979

74. Ewing DJ, Campbell IW, Clark BF: Heart rate changes in diabetes mellitus. Lancet 1:183, 1981

75. Ewing DJ, Borsey DQ, Travis P et al: Abnormalities of ambulatory 24 hour heart rate in diabetes mellitus. Diabetes 32:102, 1983

76. Ewing DJ, Campbell IW, Murray A et al: Immediate heart rate response to standing: simple test for autonomic neuropathy in diabetes. Br Med J 1:145, 1978

77. Bellavere F, Ewing DJ: Autonomic control of the immediate heart rate response to lying down. Clin Sci 62:57, 1982

78. Dyrberg T, Benn J, Christiansen JS et al: Prevalence of diabetic autonomic neuropathy measured by simple bedside tests. Diabetologia 20:190, 1981

79. Hume l, Ewing DJ, Campbell IW et al: Heart rate response to sustained handgrip: comparison of the effects of cardiac autonomic blockade and diabetic autonomic neuropathy. Clin Sci 56:287, 1979

80. Sundkvist G, Lilja B, Almer LO: Abnormal diastolic blood pressure and heart rate reactions to tilting in diabetes mellitus. Diabetologia 19:433, 1980

81. Hulper B, Willms B: Investigations of autonomic diabetic neuropathy of the cardiovascular system. p. 77. In Gries FA, Freund HJ, Rabe F, Berger H (eds): Aspects of Autonomic Neuropathy in Diabetes. George Thieme Verlag, Stuttgart, 1980

82. Hilsted J, Galbo H, Christiansen NJ: Impaired cardiovascular responses to graded exercise in diabetic autonomic neuropathy. Diabetes 28:313, 1979

83. Low PA, Walsh JC, Huang CY et al: The sympathetic nervous system in diabetic neuropathy—a clinical and pathological study. Brain 98:341, 1975

84. Howard BV: Lipoprotein metabolism in diabetes mellitus: J Lipid Res 28:613, 1987

85. Kannel WB: Lipids, diabetes and coronary artery disease: insights from the Framingham study. Am Heart J 110:1100, 1985

86. Jensen T, Borch-Johnsen K, Kofoed-Enevoldsen A et al: Coronary heart disease in young type 1 (insulin-dependent) diabetic patients with and without diabetic nephropathy: incidence and risk factors. Diabetologia 30:144, 1987

87. Krolewski AS, Kosinski EJ, Warram JH et al: Magnitude and determinants of coronary artery disease in juvenile onset insulin dependent diabetes mellitus. Am J Cardiol 59:750, 1987

88. Barrett-Connor E, Orchard TJ: Insulin dependent diabetes mellitus and ischemic heart disease. Diabetes Care 8:65, 1985

89. Eschwege E, Richard JL, Thibault N et al: The Paris Prospective Study—10 years later. Horm Metab Res 15:43, 1985

90. Butler WJ, Ostrander LD, Jr, Carman WJ et al: Mortality from coronary heart disease in the Tecumseh study—Long term effects of diabetes mellitus, glucose tolerance and other risk factors. Br Med J 291:303, 1985

91. Pan WH, Cedres LB, Liu K et al: Relationship of clinical diabetes and asymptomatic hyperglycemia to risk of coronary heart disease mortality in men and women. Am J Epidemiol 123:504, 1986

92. Wilson PWF, Cupples LA, Kannel WB: Is hyperglycemia associated with cardiovascular disease? The Framingham study. Am Heart J 121:586, 1991

93. Niakan E, Harati Y, Rolak LA et al: Silent myocardial infarction and diabetic cardiovascular autonomic neuropathy. Arch Intern Med 146:2229, 1986

94. Theron HD, Steyn AF, du Raan HE et al: Autonomic neuropathy and atypical myocardial infarction in a diabetic clinic population. S Afr Med J 72:253, 1987

95. Yoshino H, Matsuoka K, Nishimura F et al: Painless myocardial infarction in diabetes. Tohuko J Exp Med, suppl. 141:547, 1983

96. Goldmann L, Caldera LD, Nussbaum SR et al: Multifactorial index of cardiac risk in noncardiac surgical procedures. N Engl J Med 297:845, 1977

97. Nesto RW, Phillips RT, Kett KG et al: Angina and exertional myocardial ischemia in diabetic and nondiabetic patients: assessment by exercise thallium scintigraphy. Ann Intern Med 108:170, 1988

98. Chiariello M, Indolfi C, Cotecchi MR et al: Asymptomatic transient ST changes during ambulatory ECG monitoring in diabetic patients. Am Heart J 110:529, 1985

99. Hultgren HN, Peduzzi P: Relation of severity of symptoms to prognosis in stable angina pectoris: Am J Cardiol 54:988, 1984

100. Weiner DA, Ryan TJ, McCabe CH et al: Significance of silent myocardial ischemia during exercise testing in patients with coronary artery disease. Am J Cardiol 59:725, 1987

101. Smith JW, Marcus FI, Serokman R et al: Prognosis of patients with diabetes mellitus after acute myocardial infarction. Am J Cardiol 54:718, 1984

102. Kannel WB, Abbott RD: Incidence and prognosis of unrecognized myocardial infarction. N Engl J Med 311: 1144, 1984

103. Kessler II. Mortality experience of diabetic patients—a twenty six year follow up study. Am J Med 51:715, 1971

104. Greenland P, Reicher-Reiss H, Goldbourt U et al: In-hospital and 1-year mortality in 1524 women after myocardial infarction. Circulation 83:484, 1991

105. Murray DP, O'Brien T, Mulrooney R et al: Autonomic dysfunction and silent myocardial ischemia on exercise testing in diabetes mellitus. Diabetes Med 7:580, 1990

106. Ewing DJ, Neilson JMM: QT interval length and diabetic autonomic neuropathy. Diabetes Med 7:23, 1990

107. Chambers JB, Sampson MJ, Sprigings DC et al: QT prolongation on the electrocardiogram in diabetic autonomic neuropathy. Diabetes Med 7:105, 1990

108. Vlay SC, Mallis GI, Brown EJ et al: Documented sudden cardiac death in prolonged QT syndrome. Arch Intern Med 144:833, 1984

109. Eschwege E, Richard JL, Thibault N et al: Coronary heart disease mortality in relation with diabetes, blood glucose and plasma insulin levels. The Paris Prospective Study—10 years later. Horm Metab Res, suppl. 15:41, 1985

110. Fuller JH, Shipley MJ, Rose G et al: Mortality from coronary heart disease and stroke in relation to degree of glycemia: the Whitehall study. Br Med J 287:867, 1983

111. Pyorala K, Savolainen E, Kaukola S et al: Plasma insulin as coronary heart disease risk factor: relationship to other risk factors and predictive value during 9 ½ year follow up of the Helsinki Policemen Study population. Acta Med Scand, suppl. 701:38, 1985

112. Yudkin JS, Oswald GA: Determinants of hospital admission and case fatality in diabetic patients with myocardial infarction. Diabetes Care 11:351, 1988

113. Oswald GA, Corcoran S, Yudkin JS: Prevalence and risks of hyperglycemia and undiagnosed diabetes in patients with acute myocardial infarction. Lancet 1:1264, 1984

114. Rytter L, Troelsen S, Beck-Nelson: Prevalence and mortality of acute myocardial infarction in patients with diabetes. Diabetes Care 8:230, 1985

115. Ulvenstam G, Aberg A, Bergstrand R et al. Long term prognosis after myocardial infarction in men with diabetes. Diabetes 34:787, 1985

116. Clark RS, English M, McNeill GP et al: Effect of intravenous infusion of insulin in diabetics with acute myocardial infarction. Br Med J 291:303, 1985

117. Savage MP, Krolewski AS, Kenien GG et al: Acute myocardial infarction in diabetes mellitus and significance of congestive heart failure as as prognostic factor. Am J Cardiol 62:665, 1988

118. Stone PH, Muller JE, Hartwell T et al: The effect of diabetes mellitus on prognosis and serial left ventricular function after acute myocardial infarction: contribution of both coronary disease and left ventricular dysfunction to the adverse prognosis. J Am Coll Cardiol 14:49, 1989

119. McBride W, Lange RA, Hillis DL: Restenosis after successful coronary angioplasty. N Engl J Med 318:1734, 1988

120. Batist G, Blaker M, Kosinski E et al: Coronary bypass surgery in juvenile onset diabetics. Am Heart J 106:51, 1980

121. Lawrie GM, Morris GC, Jr, Glaeser DH: Influence of diabetes mellitus on the results of coronary bypass surgery. JAMA 256:2967, 1986

122. Salomon N, Page US, Okies JE et al: Diabetes mellitus and coronary artery bypass. J Thorac Cardiovasc Surg 85:264, 1983

123. Johnson WD, Pedraza P, Kayser KL: Coronary artery surgery in diabetics: 261 consecutive patients followed four to seven years. Am Heart J 104:823, 1982

124. Clement R, Rousou JA, Engleman RM et al: Perioperative morbidity in diabetics requiring coronary artery bypass surgery. Ann Thorac Surg 46:321, 1988

125. Jacoby RM, Nesto RW: Effective management of acute MI in diabetic patients. J Crit Illness 5:1109, 1990

126. Walden CE, Knopp RH, Wahl PW et al: Sex differences in the effect of diabetes mellitus on lipoprotein triglyceride and cholesterol concentrations. N Engl J Med 311: 953, 1984

127. Barrett-Connor EL, Cohn BA, Wingard DL et al: Why is diabetes mellitus a stronger risk factor for fatal ischemic heart disease in women than in men? JAMA 265: 627, 1991

128. Moy CS, LaPorte RE, Dorman JS et al: Insulin dependent diabetes mellitus mortality: The risk of cigarette smoking. Circulation 82:37, 1990

129. Rubler S, Gerber D, Reitano J et al: Predictive value of clinical and exercise variables for detection of coronary artery disease in men with diabetes mellitus. Am J Cardiol 59:1310, 1987

130. Felsher J, Meissner MD, Hakki AH et al: Exercise thallium imaging in patients with diabetes mellitus. Arch Intern Med 147:313, 1987

131. Castelli WP: Epidemiology of CHD: The Framingham Study. Am J Med 76(2A):4, 1984

6

The Role of Physicians in Primary Prevention of Coronary Heart Disease

Sally E. McNagny
Nanette Kass Wenger

Coronary heart disease (CHD) is a major cause of mortality in the industrialized world. The goal of primary prevention is to decrease the incidence of CHD by reducing its risk factors before the onset of clinical evidence of disease; physicians have a pivotal role in this primary prevention. The strategies suggested in this chapter enable physicians to provide cost-effective preventive care at routine clinical encounters. The resulting favorable outcomes in risk reduction should prove rewarding to both patients and their physicians. The following overview of evidence of the coronary risk imparted by hypercholesterolemia, hypertension, and cigarette smoking, as well as the benefits attributable to risk reduction, provides physicians with the scientific basis for the efficacy of coronary risk modification.

THE SCIENTIFIC BASIS FOR CORONARY RISK REDUCTION

Observational Evidence

Two large prospective epidemiologic projects, begun during the 1940s, identified factors associated with an increased likelihood of CHD: the Framingham Heart Study[1] and the Minnesota Businessmen Study.[2] During the next two decades, these and other popula-

tion studies confirmed a strong association between CHD and elevated serum cholesterol levels, hypertension, and cigarette smoking.[1-4] Comparative population surveys also lent support to the direct predictive association between risk factor status and CHD incidence. Surveys of CHD incidence documented widely differing rates of occurrence of CHD among different countries.[5-8] When potential coronary risk factors were examined, the prevalence of elevated serum cholesterol levels, hypertension, and smoking also varied significantly among populations.[5-8] Importantly, high CHD rates in specific countries were associated with a greater prevalence of these three major coronary risk factors.[4-6]

Since CHD death rates have changed dramatically over time periods as short as 5 to 10 years,[9,10] population differences in CHD are unlikely to be due to genetic factors. For example, Japanese persons living in the United States were noted to have both increased dietary intake of cholesterol and higher average serum cholesterol level, with a concomitant higher incidence of CHD, in comparison to those living in Japan who were eating a traditional Japanese diet.[11] This evidence highlights the potential role of modifying risk factors, such as dietary behaviors, to achieve CHD reduction.[11]

Epidemiologic studies also underscored the significant interrelationships and cumulative effects among these three major coronary risk factors. Cigarette smoking was significantly associated with lower serum high-density lipoprotein (HDL) levels.[12] Hypertension had an especially strong impact on increasing the relative risk of CHD when there was coexistent hypercholesterolemia.[13] Persons with all three risk factors were at substantially greater risk for CHD than would be expected if the risks were simply additive.[14,15] The early prospective studies strengthened the link between these major risk factors and CHD incidence by documenting a clear graded effect, with the relative risk of CHD increasing with increasing severity of the three major coronary risk attributes.[1-4] Interventional studies were then undertaken to confirm the hypothesis that CHD incidence could be lowered by favorably modifying these three major coronary risk factors.

Interventional Studies: Coronary Heart Disease Prevention

Within the research community, two different but complementary prevention strategies have emerged.[16,17] The "clinical" approach is modeled after the physician-patient relationship in which physicians are responsible for detecting coronary risk factors and instituting risk modification through counseling or medication, or both. In this model, patients at highest risk are usually selected for intervention. The "population" approach attempts to alter coronary risk factors in individuals by intervening to change community values and societal norms. By decreasing the overall risk profile of a community, the potential benefits of risk intervention are expanded to the entire population.

Interventional studies using the *clinical approach* provided information about methods that enabled major risk factors to be modified to lower the incidence of CHD. On the basis of on these findings, medical advisory boards of national professional societies and governmental agencies established screening guidelines and recommendations for modification of hypercholesterolemia, hypertension and cigarette smoking behavior.[18-24] The selected interventional studies summarized below provide for the practicing physician highlights of the scientific evidence that supports primary preventive guidelines and strategies for coronary risk reduction.

Hypercholesterolemia

In two large primary prevention trials involving high-risk men, treatment with the lipid-lowering medications cholestyramine and gemfibrozil was associated with a decrease in mortality and morbidity from CHD.[25-27] On the basis of these and other studies, the National Cholesterol Education program asserts that the incidence of coronary events in such men can be decreased by an average of 2% for every 1% reduction in serum cholesterol concentration. The positive impact of lipid lowering was further strengthened by the angiographic demonstration of regression and/or lack of progression of atherosclerotic coronary artery lesions after cholesterol lowering with lipid-reducing medications.[28,29]

Lowering of serum cholesterol levels by modifying patients' dietary intake of saturated fat and cholesterol, although extensively studied, has had variable success,[30-37] largely dependent on the regimen used and the duration of intervention. When the results of all randomized dietary trials are combined, a significant trend emerges: a 10% reduction in serum cholesterol level through dietary modification is associated with a reduction of 13% ± 6% in CHD incidence.[38] The American Heart Association,[39] the National Heart, Lung, and Blood Institute,[40] and other national and international professional and governmental organizations have all recommended comparable dietary guidelines to lower the daily consumption of saturated fat and cholesterol.[18,21,22,41,42]

Hypertension

In the landmark Veterans Administration (VA) Cooperative studies on antihypertensive agents, control of moderate and severe hypertension was demonstrated conclusively to decrease the risk of heart failure, stroke, and total mortality.[43,44] Universal acceptance of these results was rapid, but the VA studies did not fully establish whether there was benefit from treatment of mild diastolic hypertension or whether hypertension control lowered the incidence of CHD.[43,44] A more recent study that included a larger and elderly population showed a significant decrease in fatal myocardial infarction in subjects receiving treatment for diastolic hypertension of 90 to 119 mmHg.[45] Although other individual trials did not clearly show benefit from treatment of mild hypertension,[33,46-48] combining the results of nine treatment trials provided sufficient statistical power to reveal that the treated group had a significant 38% reduction in fatal stroke, and a 11% reduction in total mortality.[49] Coronary heart disease mortality was 8% lower in the drug treatment than in the control groups but this difference was not significant.[49]

In evaluating the relationship between incidence of CHD and the treatment of severe hypertension, defined as diastolic blood pressures of >115 mmHg, the Göteborg Study established that treatment with β-blocking medications significantly decreased the pooled incidence of fatal and nonfatal CHD in middle-aged men.[50] Treatment of moderate diastolic hypertension with β-blockade in middle-aged subjects in the International Prospective Primary Prevention Study in Hypertension (IPPPSH), however, failed to demonstrate a significant decrease in CHD mortality.[51] Combined data from 14 treatment trials of mild, moderate, and severe hypertension demonstrated that an average decrease of 5 to 6 mmHg in diastolic blood pressure over long-term follow-up was associated with about 35 to 40% less stroke and 20 to 25% less CHD.[52] Only one-half the reduction in CHD incidence was apparent within the first 3 years after initiation of antihypertensive medications, whereas the benefit in stroke reduction occurred within the first 2 to 3 years of treatment.[52] Thus, one reason that individual treatment studies might not have demonstrated a reduction in CHD from antihypertensive treatment was the relatively short duration of follow-up. In addition, isolated reduction of elevated blood pressure, without control of other coronary risk characteristics,[53] and the adverse effects of some antihypertensive agents on serum lipid,[54] potassium,[33] and glucose levels may also have limited the potential benefit in CHD prevention from pharmacologic control of blood pressure.

Associations between hypertension and dietary sodium intake, obesity, a sedentary life-style, excessive alcohol intake, and stress are described in a number of research studies.[55-57] Nonpharmacologic interventions to alter these predisposing factors have shown promising results. For example, rapid regression of alcohol-associated hypertension was described with abstinence from alcoholic intake.[57] In a small randomized trial to lower stress, relaxation and biofeedback appeared to control mild hypertension.[58] Future clinical trials of these and other nonpharmacologic interventions will better define their role in blood pressure control.

Cigarette Smoking

Epidemiologic studies have had a greater role than have interventional trials in establishing that cigarette smoking predisposes to coronary heart disease, lung cancer, and occlusive peripheral arterial disease.[59] Several prospective studies have documented that death rates increase with the number of cigarettes smoked[59]; that persons who give up cigarette smoking have a lower death rate than those who continue to smoke[59,60]; and that low-tar, low-nicotine, or filtered cigarettes do not lessen the coronary risk of smoking.[61] Multifactorial risk intervention trials such as the Multiple Risk Factor Intervention Trial[33] and the Oslo Primary Prevention Study[32] documented benefit from never smoking compared with smoking and found that former smokers had a significantly lower risk of myo-

cardial infarction and coronary death than did subjects who continued to smoke. Thus, the coronary risk of smoking appears to be reversible and noncumulative.[62,63]

The Population Approach to Risk Reduction

The *population approach* is based on the observation that most CHD events attributed to coronary risk factors occur among a large subset of the population with only modest abnormalities of several risk characteristics, rather than from the extremely high risk component of the population, comprising few individuals. This is illustrated in Figure 6-1, which compares the relative risk of CHD mortality and the attributable risk at different concentrations of serum cholesterol.[16,64] The relative risk rises sharply with increasing cholesterol concentrations, but for persons with high serum cholesterol levels whose risk is highest, their prevalence is quite low. Thus, the attributable deaths from the excess risk of high serum cholesterol concentrations, shown above each bar, add up to only to 3 per 1,000 men over a 10-year period for those with cholesterol levels in excess of 310 mg/dl. By contrast, 26 of the excess risk events occurred in men with serum cholesterol levels of 220 to 310 mg/dl, where the relative risk is lower. These 26 cases constitute 76% of all excess events attributable to elevated serum cholesterol levels. These data highlight a fundamental issue in prevention: a large number of people exposed to a modest risk will result in more events than will a small number of people exposed to a high risk.[16] Thus, even relatively small improvements in population risk profiles would have greater impact in coronary risk reduction than would comparable efforts toward the treatment of only the small percentage of people at highest risk and should result in substantial improvement in population rates of CHD.[4,7,16,65]

Public health and community research studies were initiated during the early 1970s[66-71] to test the feasibility of CHD prevention through modification of population risk characteristics. A model community-based intervention study is the 14-year Stanford Five City Project.[70,71] This study was designed to ascertain whether community-wide health education could improve knowledge of coronary risk factors; lower average serum cholesterol levels, blood pressure levels, and smoking habits; and reduce the incidence of stroke and cardiovascular events. Two cities received community-wide educational programs through television, radio, newspaper, voluntary agencies, and school-based programs about nutrition, exercise, and smoking; two control cities received no intervention; the fifth city was being monitored for morbidity and

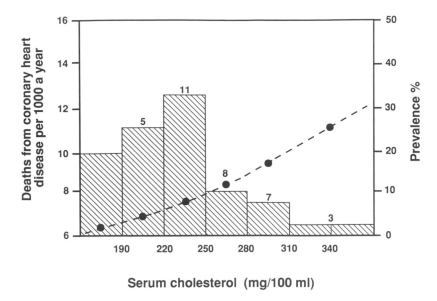

Fig. 6-1. Prevalence distribution of serum cholesterol concentration related to coronary heart disease mortality (---) in men aged 55–64. Number above each bar represents estimate of attributable deaths per 1,000 population per 10 years. Based on the Framingham Study.[64] (Modified from Rose,[16] with permission.)

mortality only and did not contribute data for this part of the study. After 30 to 64 months of these educational programs, cohort samples from the intervention cities had significantly greater reductions in serum cholesterol levels, blood pressure levels and smoking rates than did cohort samples from the control cities. In this ongoing study, total CHD risk in the intervention populations was calculated to decline by about 16%, at a per capita annual cost of $4.00.[71] Thus, the Stanford Project also demonstrated the economic feasibility of effective community-based coronary risk intervention.[71]

A UNIFIED PREVENTIVE CARE STRATEGY FOR CHD

Epidemiologic observational data, coupled with the results of clinical studies in high-risk persons and population-based studies, have provided mounting scientific evidence of the importance and feasibility of primary prevention of CHD. These studies have guided the formulation of major U.S. public health policies during the past 30 years, as summarized in Table 6-1.[22,24,41,63,72–90] A unified, albeit complex, strategy has emerged, involving a combination of interventions designed to improve coronary risk profiles. A World Health Organization (WHO) report summarized the multilevel approach needed to decrease CHD incidence: "All evidence and common sense show that successful control of the epidemic of CHD needs not only

better treatment of those already sick and improved detection and care for those at high risk, but most importantly broad-based primary prevention for the whole population."[18] This and other Expert Committees[19–21,91] advocated multiple concomitant preventive approaches involving the medical community, legislative branches of government, agricultural and food industries, educational organizations, and religious groups. Consensus goals for reducing the incidence of CHD included (1) elimination of cigarette smoking; (2) control of hypertension and reduction of serum cholesterol levels, initially by diet and next with medication; (3) adjustment of calories to achieve ideal body weight, (4) moderate exercise; and (5) control of diabetes mellitus.

SUCCESS OF PRIMARY PREVENTION OF CHD IN THE UNITED STATES

After increasing for decades, mortality rates from CHD in the United States began to decline during the 1960s and continued to decline by 21% between 1968 and 1976.[9,92–94] There was a concomitant decline in the incidence of first myocardial infarctions of approximately 25%, as reflected by trends in hospital admissions[95–97] and in a large employed population.[98] Although improvements in medical and surgical care for CHD may have decreased the mortality of patients with myocardial infarction, the decline in incidence of initial myocardial infarction reflected, at least in part, the effect of favorable coronary risk modification.

TABLE 6-1. Major Steps in the Development of Public Health Policy for the Prevention of Coronary Heart Disease in the United States

1959	Statement on Arteriosclerosis; Main Cause of "Heart Attacks" and "Strokes," by a group of leading scientists[72]
1960	American Heart Association Statement on Cigarette Smoking and Cardiovascular Disease[73]
1961	American Heart Association Statement on Dietary Fat and Its Relation to Heart Attacks and Stroke[74]
1964	Report of the Advisory Committee to the Surgeon General on Smoking and Health[75]
1970	Inter-Society Commission for Heart Disease Resources: Recommendations for Primary Prevention of the Atherosclerotic Diseases[76]
1970	White House Conference on Food, Nutrition and Health[77]
1971	Task Force on Arteriosclerosis of the National Heart and Lung Institute[78]
1971	Inter-Society Commission for Heart Disease Resources: Guidelines for the Detection, Diagnosis and Management of Hypertensive Populations[79]
1972	National High Blood Pressure Education Program launched
1977	Select Committee on Nutrition and Human Needs. U.S. Senate Dietary Goals for the United States[80]
1977	Report of the Joint National Committee on Detection, Evaluation, and Treatment of High Blood Pressure[81]
1979	The Surgeon General's Report on Health Promotion and Disease Prevention[82]
1980	U.S. Department of Agriculture and U.S. Department of Health, Education and Welfare: Nutrition and Your Health[83]
1980	Bethesda Conference on Prevention of Coronary Heart Disease, sponsored by the American College of Cardiology, American Heart Association, Center for Disease Control, National Heart, Lung, and Blood Institute[84]
1981	Report of the Working Group on Arteriosclerosis of the National Heart, Lung, and Blood Institute[95]
1984	Inter-Society Commission on Heart Disease Resources: Optimal Resources or Primary Prevention of Atherosclerotic Diseases[86]
1984	Consensus Development Conference Statement: Lowering Blood Cholesterol to Prevent Heart Disease[41]
1985	National Heart, Lung, and Blood Institute Smoking Education Program launched
1988	The Surgeon General's Report on Nutrition and Health[87]
1988	Report of the National Cholesterol Education Program Expert Panel on Detection, Evaluation, and Treatment of High Blood Cholesterol in Adults[22]
1988	The 1988 Report of the Joint National Committee on Detection, Evaluation, and Treatment of High Blood Pressure[88]
1989	National Academy of Science and National Research Council Report on Diet and Health[89]
1989	Report of the U.S. Preventive Services Task Force[24]
1990	The Surgeon General's 1990 Report on the Benefits of Smoking Cessation[63]
1990	Report of the Expert Panel on Population Strategies for Blood Cholesterol Reduction[90]

(Modified from Pyörälä,[17] with permission.)

A formidable change in eating patterns has occurred in the United States in recent decades. U.S. Department of Agriculture surveys indicate that the per capita consumption of eggs decreased by 30% between 1950 and the late 1970s.[99,100] During the same time interval, butter consumption dropped 57% and margarine and chicken consumption increased by 100% and 134%, respectively.[99,100] Mean serum cholesterol levels in middle-aged men concomitantly decreased from an average of 235 mg/dl to 215 mg/dl, a reduction of approximately 8%.[95] This reduction in mean serum cholesterol level has been estimated to account for 30% of the decline in CHD mortality rates in the United States.[9]

Increased awareness of the importance of diet is currently so prevalent that it is easy to overlook that these changes are relatively new. Cookbooks now emphasize low fat and low cholesterol recipes, many restaurants offer low fat and low cholesterol meals, food labeling often includes cholesterol and saturated fat content, and even radio talk shows discuss ways to avoid high fat foods. Public interest in nutrition is also evident in bookstores where there are now larger sections about food and nutrition. Physicians are no longer alone in advocating proper nutrition and some may be less informed about contemporary dietary recommendations than are their patients. These many gains have not penetrated all aspects of society. Favorable dietary modifications are less evident in the lower socioeconomic and less educated segments of U.S. society.[95]

Improved detection and treatment of hypertension was a second successful component of coronary preventive care in the United States. Although National Health Survey data do not show a change in the prevalence of hypertension between 1960 and 1970,[101] the percentage of patients with hypertension receiving treatment and attaining blood pressure control has improved.[102] By the mid-1970s, 50% of patients with known hypertension had their blood pressures successfully controlled with treatment.[103–105] Improvements are still needed, but this partial success has been estimated to contribute about 8% to the recent decline in coronary mortality in the United States.[9]

A third favorable change in health-related behavior is that fewer people in the United States now smoke cigarettes. Prior to 1900, the regular, addictive use of tobacco was not part of the societal norm[18]; rather, smoking became widespread for the first time at the beginning of the twentieth century. The prevalence of smoking in men in the Framingham Heart Study declined from 66% to 37% between 1950 and 1968.[106] The decrease in smoking prevalence has been estimated to account for 24% of the decrease in coronary mortality.[9] A less dramatic reduction in smoking, 41% to 31% from 1950 to 1968, was documented among women in the Framingham Study,[106] and an alarming increase in smoking rates among teenage girls has been evident in recent years.[95] Nevertheless, the remarkable decrease in smoking prevalence among U.S. men establishes the feasibility of changing smoking behavior, and suggests the possibility that habitual smoking could be eliminated in the coming decades.

Overall, the United States has moved toward a more favorable population coronary risk profile. The more educated segments of society have reduced cigarette use, modified their diets, and lowered their serum cholesterol and blood pressure levels. The success of these initial steps should encourage physicians to promote favorable life-style and behavioral changes in all patients, thereby further lowering CHD incidence. Based on the Pooling Project data collected from five U.S. cities, hypercholesterolemia, hypertension, and cigarette smoking were estimated to be responsible for two-thirds of all coronary events among middle-aged men during the 1960s.[4] As summarized by Stamler, "coronary rates would be lower by two-thirds if all middle-aged men had levels for these major risk factors like those of the lowest 20 percent of coronary risk in our population; . . . mean serum cholesterol level . . . about 205 mg/dl, not 235; . . . mean blood pressure . . . about 120/80 mg Hg, not 136/86; if none, or almost none of us smoked cigarettes regularly."[95]

THE PHYSICIAN'S ROLE IN CORONARY PREVENTION

The Challenge

Physicians in the United States are considered by their patients to be the most reliable and credible sources of medical information, placing them in an excellent position to help patients modify coronary risk-related behaviors. Although more physicians currently practice preventive strategies than was the norm three decades ago, many physicians still devote insufficient attention to implementing preventive approaches and educating their patients about coronary risk modification.[107–111] Physician guidelines are now available for coronary risk factor screening, and physicians are exhorted from their professional societies and from many patients to provide preventive care. Yet, only two-thirds of a recently surveyed sample of American College of Physicians members obtained information from their patients on smoking and alcohol use.[112] Younger physicians and general internists were more likely to address preventive measures than were older physicians and subspecialists.[112] The barriers to physician involvement in preventive care and suggested methods to overcome them[113–115] are addressed in the remainder of the chapter.

Education about prevention and preventive care is inadequate in the curriculum of most medical schools[116–119]; more emphasis is needed on nutrition, preventive strategies, and techniques of behavioral modification during medical education and training. Although aware of coronary risk attributes, most medical students and postgraduate medical trainees are not knowledgeable about how to change behavioral and life-style patterns. Practicing physicians report lack of confidence in their ability to succeed in altering patient behaviors,[107,112,120,121] since these skills were not taught or practiced during their medical training.

Both knowledge of coronary risk factors and familiarity with techniques for risk modification are essential to integrating preventive strategies into daily patient care. Brief tutorials have been effective in increasing physician knowledge about risks and their commitment to prevention.[122–124] Table 6-2[19,22,24,88,125–128] lists sources for guidelines for coronary risk assessment and screening that can aid physicians in appropriately implementing preventive care for different age groups in daily patient encounters. This table also includes information about educational materials designed both for physicians and their patients. The National Heart, Lung, and Blood Institute (NHLBI) Manual[126] provides an extensive list of print, audiovisual materials, and posters from varied sources, with information about ordering them. For example, excellent educational print materials of the American Heart Association are referenced in the NHLBI Manual. The Manual also identifies cardiovascular disease contact professionals in each state who can provide information about community preventive care services. Another catalog, entitled Materials for Health Promotion, offers descriptions of the print and video materials in English and in Spanish produced by the

---

TABLE 6-2. Physician Resources for Coronary Risk Assessment, Screening Guidelines, and Physician-Patient Educational Materials

I. Risk assessment and screening guidelines
  • Coronary Handbook[125]
  • Cardiovascular and Risk Factor Evaluation of Healthy American Adults[19]
  • Guide to Clinical Preventive Services[24,a]
  • Report of the National Cholesterol Education Program Expert Panel on Detection, Evaluation, and Treatment of High Blood Cholesterol in Adults[22]
  • The 1988 report of the Joint National Committee on Detection, Evaluation, and Treatment of High Blood Pressure[88]

II. Physician and patient educational materials
  • National Heart, Lung, and Blood Institute Manual A[126]   (301)951-3260
  • Materials for Health Promotion[127]   (415)723-0003
  • American Heart Association videotapes[128] (214)750-5300

---

a An extensive reference for screening recommendations.

Stanford Center for Research in Disease Prevention.[127] Both the NHLBI Manual and the Stanford Catalog resources address nutrition, smoking cessation, weight control, blood pressure control, and exercise.

Knowledge of coronary risk modification must include information about the effectiveness of such interventions and about realistic goals to be set in altering patient behaviors. Despite published evidence that physicians can favorably alter smoking and dietary behaviors,[129–132] most physicians surveyed report uncertainty about the effectiveness of patient counseling by physicians.[116,117,133,134] Medical education has traditionally addressed the goal of curing a patient's illness, rather than that of preventing disease; thus, physicians are uncertain about health promotion as a physician role. Physicians feel successful when most patients show short-term improvements but often consider themselves ineffective when only 10% of patients who receive counseling stop smoking cigarettes or improve dietary habits.[133] Given the high prevalence of coronary risk factors and CHD in the United States, physicians must realize that even such modest improvements can make a substantial impact on overall CHD reduction.

Physicians also require financial compensation for time spent in providing preventive services, and current third-party reimbursement rarely covers health promotion.[113,134,135] The recent restructuring of reimbursement policies using resource-based relative value scales[136] is designed to compensate for nonprocedure-related services but third party insurers are unlikely to add payment for new services in the near future. Physicians also perceive that they have inadequate time, staff, and resources to undertake patient counseling for risk reduction in daily practice.[116] Thus, the challenge is to develop approaches within the current structure of clinical practice that enable physicians to offer preventive care services in a cost-effective and time efficient manner.

Suggested Approach: A Model for Coronary Risk Reduction

Establishing time-efficient and cost-effective preventive care services requires development of a supporting framework for office-based interventions. One model,[137] designed for a group practice or community clinic, describes seven elements required for basic coronary risk reduction:

Establishment of Policy

The physicians and staff define specific preventive care goals and emphasize that they have high priority in the office or clinic. Goals for coronary risk reduction include individual risk assessment, smoking cessation, appropriate screening for and control of hypertension and hypercholesterolemia, exercise counseling, proper management of patients with diabetes mellitus, and nutrition counseling. These goals must be endorsed by all staff members and commitment made to attaining these goals for both patients and staff members. This commitment can be demonstrated to patients through such examples as a smoke-free office or clinic, educational materials and posters in the waiting room, as well as an informed and involved office staff.

Coordination

Either a physician or staff member, or both, must be identified to take responsibility for implementing coronary risk reduction policies. The designated coordinator updates screening guidelines and other policies as needed and reports at periodic staff meetings the office progress in preventive interventions.

Written Implementation Plan

A written implementation plan that identifies how each intervention is to be performed includes definitions of roles, analyses of financial impact, efficient methods for record-keeping, scheduling plans, and a time-table for start-up. For example, a paper flow sheet in every patient's medical record that lists screening recommendations can remind physicians to check blood pressure and cholesterol levels at appropriate intervals and enable physicians to follow changes over time. Prominent smoking status labels on each patient record can signal physicians to talk with patients about smoking cessation or congratulate those who have recently stopped smoking at each office contact.

Orientation and Training

The fourth element for implementation of the health promotion plan is orientation and training of the physicians and support staff. The coordinator should emphasize the public health philosophy of shifting patients' behaviors toward healthier life-styles, citing potential benefits of even modest changes. Staff members derive more job satisfaction if sufficient time is allotted for staff education and involvement. Physicians must be trained to deliver an unequivocal message to patients at each visit about the importance of altering unhealthy lifestyles and behaviors. This physician support for preventive practices does not require more than a few minutes and more time-consuming discussions can be effectively delegated to other health professionals and support staff. Secretaries can update flowsheets, record smoking status, and encourage patients in the waiting room to read educational materials or view audiovisual programs.

Resources

The interventional framework requires a fifth element, resources, such as educational written and audiovisual materials for both medical staff and patients. Another resource is tested flowsheets in the patient record to track coronary risk modification, as well as other preventive care concerns such as immunizations and cancer screening.[138] An example that is easily adapted to any office setting is the flowsheet form of the Tri-County Family Medicine Program.[139,140] The flowsheet is used in conjunction with a postcard reminder system to recall patients at given intervals. At each office visit, staff members identify the need for specific subsequent reminders, address postcards to the patient, and place them in a file for the month in which they are to be mailed.[139] Such postcard reminders, sent soon after a patient attempts to stop smoking, reinforces physician support of patient efforts in smoking cessation.

Progress is being made in developing computerized reminder systems for tracking health maintenance in clinical practice.[139,141–144] A survey of physicians using the North Carolina Memorial Practice computer prompting system found improved physician performance, a high level of acceptance of the system, and improved attitudes toward health promotion and disease prevention.[145] Although computer-based systems are likely to be routine in the future, most presently in operation are part of large computerized medical record systems and are not financially feasible for use in small practice settings. Adaptions of the more complex systems are under development and may become as commonplace as computerized office billing systems.[141,143,146]

Patient and physician educational materials can be easily ordered (Table 6-2). Office staff members must become familiar with all patient educational materials so they can recommend pamphlets appropriate to the educational level and needs of each patient. Excellent videotapes on such topics as smoking cessation, exercise programs, nutrition, and managing stress are available from the American Heart Association[128] and enable physicians to develop videotape libraries for patient use. Such educational materials are inexpensive, require minimal or no physician time for explanation and guidance, can educate patients and their families, and can emphasize the overall message of physician commitment to coronary prevention.

Community resources also enable physicians to refer patients for low cost health promotion counseling at health departments, recreation programs, local hospitals, YMCA/YWCAs, American Heart Association

chapters, American Cancer society chapters, and local self-help groups. Patients can be referred to smoking cessation, nutrition and exercise programs for in-depth teaching, often with greater expertise and at less cost than can be provided in the physicians' office. These referral sources assume added importance in a solo practice setting. Finally, physicians can share office organizational strategies, resources, and community contacts with each other. Mutual support among physicians can be facilitated by prevention committees of local medical societies or hospital staffs. All graduating internal medicine and family practice residents should be aware of community and other preventive care resources, the sources for necessary guidelines and materials, and should receive training in methods of establishing efficient preventive care practices.

Periodic Auditing of Progress

Secretaries can tally the percentage of adequately completed patient flowsheets and periodically present performance summaries for each medical staff member. Some clinics use smoking record cards that the list the patient's name, date of visit, and smoking status[147] at each clinical contact. Review of these cards at 6-month intervals can assess progress in smoking cessation interventions. By documenting trends in lifestyle and behavioral changes for clinic or office patients as a group, the medical staff can become aware of their positive impact on coronary risk modification among their patients.

Maintenance of the Program

Maintenance of preventive care interventions involves appropriate feedback to staff and patients at periodic reviews, repeated orientation and training, and staff meetings where preventive care goals are legitimated by emphasizing their high priority in daily patient care.

Physicians who use these seven elements to integrate preventive practices into daily patient care should be able to establish an effective program in their clinical practices. The priorities physicians set in their practices and in personal life-styles can powerfully influence patient health and patient care.[148,149] Initially, some physicians may feel overwhelmed by the multiple screening guidelines and the multiplicity of patient educational pamphlets and other materials that are available. Because few physicians will elect to review the scientific literature to critically assess differences in screening recommendations, the key is to choose an established screening approach recommended by a reputable professional association that most closely fits one's personal sense of appropriateness and to implement it in daily patient care. In selecting among multiple educational materials, the physician might review a broad selection from the NHLBI Manual or Stanford Catalog, decide which print or audiovisual materials appear most helpful and appropriate in a specific practice setting, and delegate to a staff member the responsibility of periodically sending for new materials. The physician should also arrange to receive periodic updates in national or other professional society recommendations for screening and intervention guidelines.

SUMMARY

Substantial evidence now exists that establishes hypercholesterolemia, hypertension, and cigarette smoking as powerful risk factors for coronary heart disease. In the United States, great progress has already been made in favorably altering these major coronary risk factors; this has been linked to declines in the incidence of CHD. Physicians have a pivotal role in the primary prevention of CHD and can accomplish coronary risk reduction interventions in a time-efficient and cost-effective manner in daily patient care.

REFERENCES

1. Dawber TR, Moore FE, Mann GV: Coronary heart disease in the Framingham Study. Am J Public Health 47:4, 1957
2. Keys A, Taylor HL, Blackburn H et al: Coronary heart disease among Minnesota business and professional men followed 15 years. Circulation 28:381, 1963
3. Keys A, Aravanis C, Blackburn HW et al: Epidemiological studies related to coronary heart disease: characteristics of men aged 40–59 in seven countries. Acta Med Scand, suppl. 460, 1966
4. The Pooling Project Research Group: Relationship of blood pressure, serum cholesterol, smoking habit, relative weight, and ECG abnormalities to incidence of major coronary events: final report of the Pooling Project. J Chronic Dis 31:201, 1978
5. Keys A: Seven Countries: a Multi-risk Analysis of Death and Coronary Heart Disease. Harvard University Press, Cambridge, 1980
6. Gordon T, Garcia-Palmieri M, Kagan A et al: Differences in coronary heart disease mortality in Framingham, Honolulu and Puerto Rico. J Chronic Dis 27:329, 1974
7. Report of the WHO Expert Committee: Prevention of Coronary Heart Disease. Technical Report Series No. 678. World Health Organization, Geneva, 1982
8. Kannel WB, Doyle JT, Ostfeld AM et al: Optimal resources for primary prevention of atherosclerotic diseases. Circulation 70:157A, 1984
9. Goldman L, Cook EF: The decline in ischemic heart disease mortality rates. An analysis of the comparative effects of medical interventions and changes in lifestyle. Ann Intern Med 101:825, 1984
10. Salonen JT, Puska P, Kottke TE et al: Decline in mortality from coronary heart disease in Finland from 1969 to 1979. Br Med J 286:1857, 1983
11. Robertson TL, Kato H, Gordon T et al: Epidemiologic studies of coronary heart disease and stroke in Japanese men living in Japan, Hawaii and California. Am J Cardiol 39:244, 1977
12. Brischetto CS, Connor WE, Connor SL et al: Plasma lipid and lipoprotein profiles of cigarette smokers from randomly selected families: enhancement of hyperlipidemia and depression of high-density lipoprotein. Am J Cardiol 52:675, 1983
13. Assmann G, Schulte H: The Prospective Cardiovascular Münster Study: prevalence and prognostic significance of hyperlipidemia in men with systemic hypertension. Am J Cardiol 59:9G, 1987
14. Gordon T, Kannel WB: Multiple risk functions for predicting coronary heart disease: the concept, accuracy and application. Am Heart J, suppl. 103:S1031, 1982
15. Stamler J, Wentworth D, Neaton JD: Prevalence and prognostic significance of hypercholesterolemia in men with hypertension. Prospective data on the primary screenees of the Multiple Risk Factor Intervention Trial. Am J Med, suppl. 80:33, 1986
16. Rose G: Strategy of prevention: lessons from cardiovascular disease. Br Med J 282:1847, 1981
17. Pyörälä K: Preventive cardiology: a progress report. Prev Med 19:78, 1990
18. World Health Organization: Primary prevention of coronary heart disease. Report on a WHO meeting, Anacapri, Oct. 15–19, 1984. EURO Reports and Studies 98, Geneva, 1985
19. Grundy SM, Greenland P, Heard A et al: Cardiovascular and risk factor evaluation of healthy American adults. A statement for physicians by an Ad Hoc Committee appointed by the Steering Committee, American Heart Association. Circulation 75:1339A, 1987
20. The British Cardiac Society Working Group on Coronary Prevention: Conclusions and recommendations. Br Heart J 57:188, 1987
21. Study Group, European Atherosclerosis Society: Strategies for the prevention of coronary heart disease: a policy statement of the European Atherosclerosis Society. Eur Heart J 8:77, 1987
22. The Expert Panel: Report of the National Cholesterol Education Program Expert Panel on Detection, Evaluation, and Treatment of High Blood Cholesterol in Adults. Arch Intern Med 148:36, 1988
23. Grundy SM, Goodman DS, Rifkind BM et al: The place of HDL in cholesterol management. Arch Intern Med 149:505, 1989
24. Report of the U.S. Preventive Services Task Force: Guide to Clinical Preventive Services. An Assessment of the Effectiveness of 169 Interventions. Williams & Wilkins, Baltimore, 1989
25. Lipid Research Clinics Program: The Lipid Research Clinics Coronary Primary Prevention Trial Results. I. Reduction in incidence of coronary heart disease. N Engl J Med 251:351, 1984

26. Lipid Research Clinics Program: The Lipid Research Clinics Coronary Primary Prevention Trial Results. II. The relationship of reduction in incidence of coronary heart disease to cholesterol lowering. JAMA 251:365, 1984

27. Frick MH, Elo O, Haapa K et al: Helsinki Heart Study: primary-prevention trial with gemfibrozil in middle-aged men with dyslipidemia. Safety of treatment, changes in risk factors, and incidence of coronary heart disease. N Engl J Med 317:1237, 1987

28. Brown G, Albers JJ, Fisher LD et al: Regression of coronary artery disease as a result of intensive lipid-lowering therapy in men with high levels of apolipoprotein B. N Engl J Med 323:1289, 1990

29. Kane JP, Malloy MJ, Ports TA et al: Regression of coronary atherosclerosis during treatment of familial hypercholesterolemia with combined drug regimens. JAMA 264:3007, 1990

30. Dayton S, Pearce ML, Hashimoto S et al: A controlled clinical trial of a diet high in unsaturated fat in preventing complications of atherosclerosis. Circulation, suppl. 40:II-1, 1969

31. Turpeinen O: Effect of cholesterol-lowering diet on mortality from coronary heart disease and other causes. Circulation 59:1, 1979

32. Hjermann I, Holme I, Byre KV et al: Effect of diet and smoking intervention on the incidence of coronary heart disease. Report from the Oslo Study Group of a randomized trial in healthy men. Lancet 2:1303, 1981

33. Multiple Risk Factor Intervention Trial Research Group: Multiple Risk Factor Intervention Trial. Risk factor changes and mortality results. JAMA 248:1465, 1982

34. Sacks FM, Castelli WP, Donner A et al: Plasma lipids and lipoproteins in vegetarians and controls. N Engl J Med 292:1148, 1975

35. Ehnholm C, Huttunen JK, Pietinen P et al: Effect of diet on serum lipoproteins in a population with a high risk of coronary heart disease. N Engl J Med 307:850, 1982

36. Blackburn H, Jacobs D: Sources of the diet-heart controversy: confusion over population versus individual correlations. Circulation 70:775, 1984

37. National Diet–Heart Research Group: The National Diet–Heart Study Final Report. Circulation, suppl. 37: I-1, 1969

38. Lewis B, Assmann G, Mancini M et al: Handbook of Coronary Heart Disease Prevention. p. 50. Current Medical Literature Ltd., London, 1989

39. Nutrition Committee, American Heart Association: Dietary guidelines for healthy American adults. A statement for physicians and health professionals. Circulation 77:721A, 1988

40. Raab C, Tillotson JL: Heart to Heart. A Manual on Nutritional Counseling for the Reduction of Cardiovascular Disease Risk Factors. Publication No. DHHS (NIH) 83-1528. National Institutes of Health, Bethesda, MD, 1983

41. Consensus Development Panel: Consensus Conference. Lowering blood cholesterol to prevent heart disease. JAMA 253:2080, 1985

42. Department of Health and Human Services: The Surgeon General's Report on Nutrition and Health. Publ No. DHHS (PHS) 88-50211. US Government Printing Office, Washington, DC, 1988

43. Veterans Administration Cooperative Study Group on Antihypertensive Agents: Effects of treatment on morbidity in hypertension. Results in patients with diastolic blood pressure averaging 115 through 129 mmHg. JAMA 202:1028, 1967

44. Veterans Administration Cooperative Study Group on Antihypertensive Agents: Effects of treatment on morbidity in hypertension II. Results in patients with diastolic blood pressure averaging 90 through 114 mmHg. JAMA 213:1143, 1970

45. Amery A, Birkenhager W, Brixko P et al: Mortality and morbidity results from the European Working Party on High Blood Pressure in the Elderly Trial. Lancet 1:1349, 1985

46. Report by the Management Committee: The Australian Therapeutic Trial in Mild Hypertension. Lancet 1:1261, 1980

47. Hypertension Detection and Follow-up Program Cooperative Group: Five year findings of the Hypertension Detection and Follow-up Program I. Reduction in mortality of persons with high blood pressure, including mild hypertension. JAMA 242:2562, 1979

48. Hypertension Detection and Follow-up Program Cooperative Group: Five year findings of the Hypertension Detection and Follow-up Program II. Mortality by race-sex and age. JAMA 242:2572, 1979

49. Cutler JA, MacMahon SW, Furberg CD: Controlled clinical trials of drug treatment for hypertension: a review. Hypertension, suppl. 13:I-36, 1989

50. Berglund G, Wilhelmsen L, Anderson OK et al: Coronary heart disease after treatment of hypertension. Lancet 1:1, 1978

51. The IPPPSH Collaborative Group: Cardiovascular risk and risk factors in a randomized trial of treatment based on the beta-blocker oxprenolol: the International Prospective Primary Prevention Study in Hypertension (IPPPSH). J Hypertens 3:379, 1985

52. Collins R, Peto R, MacMahon S et al: Blood pressure, stroke and heart disease: part 2, short-term reduction in blood pressure: overview of randomised drug trials in their epidemiological context. Lancet 335:827, 1990

53. Heyden S, Schneider KA, Fodor GJ: Failure to reduce cholesterol as explanation for the limited efficacy of antihypertensive treatment in the reduction of CHD. Examination of the evidence from six hypertension intervention trials. Klin Wochenschr 65:828, 1987

54. Lardinois CK, Neuman SL: The effects of antihypertensive agents on serum lipids and lipoproteins. Arch Intern Med 148:1280, 1988

55. Arkwright PD, Beilin LJ, Rouse I et al: Effects of alcohol use and other aspects of lifestyle on blood pressure levels and prevalence of hypertension in a working population. Circulation 66:60, 1982

56. Stamler J, Farinaro E, Majonnier LM et al: Prevention and control of hypertension by nutritional-hygienic means. Long-term experience of the Chicago Coronary Prevention Evaluation Program. JAMA 243:1819, 1980

57. Klatsky AL, Friedman GD, Armstrong MA: The relation-

ships between alcoholic beverage use and other traits to blood pressure: a new Kaiser Permanente study. Circulation 73:628, 1986

58. Patel C, Marmot MG, Terry DJ et al: Trial of relaxation in reducing coronary risk: four year follow up. Br Med J 290:1103, 1985

59. Kannel WB: Update on the role of cigarette smoking in coronary artery disease. Am Heart J 101:319, 1981

60. Gordon T, Kannel WB, McGee D: Death and coronary attacks in men after giving up cigarette smoking. A report from the Framingham Study. Lancet 2:1345, 1974

61. Kaufman DW, Helmrich SP, Rosenberg L et al: Nicotine and carbon monoxide content of cigarette smoke and the risk of myocardial infarction in young men. N Engl J Med 308:409, 1983

62. Kannel WB, D'Agostino RB, Belanger AJ: Fibrinogen, cigarette smoking, and risk of cardiovascular disease: insights from the Framingham Study. Am Heart J 113:1006, 1987

63. Centers for Disease Control: The Surgeon General's 1990 Report on the health benefits of smoking cessation (Executive Summary). MMWR 39:7, 1990

64. Shurtleff D: Some characteristics related to the incidence of cardiovascular disease and death: Framingham Study, 16-year follow-up. Table 13 3B. In Kannel WB, Gordon T (eds): The Framingham Study. An Epidemiological Investigation of Cardiovascular Diseases. Section 26. US Government Printing Office, Washington, DC, 1970

65. Blackburn H, Watkins LO, Agras WS et al: Task Force: primary prevention of coronary heart disease. Circulation, suppl. 76:I-165, 1987

66. Farquhar JW, Maccoby N, Wood PD et al: Community education for cardiovascular health. Lancet 1:1192, 1977

67. Puska P, Tuomilehto J, Salonen J et al: Changes in coronary risk factors during comprehensive five-year community programme to control cardiovascular diseases (North Karelia Project). Br Med J 2:1173, 1979

68. Elder JP, McGraw SA, Abrams DB et al: Organizational and community approaches to community-wide prevention of heart disease: the first two years of the Pawtucket Heart Health Program. Prev Med 15:107, 1986

69. Mittelmark MB, Luepker RV, Jacobs DR et al: Community-wide prevention of cardiovascular disease: education strategies of the Minnesota Heart Program. Prev Med 15:1, 1986

70. Farquhar JW, Fortmann SP, Maccoby N et al: The Stanford Five-City Project: design and methods. Am J Epidemiol 122:323, 1985

71. Farquhar JW, Fortmann SP, Flora JA et al: Effects of communitywide education on cardiovascular disease risk factors. JAMA 264:359, 1990

72. White PD, Sprague HB, Stamler J et al: A statement on arteriosclerosis. Main cause of "heart attacks" and "strokes." National Health Education Committee, New York City, 1959

73. Ad Hoc Committee on smoking and cardiovascular disease, American Heart Association: Cigarette smoking and cardiovascular diseases. Circulation 22:160, 1960

74. American Heart Association, Central Committee for Medical and Community Program: Dietary fat and its relation to heart attacks and strokes. American Heart Association, New York City, 1961

75. Smoking and Health: Report of the Advisory Committee to the Surgeon General of the Public Health Service, U.S. Department of Health, Education and Welfare, Public Health Service Publ 1103. US Government Printing Office, Washington, DC, 1964

76. Inter-Society Commission for Heart Disease Resources. Atherosclerosis Study Group and Epidemiology Study Group: Primary prevention of the atherosclerotic diseases. p. 15. In: Wright IS, Fredrickson DT (eds): Cardiovascular Diseases: Guidelines for Prevention and Care. US Government Printing Office, Washington, DC, 1974

77. White House Conference on Food, Nutrition and Health—Final report to the President. The White House, Washington, DC, 51:1970

78. Task Force on Arteriosclerosis of the National Heart and Lung Institute: Arteriosclerosis. Vol. 1:72. US Department of Health, Education and Welfare, Public Health Service, Washington, DC, 1971

79. Inter-Society Commission for Heart Disease Resources: Guidelines for the detection, diagnosis and management of hypertensive populations. p. 186. In Wright IS, Fredrickson DT (eds): Cardiovascular Diseases: Guidelines for Prevention and Care. 186. US Government Printing Office, Washington, DC, 1974

80. Select Committee on Nutrition and Human Needs: U.S. Senate Dietary Goals for the United States. 2nd Ed. US Government Printing Office, Washington, DC, 1977

81. Report of the Joint National Committee on Detection, Evaluation, and Treatment of High Blood Pressure: A cooperative study. JAMA 237:255, 1977

82. US Department of Health, Education, and Welfare: Healthy People. The Surgeon General's Report on Health Promotion and Disease Prevention. DHEW (PHS) Publ No. 79-55071. US Government Printing Office, Washington, DC, 1979

83. US Department of Agriculture and U.S. Department of Health, Education and Welfare: Nutrition and your Health—Dietary Guidelines for Americans. USDA–DHEW. US Government Printing Office, Washington, DC, 1980

84. Eleventh Bethesda Conference. Prevention of Coronary Heart Disease, September 27–28, 1980, Bethesda, MD. Am J Cardiol 47:713, 1981

85. Working Group on Arteriosclerosis of the National Heart, Lung, and Blood Institute. Prevention: Report of the Working Group on Arteriosclerosis of the National Heart, Lung, and Blood Institute. p. 261. NIH Publ No. 81-2035. US Department of Health and Human Services, National Institutes of Health, Bethesda, MD, 1981

86. Inter-Society Commission on Heart Disease Resources: Atherosclerosis Study Group. Optimal resources for primary prevention of atherosclerotic diseases. Circulation 70:153A, 1984

87. US Department of Health and Human Services: The Surgeon General's Report on Nutrition and Health. DHHS (PHS) Publ No. 88-50210. US Government Printing Office, Washington, DC, 1988

88. 1988 Joint National Committee: The 1988 report of the

Joint National Committee on Detection, Evaluation, and Treatment of High Blood Pressure. Arch Intern Med 148:518, 1988

89. National Research Council: Diet and Health: Implications for Reducing Chronic Disease Risk. National Academy Press, Washington, DC, 1989

90. The National Cholesterol Education Program: Report of the Expert Panel on Population Strategies for Blood Cholesterol Reduction. NIH Publ No. 90-3046. US Department of Health and Human Services (NHLBI), Bethesda, MD, 1990

91. Inter-society Commission for Heart Disease Resources: Optimal resources for primary prevention of atherosclerotic diseases. Circulation 70:153A, 1984

92. Cooper R, Stamler J, Dyer A et al: The decline in mortality from coronary heart disease, U.S.A., 1968–1975. J Chronic Dis 31:709, 1978

93. Stern MP: The recent decline in ischemic heart disease mortality. Ann Intern Med 91:630, 1979

94. National Center for Health Statistics: Vital Statistics of the United States, 1978, Vol. II, Part A, Section 1, p. 7. DHHS Publ No. (PHS) 83-1101. US Government Printing Office, Washington, DC, 1982

95. Stamler J: Primary prevention of coronary heart disease: the last 20 years. Am J Cardiol 47:722, 1981

96. Friedman GD: Decline in hospitalizations for coronary heart disease and stroke: the Kaiser Permanente experience in Northern California, 1971–1977. p. 109. In Havlik RJ, Feinleib M (eds): Proceedings of the Conference on the Decline in Coronary Heart Disease Mortality. NIH Publ No. 79-1610. US Department of Health, Education, and Welfare, Bethesda, MD, 1979

97. Strong J, Guzmán MA: Decrease in coronary atherosclerosis in New Orleans. Lab Invest 43:297, 1980

98. Pell S, Fayerweather WE: Trends in the incidence of myocardial infarction and in associated mortality and morbidity in a large employed population, 1957–1983. N Engl J Med 312:1005, 1985

99. US Bureau of the Census: Statistical Abstract of the United States: 1975. 96th Ed. p. 92. US Government Printing Office, Washington, DC, 1975

100. US Bureau of the Census: Statistical Abstract of the United States: 1979. 100th Ed. p. 127. US Government Printing Office, Washington, DC, 1979

101. Roberts J, Maurer K: Blood pressure levels of person 6–74 years: United States, 1971–1974. p. 24. In National Center for Health Statistics. Series 11, No. 203. DHEW Publ No. 78-1648. National Center for Health Statistics, Hyattsville, MD, 1977

102. Borhani NO: Mortality trend in hypertension, United States, 1950–1976. p. 218. In Havlik RJ, Feinleib M (eds): Proceedings of the Conference on the Decline in Coronary Heart Disease Mortality. NIH Publ No. 79-1610. US Department of Health, Education, and Welfare, Bethesda, MD, 1979

103. Schoenberger JA, Stamler J, Shekelle RB et al: Current status of hypertension control in an industrial population. JAMA 222:559, 1972

104. Hypertension Detection and Follow-Up Program Cooperative Group: Blood pressure studies in fourteen communities: a two-stage screen for hypertension. JAMA 237:2385, 1977

105. Stamler J, Stamler R, Riedlinger WF et al: Hypertension screening of 1 million Americans: Community Hypertension Evaluation Clinic (CHEC) Program, 1973 through 1975. JAMA 235:2299, 1976

106. Gordon T, Shurtleff D: Means at each examination and inter-examination variation of specified characteristics: Framingham Study, Exam 1 to Exam 10. Table A-12. In Kannel WB, Gordon T (eds): The Framingham Study. An Epidemiological Investigation of Cardiovascular Diseases. Section 29. DHEW Publ No. (NIH) 74-478. US Government Printing Office, Washington, DC, 1973

107. Wechsler H, Levine S, Idelson RK et al: The physician's role in health promotion—a survey of primary care practitioners. N Engl J Med 308:97, 1983

108. Anda RF, Remington PL, Sienko DG et al: Are physicians advising smokers to quit? The patient's perspective. JAMA 257:1916, 1987

109. Romm FJ, Fletcher SW, Hulka BS: The periodic health examination: comparison of recommendations and internists' performance. South Med J 74:265, 1981

110. Wells KB, Lewis CE, Leake B et al: The practices of general and subspecialty internists in counseling about smoking and exercise. Am J Public Health 76:1009, 1986

111. Woo B, Woo B, Cook EF et al: Screening procedures in the asymptomatic adult: comparison of physicians' recommendations, patients' desires, published guidelines, and actual practice. JAMA 254:1480, 1985

112. Schwartz JS, Lewis CE, Clancy C et al: Internists' practices in health promotion and disease prevention. Ann Intern Med 114:46, 1991

113. Becker, MH, Janz NK: Practicing Health Promotion: the doctor's dilemma. Ann Intern Med 113:419, 1990

114. Kottke TE, Blackburn H, Brekke ML et al: The systematic practice of preventive cardiology. Am J Cardiol 59:690, 1987

115. Orlandi MA: Promoting health and preventing disease in health care settings: an analysis of barriers. Prev Med 16:119, 1987

116. Taylor KB: Preventive medicine in general practice. Br Med J 284:921, 1982

117. Weinberger M, Mazzuca SA, Cohen SJ et al: Physicians' ratings of information sources about their preventive medicine decisions. Prev Med 11:717, 1982

118. Bartlett EE: Teaching health education in medical education: selected perspectives. Prev Med 13:100, 1984

119. Cardullo AC: Nutrition education in the medical curriculum. J Med Educ 57:372, 1982

120. Valente CM, Sobal J, Muncie HL et al: Health promotion: physicians' beliefs, attitudes, and practices. Am J Prev Med 2:82, 1986

121. Orleans CT, George LK, Houpt JL et al: Health promotion in primary care: a survey of US family practitioners. Prev Med 14:636, 1985

122. Maiman LA, Becker MH, Liptak GS et al: Improving pediatricians' compliance-enhancing practices. Am J Dis Child 142:773, 1988

123. Inui TS, Yourtee EL, Williamson JW: Improved outcomes in hypertension after physician tutorials. Ann Intern Med 84:646, 1976

124. Weinberg A, Andrus PL: Continuing medical education: does it address prevention? J Community Health 7:211, 1982

125. American Heart Association: Coronary Risk Handbook: Estimating Risk of Coronary Disease in Daily Practice. American Heart Association, Dallas, 1986

126. NHLBI Education Program: The Right Moves: Manual A. Information for Program Planners, NHLBI Kit '90. US Department of Health and Human Services, Bethesda, MD, 1990

127. Health Promotion Research Center: Materials for Health Promotion Catalog, 1990–1991. Stanford Center for Research in Disease Prevention, Palo Alto, CA, 1990

128. American Heart Association: Active Partnerships. American Heart Association, Dallas, 1990

129. Janz NK, Becker MH, Kirscht JP et al: Evaluation of a minimal-contact smoking cessation intervention in an outpatient setting. Am J Public Health 77:805, 1987

130. Ockene JK: Smoking intervention: the expanding role of the physician. Am J Public Health 77:782, 1987

131. McAlister A: Helping people quit smoking: current progress. p. 147. In Enelow AJ, Henderson JB (eds): Applying Behavioral Science to Cardiovascular Risk, Proceedings of a Conference. American Heart Association, New York, 1975

132. Wilson D, Wood G, Johnston N et al: Randomized clinical trial of supportive follow-up for cigarette smokers in family practice. Can Med Assoc J 126:127, 1982

133. Zifferblatt SM: Health habits and behavior change: realigning expectations with reality. p. 254. In Podell RN, Stewart MM (eds): Primary Prevention of Coronary Heart Disease: A Practical Guide for the Clinician. Addison-Wesley, Menlo Park, CA, 1983

134. Rosen MA, Logsdon DN, Demak MM: Prevention and health promotion in primary care: baseline results on physicians from the INSURE project on lifecycle preventive health services. Prev Med 13:535, 1984

135. Relman AS. Encouraging the practice of preventive medicine and health promotion. Public Health Rep 97:216, 1982

136. Hsiao WC, Braun P, Dunn D et al: Results and policy implications of the resource-based relative value study. N Engl J Med 319:881, 1988

137. Kottke TE, Leif I, Solberg LI et al: Smoking cessation intervention strategies for the clinician. Qual Life Cardiovasc Care 1:86, 1990

138. Podell RN: Organizing the office for health promotion. p. 226. In Podell RN, Stewart MM (eds): Primary Prevention of Coronary Heart Disease: A Practical Guide for the Clinician. Addison-Wesley, Menlo Park, CA, 1983

139. Frame PS: Can computerized reminder systems have an impact on preventive services in practice? J Gen Intern Med, suppl. 5:S112, 1990

140. Frame PS: A critical review of adult health maintenance. Part I. Prevention of atherosclerotic disease. J Fam Pract 22:341, 1986

141. Campbell JR, Tierney WM: Information management in clinical prevention. Prim Care 16:251, 1989

142. McDonald CJ, Blevins L, Tierney WM et al: The Regenstrief Medical Records. MD Computing 5:34, 1988

143. McDonald CJ, Tierney WM: Computer-stored medical records. JAMA 259:3433, 1988

144. McDonald CJ, Hui SL, Smith DM et al: Reminders to physicians from an introspective computer medical record. Ann Intern Med 100:130, 1984

145. Knight BP, O'Malley MS, Fletcher SW: Physician acceptance of a computerized health maintenance prompting program. Am J Prev Med 3:19, 1987

146. McDonald CJ: Computers. JAMA 261:2834, 1989

147. American Academy of Family Physicians: AAFP Stop Smoking Program. Physician and Office Staff Manual. American Academy of Family Physicians, Kansas City, MO, 1987

148. Wells K, Lewis CE: The relation of physicians' personal health habits and attitudes to patient counseling, abstracted. Clin Res 29:327A, 1981

149. Lewis CE, Clancy C, Leake B et al: The counseling practices of internists. Ann Inter Med 114:54, 1991

Section II

RISK ASSESSMENT AND PROGNOSIS OF CORONARY HEART DISEASE

7

Single Vessel Coronary Artery Disease

David T. Kelly

With the reported good outcome of medical treatment in patients with single vessel disease (SVD), the ever-increasing use of angioplasty, and the relative reluctance to perform bypass surgery, it is important to define the incidence and natural history and to review the data on SVD of each of the three main coronary arteries.

Clinical predictors that may separate single vessel from multivessel disease are younger patients with few risk factors, a short history of chest pain or those who present with myocardial infarction and no previous symptoms. Many present with stable angina or atypical chest pain.[1] The percentage of women tends to be higher, reflecting their lesser susceptibility to coronary disease.[2] Overall clinical assessment is at best an enlightened guess.

INCIDENCE

The incidence of SVD varies with the different sample populations studied. The lower the mean age of the patient sample, the higher the percentage of SVD. In several series, SVD in patients studied after myocardial infarction occurs in a significant proportion of cases and may have a higher incidence than multivessel disease (Table 7-1).

All the series cited in Table 7-1 have approximately the same mean age, but the incidence of SVD varies considerably. This is due to sample selection. In Taylor's series, only 39% of eligible patients had catheterization versus 87% in Roubin's. If women are excluded, as in Sanz's series, this may decrease the number of

patients with SVD. Most such studies are from tertiary institutions who receive a referral population because of complications rather than from the surrounding area which should reflect better the community incidence, and when this is accounted for the incidence appears to be higher.[3] One of the first studies, in patients presenting with angina rather than infarction with a similar mean age, shows a similar incidence, 40% of SVD[7] (Fig. 7-1). In the Coronary Artery Surgery Study (CASS), conducted in patients with stable angina, 60% had suffered previous myocardial infarction and the incidence of SVD was 28%. This is a highly selected series as only 12.7% of the total registered were randomized.[8] In the older age groups, the incidence, although less, is not well documented.

The distribution of SVD in the three major coronary arteries varies in different series, again attributable to different sample populations studied. Various series are shown in Table 7-2 with overall mean figures for left anterior descending artery (LAD), left circumflex (CX), and right coronary artery disease.

LEFT ANTERIOR DESCENDING ARTERY DISEASE

The LAD was described by Herrick in 1912 as the widow maker's artery and the passage of time has not ameliorated its ominous significance.[13] LAD disease has been divided either into disease from the origin to the first septal branch (LAD_1), from the first septal to the first diagonal (LAD_2), or the remainder of the left

TABLE 7-1. Number of Patients After Myocardial Infarction

Age Limit	Mean Age	% Female	No. of Patients	% SVD	Reference
60	51	15	229	58	Roubin et al.[3]
65	49	26	106	26	Taylor et al.[4]
65	51	13	140	39	Gibson et al[5]
60	51	Nil	259	34	Sanz et al.[6]

anterior descending (LAD₃). The major prognostic difference is found when there is obstruction prior to the first septal branch (Fig. 7-2). When infarction occurs, this is associated with a higher mortality acutely from shock and left ventricular failure, and it is a long-term problem because of the greater impairment of left ventricular function.[14] Many of the survival curves of LAD disease that describe later outcome may not differ much from SVD in other arteries because the early in-hospital mortality is not considered. It is not only the site of the obstruction of the LAD, but also its degree, that is important in outcome. The CASS showed when the most severe stenosis is less than 50% the risk of infarction is 2% over a 3-year period; when it is 50 to

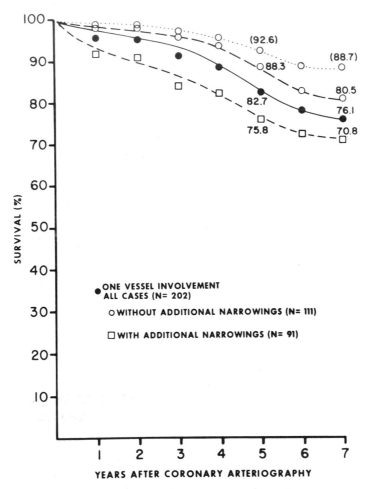

Fig. 7-1. Survival curves in patients with angina and single-vessel disease with and without additional moderate (>30% and <50%) stenosis. The top survival curve represents patients without significant coronary disease. (From Bruschke et al.,[7] with permission.)

TABLE 7-2. Distribution of Single Vessel Disease

Age Limit	Age Range	No. of Patients	% Female	% LAD	% RCA	% LCX	Reference
None	Not specified	54	0	48	39	13	Feit et al.[9]
None	24–81	354	46	51	35	14	Hillis and Winniford[10]
None	20–79	58	11	52	39	9	Diethrich et al.[11]
None	24–77	215	12	61	19	20	Garcia-Rubira et al.[12]

Abbreviations: LAD, left anterior descending; RCA, right coronary artery; LCX, left circumflex artery.

90% the risk of infarction is 6 to 9%; and when the stenosis is greater than 90% this risk is approximately 10%. Also multiple stenoses of greater than 50% in the LAD increase this risk.[15] Luminal roughness and the length of the lesion enhance the risk as well.[16]

In addition, mortality has been shown to be associated more with total occlusion of the LAD.[17] In a series of patients followed up for a mean of 45 months, 11% or 16 of 144 patients with total occlusion of the LAD and extensive left ventricular damage died most suddenly. The importance of total occlusion has also been confirmed in the recent thrombolytic trials. Outcome is better when the artery is recanalized rather than left totally occluded. Thus, site and severity of stenosis have been shown to reflect outcome in patients with LAD disease. This is relevant in assessment particularly if the patient presents with angina and has not suffered from infarction. It is important to ascertain the area of the anterior left ventricular myocardium that is at risk. This can be done by exercise gated blood pool scan or a thallium reperfusion scan.[18,19] Both studies suggest that, if ventricular function decreases on exercise or the area of reperfusion is large, the event rate in terms of infarction or limiting angina is significant, and angioplasty or bypass surgery may be warranted in asymptomatic cases. If a proximal lesion is excluded, the outcome over 1 to 2 years is good.

In summary, LAD disease is common. Acute occlusion proximally can result in early or late mortality. Outcome is related not only to the site of the obstruction but also its severity and the number of stenoses in the artery and is worst with residual total occlusion after infarction. When angina occurs with LAD disease, the extent of the area of risk should be quantified by nuclear scanning or other techniques and if there is a large area of reversible ischemia it is associated with a higher event rate.

CIRCUMFLEX ARTERY DISEASE

CX disease is relatively uncommon, occurring in only 2.4% of patients studied at angiography for various reasons, and constitutes approximately 15 to 20% of patients with SVD.[20] Dunn et al.[20] reviewed 84 patients with CX disease with a mean age of 50 years

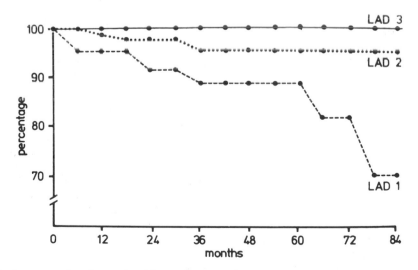

Fig. 7-2. Survival curves of patients classified according to the site of the most proximal anterior descending artery obstruction. (From Brooks et al.,[14] with permission.)

(10% females), 60% of whom had suffered myocardial infarction. Left ventricular function was abnormal in only 22% of cases. Approximately one-half the stenoses were proximal and one-half were peripheral.[20] Location does not seem to be important in survival.[2] The patterns of infarction are usually found in the inferior leads II to III AVF, plus V5 and V6; the anterolateral leads I, AVL, V5, and V6; and the RV pattern, dominant R wave in V1 and V2. These patterns can occur with isolated disease to the right coronary artery, but the lateral and RV patterns tend to be more specific for CX disease.[20]

Thallium scanning may more precisely identify CX disease and, allowing for the wide variation in coronary artery distribution, can suggest whether the stenosis is peripheral or distal in the CX segment. The prognosis is excellent as 97.5% of patients with isolated CX disease are reported to survive a mean of 2.5 years.[20] Another study suggested CX disease had a mortality of 2% per year, approximately the same as that of right coronary disease.[21] Califf et al.[2] reported the outcome is worse than right coronary artery disease but less than LAD.

In summary, isolated CX disease is less common than right or LAD disease. It may be suspected on electrocardiographic (ECG) criteria but cannot be diagnosed definitely. Thallium scanning may precisely outline the area and extent of myocardial involvement. There is a good prognosis and a good response to medical therapy. CX artery-related infarction is less likely to result in acute ECG changes because of its posterior location, although it may occur in the lateral leads. The abnormal R-wave in V1 is a specific but insensitive marker for CX related coronary infarction and indicates a larger area of myocardial damage.

RIGHT CORONARY ARTERY DISEASE

Right coronary artery (RCA) disease is usually only included in SVD when the RCA is dominant, which it is in approximately 80% of patients.[22] Approximately 35% of patients with SVD have RCA disease (Table 7-1). The distribution of the RCA varies considerably. Both the area of ischemia and the extent of damage after infarction depend on the amount of the left ventricle supplied by the RCA. The location of the stenosis has not been shown to determine prognosis.[2] After infarction, T-wave inversion in the lateral chest leads indicates left ventricular distribution and an accordingly worse prognosis. The conduction system is often damaged after infarction and partial or complete infarction may occur because the RCA supplies the sinus node and partially the atrioventricular (AV) node.

Many reports suggest methods to separate RCA and CX disease and, although helpful, the wide individual variation in distribution of these arteries tends to decrease the specificity of these procedures.[23] Electrocardiographic (ECG) Q waves in leads II, III, and AVF suggest RCA disease. Regional defects on thallium scanning may separate RCA and CX disease. Thallium defects in the inferior segment of the anterior view tend to predict RCA disease, and in the lateral segment of the 40-degree anterior oblique view CX disease. In patients with CX disease, 68% had a perfusion defect in the lateral segment, but only 5% with single RCA disease had a similar defect. Inferior segment defects predicted RCA with an accuracy of 89% and a specificity of 92. Lateral defects predicted CX disease with 90 percent accuracy and a specificity of 96%.[23] Trappe et al.[17] showed that in patients with totally occluded RCA and arrhythmias with left ventricular dysfunction the mortality is higher.

In summary RCA disease is common. Outcome depends on how much the left ventricle depends on RCA supply. The region of ischemia or infarction can be defined by thallium scanning.

PROGNOSIS OF SINGLE VESSEL DISEASE

In 97 patients following infarction, Wilson et al.[19] found 32% experienced events, 6% nonfatal reinfarction, and 26% unstable angina over a mean time of 39 months. All patients had had coronary arteriography, exercise testing, and Thallium scanning. Thallium scanning on exercise showed redistribution was the best predictor of events.

With the exception of proximal LAD disease prognosis is overall good for SVD of all three major coronary arteries. The CASS overall showed a 93% 5-year survival in patients who were 65 years or younger.[8] The design of this study tended to exclude patients with severe left ventricular dysfunction; however, it showed that, in patients with SVD, the prognosis was accordingly worse as left ventricular function deteriorated. The 4-year survival figures were as follows: a normal ejection fraction was associated with 94% survival; an ejection fraction of 49 to 35% was associated with 83% survival; and an ejection fraction of less than 35% percent, with 58% survival. At the time of publication, which was before the widespread application of angioplasty influenced the management of SVD, there was no difference in mortality over 4 years between medical and surgical management. A more recent publication from the CASS has shown that mortality in medically versus surgically treated patients is similar at 10 years, 85% and 82% and the reinfarction rate the same, 28% and 30%, illustrating that the long-term picture is good, and there is no difference between medical and surgical management[24] (Fig. 7-3). Although these data have now been accepted, it probably

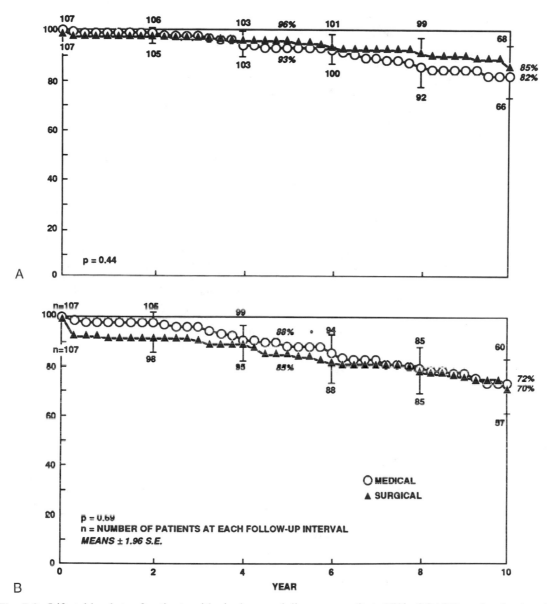

Fig. 7-3. Life-table plots of patients with single-vessel disease constitute 27% of CAST randomized patients. There are no significant differences in survival (**A**) or event rates (**B**). The proportion of patients who are survivors remaining free of infarction is influenced by the incidence of early perioperative infarction, a subsequent plateau phase, and a slight insignificant late trend toward increased survival in surgically treated patients. (From Alderman et al.,[24] with permission.)

does not influence management significantly because of the availability of angioplasty. With the exception of proximal LAD disease, when bypass surgery with the internal mammary artery must be considered, angioplasty is recommended in patients with severe angina, a large area of reversible ischemia or greater than 90% lesion or an eccentric graft lesion.[24] In practice, most patients would seem to be referred for angioplasty despite the prevalence of data suggesting other patients have a good prognosis and respond to medical therapy.[25]

Stone et al.[26] showed in patients presenting with acute myocardial infarction direct angioplasty without thrombolytic therapy results in a 50% improvement in left ventricular function, and a 92% 3-year cardiac survival with 77 percent of patients symptom free.[26] Similar results had been shown with acute coronary artery bypass grafting (CABG) in patients with infarction many years earlier.[27] The decision about management in patients with SVD therefore depends on the particular characteristics of the individual. The decision to do angioplasty is compelling; not to do so is difficult, but this should not be regarded as negative therapy, as medical treatment in many of the patients is comparable.

Although the prognosis of SVD is generally satisfactory, over many years the picture may be altered by the development of multivessel disease, owing to the progressive nature of coronary atherosclerosis.

REFERENCES

1. CASS Principal Investigators et al: Coronary Artery Surgery Study (CASS): A randomized trial of coronary artery bypass surgery: quality of life in patients randomly assigned to treatment groups. Circulation 68:951, 1983
2. Califf RM, Tomabechi Y, Lee KL et al: Outcome in one-vessel coronary artery disease. Circulation 67:283, 1983
3. Roubin GS, Harris PJ, Bernstein L, Kelly DT: Coronary anatomy and prognosis after myocardial infarction in patients 60 years of age and younger. Circulation 67:743, 1983
4. Taylor GJ, Humphries JO, Melletis ED et al: Predictors of clinical course, coronary anatomy and left ventricular function after recovery from acute myocardial infarction. Circulation 62:960, 1980
5. Gibson RS, Watson DD, Craddock GB et al: Prediction of cardiac events after uncomplicated myocardial infarction: a prospective study comparing predischarge exercise thallium-201 scintigraphy and coronary angiography. Circulation 68:321, 1983
6. Sanz G, Castaner A, Betriu A et al: Determinants of prognosis in survivors of myocardial infarction. N Engl J Med 306:1065, 1982
7. Bruschke AVG, Proudfit WL, Sones FM: Progress study of 590 consecutive nonsurgical cases of coronary disease followed 5–9 years: arteriographic correlations in CD. Circulation 47:936, 1973
8. CASS Principal Investigators et al: Coronary Artery Surgery Study (CASS): A randomized trial of coronary artery bypass surgery: survival data. Circulation 68:939, 1983
9. Feit FA, Khan R, El-Sherif N, Reddy C: Nonrandom occurence of single-vessel coronary artery disease. Am J Med 77:683, 1984
10. Hillis LD, Winniford MD: Frequency of severe (70% or more) narrowing of the right, left anterior descending, and left circumflex coronary arteries in right dominant circulations with coronary artery disease. Am J Cardiol 59:358, 1987
11. Diethrich EB, Liddicoat JE, Kinard SA et al: Surgical significance of angiographic patterns in coronary arterial disease. Circulation, suppl 1. 35/36:155, 1967
12. Garcia-Rubira JC, Galvez CP, Garcia JC: Is the prevalence of severe stenoses of left circumflex different from that of the right coronary artery? Int J Cardiol 26:114, 1990
13. Herrick JF: Coronary arteries. JAMA 59:2015, 1912
14. Brooks N, Cattell M, Jennings K et al: Isolated disease of left anterior descending coronary artery: angiocardiographic and clinical study of 218 patients. Br Heart J 47:71, 1982
15. Ellis S, Alderman E, Cain K et al: Prediction of risk of anterior myocardial infarction by lesion severity and measurement method of stenoses in the left anterior descending coronary distribution: a CASS registry study. J Am Coll Cardiol 11:908, 1988
16. Ellis S, Alderman EL, Cain K et al: Morphology of left anterior descending coronary territory lesions as a predictor of anterior myocardial infarction: a CASS registry study. J Am Coll Cardiol 13:1481, 1989
17. Trappe HJ, Lichtlen PR, Klein H et al: Natural history of single vessel disease: risk of sudden coronary death in relation to coronary anatomy and arrhythmia profile. Eur Heart J 10:514, 1989
18. Leong KH, Jones RH: Influence of the location of left anterior descending coronary artery stenosis on left ventricular function during exercise. Circulation 65:109, 1982
19. Wilson WW, Gibson RS, Nygaard TW et al: Acute myocardial infarction associated with single vessel coronary artery disease: an analysis of clinical outcome and the prognostic importance of vessel patency and residual ischemic myocardium. J Am Coll Cardiol 1:223, 1988
20. Dunn RF, Newman HN, Bernstein L et al: The clinical features of isolated left circumflex coronary artery disease. Circulation 69:477, 1984
21. Huey BL, Beller GA, Kaiser DL, Gibson RS: A comprehensive analysis of myocardial infarction due to left circumflex artery occlusion: comparison with infarction due to right coronary artery and left anterior descending artery occlusion. J Am Coll Cardiol 12:1156, 1988
22. James TN: Anatomy of the Coronary Arteries. Paul B Hoeber, New York, 1961
23. Newman HN, Dunn RF, Harris PJ et al: Differentiation between right and circumflex coronary artery disease on Thallium myocardial perfusion scanning. Am J Cardiol 51:1052, 1983
24. Alderman EL, Bourassa MG, Cohen LS et al: Ten-year follow up of survival and myocardial infarction in the

randomized coronary artery surgery study. Circulation 82:1629, 1990

25. Kramer JR, Proudfit WL, Loop FD et al: Late follow-up of 781 patients undergoing percutaneous transluminal coronary angioplasty or coronary artery bypass grafting for an isolated obstruction in the left anterior descending coronary artery. Am Heart J 118:1144, 1989

26. Stone GW, Rutherford BD, McConahay DR et al: Direct coronary angioplasty in acute myocardial infarction: outcome in patients with single vessel disease. J Am Coll Cardiol 15:534, 1990

27. Berg R, Kendall RW, Duvoisin GE et al: Acute myocardial infarction: a surgical emergency. J Thorac Cardiovasc Surg 70:432, 1975

8
Risk Assessment and Prognosis of Patients With Left Main Coronary Artery Disease

Michael B. Jorgensen
Amar S. Kapoor

Left main coronary artery stenosis is the most severe manifestation of coronary artery disease. Delays in securing the diagnosis increase the risk of significant myocardial infarction or sudden death. With the knowledge that surgical therapy improves survival in these patients, the clinician must be familiar with this entity. Increased awareness raises the physician's ability to screen patients for those features that suggest the presence of significant left main coronary artery stenosis, results in expeditious evaluation and treatment, and improves the patient's prognosis.

ETIOLOGY

Stenosis of the left main coronary artery has a variety of etiologies, the most common of which is atherosclerosis. An array of other causes of left main stenosis have been identified, including syphilis, radiation, Takayasu's disease, congenital stenosis, and iatrogenic causes. These are important to consider when evaluating a patient with left main stenosis. Syphilitic involvement of the aorta is rare today as a cause of coronary stenosis. In the past, syphilitic aortitis led to ostial stenosis in 17 to 26% of autopsied cases.[1,2]

Mediastinal radiation therapy causes intimal fibrosis and may contribute to accelerated atherosclerosis.[3] The effects of ionizing radiation on the vascular system were initially described in 1942.[4] Reports since then have documented the development of left main coronary artery stenosis in patients subjected to radiation therapy who lack other coronary risk factors.[5,6] Stenosis as a result of radiation therapy frequently involves the ostium of the left main coronary artery.[5,7]

Takayasu's disease is an arteritis that involves the arch of the aorta and its major branches. This involvement of the arterial branches of the aorta can lead to stenosis or occlusion. Angina is common in these patients as a result of encroachment on the coronary arteries by the arteritis.[8-10] Involvement of the left main coronary artery frequently results in ostial stenosis.[10-12]

Congenital hypoplasia or atresia of the left main coronary artery is a rare cause of stenosis.[13-15] In these cases, the ostial tissue histologically is composed of normal aortic tissue.[14] This is consistent with a failure of normal canalization of the coronary arteries during embryologic development.[16,17]

Injury to the left main coronary artery from selective coronary perfusion during cardiac surgical procedures can lead to the development of coronary stenosis. First described in 1969,[18] the incidence is 1.6 to 5%.[19–21] The stenosis occurs at the ostium. The left main coronary artery is particularly susceptible to the subsequent development of stenosis after selective cannulation and perfusion of the right and left coronary arteries during surgery.[22] This causes angina within the first 5 to 6 months after the procedure.[21,22] Endothelial injury caused by the perfusion catheter results in intimal fibrosis in some patients, which narrows the ostium.[23] The process, most often seen following aortic valve replacement may occur in any patient having selective cannulation of the coronary arteries during cardiac surgery.[24]

Accelerated development of acquired left main coronary artery stenosis is a rare outcome after coronary angioplasty. It occurs in approximately 0.33 to 1.7% of patients undergoing percutaneous transluminal coronary angioplasty (PTCA) in the left coronary system[25,26] and results from a fibrocellular proliferation in the left main coronary artery.[27] Histologic analysis of left main coronary arteries at necropsy in patients who died within 72 hours after angioplasty has shown a focal loss of the endothelium.[27] This intimal damage in the left main coronary artery is caused by guiding catheter manipulation, guide wires, angioplasty balloons, or a combination of these factors.[27] This denuding of the endothelium may be the stimulus for the development of the fibrocellular proliferation. Symptoms of angina resulting from the development of left main coronary artery stenosis after angioplasty occur within 4 to 5 months.[25–30]

INCIDENCE

At the Kaiser Permanente Medical Center, Los Angeles, from 1978 to 1988, we identified 393 patients with 50% or greater stenosis of the left main coronary artery among those undergoing cardiac catheterization. The findings of this 10-year experience closely parallel the data reported in the literature (Table 8-1). The incidence ranges from 2.4 to 14.8%.[31–34] No specific clinical variables have been shown to correlate with the presence of left main coronary artery stenosis.[41]

NONINVASIVE EVALUATION

Exercise testing is widely used in the diagnosis of coronary artery disease. Numerous exercise test variables have been analyzed to determine whether patients with left main coronary artery stenosis can be identified noninvasively. Unfortunately, this diagnosis cannot be made with any certainty on the basis of exercise testing alone. Exercise treadmill testing was per-

TABLE 8-1. Clinical Variables in Patients with Left Main Coronary Artery Disease

	Kaiser Medical Center	Previous Literature
Incidence	3.7%	2.4–14.8%[31–34]
Stenosis of other coronaries	—	2.7–2.9[35,36]
Angina	96%	85–100%[37–40]
Dyspnea with angina		9–18%[37,39]
Previous myocardial infarction	34%	36–63%[38,40]
Male:female	5.7:1	5:1[38,40]
Hypertension	50%	33%[38]
Diabetes mellitus	21%	
Smoking history	51%	
Hypercholesterolemia	30%	35–43%[35,38]

formed on 52% of patients with left main coronary artery stenosis at the Kaiser Medical Center; this experience follows the data reported in the literature (Table 8-2). Individually, each of the exercise test variables is not adequate to predict the presence of left main stenosis in patients with any degree of certainty.[44] Attempts have been made to define a markedly positive exercise test response to improve the predictive value and, although definitions vary slightly between studies, a markedly positive treadmill response demonstrates either ≥2 mm ST depression, ST changes in stage 1, termination of exercise in stage 1 or 2, or exercise-induced hypotension.[41] Among our patients, 92% of those undergoing treadmill testing demonstrated a markedly positive response. Similarly, 88% of patients tested in one series showed a markedly positive response.[41] When combining exercise test variables that define a markedly positive response, the predictive value of an exercise test to identify patients with left main coronary artery disease is approximately 32%.[41]

Myocardial perfusion scintigraphy is also an important tool in the diagnosis of coronary artery disease. As exercise testing is not sufficiently sensitive to identify

TABLE 8-2. Exercise Stress Test Variables in Patients with Left Main Coronary Artery Disease

	Kaiser Medical Center	Previous Literature
Angina on exertion	86%	53–83%[41–43]
Hypotension with exertion	13%	23%[40]
ST depression >1 mm	97%	77–93%[41,42]
ST depression >2 mm	80%	52–85%[42,44,45]
Persistent ST depression in recovery	13%	71–83%[41,42]

patients with left main coronary artery stenosis correctly, stress thallium studies have been used to improve the sensitivity. Identification of these patients among all patients undergoing thallium imaging requires the definition of a characteristic left main scintigraphic image. Left main coronary artery stenosis should be suspected when perfusion abnormalities are present in the anterolateral, septal, and posterolateral left ventricular areas on an individual test. Although 92 to 100% of patients with left main coronary artery disease have positive stress perfusion scintigrams, not all of these patients will be correctly identified as having left main coronary artery stenosis because of the lack of the characteristic pattern of the left main coronary artery.[46–48]

Of the 21% of the patients at the Kaiser Permanente Medical Center with left main stenosis who had stress perfusion scintigraphy, 100% were identified as having coronary artery disease; however, only 6.1% demonstrated the characteristic left main pattern. When the scintigraphy data were combined with the treadmill results that were markedly positive during the stress phase, 70% of the tests suggested left main coronary artery disease.

Indeed, stress thallium imaging has a 15 to 33% sensitivity for detecting the presence of left main stenosis.[46,47] The sensitivity is increased to 67 to 77% when the thallium imaging is considered together with variables from the exercise test that suggest significant disease.[46,47] There are several explanations for this lack of sensitivity. Patients with left main coronary artery disease usually have associated severe disease in the other coronary arteries.[35,36] When the right coronary artery is severely stenosed in combination with the left main coronary artery stenosis, a scintigraphic image consistent with three vessel disease can result.[46] The presence of collaterals in patients with left main coronary artery disease can affect the scintigraphy, producing an image that does not suggest left main coronary artery stenosis. It is important to recall that thallium imaging is a relative test, and a myocardial segment that shows the most activity might not have normal perfusion.[49] This will alter the ability to detect left main coronary artery stenosis.

Echocardiography is a noninvasive imaging technique that can be used to visualize the left main coronary artery. Since the first description of this method in 1976,[50] interest in the use of echocardiography to diagnose or exclude the presence of left main coronary artery stenosis has grown. The left main coronary artery can be visualized by the transthoracic method in 71 to 92% of patients.[51–53] The sensitivity of this technique for the detection of left main coronary artery stenosis ranges from 67% to 100%.[52,54,55] This variation can be partially accounted for by the technical demands of attempting to visualize the left main coro-

nary artery as it moves continuously during the cardiac cycle. Inadequate orientation of the scan beam relative to the course of the left main coronary artery can increase false-negative results.[50] In up to 66% of patients, only the proximal and midportion of the vessel can be clearly visualized.[53] The distal left main coronary artery is the most likely area to be inadequately seen.[51,53] The specificity ranges from 92 to 96%.[51–54] False-positive studies are rare but occur in a few clinical situations. Patients with aortic stenosis can appear to have proximal stenosis of the left main coronary artery because of increased echoes originating from the valve.[52,54] Proximal left anterior descending artery (LAD) stenosis can appear to be a distal left main coronary artery stenosis if the location of the bifurcation of the LAD and the circumflex (CX) artery is not clearly identified.[52,54]

Transesophageal echocardiography can improve the ability to visualize the left main coronary artery. Images of the entire left main coronary artery have been obtained in 90% of patients studied.[56] There was a 91% sensitivity for the detection of left main coronary artery stenosis with this technique and 100% specificity.[55] The superiority of transesophageal echocardiography in visualizing the left main coronary artery arises from its improved echocardiographic window leading to a marked improvement in its imaging capability. Certainly more investigation into this modality is necessary to define its value fully in the evaluation of a patient with suspected left main coronary artery stenosis.

INVASIVE EVALUATION AND RISK OF CORONARY ANGIOGRAPHY

Fluoroscopic examination in patients undergoing coronary angiography can demonstrate calcification in the region of the left main coronary artery. Calcification in this area was previously thought to be an important sign indicating the probable presence of left main coronary artery stenosis.[38] It has been subsequently demonstrated that calcification in the proximal left arterial system does not correlate with the presence of left main coronary artery disease.[31] Rather, it correlates best with the age of the patient than with a particular anatomic subset.[31]

Definitive evaluation of the patient with suspected coronary artery disease requires coronary angiography. This procedure is particularly important in quantifying left main coronary artery stenosis and in delineating possible surgical targets. The procedure, however, presents unique challenges and hazards in this subset of patients.

Damping of the arterial pressure waveform upon introduction of the diagnostic catheter tip into the left main alerts the angiographer to the possibility of proximal or ostial left main coronary artery stenosis.[31,57] (Fig. 8-1). Pressure damping can also be seen in patients with short left main coronary arteries where the catheter tip touches the left main bifurcation[31] or is subselectively engaged in either the LAD or the CX coronary arteries.[57] The occurrence of pressure damping requires immediate withdrawal of the catheter from the ostium because of the obstruction to coronary flow, which can lead to profound ischemia. In the absence of pressure damping, proximal or ostial left main coronary artery stenosis is also suspected when there is a lack of reflux of contrast into the aorta with injection. After the catheter has been withdrawn in these situations, the tip should be placed outside the coronary ostium in preparation for a cusp injection, which will visualize the proximal left main coronary artery and define the presence or absence of stenosis.[31]

Precise determination of the anatomy requires optimal angiographic definition. Shallow left and right anterior oblique views as well as anteroposterior (AP) views have been shown to best visualize the left main coronary artery.[31,38,57] The location of the stenosis has also been shown to influence which projection defines it best. Proximal stenoses are optimally visualized in the shallow left anterior oblique projection.[31] Distal stenoses are frequently seen best in the shallow right anterior oblique or AP view[31] (Fig. 8-2). Tight coning improves the image definition in all views but is especially critical when visualizing over the spine.[31]

Contrast agents have several deleterious effects on the cardiovascular system that are important to consider in angiography of left main coronary artery disease. Left ventriculography performed with high osmolality contrast material causes more severe hemodynamic alterations than with low osmolality contrast. The left ventricular end diastolic pressure rises and arterial systolic pressure falls to a greater extent with the use of high osmolality contrast.[58-61] The increase in end-diastolic pressure and the decrease in arterial pressure can potentially cause hemodynamic instability in patients with left main coronary artery stenosis. It is prudent in patients with

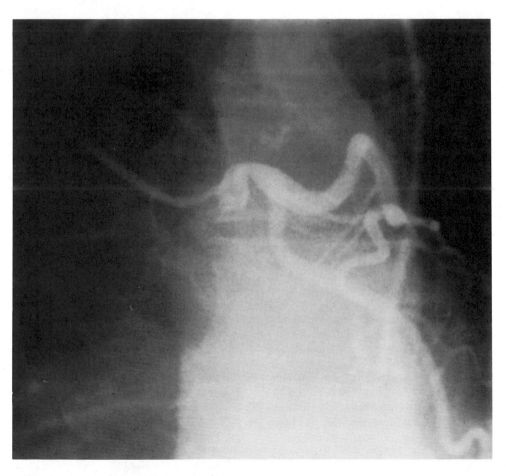

Fig. 8-1. Cineangiographic demonstration of an ostial left main coronary artery stenosis.

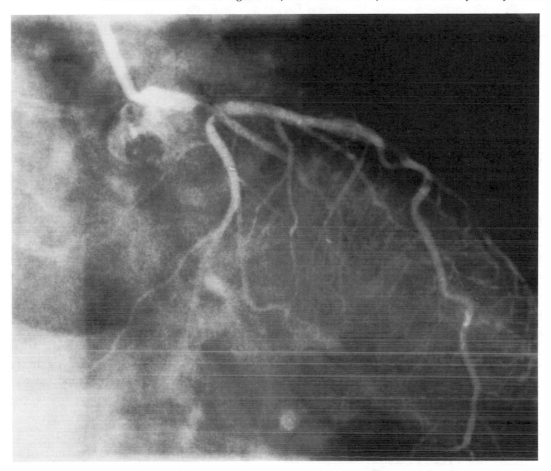

Fig. 8-2. Cineangiogram showing a distal stenosis of the left main coronary artery in a shallow right anterior oblique view.

suspected left main coronary artery stenosis to perform coronary angiography first. Subsequently, performance of left ventriculography can be weighed against the risks of hemodynamic alterations caused by the contrast. If left ventriculography is performed in patients with left main coronary artery disease, it is wise to use low osmolality contrast.

Coronary angiography using high osmolality contrast can cause potentially serious hemodynamic changes compared with low osmolality contrast. Significant decreases in systolic and diastolic pressure occur with the use of high osmolality contrast compared with low osmolality contrast.[58,60–62] High osmolality contrast also causes larger decreases in heart rate when used in coronary angiography.[58–61] The hemodynamic alterations induced by high osmolality contrast could lead to dangerous hypotension or bradycardia. Low osmolality contrast should be used in coronary angiography to minimize this risk when left main coronary artery disease is suspected. When left main coronary artery stenosis is noted during a proce-

dure, it is wise to change to low osmolality contrast for the duration of the procedure. It is also critical to limit the number of injections to the minimum number that adequately demonstrate the surgical targets. In the past, mortality with cardiac catheterization in patients with left main coronary artery stenosis was 10 to 19%.[38,43,63] Improved angiographic techniques have resulted in a decrease in mortality to 0 to 2.8%.[31,64,65]

MEDICAL THERAPY

Patients with greater than 50% stenosis of the left main coronary artery have an ominous prognosis when treated medically (Table 8-3). Survival is adversely affected by the increasing severity of the left main coronary artery stenosis. Patients with 50 to 70% stenosis had a survival of 66% at 3 years, compared with 41% survival in those with greater than 70% stenosis.[71] In another series, patients with increasing de-

TABLE 8-3. Survival with Medical Therapy

Investigators	Percentage Surviving Per Year				
	1 yr	2 yr	3 yr	4 yr	5 yr
DeMots et al.[66]	—	56%	—	42%	—
Cohen and Gerlin,[67]	—	56.4%	48.9%	29.4%	—
Oberman et al.[68]	73%	65%			
Takaro et al.[69]	—	—	64%	—	—
Chaitman et al.[70]	—	—	69%	63%	—
Lim et al.[39]	—	—	—	—	49%

grees of left main coronary artery stenosis had incrementally worse survival rates[70] (Fig. 8-3). Survival is also decreased with worsening left ventricular function.[70,72] A worse prognosis has been associated with the combination of right coronary artery stenosis and left main coronary artery disease.[72] The addition of left ventricular dysfunction to the combination of right coronary and left main coronary artery stenosis results in a more unfavorable prognosis.[70] Other factors associated with an increase in mortality in patients with left main coronary artery stenosis who are treated medically are chest pain at rest, cardiomegaly on chest radiography, a history of congestive heart fail-

ure, (CHF), and ST-T-wave changes on the resting electrocardiogram (ECG),[71] as well as increasing age, hypertension, and left coronary artery dominance.[70]

SURGICAL THERAPY

It is clear that medical therapy for left main coronary artery disease is not efficacious. Many studies have demonstrated that surgical intervention results in greatly improved survival in this subset of patients[66–70,73–76] (Table 8-4). A higher survival rate has been demonstrated with increasing numbers of coronary bypasses performed during surgery.[76] Survival is enhanced to a greater degree in those patients with better left ventricular function.[70,75] Long-term survival after surgery may also be adversely affected by an increase in the severity of the left main coronary artery stenosis.[70,77,78] It appears that the difference in survival is due to the increasing operative mortality with increasing severity of left main stenosis.[77] The difference in survival is therefore established at surgery and remains relatively unchanged during follow-up.[70,76]

Early in the surgical experience with left main

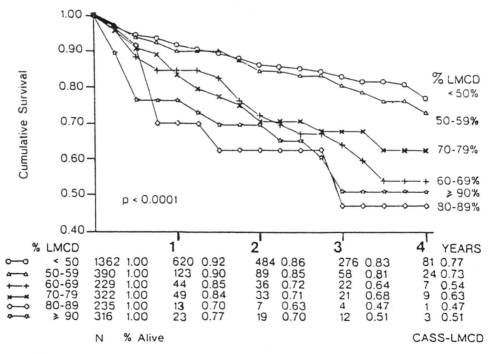

Fig. 8-3. Cumulative survival rates of nonsurgically treated patients with left main coronary artery disease stratified by percent intraluminal narrowing. (From Chaitman et al.,[70] with permission.)

TABLE 8-4. Survival after Coronary Artery Bypass Graft Surgery

	Percentage Surviving Per Year					
Investigators	1 y	2 y	3 y	4 y	5 y	6 y
DeMots et al.[66]	—	73%	70%	—	—	—
Cohen and Gorlin[67]	—	—	—	87.5%	—	—
Oberman et al.[68]	—	86%	—	—	—	—
Takaro et al.[69]	—	—	80%	—	—	—
Chaitman et al.[70]	—	—	91%	88%	—	—
Loop et al.[75]	—	—	—	—	88.2%	87.1%
Killen et al.[76]	—	—	—	—	88.8%	—

stenosis, the operative mortality was 7 to 18%.[66,67,69,72,74,77,78] More recent studies have demonstrated an improved operative mortality of 1.5 to 4.3%.[68,70,75–77,79–83] The mortality prior to discharge after bypass surgery at the Kaiser Permanente Medical Center was 2.6%. The improvement in operative mortality is due to better myocardial protection, improved anesthesia, and superior surgical techniques.[84] There are certain subsets of patients with an increased operative mortality. Women have an increased operative mortality compared with men.[70,75,82–84] An increase in the operative mortality has also been noted in older patients,[70,79,80,82,83] in patients with left dominant coronary circulation,[70,82,83] in those requiring emergency bypass surgery,[72,83,84] in patients with left ventricular dysfunction,[74,77,80,83] and in those with unstable angina.[82,83] Increases in operative mortality are also seen with longer durations of cardiopulmonary bypass.[80,83]

Coronary artery bypass surgery has been noted to result in an improved functional status in patients with left main coronary artery stenosis.[69,74,77,80] In one series, 89% were without angina after 1 year,[80] and 70 to 76% were angina free after 2 years.[74,77] Myocardial infarction during the perioperative period occurs in 1.5 to 4.8% of cases.[75,78,82] Routine use of intra-aortic balloon counterpulsation has been advocated as a way to decrease the possibility of ischemia and resultant infarction during anesthetic induction and placement of the patient on cardiopulmonary bypass.[85–88] Careful induction of anesthesia with control of the heart rate and blood pressure and rapid placement of cardiopulmonary bypass has been shown to result in low operative mortality and low perioperative myocardial infarction rate.[81,82,89] Use of intra-aortic balloon counter pulsation is therefore reserved for those patients with unstable angina not controlled with medical therapy prior to surgery.[82,89] Among the patients having bypass surgery at the Kaiser Permanente Medical Center intra-aortic balloon counterpulsation was required preoperatively due to lack of stabilization with medical therapy in only 3% of cases.

A unique surgical challenge is seen in those patients with isolated left main ostial stenosis. Consistent with its rarity, at the Kaiser Permanente Medical Center only two patients with isolated ostial stenosis out of 17 patients with ostial stenosis were identified out of 393 patients with left main coronary artery disease. In the absence of distal coronary stenosis, the establishment of a widely patent ostium would result in normalization of the coronary circulation and would obviate the need for bypass grafting. This would avoid subjecting the patient to the limited life expectancy of saphenous vein grafts and offers an option to internal mammary grafts. The procedure of direct ostioplasty was initially described in patients with ostial stenosis caused by syphilitic aortitis, in whom the obstructing tissue was directly resected.[90,91] Left main ostioplasty has also been performed using a pericardial autograft to enlarge the ostium.[92] Recent reports have demonstrated the effectiveness of saphenous vein patch angioplasty for isolated ostial stenosis of the left main coronary artery.[93,94] One of the two patients with isolated ostial stenosis at the Kaiser Permanente Medical Center underwent direct ostioplasty of the left main coronary artery for a 70% stenosis. Through an aortotomy, a ridge of tissue obstructing the left main ostium was resected. The intima of the left main coronary artery was then sutured to the intima of the ascending aorta, to establish an intact endothelium. Postoperatively the heart rate and blood pressure were rigidly controlled, and the patient had an uneventful recovery. Coronary angiography 1 year later showed the left main coronary artery to be widely patent.[95]

PROGNOSIS

Patients with left main coronary artery stenosis have a dismal prognosis when treated medically. The 42-month survival among medically treated patients in the Veterans Administration (VA) Cooperative Study was 65% compared with 88% in the surgically treated group (p = 0.016).[69] Similarly, in the Coronary Artery Surgery Study (CASS) data, medically treated patients had a 69% 3-year survival compared with 91% in the surgically treated group (p < 0.0001).[70] In the European Coronary Surgery Study, the 5-year survival was 68% with medical treatment and 86% with surgical therapy (p = 0.11).[73] There is strong evidence from randomized as well as nonrandomized studies that survival is significantly improved with surgical revascularization compared with medical therapy in patients with hemodynamically significant left main coronary artery stenosis.

CONCLUSION

Surgical revascularization improves the prognosis of patients with left main coronary artery stenosis. Identification of a markedly positive treadmill response or a left main coronary artery pattern on stress perfusion scintigraphy suggests left main coronary artery disease, but the ability to predict the presence of left main coronary artery stenosis with any degree of certainty is imprecise. Coronary angiography remains the definitive method to diagnose left main coronary artery stenosis. The test must be performed with caution, using low osmolality contrast agents and minimizing the number of coronary injections, to decrease the chance of serious hemodynamic changes. Intra-aortic balloon counterpulsation should be used preoperatively in patients whose anginal symptoms are not controlled with medical therapy. Coronary artery bypass surgery can be performed with low operative risk and improves survival in these patients. With an increased awareness of those factors that suggest left main coronary artery stenosis, the clinician can expedite evaluation of these patients so that surgery can be performed to reestablish normal hemodynamics in the coronary circulation.

REFERENCES

1. Heggtveit HA: Syphilitic aortitis. Circulation 29:346, 1964
2. Scharfman WB, Wallach JB, Angrist A: Myocardial infarction due to syphilitic coronary ostial stenosis. Am Heart J 40:603, 1950
3. Kopelson G, Herwig KJ: The etiologies of coronary disease in cancer patients. Int J Radiat Oncol Biol Phys 4:895, 1978
4. Warren S: Effects of radiation on normal tissues. Arch Pathol 34:1070, 1942
5. Radwaner BA, Geringer R, Goldman AM et al: Left main coronary artery stenosis following mediastinal irradiation. Am J Med 82:1017, 1987
6. McEniery PT, Dorosti K, Schiavone WA et al: Clinical and angiographic features of coronary disease after chest irradiation. Am J Cardiol 60:1020, 1987
7. Tommaso CL, Applefeld MM, Singleton RT: Isolated left main coronary artery stenosis and mediastinal radiotherapy as an etiologic factor. Am J Cardiol 61:1119, 1988
8. Young JA, Sengupta A, Khaja Fu: Coronary arterial stenosis, angina pectoris and atypical coarctation of the aorta due to non-specific arteritis. Am J Cardiol 32:356, 1973
9. Cipriano PR, Silverman JF, Perlroth MG et al: Coronary arterial narrowing in Takayasu's aortitis. Am J Cardiol 39:744, 1977
10. Kaul U, Reddy KS, Narula J et al: Angiographic recognition of coronary ostial stenosis in non-specific aorto-arteritis. Cathet Cardiovasc Diagn 14:175, 1988
11. Morgan JM, Honey M, Gray HH et al: Angina pectoris in a case of Takayasu's disease: revascularization by coronary ostioplasty and bypass grafting. Eur Heart J 8:1354, 1987
12. Chun PKC, Jones R. Rabinowitz M et al: Coronary ostial stenosis in Takayasu's arteritis. Chest 78:330, 1980
13. Mullins CE, El Said G, McNamara DG: Atresia of the left coronary ostium. Circulation 46:989, 1972
14. Josa M, Danielson GK, Weidman WH, Edwards WD: Congenital ostial membrane of the left main coronary artery. J Thorac Cardiovasc Surg 81:383, 1981
15. Head GB, Parmley LF, Hightower BM: Left main coronary artery disease in a 19 year old woman. Am J Med 76:324, 1984
16. Grant RT: Development of cardiac coronary artery vessels in the rabbit. Heart 13:261, 1926
17. Fortuin NJ, Roberts NC: Congenital atresia of the left main coronary artery. Am J Med 50:385, 1971
18. Trimble AS, Bigelow WG, Wigle ED, Silver MD: Coronary ostial stenosis. J Thorac Cardiovasc Surg 57:792, 1969
19. Reed GE, Spencer FC, Boyd AD et al: Late complications of intraoperative coronary artery perfusion. Circulation, suppl. 48:III–80, 1973
20. Hazan E, Rioux C, Dequirot A, Mathey J: Postperfusion stenosis of the common left coronary artery. J Thorac Cardiovasc Surg 69:703, 1975
21. Yates JD, Kirsh MM, Soderman Tm et al: Coronary ostial stenosis: a complication of aortic valve replacement. Circulation 49:503, 1974
22. Midell AI, DeBoerA, Bermudez G: Postperfusion coronary ostial stenosis: incidence and significance. J Thorac Cardiovasc Surg 72:80, 1976
23. Nakhjavan FK, Maranhao V, Goldberg H: Iatrogenic stenosis of the proximal portion of the coronary arteries. Am Heart J 83:318, 1972
24. Coplan NL, Estioko MR, Ambrose JA: Ostial left main stenosis following repair of a ruptured sinus of Valsalva aneurysm. Chest 88:471, 1985
25. Kells KM, Miller RM, Henderson MA et al: Left main coronary artery disease progression after percutaneous transluminal coronary angioplasty. Am J Cardiol 65:513, 1990
26. Vardhan IN, Aharonian VJ, Gordon S, Mahrer PR: A rare complication of percutaneous transluminal coronary angioplasty; left main disease. Am Heart J 121:902, 1991

27. Waller BF, Pinkerton CA, Foster LN: Morphologic evidence of accelerated left main coronary artery stenosis: a late complication of percutaneous transluminal balloon angioplasty of the proximal left anterior descending coronary artery. J Am Coll Cardiol 9:1019, 1987

28. Wayne VS, Harper RW, Pitt A: Left main coronary artery stenosis after percutaneous transluminal coronary angioplasty. Am J Cardiol 61:459, 1988

29. Hamad N, Pichard A, Oboler A, Lindsay J: Left main coronary artery stenosis as a late complication of percutaneous transluminal coronary angioplasty. Am J Cardiol 60: 1183, 1987

30. Haraphongse M, Rossall RE: Subacute left main stenosis following percutaneous transluminal coronary angioplasty. Cathet Cardiovasc Diagn 13:401, 1987

31. Lipton MJ, Pfeifer JF, Murphy ML, Hultgren HN: Dangers of left main coronary artery lesions: angiographic technique and evaluation. Invest Radiol 12:447, 1977

32. Rosch J, DeMots H, Antonvic R et al: Coronary arteriography in left main coronary artery disease. AJR 121:583, 1974

33. Takaro T, Hultgren HN, Lipton MJ, Detre KM: VA cooperative randomized study of surgery for coronary arterial occlusive disease: subgroup with significant left main lesions. Circulation, suppl. 54:III–107, 1976

34. Green GS, McKinnon CM, Rosch J, Judkins MP: Complications of selective percutaneous transfemoral coronary arteriography and their prevention. Circulation 45:552, 1972

35. Bulkley BH, Rogers WC: Atherosclerotic narrowing of the left main coronary artery. Circulation 53:823, 1976

36. Moore CH, Lombardo TR, Allums JA, Gordon FT: Left main coronary artery stenosis: hemodynamic monitoring to reduce mortality. Ann Thorac Surg 26:445, 1978

37. Khaja FU, Sharma SD, Easley RM et al: Left main coronary artery lesions. Circulation, suppl. 49:II–136, 1974

38. Lavine P, Kimbris D, Segel BL, Linhart JW: Left main coronary artery disease. Am J Cardiol 30:791, 1972

39. Lim JS, Proudfit WL, Sones FM: Left main coronary arterial obstruction: long term follow-up of 141 non-surgical cases. Am J Cardiol 36:131, 1975

40. Cohen MV, Gorlin R: Main left coronary artery disease: clinical experience from 1964–1974. Circulation 52:275, 1975

41. Weiner DA, McCabe CH, Ryan TJ: Identification of patients with left main and three vessel coronary disease with clinical and exercise test variables. Am J Cardiol 46: 21, 1980

42. Stone PH, Lafollette BA, Cohn K: Patterns of exercise treadmill test performance in patients with left main coronary artery disease. Am Heart J 104:13, 1982

43. Cohen MV, Cohn PF, Herman MV: Diagnosis and prognosis of left main coronary obstruction. Circulation, suppl. 45:I–57, 1972

44. Nixon JV, Lipscomb K, Blomquist CG, Shapiro W: Exercise testing in men with significant left main coronary artery disease. Br Heart J 42:410, 1979

45. Sharma S, Khaja F, Heinle R, Goldstein S, Easley R: Left main coronary artery lesions: risk of cath, exercise testing, and surgery, abstracted. Circulation, suppl. 47/48: IV–53, 1973

46. Maddaha J, Abdullah A, Garcia EV et al: Noninvasive identification of left main and triple vessel coronary artery disease: improved accuracy using quantitative analysis of regional myocardial stress distribution and washout of thallium 201. J Am Coll Cardiol 7:53, 1986

47. Dash H, Massie BM, Botvinick EH, Brundage BH: Noninvasive identification of left main and three vessel coronary artery disease by myocardial stress perfusion scintigraphy and treadmill exercise electrocardiography. Circulation 60:276, 1979

48. Rehn T, Griffith L, Achuff S et al: Rest and stress thallium 201 imaging in left main coronary disease, sensitive but not specific. Am J Cardiol 41:413, 1978

49. Botvinick EH, Taradash MR, Shames DM, Parmley WW: Thallium 201 myocardial perfusion scintigraphy for the clarification of normal, abnormal, and equivocal electrocardiographic stress tests. Am J Cardiol 41:43, 1978

50. Weyman AE, Feigenbaum H, Dillon JC et al: Non-invasive visualization of the left main coronary artery by cross sectional echocardiography. Circulation 54:169, 1976

51. Chen CC, Morganroth J, Ogawa S, Mardell TJ: Detecting left main coronary artery disease by apical cross sectional echocardiography. Circulation 62:288, 1980

52. Ryan T, Armstrong WF, Feigenbaum H: Prospectiv evaluation of the left main coronary artery using digital 2-dimensional echocardiography. J Am Coll Cardiol 7:807, 1986

53. Vered Z, Katz M, Rath S et al: Two dimensional echocardiographic analysis of proximal left main coronary artery in humans. Am Heart J 112:972, 1986

54. Rink LD, Feigenbaum H, Godley RW et al: Echocardiographic detection of left main coronary artery obstruction. Circulation 65:719, 1982

55. Ronderos R, Sakedo EE, Kramer JR et al: Value and limitation of two dimensional echocardiography for the detection of left main coronary artery disease. Cleve Clin J Med 51:7, 1984

56. Yoshida K, Yoshikawa J, Hozumi T et al: Detection of left main coronary artery stenosis by transesophageal color doppler and two dimensional echocardiography. Circulation 81:1271, 1990

57. Kern MJ: Approach to the patient with left main coronary artery stenosis. Cathet Cardiovasc Diagn 18:181, 1989

58. Gertz EW, Wisneski JA, Chiu D et al: Clinical Superiority of a new nonionic contrast agent for cardiac angiography. J Am Coll Cardiol 5:250, 1985

59. Hirshfeld JW, Wieland J, Davis CA et al: Hemodynamic and electrocardiographic effects of ioversol during cardiac angiography. Invest Radiol 24:138, 1989

60. Bettman MA, Bourdillon PD, Barry WH et al: Contrast agents for cardiac angiography: effects of a nonionic agent vs. a standard ionic agent. Radiology 153:583, 1984

61. Bettman MA, Higgins CB: Comparison of an ionic with a nonionic contrast agent for cardiac angiography. Invest Radiol 20:572, 1985

62. Cooper MW, Reed PJ: Comparison of ionic and nonionic contrast agents in cardiac catheterization. Cathet Cardiovasc Diagn 22:267, 1991

63. Wolfson S. Grant D, Ross AM: Risk of death related to

coronary arteriography: role of left coronary arterial lesions. Am J Cardiol 37:210, 1976

64. Gordon PR, Abanms C, Gash AK, Carabello BA: Pericatheterization risk factors in left main coronary artery stensosis. Am J Cardiol 59:1080, 1987
65. Davis K, Kennedy JW, Kemp HG et al: Complications of coronary arteriography from the collaborative study of coronary artery surgery. Circulation 59:1105, 1979.
66. DeMots H, Bonchek LI, Rosch J et al: Left main coronary artery disease. Am J Cardiol 36:136, 1975
67. Cohen MV, Gorlin R: Main left coronary disease. Circulation 52:275, 1975
68. Oberman A, Harrell RR, Russell RO et al: Surgical versus medical treatment in disease of the left main coronary artery. Lancet 1:591, 1976
69. Takaro T, Hultgren HN, Lipton MJ, Detre KM: VA cooperative randomized study of surgery for coronary arterial occlusive disease. Circulation, suppl. 54:III–107, 1976
70. Chaitman BR, Fisher LD, Bourossa MG et al: Effect of coronary bypass surgery on survival patterns in subsets of patients with left main coronary artery disease. Am J Cardiol 48:765, 1981
71. Conley MJ, Ely RL, Kisslo J et al: Prognostic spectrum of left main stenosis. Circulation 57:947, 1978
72. Hind CRK, Oldershaw PJ, Miller GAH: Left main coronary artery stenosis. J Cardiovasc Surg 23:394, 1982
73. European Coronary Surgery Study Group: Coronary artery bypass surgery in stable angina pectoris. Lancet 1:889, 1979
74. Zeft HJ, Manley JC, Husto JH: Left main coronary artery stenosis: results of coronary bypass surgery. Circulation 48:68, 1974
75. Loop FD, Lyttle BW, Cosgrove DM et al: Atherosclerosis of the left main coronary artery: 5 year results of surgical treatment. Am J Cardiol 44:195, 1979
76. Killen DA, Reed WA, Kindred L et al: Surgical therapy for left main coronary artery disease. J Thorac Cardiovasc Surg 80:255, 1980
77. Farinha JB, Kaplan MA, Harris CN et al: Disease of the left main coronary artery. Am J Cardiol 42:124, 1978
78. Lawrie GM, Morris GC, Howell JF et al: Improved survival beyond 5 years after coronary bypass surgery in patients with left main coronary artery disease. Am J Cardiol 44:612, 1979
79. Jeffery DL, Vijayanagar RR, Bognolo DA et al: Coronary bypass for left main disease in patients over 70 years of age. J Cardiovasc Surg 26:212, 1985
80. Rittenhouse EA, Sauvage LR, Mansfield PB et al: Severe left main coronary arterial stenosis with right coronary occlusion. Am J Cardiol 49:645, 1982
81. Brandt B, Wright CB, Doty DB et al: Surgical treatment of left main coronary artery disease: operative risk. Surgery 87:436, 1980
82. Jeffery DL, Vijayanagar R, Bognolo DA et al: Surgical treatment of 200 consecutive patients with left main coronary artery disease. Ann Thorac Surg 36:193, 1983
83. Chaitman BR, Rogers WJ, Davis K et al: Operative risk in patients with left main coronary artery disease. N Engl J Med 303:953, 1980
84. Gomberg J, Klein LW, Seelaus P et al: Surgical revascularization of left main coronary artery stenosis: determinants of perioperative and long term outcome in the 1980's. Am Heart J 116:440, 1988
85. Anderson RP, Li W, Baltour RI: Surgical management of left main coronary artery stenosis and ischemic left ventricular dysfunction. J Thorac Cardiovasc Surg 77:369, 1979
86. McConahay DR, Killin DA, McCallister BD: Coronary artery bypass surgery for left main coronary artery disease. Am J Cardiol 37:885, 1976
87. Tahan SR, Geha AS, Hammond GL: Bypass surgery for left main coronary artery disease; reduced perioperative myocardial infarction with preoperative intra-aortic balloon counterpulsation. Br Heart J 43:191, 1980
88. Cooper GN, Singh AK, Christian FC et al: Preoperative intra-aortic balloon support in surgery for left main coronary stenosis. Ann Surg 185:242, 1977
89. Miller DW, Tobis FM, Ivey TD, Rubenstein SA: Risk of coronary arteriography and bypass surgery in patients with left main coronary artery stenosis. Chest 79:387, 1981
90. Connolly JE, Eldridge FL, Calvin JW, Stemmer EA: Proximal coronary artery obstruction. N Engl J Med 271:213, 1964
91. DuBost PB, Piwnica A, Weiss M et al: Syphilitic coronary obstruction: correction under artificial heart-lung and profound hypothermia. Surgery 48:540, 1960
92. Sabiston DC, Ebert PA, Friesinger GC et al: Proximal endarterectomy, arterial reconstruction for coronary occlusion at the aortic origin. Arch Surg 91:758, 1965
93. Sullivan JA, Murphy DA: Surgical repair of stenotic ostial lesions of the left main coronary artery. J Thorac Cardiovasc Surg 98:33, 1989
94. Deuvaert FE, Paepe JD, VanNooten G et al: Transaortic saphenous patch angioplasty for left main coronary artery stenosis. J Cardiovasc Surg 29:610, 1988
95. Jorgensen MB, Kapoor A, Aharonian V et al: Left main ostial stenosis and management with ostioplasty or multi-vessel bypass grafting. Chest, suppl. 98:88S, 1990

9

Unstable Angina: Prognosis and Risk Factors

Pierre Théroux

This book on the prognosis of cardiovascular disease answers a need, since no equivalent exists. It represents, however, the major challenge of gathering together information derived from studies with often limited sample sizes, of patients with various characteristics and with different clinical expression of the disease. These studies have been performed during decades of constant progress in the application of clinical and laboratory diagnostic methods and in advances in medical and surgical therapy. In a way this book on the assessment of prognosis marks a halt; to fulfill its expectations and to keep pace with the growing progress of cardiology, it will require constant updating.

Unstable angina typically illustrates the challenge of this book. This clinical syndrome incorporates various clinical manifestations expressing pathophysiologic mechanisms of different nature and intensity. The prognosis has been learned from various series published over a period of 40 years that have progressively incorporated the progresses made in the therapy of cardiovascular diseases. It has only lagged behind by a lack of diagnostic procedures and, until recently, the laboratory investigation was confined almost exclusively to 12-lead electrocardiography (ECG) and to coronary angiography.

In this chapter, unstable angina is first located in its historical perspective. Data on natural history are then reviewed, followed by a discussion of the various approaches used for risk stratification. The influence on the prognosis of the various medical and surgical

therapeutic measures is then discussed. This approach should lead us to a projection in the near future.

HISTORICAL PERSPECTIVES

The syndrome of unstable angina originated from early retrospective observations of a high rate of prodromal symptoms preceding an acute myocardial infarction (AMI). These prodromal symptoms were first clearly described in 1937 as prolonged chest pain or progressively severe exertional angina or angina attacks unrelated to effort and emotion. They were found in more than 50% of patients hospitalized for AMI.[1,2] Subsequent retrospective reviews of medical records and administration of structured questionnaires to large series of patients hospitalized for AMI confirmed the variable but consistently high frequency of these premonitory symptoms.[3-5] These observations have led to prospective evaluation of patients presenting with a changing pattern of chest pain. The first of these studies, by Levy[6] in 1956, reported an incidence of MI of 38% and of mortality of 32% after a 3-month follow-up of 158 patients with an unstable pattern of angina. Subsequently in 1961, Vakil[7] described 251 patients with chest pain of 15 minutes or more duration with electrocardiographic (ECG) signs of ischemia but no evidence of an MI: MI had occurred in 37% of patients at 3 months and mortality in 0.8%.

The clinical investigation of unstable angina can be divided into three decades of progress with some overlap between each. From 1960 to 1970, the natural history of the disease was described and a search made for a proper definition. Treatment was introduced, consisting mainly of anticoagulants and clinical observations made on its efficacy. From 1970 to 1980, the disease was defined, classified, risk stratified, and applied the new treatment forms available for the management of coronary artery disease, including β-blockers and coronary revascularization. The latter part of this decade also saw an attempt at defining and investigating the pathophysiologic mechanisms involved. Between 1980 and 1990, considerable insight was gained in an understanding of the causes of the disease, helped by pathologic studies and new diagnostic procedures, such as qualitative coronary angiography, coronary angioscopy, and laboratory measures of activation of the blood factors. The art of recent sophisticated clinical trials was also used to define the most useful forms of treatment; the efficacy of calcium antagonists, platelet active drugs, and antithrombotic treatment was tested. In the early 1990s, the challenge of unstable angina remains more lively than ever.

PROGNOSIS OF UNSTABLE ANGINA

Clearly, unstable angina carries a higher risk of myocardial infarction and death than stable angina. Table 9-1 shows the results of some of the studies published. It is not intended to be complete, but to give a general overview. Krauss et al.[8] reported the occurrence of MI in 7% of patients during hospitalization and in 20% at 1 year; mortality was 1% and 15%, respectively. In a study of 175 patients conducted by Fulton et al.,[9] most of whom were not hospitalized, the incidence of MI at 3 months was 16% and the incidence of mortality 2%. Gazes et al.[10] obtained a long-term follow-up in 140 patients; at 3 months, MI had occurred in 21% of patients and mortality in 10%; the mortality rate at 1 year had increased to 18%, at 5 years to 39%, and at 10 years to 52%.[10] In a report by Heng et al.,[11] the infarction rate at 3 weeks was 13% and the mortality rate 4% with a subsequent increase in the mortality rate of 5% per year for the next 6 years. Duncan et al.[12] published their follow-up of 251 patients who were not hospitalized; MI had occurred in 12% of the patients at 6 months and mortality in 4%. From these so-called natural history studies, the average incidence of MI at 1 year can be estimated to be 15 to 20% and of mortality 4 to 15%. It is important to stress that most events occur early, within the first few months after diagnosis.

Notwithstanding these results, the reported prognosis of unstable angina is variable with extremes described. Thus, in earlier series, when medical therapy was minimal or when patients not treated by anticoagulant therapy were considered controls, incidences of MI as high as 80% were reported by Beamish and Storrie[13] and of 22% by Wood.[14] By contrast, more recent series using minimal therapy, have reported a 12%

TABLE 9-1. Natural History Studies in Unstable Angina

Investigators/Year	No. of Patients[a]	Duration of Follow-up	Myocardial Infarction	Mortality
Early studies				
Levy (1956)[6]	158	3 mo	39.2%	32.3%
Beamish and Storrie (1960)[13]	15	6 wk	80.0%	60.0%
Vakil (1961)[7]	251	3 mo	37.1%	0.8%
Wood (1961)[14]	50	2 mo	22.0%	16.0%
Natural history studies				
Krauss et al. (1972)[8]	100	1 mo	7.0%[b]	1.0%
		12 mo	20.0%[b]	14.8%
Fulton et al. (1972)[9]	213	3 mo	16.6%	1.9%
Gazes et al. (1973)[10]	140	3 mo	20.7%	10.0%
		1 yr	—	18.0%
Heng et al. (1976)[11]	158	3 wk	13%[b]	4%
Duncan et al (1976)[12]	251	6 mo	12%[b]	4%
More recent studies				
Mulcahy et al. (1981)[15]	101	28 d	9%	4%
		1 yr	12%	10%
Telford and Wilson (1981)[102]	114	7 d	14.9%	1.7%
Lewis et al. (1983)[96]	641	3 mo	7.8%[b]	3.3%
Cairns et al. (1985)[97]	279	18 mo	14.7%[b]	9.6%
Théroux et al. (1988)[98]	118	5 d	11.8%[b]	1.7%
RISC Study Group (1990)[99]	199	90 d	17.1%[b]	—
Balsano et al. (1990)[100]	338	6 mo	10.9%[b]	4.7%

[a] Refers to the control population in drug intervention trials.
[b] Includes fatal and nonfatal myocardial infarction.

nonfatal MI and 12% mortality rates at 1 year.[15] Also, the vast majority of patients with unstable angina will become clinically stable after a few days, often without recurrence of symptoms.[8]

The variability in these results stresses the importance of risk evaluation in patients with unstable angina. The classic approach to risk stratification is performed using clinical characteristics and angiographic findings. The clinical characteristics include a previous history of angina, the clinical presentation of unstable angina, the presence of ECG changes, and the early in-hospital clinical evolution. Angiographic characteristics have stressed the presence and extent of coronary artery disease and of left ventricular dysfunction. More recent investigations however have opened the field to a new area of risk evaluation, which include perfusion scintigraphic studies, quantitative coronary angiography, Holter monitoring, and assessment of the markers of activation of platelets and of coagulation factors related to thrombus formation.

Clinical Presentation of Unstable Angina

The term *unstable angina* proposed by Fowler[16] in 1971 and by Conti et al.[17] is now largely accepted. Also, the classification described by Gazes et al.[9] in 1973 remains classic and is widely used to stratify risk. This classification defines three subgroups: (1) new-onset angina in patients previously free of symptoms; (2) crescendo angina with more frequent or more severe chest pain, occurring at rest or with minimal exercise; and (3) prolonged chest pain, poorly relieved with nitroglycerin without enzymatic or ECG evidence of MI.

Other subgroups of patients with unstable coronary syndromes have since been recognized that could be included in a broader classification of unstable angina.[18] These are unstable angina occurring early after MI, so-called early postinfarction ischemia, unstable angina occurring after coronary angioplasty and after coronary artery bypass surgery, non-Q-wave MI, and Prinzmetal's variant angina (Table 9-2).

This broad classification could be useful, as it accounts for the signs and symptoms of the disease and can serve for early risk stratification and orientation of patients. The classification can further be sophisticated to include the presence of ECG changes during pain[19]—or of other objective markers of ischemia. The classification should also be updated on a day-to-day basis, to account for the presence or absence of recurrent chest pain, and of other objective evidence of myocardial ischemia.

New Onset of Angina

Most investigators have included angina of recent onset in their study groups, but requiring that a progressive pattern in the severity of angina be pres-

TABLE 9-2. Description of Unstable Angina

Clinical presentation
  New-onset angina
    Stable
    Progressive
  Crescendo angina
  Acute coronary insufficiency
  Non-Q-wave myocardial infarction
  Early postinfarction angina
  Unstable angina after coronary angioplasty
  Unstable angina after coronary artery bypass surgery
  Prinzmetal's variant angina
Objective evidences of ischemia
  Electrocardiographic changes
  Other markers of ischemia
Clinical evolution
  Recurrent ischemia

ent.[8–11,20] This progressive pattern could consist of angina occurring both at rest or during exercise or of angina provoked by minimal exercise. New-onset angina restricted to heavy exercise and resulting in only slight limitation of functional capacity (Canadian Cardiovascular Society class 1 and 2) and without an element of progression should probably be diagnosed as stable rather than unstable angina.

The prognosis reported in these patients with new-onset angina has varied but, in general, has approached the prognosis described for unstable angina. Some studies have suggested a better prognosis when no previous chronic stable angina was present.[9,10,20] One study has shown a worse prognosis with more prolonged chest pain.[21] In a retrospective analysis of 329 patients with new-onset angina and of 1,398 control patients with chronic stable angina, cardiac events at 1 year had occurred in 16% of patients in the former group compared with 7% in the latter.[22]

Clearly, new-onset angina includes a heterogeneous class of patients. Prognosis may be better in some owing to different pathophysiologic mechanisms unrelated to an acute thrombotic process; the prognosis could also be better because some patients without previous angina have less extensive coronary artery disease and are more likely to benefit from treatment. It is generally suggested that patients with new-onset angina be promptly considered as unstable as soon as one clinical feature of instability is recognized.

Acute Coronary Insufficiency Versus Crescendo Angina

These clinical forms represent the classic presentation patterns of unstable angina. Prognosis is generally believed to be worse with acute coronary insufficiency than with crescendo angina. Bertolasi et al.[23] reported an incidence of myocardial infarction of 32% in patients with acute coronary insufficiency compared with 7% in patients with crescendo angina in a 32-month follow-up study; respective mortality rates during that period were 46 and 7%. The reported incidences of MI in patients with acute coronary insufficiency differ considerably, from 3%[24] to 62%[25] but most complications consistently occur early.[21] These differences in prognosis can partly be related to various characteristics of patients included and various sample sizes and to different treatments used. It is also likely that a variable proportion of patients with non-Q-wave myocardial infarction have been included in the various series.

Non-Q-Wave Myocardial Infarction

Numerous studies have documented that non-Q wave myocardial infarction carries a high risk of MI and death during hospitalization and during follow-up. Indeed, the better prognosis observed acutely, as compared with patients with Q-wave MI, is rapidly lost during follow-up, stressing the unstable coronary artery status of these patients.[26-29] Early reinfarction rates of 9% and mortality rates as high as 17% have been documented.[28-31]

The clinical distinction between non-Q-wave MI and acute coronary insufficiency is somewhat artifactual and is more quantitative than qualitative. It is based mainly on the results of the cardiac enzyme determinations; these are obtained at various times after chest pain, using different laboratory techniques for measurements and different cutpoints for the diagnosis of MI. Most patients with non-Q-wave MI should be considered patients with acute coronary insufficiency, accounting for a similar pathophysiology and a similar prognosis. The differences in prognosis between the two conditions are more likely conditioned by the intrinsic activity of the disease process, the extent of coronary artery disease and of left ventricular function, rather than by the basic pathophysiologic process itself.

Early Postinfarction Ischemia

Early postinfarction ischemia defines patients with recurrent chest pain 24 hours or more after an AMI.[32] This syndrome occurs in 18% of patients with a recent MI and is often associated with more severe and more extensive coronary artery disease or with persistent viable myocardium in an infarct zone remaining in jeopardy by a critical coronary artery stenosis.[33] It carries a 28% risk of early in-hospital myocardial infarct extension, as compared with a 2% risk when absent.[32,33] Postdischarge prognosis is also impaired and, in one study, the mortality rate was 56% at 6 months.[32] In another study, the risk of fatal or nonfatal MI was 33% after a mean follow-up of 14 months, compared with 19% in the absence of early ischemia.[33]

Unstable Angina After Coronary Angioplasty

Recurrent angina occurs in as much as 20% of patients in the follow-up of coronary angioplasty, mostly during the first 6 months after the procedure.[34] This high incidence is a direct consequence of the high 30 to 40% restenosis rate occurring during that period.[35,36] The prognosis is favorable, however, and angina in these circumstances, although at times severe and occurring at rest, is only exceptionally associated with more severe complications. When angina occurs later than 6 months after the procedure, it is more likely related to a new active lesion than to restenosis at the site of the previous dilation.[37]

These findings following coronary angioplasty emphasize the pathophysiologic mechanisms involved in unstable angina. The procedure by itself can be considered an unstable state, since the catheter and balloon-induced endothelium damage can trigger an acute thrombosis. Past the acute phase, however, and within the first 6 months, restenosis per se can cause exertional and rest angina but is rarely associated with the more serious complications of MI and death, indicating that the basic problem is mechanical impairment of blood flow delivery, and not a thrombogenic process with the inherent risk of acute occlusion. Past this period of restenosis, the usual diagnostic is a new active lesion and these patients should be considered as typical unstable angina patients and managed appropriately.

Unstable Angina After Coronary Artery Bypass Surgery

Unstable angina in patients with previous bypass surgery is a current medical problem, representing in active cardiology centers as much as 20% of all patients admitted for unstable angina.[38] Twenty-one percent of patients with vein graft implants had experienced angina a mean of 7 years after surgery and 17% a nonfatal MI.[39] The early in-hospital clinical course of these patients is similar to that of patients with unstable angina without previous bypass surgery. The long-term prognosis is worse, however, and as many as twice the patients experience a new acute coronary event or more severe angina. The explanation proposed for this unfavorable prognosis is that the patients with previous bypass surgery are less amenable to a corrective revascularization procedure.[40] It would thus seem that the acute thrombotic process can be controlled but not the basic disease process that had triggered this acute process.

Clinical Evolution

The early hospital course has long been recognized early as an important determinant of prognosis.[8,10,11] Chest pain persisting for more than 48 hours after hospitalization in the study by Gazes et al.,[10] occurred in 54 patients and was associated with a mortality at 1 month of 20% and at 1 year of 43% in contrast with a 1-year 2% mortality in the 86 patients with no early angina mortality. In the study by Krauss et al.,[8] chest pain after 12 hours identified 86% of patients who experienced in-hospital MIs. The prognostic implication of persisting chest pain was also observed by Heng et al.[11] with a threefold increase in the risk of MI or death during hospitalization.

This prognostic significance of early recurrent chest pain is also recognized in recent studies and often dictates the medical management of patients. In a natural history study, Mulcahy et al.[15] identified early chest pain as the only predictive feature of subsequent cardiac events; they occurred in 35% of patients when present as compared with 13% when absent. In a study including a multivariate analysis of clinical, ECG, and angiographic characteristics, the recurrence of chest pain was retained as the single most powerful predictor of subsequent prognosis.[41]

The current understanding is that recurrent angina indicates no or incomplete control of the disease process and ongoing disease activity with the inherent risk of complications. This prognostic value of recurrent chest pain should be attenuated in the future as new and more efficient therapeutic will be developed. For these reasons, persistent ischemia can be regarded as a valid endpoint in clinical trials testing the efficacy of therapeutic interventions.

Electrocardiographic Changes

Ischemic ST-T changes present on the basal 12-lead ECG or on the ECG obtained during chest pain imply a worse prognosis. The changes could be ST-segment elevation, ST-segment depression, inversion of the T waves or pseudonormalization of a previously negative T wave. A particular pattern of ST-T changes in the anterior leads has been associated with a proximal left anterior descending coronary artery disease and an unfavorable clinical outcome.[42] ECG changes can be observed on the basal electrocardiogram. When present during chest pain, they add further discriminative power.[10] In one study, the combination of ischemic ECG changes and ongoing angina was associated with a risk of death of 23% at 1 month and of 42% at 1 year, as opposed to a risk of 5% at 2 years when absent.[43] This prognostic significance of ST-T changes is likely related to a greater likelihood of significant coronary artery disease to an ischemic zone that could be more extensive and to coronary artery lesions that could be more critical.

The information obtained from the ECG during chest pain, in addition to their prognostic significance, can also help in specific clinical situations, such as decision-making for coronary angioplasty and the diagnosis of early postinfarction ischemia. Schuster and Bulkley[32] distinguished ischemia in the infarct zone and ischemia at a distance. In the former, the transient ECG changes are located in the same leads as the original infarct, and in the latter, they are located in leads away from the original infarct. Ischemia in the infarct zone, as compared with ischemia at a distance, is more frequent in non-Q-wave MI (61% versus 36% of patients) and in anterior MI (63% versus 21%); it is less often associated with total occlusion coronary artery occlusion of the infarct-related artery (47% versus 71%). The pathophysiologic basis for ischemia in the infarct zone is thrombus formation, thrombolysis, and a residual significant stenosis.[44] On the other hand, ischemia at a distance is associated with more extensive coronary artery disease (2.6 ± 0.6 diseased vessel per patient versus 1.9 ± 0.7 with ischemia in the infarct zone). The underlying mechanism may be thrombotic coronary occlusion associated with multivessel disease and abrupt changes in the collateral circulation.[33] Chest pain when not associated with ECG signs of ischemia implies a better prognosis, close to the prognosis of patients without early postinfarction angina.[45]

Coronary Angiography

Coronary angiography, when analyzed in the traditional terms of extent and severity of the coronary artery lesions, shows a similar pattern of disease in unstable angina and in chronic stable angina. In both conditions, more extensive disease is associated with a worse prognosis. Eleven of the 12 patients who experienced either MI or death, or both, in a study of 188 patients by Alison et al.[40] had triple vessel disease and six had left main disease. Bertolasi et al.[23] reported no deaths in patients with single vessel disease during a 32-month follow-up study.

In an observational study of 217 patients with chest pain at rest and with ST-T changes,[46] the angiographic data were the most powerful predictors of mortality at 3 years; three of all variables analyzed were independent predictors of prognosis: left main disease, number of diseased vessels, and left ventricular end-diastolic pressure. The use of these three variables permitted subgroup risk estimates of death with respective mortality of 2%, 18% and 42% at 3 years. Fifty-nine percent of the patients included in this study had ST-segment elevation during chest pain, limiting extrapolation of the results to other populations.

The predictive value of the angiographic findings is

not however as transparent in all studies. Thus, the National Cooperative Study reported an inverted correlation between mortality and the number of diseased vessel.[47] In hospital, mortality was 6% with single vessel disease, 4% with two vessel disease and 0% with three vessel disease. This surprising trend persisted during follow-up with mortality rates of 11%, 6%, and 5%, respectively. In a recent prospective study of patients with recent-onset angina followed for a mean of 3 years, the clinical risk factors were the only predictors of new coronary events without a difference between subsets of patients with one, two, and three vessel disease. The extent of coronary artery disease was predictive only of more frequent bypass surgery. In this study, as in others, most of coronary events also occurred early after the acute episode of unstable angina.[48]

These results emphasize the limitations of the traditional analytic method of the coronary angiogram in unstable angina. The nonreproducible results noted, at least in the prediction of short-term prognosis, can be explained by the pathophysiologic mechanisms involved in unstable angina. The unstable state is a transient clinical state with an identifiable culprit coronary artery lesions, poorly described by the extent of coronary artery disease and better by the characteristics of the lesion; the site of the coronary lesion can, however, have an independent prognostic implication if it involves a substantial area of jeopardized myocardium; examples are left main or proximal left anterior descending coronary artery involvement. Following the acute phase, prognosis may be more influenced by the factors influencing the long-term prognosis of coronary artery disease.

The new approach for the interpretation of coronary angiography using quantitative angiography and morphologic and dynamic description of the culprit lesions have provided new insights on the pathophysiology and prognosis of unstable angina. These will be discussed in a following section.

Left Ventricular Function

Studies on left ventricular (LV) function have focused mainly on the angiographic findings and have suffered from the same limitations as coronary angiographic studies. As in coronary artery disease at large, a poorer LV function is associated with a worse prognosis, particularly in patients with more extensive coronary artery disease.[23,49] In one study of patients with vasospastic disease, a higher end-diastolic pressure was an independent predictor of prognosis.[46] In the Veterans Administration Cooperative Study for treatment of patients with unstable angina, LV function was an independent risk factor for long-term survival in medically treated patients; surgically treated patients had a better prognosis.[50] By contrast, in one other large nonrandomized study of surgically treated patients with unstable angina, LV function was not a significant independent risk factor of mortality.[51,52] Unstable angina is frequently associated with recurrent ischemia representing an ideal setting for the serial and noninvasive study of acute phase regional myocardial function and of the mechanisms involved in various pathophysiologic phenomena that remain to be investigated, such as the stunned and the hibernating myocardium.

NEWER INVESTIGATIONAL PROCEDURES AND PROGNOSIS

Recent insight gained in the understanding of the pathophysiologic mechanisms of unstable angina has stimulated the use of new investigational tools and diagnostic procedures. These have further contributed to our understanding of the mechanisms of the disease.

Unstable angina is the direct consequence of a primary decrease in coronary blood flow which is provoked by an abrupt progression in lumen obstruction at the site of an atherosclerotic coronary artery lesion. This rapid progression is caused by thrombus formation at the site of a plaque fissure or rupture.[53,54] Rarely, the abrupt occlusion will be caused by a coronary artery spasm.[55] This new understanding of the disease process has led to morphologic analysis of the culprit lesion using coronary angiography and coronary angioscopy, and to the study of blood markers of platelet aggregation of thrombus formation. Also better markers of myocardial ischemia have been investigated using 24-hour Holter monitoring and radionuclide imaging techniques.

Coronary Angiography and Coronary Angioscopy

Unstable angina is associated with angiographic evidence of rapid progression of coronary artery disease,[56,57] providing an explanation for the low predictive value of coronary angiography often reported previously. Culprit lesions are now identified that are complex, eccentric, irregular,[58] and often with intraluminal filling defect caused by intraluminal thrombi.[59] The presence of these complex lesions on the coronary angiogram are associated with more frequent and more severe episodes of ischemia and with an impaired early prognosis[58,60,61] independent of the presence of either multivessel or of minimal coronary artery disease; they often require an urgent revascularization procedure because of recurrent symptoms or because of the occurrence of in-hospital cardiac events.[60,61] The resolution of coronary angiography for the detection of the presence of intracoronary thrombosis remains not optimal and low[59]; it is expected that in the near future new techniques, such as coronary angioscopy and intravascular echography, will improve our diagnostic capability.

Holter Monitoring

The prognostic significance of recurrent myocardial ischemia, until recently based on the presence of chest pain, is now being expanded to a concept of total ischemic load that also includes the presence of silent ischemia. Ischemia is more often asymptomatic than symptomatic, as in stable angina. In one study of 135 patients studied with 24-hour Holter monitoring, a mean of 6.5 ±5.9 hours after the qualifying chest pain episode, ST-segment shifts were recorded in 66% of patients, with 92% of the 593 episodes being asymptomatic. The outcome was unfavorable in 48% of patients with ST-segment shifts compared with 20% of the patients without.[62] Other studies have also documented an unfavorable 1- and 6-month outcome with the presence of ≥1 hour of silent ischemia.[63–65] The variability in the incidence of ST-segment shift and in its prognostic value may however be greater in patients with unstable angina because of the unexpected course of the disease; thus, in some studies, the sensitivity of ST-segment shifts to detect subsequent coronary events was low.[66]

Radionuclide Perfusion Imaging

Radionuclide perfusion imaging with thallium-201 or with 99m-technetium Sestamibi can enhance the sensitivity of the electrocardiogram to detect the presence of myocardial ischemia, providing additional information in unstable angina. In patients with suspected unstable angina, single photon emission computed tomography (SPECT) studies obtained following the injection of 99m-technetium Sestamibi during an episode of chest pain had a sensitivity of 96% and a specificity of 79% for the detection of coronary artery disease as compared with sensitivities of 63% for the basal ECG and of 35% for the ECG obtained during pain.[67] Exercise thallium 201 perfusion defect and abnormal exercise test ECG are related to future MI and cardiac death in patients admitted with suspected MI but no cardiac enzyme elevation.[68] In stabilized patients with unstable angina, exercise thallium-201 is useful to evaluate long-term prognosis. In one study, 15 of 19 patients with thallium 201 developed MI or class 3 or 4 angina 12 weeks after discharge as compared with only two of 18 patients without redistribution defect.[69] A multivariate analysis which included clinical, electrocardiographic, and coronary angiographic data identified thallium 201 redistribu-

tion as the only independent significant predictor of cardiac death or nonfatal MI at 39 months, optimizing the prognostic value observed when considering the exercise test alone.[70] Another multivariate analysis including the results of 24-hour Holter monitoring obtained at admission and of coronary angiography at 5 days also retained the presence of a reversible exercise thallium perfusion defect predischarge as the only predictor of an unfavorable outcome at 6 months in patients without a previous MI. When patients with a previous MI were included, follow-up events could be better predicted by the size of the perfusion defect.[71]

The prognostic value of exercise testing and of scintigraphic studies are likely related to the high sensitivity of these tests to detect the presence and extent of coronary artery disease.[72] Dipyridamole scintigraphy may be an alternative to exercise scintigraphy in disabled patients or in patients at higher risk for dynamic exercise.[73] The procedure is safe and useful as a guide to diagnosis and probably to prognosis and management as well. Much remains to be learned, however, on the potential of radionuclide techniques for the evaluation of unstable angina. Thus a large proportion of patients shows perfusion defects on the scintigraphic studies obtained when pain free.[67] The significance of these defects and their natural history remain to be investigated.

Surrogate Markers of Blood Activation

In accordance with its thrombogenic pathogenesis, unstable angina is associated with in vivo evidences of platelet activation, thrombin generation and endogenous fibrinolysis.[74–76] Increases in fibrinopeptide A blood levels[77] and in the urinary metabolites of prostacyclin and of thromboxane A_2 have been correlated with the clinical activity of the disease.[74] A reduced blood activity of the tissue plasminogen activator with elevated levels of its rapid inhibitor was also found in patients with recurrent MI in long term studies.[78,79] The information that can be learned with the study of the blood markers of intravascular thrombus formation remain to be investigated. Potential exists for a better evaluation of the diagnosis, of the severity of the disease process, of the natural history and of the influence of treatment.[80]

INFLUENCE OF TREATMENT ON PROGNOSIS

The clinical application of the various forms of treatment in unstable angina patients has generally followed the demonstration of their efficacy in patients with stable angina pectoris and with AMI. Greater caution has generally been used because of the unstable state. However, the progress made in the aggressive investigation and management of acute coronary patients has accelerated the application of new treatment forms.

From an historical perspective, oral anticoagulants have first been used. Then, in a semisequential order, β-blockers, coronary artery bypass surgery, intravenous nitroglycerin, calcium antagonists, coronary angioplasty, heparin, and fibrinolytic agents have been evaluated. Variable influence on prognosis has been described with these interventions but not all have been adequately tested.

Antianginal Therapy

Nitrates

Although nitrates have been used early in unstable angina, the continuous intravenous use has been advocated only since 1979.[81] Many studies have now documented the benefit of the intravenous infusion for controlling chest pain episode; complete relief of pain occurs in two-thirds of patients.[82-84] However, none of the studies has documented a benefit in preventing MI and death.

The precise mechanisms leading to improvement are unclear but may be related to the hemodynamic, coronary vasodilating, and antiplatelet effects of nitroglycerin.[85] All these properties offer a potential for benefit. The side effects of nitroglycerin, including hypotension and headache, are easily controlled by titrating the perfusion rate. The rapid hemodynamic tachyphylaxis limiting the usefulness of continuous application of nitroglycerin in stable angina may not be as a limiting factor in unstable angina. Indeed, paradoxically, recurrence of chest pain is frequently observed following discontinuation of nitroglycerin, even after prolonged use; the mechanisms for this apparent rebound are not known. Also the observations that nitroglycerin could increase the required dose of heparin remains controversial.[86] Much remains to be learned on the role and mechanisms of benefit of nitroglycerin in unstable angina.

β-Blockers

Despite their wide use, only few studies have objectively documented the benefit of β-blockers in unstable angina. However, many decades of clinical experience and a few controlled studies have shown that they can reduce the rate of recurrent angina and possibly of MI. In one study, events occurred in 5 of 35 patients administered propranolol compared with 14 of 33 receiving placebo.[87] A few reports have suggested that β-blockers could exacerbate chest pain in patients

with Prinzmetal's variant angina, cautioning against their use in this syndrome. Their well-documented protective effect in AMI, however, strongly supports their use in other acute ischemic syndromes. Indeed, many of the trials published on AMI have included patients with "threatened myocardial infarction" and acute coronary insufficiency. A pooling of the results of these trials has suggested a 13% reduction in the risk of MI with the use of β-blockers.[89]

Calcium Antagonists

Calcium antagonists have been studied more extensively because of their property to relieve coronary artery spasm and the potential role of spasm in unstable angina that has been much emphasized during the late 1970s and early 1980s.[55] Many trials have shown that verapamil, nifedipine, and diltiazem could efficiently control the recurrence of coronary artery spasm in Prinzmetal's angina and the recurrence of chest pain in unstable angina. However, these drugs have generally failed to reduce the rate of MI and death.[90] In one study, diltiazem and propranolol had the same efficacy to control recurrent ischemia and to prevent cardiac events.[91] Other studies with nifedipine have shown an unfavorable trend,[92-94] but its combined use with a β-blocker was superior to either drug alone to prevent angina.[94] In one study involving patients with non-Q-wave MI, diltiazem reduced the incidence of early recurrent infarction.[31]

Intra-aortic Balloon Counterpulsation

Intra-aortic balloon counterpulsation is indicated in patients with recurrent symptoms, despite optimal medical therapy, and in hemodynamically unstable patients. It is usually used as a bridge to more definitive corrective therapy with coronary angioplasty or bypass surgery, although short-term use may favorably influence the longer term evolution on medical therapy.

Clot-Specific Treatment

Oral Anticoagulants

Four early uncontrolled, open-labeled trials have studied the effects of anticoagulants.[7,13,14,95] Although the four trials have suggested striking benefit, none should be judged as conclusive using actual criteria. The studies have however historical interest and the merit of suggesting a working hypothesis for future trials. In the study by Nichol et al.[95] of 318 patients treated with anticoagulants, the 30-day infarction rate was 6.6% and the mortality 1.6%. Beamish and Storrie[13] compared the follow-up at six months of 85 hospitalized patients treated with anticoagulants and 15 not hospitalized control patients. Two of the 85 treated patients suffered a myocardial infarction and none died; 12 of the 15 control patients experienced infarction and nine died. Wood[14] published 150 patients treated alternatively by admission sequence with or without anticoagulants. This study was stopped prematurely after the first 40 patients had been enrolled because of the benefit observed with the anticoagulants; the subsequent control patients were selected on the basis of a contraindication to the use of anticoagulants. After a follow-up of 2 months, myocardial infarction had occurred in 3% and death in 2% of the 100 treated patients, compared with 22% and 16%, respectively of the 50 control patients. In a study of 360 patients, Vakil[7] found that the 3-month incidence of MI was 36.3 in patients treated with anticoagulants and 49.4 in controls; mortality rates were 9.5% and 23.7%.

Antiplatelet Drugs

Four major trials have conclusively documented that aspirin can reduce the incidence of MI and of mortality in patients with unstable angina[96-98] (Table 9-3). One trial has shown similar benefit with another antiplatelet agent, ticlopidine.[99] The benefit is significant in the acute (less than 24 hours),[98] subacute (2 days to 3 months)[96,99] and more chronic phase (7 days to 3 years)[97] of the disease. The rate of combined fatal and nonfatal MI, with aspirin compared with placebo, was significantly reduced acutely from 12% to 3%, subacutely from 10% to 5%[96] and from 17% to 7%[99] and long-term from 17% to 9%. Thus, the relative benefits observed in the various studies are within the same range despite the differences in protocol design, patient characteristics, and doses of aspirin used. With ticlopidine, the benefit was similar with an event rate

of 7% compared with 13% with placebo after a follow-up of 6 months. Not all antiplatelet drugs share this benefit of aspirin, and no gain was apparent in trials using sulfinpyrazone[97] and prostacyclin.[101]

Heparin

The usefulness of heparin has also been documented in the acute phase of unstable angina (Table 9-3); in one study comparing β-blockers and heparin, the incidence of fatal and nonfatal MI was reduced from 16.7% with β-blockers to 3% with heparin[102]; in a second study, heparin reduced the event rate from 13.7% to 5.9%[103] and in another from 12% to 0.8%, providing additional benefit compared with aspirin.[98] Heparin and not aspirin can control severe recurrent ischemia.[98,104] In one study in which treatment was initiated relatively late, heparin significantly influenced the incidence of fatal and nonfatal MI only when combined with aspirin.[99]

Fibrinolytic Therapy

The role of fibrinolytic therapy in unstable angina remains to be more accurately defined and more specifically which patients will benefit from therapy. An early clinical study of 40 patients has suggested that fibrinolysis could be useful.[105] Other studies have shown fewer recurrent chest pain[106] with recombinant tissue plasminogen activator and improvement in anginal threshold but no differences in clinical outcome.[107] Overall a minority of patients, 10 to 20%, benefits clinically from therapy.[38] Control of symptoms is more apparent during the first 24 hours, with less benefit thereafter.[104]

Angiographic studies, however, have suggested more beneficial effects with a lower incidence of intracoronary thrombus.[106] The severity of the culprit, coronary artery stenosis, was significantly reduced from

TABLE 9-3. Specific Therapy in Unstable Angina

Investigators/Year	No. of Patients	Time of Entry[a] Early	Time of Entry[a] Late	Duration of Follow-up	Relative Risk	95% Confidence Limits
Antiplatelet drugs						
Lewis et al. (1983)[96]	1,266	—	X	3 mo	0.45	0.28–0.73
Cairns et al. (1985)[97]	555	—	X	18 mo	0.48	0.28–0.82
Théroux et al. (1988)[98]	479	X	—	5 d	0.29	0.08–0.80
RISC Study Group (1990)[99]	794	—	X	90 d	0.34	0.22–0.54
Balsano et al. (1990)[100]	657	—	X	6 mo	0.44	0.24–0.79
Heparin						
Telford and Wilson (1981)[102]	1,214	X	—	7 d	0.12	0.02–0.61
Théroux et al. (1988)[98]	479	X	—	5 d	0.06	0.01–0.49
RISC Study Group (1990)[99]	794	—	X	90 d	0.68	0.32–1.4

[a] See text for discussion.

$65 \pm 22\%$ to $51 \pm 19\%$ in one study[108] and nonsignificantly from $82 \pm 7\%$ to $73 \pm 10\%$ in another.[107] This improvement in angiographic findings in patients recatheterized 24 to 48 hours after treatment was no better, however, with fibrinolysis than with standard therapy with aspirin and heparin.[109]

A possible explanation for the relative failure of fibrinolysis in unstable angina is a transient beneficial effect outlasted by an ongoing active disease process; also, clot bound thrombin, exposed by partial fibrinolysis, could lead to further platelet aggregation and thrombus formation.

Revascularization Procedure

Coronary Artery Bypass Surgery

Coronary artery bypass surgery can be performed safely in unstable angina and can alleviate symptoms.[51,52] In hospitalized patients with recurrent symptoms on medical treatment, an attempt to a myocardial revascularization procedure is usually indicated. Bypass surgery can also provide long-term relief of angina; indeed, randomized trials comparing medical and surgical treatment have observed a better control of angina in surgically treated patients[47] and a better quality of life.[110] Furthermore, as many as 43% of medically treated patients in the various randomized trials have crossed over to surgery during follow-up because of recurrent angina.[47,111] Bypass surgery in these trials has nevertheless failed to reduce the rate of fatal and nonfatal MI,[47,112] except in subsets of patients. These subsets include patients with left main coronary artery disease (CAD) and patients with three vessel disease and impaired LV function.[50,111] The same subsets of patients with stable angina are helped by surgery, suggesting that the mechanisms for long-term improvement are more related to correction of the severity of the underlying CAD more than to the correction of the unstable angina process per se. Survival in patients with recurrent unstable angina in hospital despite optimal medical treatment is also probably improved by surgery; a randomized study is not possible in these patients, since they should have a revascularization procedure whenever possible to correct the recurrence of chest pain.

Coronary Angioplasty

Coronary angioplasty is now a valuable revascularization procedure that can relieve symptoms in unstable angina; the risk of major procedure-related complications is increased, however, as compared with patients with stable angina. This risk was initially reported to be 10%.[113] A recent report comparing the results of angioplasty in 406 stable angina and in 202 unstable angina patients confirmed the greater acute complication rate and also showed a higher cardiac event during the first week, 10.4% compared with 1.7% in patients with stable angina. Long-term quality of life was also worse in unstable angina patients with more frequent residual angina and more intensive medical treatment required.[114] The complication rate of coronary angioplasty in unstable angina can be reduced when the procedure is deferred 1 to 2 weeks after the acute episode.[115] These observations suggest that the mechanical intervention involved in coronary angioplasty could stimulate the pathophysiologic process triggering unstable angina resulting in an increased risk of acute thrombotic occlusion. Whether additional preventive measures in these patients could reduce the complication rate remain to be investigated. Studies have suggested that adjunctive treatment with a fibrinolytic agent could be useful in this regard.[116] A widely used approach is to defer the procedure of angioplasty of high risk lesion until after 1 week of treatment with heparin. The high primary success rate of angioplasty using low-profile balloon catheters and steerable guide wires is attractive for the management of unstable angina. Studies are now being conducted to test the efficacy of an aggressive management with surgery or angioplasty with and without fibrinolysis, by the Thrombolysis in Myocardial Ischemia (TIMI) study group.

PERSPECTIVES FOR THE FUTURE

The results published so far on the prognosis of unstable angina and the influence of treatment may appear somewhat confusing. When they are considered together with our new understanding of the mechanisms of the disease, however, a general overview can be drawn, and this overview can help orient future developments.

Clearly, unstable angina is an acute process complicating the course of a chronic disease. This acute process is associated with an immediate risk of thrombotic occlusion directly related to the instability of the coronary atherosclerotic plaque. Ongoing active disease is clinically manifested by recurrent ischemia and myocardial infarction. The risk of death is greater if a large coronary artery is involved and the amount of jeopardized myocardium extensive, compromising left ventricular function. Past the acute phase, prognosis is more related to the prognostic factors of CAD in general and influenced by the extent of CAD, LV function, and presence of risk factors. This distinction between the acute and chronic phases of the disease should be remembered when assessing prognosis of unstable angina and the influence of treatment. As discussed by Lubsen,[117] early entry trials differ from late entry trials and address different issues, different prognostic factors, and therefore different therapeutic interventions.

Early-entry trials deal with an acute thrombotic process. Valid endpoints are recurrent ischemia, myocardial infarction, and death. Few trials have specifically addressed these acute specific issues; fibrinolytic therapy is of limited benefit, aspirin is useful and reduces the rate of AMI, and heparin offers additional benefit to prevent MI and also prevents recurrent angina. The failure of angioplasty is not surprising, considering that the obstructive lesion is mainly thrombotic. At a later stage of the disease, the prognosis is more likely influenced by measures of secondary prevention and by correction of the obstructive coronary artery lesions. The successes of angioplasty and of surgery are not surprising in this regard.

A subacute phase of the disease can also be defined that shares the prognostic factors associated with both the acute and more chronic phases. Prognosis is then influenced by the severity of the CAD and by the instability of the plaque; this instability may persist for many days and may lead to rapid progression of coronary atherosclerosis. Prognosis could then be influenced by antiplatelet therapy and by myocardial preservation measures with β-blockers therapy and revascularization procedures. Other forms of therapy could also be useful. Future research in unstable angina will concentrate more on the acute and subacute disease processes. Standard treatment with aspirin and heparin too often fails defining a need for the investigation of more active and more specific antithrombotic therapy. Potent agents are now under development or at the early stages of clinical investigation. The most promising of these agents are the specific inhibitor of platelet receptors, IIIB-IIA and the specific thrombin inhibitors such as hirudin and related peptides. How these agents and others will influence the rapid progression of atherosclerosis associated with unstable angina remains an exciting field for future clinical investigation.

REFERENCES

1. Sampson JJ, Eliaser M, Jr: The diagnosis of impending acute coronary artery occlusion. Am Heart J 13:675, 1937
2. Feil H: Preliminary pain in coronary thrombosis. Am J Med Sci 193:42, 1937
3. Master AM, Dack S, Jaffe HL: Premonitory symptoms of acute coronary occlusion; a study of 260 cases. Ann Intern Med 14:115, 1941
4. Mounsy P: Prodromal symptoms in myocardial infarction. Br Heart J 13:215, 1951
5. Smith FJ, Keyes JW, Denham RM: Myocardial infarction: a study of the acute phase in 920 patients. Am J Med Sci 221:508, 1951
6. Levy H: The natural history of changing pattern of angina pectoris. Ann Intern Med 44:1123, 1956
7. Vakil RJ: Intermediate coronary syndrome. Circulation 24:557, 1961
8. Krauss KR, Hutter AM, De Sanctis RW: Acute coronary insufficiency course and follow-up. Circulation, suppl I 45:I-66, 1972
9. Fulton M, Lutz W, Donald KM et al: Natural history of unstable angina. Lancet 1:800, 1972
10. Gazes PC, Mobly FM, Faris HM et al: Pre-infarctional (unstable angina)—a prospective study—10 year follow-up. Prognostic significance of electrocardiographic changes. Circulation 48:331, 1973
11. Heng MK, Norris RM, Singh BN et al: Prognosis in unstable angina. Br Heart J 38:921, 1976
12. Duncan B, Fulton M, Morrison SL et al: Prognosis of new and worsening angina pectoris. Br Med J 1:981, 1976
13. Beamish RE, Storrie VM: Impending myocardial infarction. Recognition and management. Circulation 21:1107, 1960
14. Wood P: Acute and subacute coronary insufficiency. Br Med J 1:1779, 1961
15. Mulcahy R, Daly L, Graham L et al: Unstable angina: natural history and determinants of prognosis. Am J Cardiol 48:525, 1981
16. Fowler NO: "Preinfarctional" angina: a need for an objective definition and for a controlled clinical trial of its management. Circulation 44:755, 1971
17. Conti CR, Greene B, Pitt B et al: Coronary surgery in unstable angina pectoris, abstracted. Circulation, suppl II 44:II-154, 1971
18. Théroux P: A pathophysiologic basis for the clinical classification and management of unstable angina. Circulation, suppl V. 75:V-103, 1987
19. Braunwald E: Unstable angina. A classification. Circulation 80:410, 1989
20. Alison HW, Russell RO, Martle JA et al: Coronary anatomy and arteriography in patients with unstable angina. Am J Cardiol 41:204, 1978
21. Skjaeggestad O: The natural history of intermediate coronary syndrome. Acta Med Scand 193:533, 1973
22. Roberts KB, Califf RM, Harrell FE, Jr, et al: The prognosis for patients with new onset angina who have undergone cardiac catheterization. Circulation 68:970, 1983
23. Bertolasi CA, Tronge JE, Ricittelli MA et al: Natural history of unstable angina with medical or surgical therapy. Chest 70:596, 1976
24. Plotnic GD, Conti DR: Unstable angina: angiography, short and long term morbidity, mortality and symptomatic status of medically treated patients. Am J Med 63:870, 1977
25. Berk G, Kaplitt M, Padmanablan V et al: Management of preinfarction angina evaluation and comparison of medical vs surgical therapy in 43 patients. J Thorac Cardiovasc Surg 71:110, 1976
26. Cannon DS, Levy W, Cohen LS: The short- and long-term prognosis of patients with transmural and non-

transmural myocardial infarction. Am J Med 61:452, 1976

27. Hutter AM, Jr, De Sanctis RW, Flynn T, Yeatman LA: Nontransmural myocardial infarction: a comparison of hospital and late clinical course of patients with that of matched patients with transmural anterior and transmural inferior myocardial infarction. Am J Cardiol 48:595, 1981

28. Marmor A, Sobel BE, Roberts R: Factors presaging early recurrent myocardial infarction ("extension"). Am J Cardiol 48:603, 1981

29. Gibson RS, Beller GA, Gheorghiade M et al: The prevalence and clinical significance of residual myocardial ischemia 2 weeks after uncomplicated non-Q wave infarction: a prospective natural history study. Circulation 73:1186, 1986

30. Eisenberg PR, Lee RB, Biello DR et al: Chest pain after non-transmural myocardial infarction: the absence of remediable coronary spasm. Am Heart J 110:515, 1985

31. Gibson RS, Boden WE, Théroux P et al: Diltiazem and reinfarction in patients with non-Q wave myocardial infarction. Results of a double-blind, randomized multicenter trial. N Engl J Med 315:423, 1986

32. Schuster EH, Bulkley B: Early post-infarction angina: ischemia at a distance and ischemia in the infarct zone. N Engl J Med 305:1105, 1981

33. Bosch X, Théroux P, Waters D et al: Early postinfarction ischemia: clinical, angiographic, and prognostic significance. Circulation 75:988, 1987

34. Meyer J, Schmitz H, Kiesslich T et al: Percutaneous transluminal coronary angioplasty in patients with stable and unstable angina pectoris: analysis of early and late results. Am Heart J 106:973, 1983

35. Leimgruber PP, Roubin GS, Hollman J et al: Restenosis after successful coronary angioplasty in patients with single vessel. Circulation 73:710, 1986

36. Johnson MR, Brayden GP, Erickssen EE et al: Changes in cross-sectional area of coronary lumen in the 6 months after angioplasty: a quantitative analysis of the variable response to percutaneous transluminal angioplasty. Circulation 73:467, 1986

37. Rupprecht HJ, Brenneke R, Rottmeyer M et al: Short- and long-term outcome after PTCA in patients with stable and unstable angina. Eur Heart J 11:964, 1990

38. Lambert M, Kouz S, Campeau L: Preoperative and operative predictive variables of late clinical events following saphenous vein coronary artery bypass graft surgery. Can J Cardiol 5:87, 1989

39. Théroux P, Waters D: Unstable angina: special considerations in the post-bypass patient. p. 169. In Waters D, Bourassa MG, Brest AN (eds): Care of the Patient with Previous Coronary Bypass Surgery. Cardiovascular Clinics. FA Davis, Philadelphia, 1991

40. Waters DD, Walling A, Roy D et al: Previous coronary artery bypass grafting as an adverse prognostic factor in unstable angina pectoris. Am J Cardiol 58:465, 1986

41. Théroux P, Ouimet H, Latour JG et al: Prediction and prevention of myocardial infarction during the acute phase of unstable angina, abstracted. J Am Coll Cardiol 13:192A, 1989

42. de Zwaan C, Bär FW, Janssen JHA et al: Angiographic

and clinical characteristics of patients with unstable angina showing an ECG pattern indicating critical narrowing of the proximal LAD coronary artery. Am Heart J 117:657, 1989

43. Olson HG, Lyons KP, Aronow WS et al: The high risk angina patient. Identification by clinical features, hospital course, electrocardiography and technetium-99m stanneous pyrophosphate scintigraphy. Circulation 64:674, 1981

44. Boden WE, Bough EW, Benham I, Shulman RS: Unstable angina with episodic ST segment elevation and minimal creatine kinase release culminating in extensive, recurrent infarction. J Am Coll Cardiol 2:11, 1983

45. Bosch X, Théroux P, Pelletier GB et al: Clinical and angiographic features and prognostic significance of early postinfarction angina with and without electrocardiographic signs of transient ischemia. Am J Med 91:493, 1991

46. De Servi S, Berzuini C, Poma E et al: Long-term survival and risk stratification in patients with angina at rest undergoing medical treatment. Int J Cardiol 22:43, 1989

47. Russell RO, Moraski RE, Kouchoukos N et al: Unstable angina pectoris: National Cooperative Study Group to compare surgical and medical therapy. II. In-hospital mortality and initial follow-up results in patients with one, two and three vessel disease. Am J Cardiol 42:834, 1978

48. Castaner A, Roig E, Serra A et al: Risk stratification and prognosis of patients with recent onset angina. Eur Heart J 11:868, 1990

49. Plotnic GD, Conti DR: Unstable angina: angiographic, short and long term morbidity, mortality and symptomatic status of medically treated patients. Am J Med 63:870, 1977

50. Scott SM, Luchi RJ, Deupree RH and the Veterans Administration Unstable Angina Cooperative Study Group: Veterans Administration Cooperative Study for treatment of patients with unstable angina. Results in patients with abnormal left ventricular function. Circulation, suppl I. 78:I-113, 1988

51. McCormick JR, Schick EC, Jr, McCabe OH et al: Determinants of operative mortality and long-term survival in patients with unstable angina: the CASS experience. J Thorac Cardiovasc Surg 89:683, 1985

52. Rahimtoola SH, Nunley D, Grunkemeier G et al: Ten-year survival after coronary bypass surgery for unstable angina. N Engl J Med 308:676, 1983

53. Davies MJ, Thomas AC: Plaque fissuring—the cause of acute myocardial infarction, sudden ischemic death, and crescendo angina. Br Heart J 53:363, 1985

54. Falk E: Plaque rupture with severe pre-existing stenosis precipitating coronary thrombosis: characteristics of coronary atherosclerotic plaques underlying fatal occlusive thrombi. Br Heart J 50:127, 1983

55. Maseri A, L'Abbate A, Baroldi G et al: Coronary vasospasm as a possible cause of myocardial infarction: a conclusion derived from the study of "preinfarction" angina. N Engl J Med 299:1271, 1978

56. Moise A, Théroux P, Taeymans Y et al: Unstable angina and progression of coronary atherosclerosis. N Engl J Med 309:685, 1983

57. Ambrose JA, Winters SL, Arora RR et al: Angiographic evolution of coronary artery morphology in unstable angina. J Am Coll Cardiol 7:472, 1986
58. Ambrose JA, Winters SL, Stern A et al: Angiographic morphology and pathogenesis of unstable angina pectoris. J Am Coll Cardiol 5:609, 1985
59. Todd Sherman C, Litvack F, Grundfest W et al: Coronary angioscopy in patients with unstable angina pectoris. N Engl J Med 315:913, 1986
60. Williams AE, Freeman MR, Chisholm RJ et al: Angiographic morphology in unstable angina pectoris. Am J Cardiol 62:1024, 1988
61. Bugiardini R, Pozzati A, Borghi A et al: Angiographic morphology in unstable angina and its relation to transient myocardial ischemia and hospital outcome. Am J Cardiol 67:460, 1991
62. Langer A, Freeman MR, Armstrong PW: ST segment shift in unstable angina: pathophysiology and association with coronary anatomy and hospital outcome. J Am Coll Cardiol 13:1495, 1989
63. Gottlieb SO, Weisfeldt ML, Ouyang P et al: Silent ischemia as a marker for early unfavorable outcomes in patients with unstable angina. N Engl J Med 314:1214, 1986
64. Nademanee K, Intarachot V, Josephson MA et al: Prognostic significance of silent myocardial ischemia in patients with unstable angina. J Am Coll Cardiol 10:1, 1987
65. Arnim RV, Gerbig HW, Krawietz W, Höfling B: Prognostic implications of transient—predominantly silent—ischaemia in patients with unstable angina pectoris. Eur Heart J 9.435, 1988
66. Wilcox I, Freedman SB, Kelly DT, Harris PJ: Clinical significance of silent ischemia in unstable angina pectoris. Am J Cardiol 65:1313, 1990
67. Bilodeau L, Théroux P, Grégoire J et al: Technetium-99m Sestamibi tomography in patients with spontaneous chest pain: correlations with clinical, electrocardiographic, and angiographic findings. J Am Coll Cardiol 18:1684, 1991
68. Madsen JK, Stubgaard M, Utne HE et al: Prognosis and thallium-201 scintigraphy in patients admitted with chest pain without confirmed acute myocardial infarction. Br Heart J 59:184, 1988
69. Hillert MC, Narahara KA, Smitherman TC et al: Thallium-201 perfusion imaging after the treatment of unstable angina pectoris: relationship to clinical outcome. West J Med 145:335, 1986
70. Brown KA: Prognostic value of thallium-201 myocardial perfusion imaging in patients with unstable angina who respond to medical treatment. J Am Coll Cardiol 17:1053, 1991
71. Marmor JD, Freeman MR, Langer A, Armstrong PW: Prognosis in medically stabilized unstable angina: early Holter ST segment monitoring compared with pre-discharge exercise thallium tomography. Ann Intern Med 113:575, 1990
72. Freeman MR, Chisholm RJ, Armstrong PW: Usefulness of exercise electrocardiography and thallium scintigraphy in unstable angina pectoris in predicting the extent and severity of coronary artery disease. Am J Cardiol 62:1164, 1988
73. Zhu YY, Chung WS, Botvinick EH et al: Dipyridamole perfusion scintigraphy: the experience with its application in one hundred seventy patients with known or suspected unstable angina. Am Heart J 121:33, 1991
74. Fitzgerald DJ, Roy L, Catella F, Fitzgerald GA: Platelet activation in unstable coronary artery disease. N Engl J Med 315:983, 1986
75. Théroux P, Latour JG, Léger-Gauthier C, deLara J: Fibrinopeptide A and platelet factor levels in unstable angina pectoris. Circulation 75:156, 1987
76. Soria C, Soria J, Mirshahi M et al: Dynamic coronary fibrinolysis evaluation in patients with myocardial infarction and unstable angina by specific plasma fibrin degradation product determination. Thromb Res 45:383, 1987
77. Neri-Serneri GG, Gensini GI, Carnovali M et al: Association between time of increased fibrinopeptide A levels in plasma and episodes of spontaneous angina: a controlled prospective study. Am Heart J 113:672, 1987
78. Hamsten A, Wiman B, de Faire U, Blombäck M: Increased plasma levels of a rapid inhibitor of tissue plasminogen activator in young survivors of myocardial infarction. N Engl J Med 313:1557, 1985
79. Gram J, Jespersen J: A selective depression of tissue plasminogen activator (t-PA) activity in euglobulins characterizes a risk group among survivors of acute myocardial infarction. Thromb Haemost 57:137, 1987
80. Grande P, Grauholt AM, Madsen JK: Unstable angina pectoris. Platelet behavior and prognosis in progressive angina and intermediate coronary syndrome. Circulation, suppl I. 81:I–16, 1990
81. Dauwe F, Affaki G, Waters DD et al: Intravenous nitroglycerin in refractory unstable angina. Am J Cardiol 43. 416, 1979
82. Curfman GD, Heinsimer JA, Lozner EC et al: Intravenous nitroglycerin in the treatment of spontaneous angina pectoris: a prospective randomized trial. Circulation 67:276, 1983
83. Kaplan K, Davidson R, Parker M et al: Intravenous nitroglycerin for the treatment of angina at rest unresponsive to standard nitrate therapy. Am J Cardiol 51:694, 1983
84. Flaherty JT: Usefulness of intravenous and transdermal nitroglycerin therapy in patients with unstable angina. Am Heart J 112:220, 1986
85. Diodati J, Théroux P, Latour JG et al: Effects of nitroglycerin at therapeutic doses on platelet aggregation in unstable angina pectoris and acute myocardial infarction. Am J Cardiol 66:683, 1990
86. Bode V, Welzel D, Franz G, Blensky U: Absence of drug interaction between heparin and nitroglycerin: randomized, placebo-controlled crossover study. Arch Intern Med 150:2117, 1990
87. Mizgala HF, Tinmouth AC, Waters DD et al: Prospective controlled trial of long term propranolol on acute coronary events in patients with unstable coronary artery disease, abstracted. Circulation, suppl III. 50:III–933, 1974
88. Robertson D, Alastair JJ, Vaughn WK, Robertson RM: Exacerbation of vasotonic angina pectoris by propranolol. Circulation 62:281, 1982

89. Yusuf S, Peto R, Lewis J et al: Betablockade during and after myocardial infarction: an overview of randomized trials. Prog Cardiovasc Dis 27:335, 1985

90. Held PH, Yusuf S, Furberg CD: Calcium channel blockers in acute myocardial infarction and unstable angina: an overview. Br Med J 299:1187, 1989

91. Théroux P, Taeymans Y, Morissette D et al: A randomized study comparing propranolol and diltiazem in unstable angina. J Am Coll Cardiol 5:717, 1985

92. Gerstenblith G, Ouyang P, Achuff SC et al: Nifedipine in unstable angina: a double-blind randomized trial. N Engl J Med 306:885, 1982

93. Muller JE, Turi ZG, Pearle DF et al: Nifedipine and conventional therapy for unstable angina pectoris. Circulation 69:728, 1984

94. Holland Interuniversity Nifedipine-Metoprolol trial (HINT) Research Group: Early treatment of unstable angina in the coronary care unit: a randomized, double-blind placebo-controlled comparison of recurrent ischemia in patients treated with nifedipine or metoprolol or both. Br Heart J 56:400, 1986

95. Nichol ES, Phillips WC, Casten GL: Virtue of prompt anticoagulant therapy in impending myocardial infarction: experiences with 318 patients during a 10-year period. Ann Intern Med 50:1158, 1959

96. Lewis HD, Davis JW, Archibald GD et al: Protective effects of aspirin against acute myocardial infarction and death in men with unstable angina. N Engl J Med 309:396, 1983

97. Cairns JA, Gent M, Singer J et al: Aspirin, sulfinpyrazone, or both in unstable angina. N Engl J Med 313:1369, 1985

98. Théroux P, Ouimet H, McCans J et al: Aspirin, heparin, or both to treat acute unstable angina. N Engl J Med 319:1105, 1988

99. RISC Study Group: Risk of myocardial infarction and death during treatment with low dose aspirin and intravenous heparin in men with unstable coronary artery disease. Lancet 2:827, 1990

100. Balsano F, Rizzon P, Violi F et al: Antiplatelet treatment with ticlopidine in unstable angina. A controlled multicenter clinical trial. Circulation 82:17, 1990

101. Théroux P, Latour JG, Diodati J et al: Hemodynamic, platelet and clinical responses to prostacyclin in unstable angina pectoris. Am J Cardiol 65:1084, 1990

102. Telford AM, Wilson C: Trial of heparin versus atenolol in prevention of myocardial infarction in intermediate coronary syndrome. Lancet 1:1225, 1981

103. Williams DO, Kirby MG, McPherson K, Phear DM: Anticoagulant treatment of unstable angina. Br J Clin Pract 10:114, 1986

104. Neri Serneri GG, Gensini GR, Poggesi L et al: Effect of heparin, aspirin, or alteplase in reduction of myocardial ischemia in refractory unstable angina. Lancet 1:615, 1990

105. Lawrence JB, Shepard JT, Bone I et al: Fibrinolytic therapy in unstable angina pectoris—a controlled clinical trial. Thromb Res 17:767, 1990

106. Gold HK, Johns JA, Leinbach RC et al: A randomized, blinded, placebo-controlled trial of recombinant tissue-type plasminogen activator in patients with unstable angina. Circulation 75:1192, 1987

107. Nicklas JM, Topol EJ, Kander N et al: Randomized, double-blind, placebo-controlled trial of tissue plasminogen activator in unstable angina. J Am Coll Cardiol 13:434, 1989

108. de Zwaan C, Bar I, Jansen H et al: Effect of thrombolytic therapy in unstable angina pectoris: clinical and angiographic results. J Am Coll Cardiol 12:301, 1988

109. Williams DO, Topol EJ, Califf RM et al: Intravenous recombinant tissue-type plasminogen activator in patients with unstable angina pectoris. Circulation 82:376, 1990

110. Booth DC, Deupree RH, Hultgren HN et al: Quality of life after bypass surgery for unstable angina. Five-year follow-up results of a Veterans Affairs Cooperative study. Circulation 83:87, 1991

111. Parisi AF, Khuri S, Deupree RH et al: Medical compared with surgical management of unstable angina. Five-year mortality and morbidity in the Veterans Administration Study. Circulation 80:1176, 1989

112. Luchi RJ, Scott SM, Deupree RH et al: Comparison of medical and surgical treatment for unstable angina. N Engl J Med 316:977, 1987

113. de Feyter PJ, Suryapranata H, Serruys PW et al: Coronary angioplasty for unstable angina: immediate and late results in 200 consecutive patients with identification of risk factors for unfavorable early and late outcome. J Am Coll Cardiol 12:324, 1988

114. Rupprecht HJ, Brennecke R, Kottmeyer M: Short- and long-term outcome after PTCA in patients with stable and unstable angina. Eur Heart J 11:964, 1990

115. Myler RK, Shaw RE, Stertzer SH et al: Unstable angina and coronary angioplasty. Circulation, suppl II. 82: II–88, 1990

116. Suryapranata H, de Feyter PJ, Serruys PW: Coronary angioplasty in patients with unstable angina pectoris: is there a role for thrombolysis. J Am Coll Cardiol 12:69A, 1988

117. Lubsen J: Medical management of unstable angina. What have we learned from the randomized trials? Circulation, suppl II. 82:II–82, 1990

10

Risk Assessment and Prognosis of Patients Admitted to the Coronary Care Unit With Suspected Myocardial Infarction

Jan Kyst Madsen

In approximately 50% of all patients admitted with suspicion of acute myocardial infarction (AMI) attributable to chest pain, AMI is not confirmed.[1-3] This group represents several subgroups of patients (e.g., unstable angina, noncardiac chest pain, angina, or possible angina). The purpose of this chapter is to describe the diagnostic possibilities, prognosis after discharge, and therapeutic consequences, with emphasis on the patients in whom the chest pain is of coronary or possible coronary origin (i.e., angina or possible angina). In this chapter, these patients are termed non-AMI patients.

NATURAL HISTORY OF CCU ADMISSIONS

Of patients admitted because of suspected AMI, several subgroups are emerging during admission:

AMI (45%)
Noncardiac chest pain (5%)
Cardiac noncoronary chest pain (5%)
Angina or possible angina, including unstable angina (45%) (non-AMI patients)

The percentages (in parentheses) denote the approximate proportion of all patients admitted to a coronary care unit (CCU) suspected of AMI.[4] These figures are the result of routine observations.

Acute Myocardial Infarction

The definition of AMI is well agreed on, but otherwise there are no published studies of systematic evaluation of all organs that may cause chest pain.

TABLE 10-1. History of Previous AMI, Angina Pectoris, and Heart Failure in Non-AMI Patients

Investigators	Previous AMI(%)	Angina Pectoris(%)	Heart Failure(%)
Dussia et al.[1]	46	—	—
Nordlander and Nyquist[12]	34	69	5
Schroeder et al.[13]	41	52	—
Madsen and Hansen[14]	29	33	19
Engby et al.[15]	38	75	—
Lindberg et al.[16]	42	69	31
Madsen et al.[2]	25	36	20
Herlitz et al.[9,20]	24	36	15
Herlitz et al.[17]	21	36	c.19

Noncardiac Chest Pain

The group with noncardiac chest pain includes patients with pneumonia, pulmonary embolism, duodenal or ventricular ulcer, back pain, thoracic facet syndrome, intercostal myoses, esophageal disorders, and other diseases. The importance of routine examinations is yet to be determined; however, there are indications that esophageal disorders are underdiagnosed.[5,6] Patients with noncardiac chest pain have no increased mortality compared with the background population[4]; however, there are no available studies on their morbidity or functional status after discharge.

Cardiac Noncoronary Chest Pain

The group with cardiac, noncoronary chest pain includes patients with arrhythmias, valve diseases, cardiomyopathies, or pericarditis. Arrhythmias are apparently the most common cause.[4,7,8]

Angina or Possible Angina, Non-AMI

The remaining group, those with angina or possible angina, non-AMI, includes patients with unstable angina that has been stabilized during admission, patients with angina or previous AMI, and patients with no history of angina, previous AMI, and no unstable angina during admission. The admission period is usually short, 2 to 4 days, with the exception of patients with severe unstable angina. The in-hospital mortality is low, less than 2%,[2,9] although not always uncomplicated, as up to 37% may require some kind of intervention.[3]

PREVALENCE OF ISCHEMIC HEART DISEASE

A history of previous AMI is found in 21 to 46% and of angina pectoris in 33 to 75% of non-AMI patients (Table 10-1). Results of noninvasive investigations are currently available from only one study.[10,11] The

TABLE 10-2. Results of Noninvasive Investigations and Subsequent 1-Year Risk of AMI or Cardiac Death

	Abnormality Present (%)	1-year risk (%) (Abnormality)		p^a
		Present	Not Present	
ECG at rest (n = 217)				
Q wave	13	11	6	0.24
Negative T wave	30	15	3	<0.001
ST depression	11	22	5	<0.01
Any abnormality	37	13	3	<0.001
Exercise ECG (n = 215)				
Abnormal ST response	27	14	3	0.009
Angina during exercise	23	12	5	0.009
ECG, rest or exercise (n = 215)	45	13	2	<0.001
Abnormal at rest, during exercise, or both				
Thallium scintigraphy (n = 158)				
Persistent defect	30	6	6	0.51
Transient defect	18	17	2	0.001
Holter monitoring (n = 198)				
Premature ventricular beats	65	12	4	0.38
Pairs of PVBs	10	20	5	0.01
Chest radiography (n = 215)				
Cardiomegaly	41	12	3	0.03
Echocardiography (n = 136)				
Mitral-septal separation >5 mm	27	15	4	0.055

[a] p values for log-rank comparison of risk curves.

TABLE 10-3. One-Year Mortality and AMI Morbidity After Discharge in Non-AMI Patients

Investigators	Mortality	AMI Morbidity	AMI or Cardiac Death	No. of Patients
Dussia et al. (1976)[1]	10.4	—	—	138
Nordlander and Nyquist (1979)[12]	19	7	—	193
Schroeder et al. (1980)[13,a]	c.6	c.10	12.6	88
Madsen and Hansen (1982)[14]	11.8	—	—	93
Engby et al. (1985)[15]	16.2	10	—	130
Lindberg et al. (1985)[16]	4	—	—	81
Madsen et al. (1987)[2]	5.1	6.7	8.7	257
Herlitz et al. (1990)[17,b,c]	5.0–6.3	5.3–8.5	—	1,274
Launbjerg et al. (1991)[18,b,c]	8.8	—	—	7,080

[a] Non-AMI defined as transient ST- or T-wave changes without the development of Q waves.
[b] Analysis of patients in multicenter intervention trial.
[c] This study distinguishes between no infarction and possible infarction.

major results from electrocardiography (ECG) at rest and during exercise, thallium scintigraphy, Holter monitoring, echocardiography, and chest radiography are shown in Table 10-2. The most sensitive parameter regarding ischemia (i.e., transient defect on thallium scintigraphy) was present in 18%.[11] The prevalence of heart failure was not well defined, as only M-mode echo and chest radiography were used. However, in general, the results indicate that approximately one-half the non-AMI patients have coronary heart disease (CHD). As discussed later in this chapter, the proportion with CHD may vary according to local circumstances.

PROGNOSIS AFTER DISCHARGE

The risk of AMI or cardiac death, after 1 year, is 4 to 19% in non-AMI patients[1,2,9,12–18] (Table 10-3). The variability between these results is partly explained by differences in patient populations. Studies that include elderly patients[12,15] or that have a high proportion of patients with previous AMI or angina pectoris[12,15] (Table 10-1) tend to find the worst prognosis (Table 10-3).

The impaired prognosis in non-AMI patients is emphasized by the close resemblance to that of AMI patients admitted during the same period. The mortality and AMI morbidity are only slightly lower in non-AMI that in AMI patients[2,13–15] (Figs. 10-1 and 10-2). The mortality in non-AMI patients, during the first year after discharge, is three to seven times higher than expected, as compared with a background population with the same age and sex distribution.[2,14,15,18] The long-term prognosis is less well described. However, as in AMI patients, the mortality in the second year and onward is less than in the first year. Compared with the background population, the mortality is increased, but not as much as in AMI patients[2,13,18,19] (Fig. 10-3).

MORBIDITY AFTER DISCHARGE

Information on morbidity, other than AMI, has only been reported in two publications.[17,20] Despite the very low mortality found in this study compared with others, the non-AMI patients had a high incidence of chest pain and after 5 years medicinal use.[20] Angina-like chest pain was experienced by 54% of patients at least once a week, and 25% daily. β-Blockers were used in 54%, calcium antagonists in 6.1%. The rate of bypass surgery was only 2.6, which, however, mainly reflects the limited use of the procedure in Sweden during the early 1980s.[20]

Chest pain and medicinal use were highest in the patients with a history of CHD. These studies emphasize that non-AMI patients with signs of CHD need close follow-up after discharge.

DEFINITION OF HIGH- AND LOW-RISK GROUPS

Most studies of non-AMI patients are retrospective or include only information from medical history and ECG without further examination. These studies indicate that non-AMI patients with a history of AMI,[12,14,15,17] angina pectoris,[12,14,17] ST-T abnormalities,[12,14,16,17] or diabetes[12,17] are at higher risk than patients without these entities. Conversely, patients without signs of CHD have an excellent prognosis.[8]

Our own detailed prospective study confirms the above findings.[2] When the prognosis is related to the results of noninvasive investigations, an increased risk is clearly associated with the presence of signs of CHD[10,11] (Table 10-2). Multivariate analysis of medical history, gender, age, and ECG on admission indicates two variables with independent significant prognostic information[2]: (1) previous AMI or angina, or both; and (2) transient or permanent ST or T abnormalities or intraventricular block on admission.

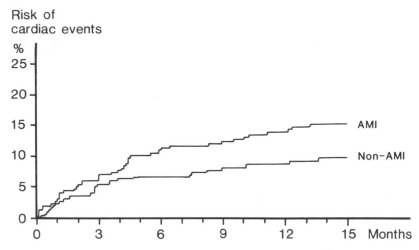

Fig. 10-1. Risk of acute myocardial infarction (AMI) or cardiac death in 275 patients with confirmed AMI and in 257 patients without confirmed AMI, with non noncardiac or cardiac noncoronary cause of chest pain (i.e., patients with coronary or possible coronary chest pain (non-AMI) (p = 0.05). (From Madsen,[4] with permission.)

High-risk groups may be identified by noninvasive investigation. Resting ECG abnormalities, angina, ST changes, and low increase in the rate-pressure product on exercise testing, transient defects on thallium scintigraphy (Fig. 10-4); couplets on Holter monitoring, increased mitral-septal separation on echocardiography, or cardiomegaly on chest radiography are all indicative of increased risk of AMI or cardiac death.[10,11]

Multivariate analysis, including variables from the medical history, admission period, and noninvasive investigations, reveals one variable with independent significant prognostic information: the combination of ECG at rest (resting ECG) and during exercise. The risk of AMI or cardiac death was increased 12-fold in patients with abnormal resting ECG (Q wave, ST deviation, negative T wave, or intraventricular block) or an abnormal ST response during exercise, compared with patients with a normal ECG during rest and exercise[10] (Fig. 10-5). When exercise testing was evaluated only in the patients with a normal resting ECG, an

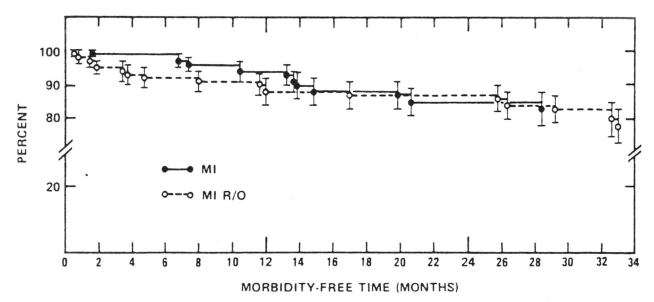

Fig. 10-2. Myocardial-infarction-free curve after discharge in 78 patients with acute myocardial infarction (AMI) (MI) and 88 patients without confirmed AMI (MI R/O). (From Schroeder et al.,[13] with permission.)

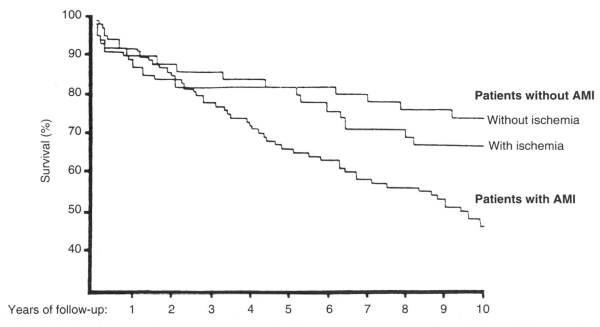

Fig. 10-3. Survival from 28 days after discharge in 175 acute myocardial infarction (AMI) and 123 non-AMI patients. (From Smyllie,[19] with permission.)

abnormal ST response had significant prognostic importance in this group too.[10]

The prognostic importance of left ventricular (LV) dysfunction may be underestimated, since precise methods such as two-dimensional echocardiography or isotope ventriculography has not been employed. Furthermore, the importance of silent ischemia on Holter monitoring has not been evaluated. The prognostic importance of risk factors has not been prospectively evaluated so far. From the above studies, it is evident that in non-AMI patients (i.e., patients admitted to a CCU with no AMI and no overt noncardiac or noncoronary cause of chest pain), high- and low-risk groups can be identified on discharge:

High-risk patients are those with signs of CHD (i.e., previous AMI, angina pectoris, permanent or transient ST changes on admission or an abnormal ECG at rest or during exercise test). Low-risk patients are those with no signs of CHD, either from history or on noninvasive investigations.

The prognosis in patients with unstable angina (i.e., angina at rest accompanied by transient ST or T

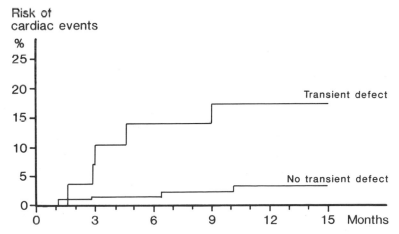

Fig. 10-4. Risk of acute myocardial infarction (AMI) or cardiac death in non-AMI patients in relation to the results of thallium scintigraphy, n = 158 (p = 0.001). (From Madsen,[4] with permission.)

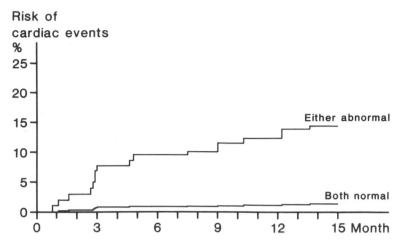

Fig. 10-5. Risk of acute myocardial infarction (AMI) or cardiac death in relationship to ECG at rest and during exercise, n = 257 (see text) (p < 0.001). (From Madsen,[4] with permission.)

changes is well described (see Chapter 9). The 1-year mortality after discharge is about 10%. Patients with unstable angina that has been stabilized during admission constituted about 14% of the non-AMI patients and accounted for 23% of later AMIs or cardiac deaths, in one study.[2] This shows that unstable angina during admission is a high-risk group, but not the only one.

MANAGEMENT OF NON-AMI PATIENTS

The "natural history" of non-AMI patients certainly depends on admission practice. In hospitals where only patients with definite ECG changes on admission are admitted to the CCU, almost all non-AMI patients will probably have CHD—and consequently a high risk following discharge. In other hospitals with a more "liberal" admission policy—more than two-thirds may be non-AMI patients, which means less patients with ischemic heart disease among these—and probably a lower risk for the whole group. However, most hospitals in North America, Europe, and the rest of the Western world use almost similar procedures; it is reasonable to assume that the prognostic information from the noninvasive investigations is about the same in all hospitals. Non-AMI patients should consequently be evaluated on discharge. Following the acute admission because of chest pain, they are usually highly motivated for necessary examinations or interventions. Furthermore, by examining non-AMI patients, a high-risk group is easily identified without the need of expensive population screening. The high-risk non-AMI patients actually present themselves to the physicians. It is advisable that all non-AMI pa-

tients be evaluated as high- or low-risk patients on discharge as described above. Medical history, resting ECG, and an exercise test are sufficient for routine purposes.

MANAGEMENT OF LOW-RISK PATIENTS

These patients should be assured of their excellent prognosis and the benign nature of their chest pain. Thus, heart neuroses and unnecessary CCU admissions or consultations may be avoided. There is no indication for any medical treatment.

MANAGEMENT OF HIGH-RISK PATIENTS

All high-risk patients should be treated with aspirin, 150 to 300 mg/day, for their lifetime in agreement with studies of "unstable angina," where a wide definition of this entity was used.[21,22] Medical treatment with antianginal drugs should be given depending on symptoms. β-Blockers[23] or calcium antagonists,[24] which lower mortality in AMI patients, may have the same effect in non-AMI patients, but this has not been shown in controlled studies and is accordingly not indicated as prophylaxis. Coronary arteriography and subsequent percutaneous transluminal coronary angioplasty (PTCA) or coronary bypass should be performed following usual guidelines according to symptoms. Risk factors should be controlled as in other patients with CHD.

CONCLUSION

Patients admitted to CCUs for chest pain, without AMI, and without an overt noncardiac or cardiac but noncoronary cause of chest pain, constitute almost 50% of all admissions. These non-AMI patients have an overall risk of AMI or cardiac death after discharge, only slightly lower than that of AMI patients. Medical history and exercise testing can easily distinguish between high- and low-risk patients.

What actually causes the pain that led to admission is uncertain. In the patients who turn out to have CHD, it may be a slight attack of unstable angina or just angina. In the remaining patients, more thorough examinations may indicate more extracardiac causes than are currently diagnosed. Low-risk non-AMI patients have no history of ischemic heart disease and a normal ECG both at rest and during exercise. They should be discharged with assurance of the benign nature of their chest pain and their excellent prognosis. High-risk patients have a history or have signs of CHD. All these patients should be followed closely after discharge and treated with aspirin. Risk factors should be controlled. Antianginal medication, PTCA, or bypass surgery should be performed according to symptoms.

REFERENCES

1. Dussia EE, Cromartie D, McCreaney J et al: Myocardial infarction with and without documentation—one year prognosis. Am Heart J 92:148, 1976
2. Madsen JK, Thomsen BL, Sørensen JN et al: Risk factors and prognosis after discharge for patients admitted because of suspected acute myocardial infarction with and without confirmed diagnosis. Am J Cardiol 59:1064, 1987
3. Fesmire FM, Wears RL, Percy RF: In hospital outcome in patients with coronary artery disease in whom myocardial infarction has been ruled out. N Engl J Med 320:1423, 1989
4. Madsen JK: Acute chest pain and prognostic aspects. p. 216. In Thygesen K, Kjekshus J (eds): Myocardial Ischaemia. Blackwell, Oxford, 1990
5. Davies HA, Jones DB, Rhodes J. "Esophageal angina" as the cause of chest pain. JAMA 248:2274, 1982
6. Launbjerg J, Fruergaard P, Jørgensen FB et al: Prognosis and diagnostic work-up in patients admitted for, but without, myocardial infarction—the value of nuclear medicine examinations. Clin Phys 10:273, 1990
7. Ahnve S: Noninfarction cases without previously known ischemic heart disease admitted to a coronary care unit. Eur J Cardiol 9:307, 1979
8. Wilcox RG, Roland JM, Hampton JR: Prognosis of patients with "chest pain? cause." Br Med J 282:431, 1981
9. Herlitz J, Hjalmarson Å, Karlson BW, Bengtson A: 5-year mortality rate in patients with suspected acute myocardial infarction in relation to early diagnosis. Cardiology 75:250, 1988
10. Madsen JK, Thomsen BL, Mellemgaard K, Hansen JF: Independent prognostic risk factors for patients admitted because of suspected acute myocardial infarction without confirmed diagnosis. Prognosis after discharge in relation to medical history and non-invasive investigations. Eur Heart J 9:610, 1988
11. Madsen JK, Stubgaard M, Utne HE et al: Prognosis and Thallium-201 scintigraphy in patients admitted with chest pain without confirmed acute myocardial infarction. Br Heart J 59:184, 1988
12. Nordlander R, Nyquist O: Patients treated in a coronary care unit without acute myocardial infarction. Br Heart J 41:647, 1979
13. Schroeder JS, Lamb IH, Hu M: Do patients in whom myocardial infarction has been ruled out have a better prognosis after hospitalization than those surviving infarction? N Engl J Med 303:1, 1980
14. Madsen JK, Hansen JF: The prognosis for patients admitted to a coronary care unit due to suspected acute myocardial infarction with and without confirmed diagnosis. Acta Med Scand 211:453, 1982
15. Engby B, Strunge P, Olsen J: The prognosis for patients referred with suspected acute myocardial infarction. Acta Med Scand 217:465, 1985
16. Lindberg K, Nyquist O, Edhag O: The significance of ST and T changes for the development of coronary events in patients with acute coronary chest pain, treated in a coronary care unit without verified acute myocardial infarction. Acta Med Scand 217:559, 1985
17. Herlitz J, Karlson BW, Hjalmarson Å: Mortality and morbidity during one year of follow-up in suspected acute myocardial infarction in relation to early diagnosis. experiences from the MIAMI trial. J Intern Med 228:125, 1990
18. Launbjerg J, Fruergaard P, Madsen JK, Hansen JF, the Danish Study Group on Verapamil in Myocardial Infarction: Three-year mortality in patients suspected of acute myocardial infarction with and without confirmed diagnosis. Am Heart J (in press)
19. Smyllie HC: Prognosis of patients discharged from a coronary care unit. Br Med J 293:541, 1986
20. Herlitz J, Hjalmarson Å, Karlson BW, Nyberg G: Long-term morbidity in patients where the initial suspicion of myocardial infarction was not confirmed. Clin Cardiol 11:209, 1988
21. Lewis HD, Davis JW, Archiebald DG et al: Protective effects of aspirin against acute myocardial infarction or death in men with unstable angina. N Engl J Med 309:396, 1983
22. Cairns JA, Gent M, Singer J et al: Aspirin, sulfinpyrazone, or both in unstable angina. N Engl J Med 313:1369, 1985
23. Beta-Blocker Heart Attack Trial Research Group: A randomized trial of propranolol in patients with acute myocardial infarction. JAMA 247:1707, 1982
24. The Danish Study Group on Verapamil in Myocardial Infarction: The effect of verapamil on mortality and major events after myocardial infarction. Am J Cardiol 66:779, 1990

11
Prognosis and Risk Assessment of Patients With Myocardial Infarction

Robin M. Norris

THE CHANGING NATURAL HISTORY OF ACUTE MYOCARDIAL INFARCTION

Mortality rates from coronary heart disease (CHD) have been falling since the mid-1960s in many Western countries, the fall in mortality being approximately 3% per year in the United States.[1] It is clear from the literature and from the personal experience of many physicians that in-hospital mortality rate from acute myocardial infarction (AMI) has been declining to a similar degree over the past 25 years. However, reports from different groups working at different hospitals with varying admission patterns make this improvement difficult to document in a quantitative way. In Auckland, New Zealand, we have a unique data set on prognosis[2–16] that spans the era of "therapeutic nihilism" that preceded the introduction of coronary care units (CCUs) on the one hand and includes the "therapeutic revolution" caused by thrombolytic therapy on the other. The data have been collected by the present author and associates, using constant criteria for the diagnosis of myocardial infarction from a group of hospitals to which admission patterns did not change to

any significant extent over the period of data collection.

The evidence from our studies that secular changes in mortality from AMI have paralleled secular changes in community mortality from CHD is summarized in Figures 11-1 and 11-2, which show, respectively, changes in acute survival from myocardial infarction (MI) in hospitals in Auckland, during five periods between 1966 and 1988, and long-term survival of patients after discharge from hospital during 1966, 1981, and 1984 to 1986.

During a 1-year period (1966 to 1967), we recorded the deaths of all 757 patients with AMI who were admitted to hospitals in Auckland,[2,3] and we followed their progress at 3 years,[5] 6 years,[7] 15 years,[8] and 20 years[9] after the index infarction. During 1966, there was no CCU in Auckland and, although six patients were resuscitated from ventricular fibrillation at one of the participating hospitals, they were considered as having died for the purposes of the mortality analysis. Twenty-six percent of these patients died in-hospital[2]; hospital mortality for patients under 70 years of age was 22%.[4] Fifty-two percent of these deaths were due to arrhythmias or presumed arrhythmias and, of these, two-thirds occurred from the fourth day of hos-

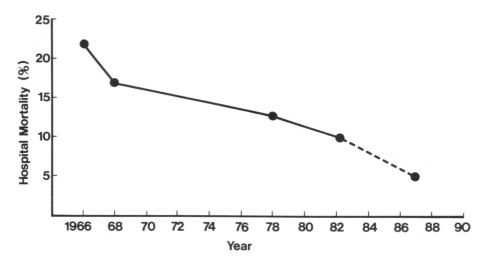

Fig. 11-1. Decline in mortality from acute myocardial infarction (AMI) in Auckland hospitals from 1966 to the present. Mortality percentages refer to patients under 70 years of age and are based on experience with (from left to right) 545 patients treated outside a coronary care unit (CCU) during 1966–1967,[3] 300 patients treated after opening of a CCU during 1967–1968,[4] 574 patients treated in a CCU during 1977–1979,[10] 719 patients treated during 1981–1984,[19] and 428 patients who received thrombolysis between 1984 and 1988.[15] The last group excludes patients with contraindications to thrombolysis (principally a known or suspected bleeding tendency) and patients diagnosed on admission to hospital as having subendocardial infarction, but does not exclude patients with cardiogenic shock. (Modified from Norris,[16] with permission.)

pital admission onward.[2] This pattern of mortality was similar to that described from other centers during the precoronary care era.[17,18]

By comparing a subsequent group of patients under 70 years of age who were treated in our CCU with the original group treated in hospital wards during the year before the CCU opened, we were able to show that hospital mortality was reduced significantly (from 31% to 12%) by coronary care for that group of patients (about one-third of the total) who had infarction of moderate severity as judged by a coronary prognostic index.[4] Overall, hospital mortality was reduced from 22% to 17% by the CCU for patients under 70 years of age. Moreover, a 3-year follow-up of 244 hospital survivors of this group of patients showed a trend toward improved long-term survival for the CCU patients compared with those who had been treated in the hospital wards.[6]

Hospital mortality for patients under 70 years of age who were treated in the CCU fell further to 13% in 1977 to 1979[10] and to 10% in 1981 to 1984.[19] The reason for this further decline did not appear to be case selection and was probably due to a combination of better treatment of arrhythmias, earlier recognition and treatment of shock and cardiac failure, and the evolution of surgical management of postinfarction angina and of the surgical complications of infarction. "Arrhythmic death," which had accounted for 52% of hospital mortality in 1966,[2] accounted for only 12% of

deaths in 1977 to 1979,[10] while mortality from shock and cardiac failure had also declined, but not significantly.

Hospital mortality for patients treated by thrombolysis in our CCU is now approximately 5% for patients under 70 years of age,[15] almost certainly because of the development of thrombolysis that has been proved to reduce mortality[20,21] and also to improve left ventricular (LV) function[22,23] for survivors of infarction. An average early mortality rate (hospital mortality or mortality at up to 6 weeks postinfarction) of 5 to 6% has also been reported for treated patients from the major trials of thrombolytic therapy.[20,21,24–32]

Our experience of secular improvement in late mortality after AMI has been no less dramatic than the improvement in early mortality. Figure 11-2 shows mortality rates for up to 20 years for patients under 70 years of age who had survived hospitalization for a MI sustained during 1966 to 1977.[5,7–9] Also shown are 3-year survival curves for 203 consecutive patients discharged from our CCU during 1981.[14] The third survival curve in Figure 11-2 shows late mortality for patients who have received thrombolysis in our own[15] and other[32–36] studies.

Figures 11-1 and 11-2 show a decline in both early and late mortality of about 70%, comparing patients treated in-hospital but outside of a CCU in 1966 with patients treated with thrombolysis during the 1980s. This decline parallels the decline of approximately

45% in age-adjusted death rates from CHD that occurred in the United States between 1965 and 1988, shown in Figure 11-3. Clearly, patients admitted to hospital are but a subset of those dying in the community of ischemic heart disease; patterns of hospital admission might have changed between 1965 and 1985, even though this had not been our clinical impression, and experience at one center does not necessarily correspond with experience in another. However, patients admitted to our hospital during 1981 had more severe MI, as judged by our coronary prognostic index[5] than did those admitted during 1966, yet their 3-year mortality rate was 44% less.[14] The conclusion seems inescapable that much of the decline in mortality from CHD is directly attributable to better treatment and secondary prevention of AMI. Whether this has been the major factor causing the decline in mortality[16,37] or merely a contributing factor, as suggested by epidemiologic studies,[38,39] will continue to be argued. Further epidemiologic research including meta-analysis of hospital and postdischarge mortality statistics to include precoronary care and post-thrombolysis studies seems fully justified and could provide further important and valuable information.

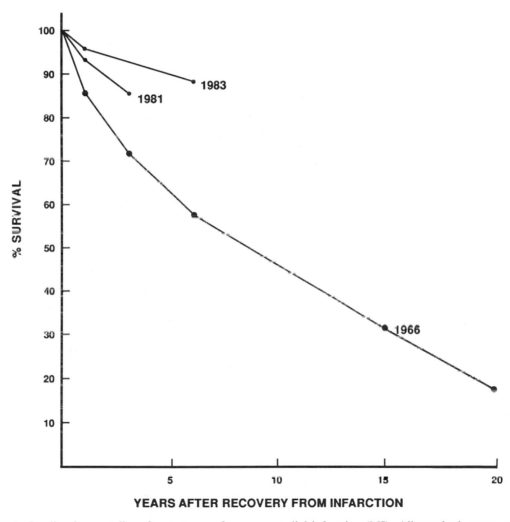

YEARS AFTER RECOVERY FROM INFARCTION

Fig. 11-2. Decline in mortality after recovery from myocardial infarction (MI). All survival curves refer to patients under 70 years of age. The bottom curve describes the fate of 413 patients admitted to Auckland Hospitals during 1966 and followed at 3 years,[5] 6 years,[7] 15 years,[8] and 20 years[9] after the index infarction. The middle curve refers to 203 patients admitted during 1981.[14] The upper curve is based on data derived from studies on patients receiving thrombolysis.[15,21,32–36] It appears that 6-year mortality after recovery from MI has been reduced by approximately 70% since 1966 for patients receiving thrombolysis. (Modified from Norris,[16] with permission.)

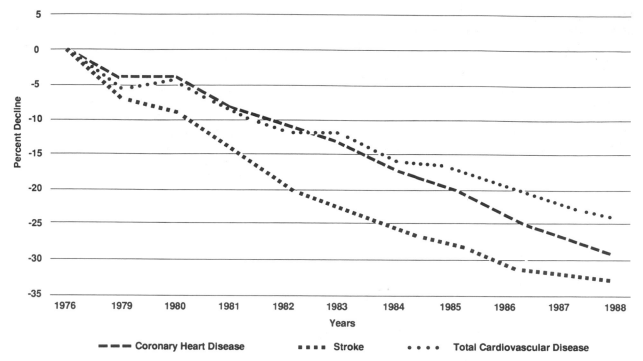

Fig. 11-3. Decline in mortality rate from coronary heart disease (From the American Heart Association,[81] with permission.)

FACTORS DETERMINING PROGNOSIS AFTER MYOCARDIAL INFARCTION

Because prognosis continues to change for the better, it is becoming increasingly difficult to prognosticate for individual patients. However, it is likely that the relative importance of factors determining prognostic is changing less than the absolute predictive power of each factor considered individually. Prognostic factors can therefore still be divided into those associated with the heart itself, the myocardium and the coronary arteries, and extracardiac factors—in other words, the primary and secondary risk factors for ischemic heart disease. Rather than following a strictly logical order, it is perhaps more useful to deal with the various factors in approximate order of importance.

Age

Every large study that has dealt with an unselected group of infarct patients from our own early studies[3,8] to the recent therapeutic "megatrials"[20,21,25] has shown that advancing age is the single most important adverse factor for short-term and long-term prognosis. The fundamental processes of aging remain ill under-

stood, but clinical experience shows that the aging myocardium tolerates ischemia poorly; moreover, elderly patients with infarction carry a greater atherosclerotic load than do younger patients. When looking for secular changes in mortality rates, it seems logical to exclude the elderly as has been done in the foregoing section of this chapter. This said, there is interesting evidence from the large thrombolytic trials[20,21] that the absolute reduction in mortality caused by thrombolysis is greater for the elderly than for the young. The practical importance of this finding is the increasing need for CCU facilities for treatment of the elderly. However, the relative increase in mortality for older compared with younger patients remains.

Myocardial Factors Associated With Prognosis

Studies of prognosis of defined subsets of patients after MI have consistently shown that infarct size, reflected in the degree of LV damage, is, apart from age, the single most important factor determining prognosis. Indirect evidence for this came originally from our coronary prognostic indices, which showed that a low systolic blood pressure on admission to hospital best predicted short-term mortality,[3] while severity of pulmonary congestion and the presence of cardiac enlargement predicted mortality at 3,[5] 6,[7] and 15 years[8] after recovery. Hypotension, cardiomegaly, and pulmonary venous congestion presumably reflected degrees of severity of LV damage from infarction. During the 1970s, data became available on angiocardiographically determined subsets of patients, angiography having been performed, in most cases, after recovery from infarction. Several reports during the early 1980s[12,40–43] described LV ejection fraction as the most important predictor of medium-term (3- to 5-year) survival. Some of these studies showed additional prognostic information from the severity of coronary arterial stenoses,[41–43] while others did not.[12,40] Our own study,[12] which showed no additional predictive power from coronary stenoses, showed that ejection fraction was of approximately equal value to the coronary prognostic index for prediction of survival for up to 6 years after recovery from first infarction for men up to 60 years of age.

Ejection fraction is an arithmetic term based on LV volume. Intuitively, it would appear that a high end-systolic or end-diastolic volume (LV dilation) would be superior to ejection fraction as an indicator of LV dysfunction and therefore of an adverse prognosis.

From the results of a multivariate analysis using the proportional hazards model of 605 patients followed for a mean of 78 months after a first or recurrent MI,[13] we found that high end-systolic volume was the most powerful predictor of an adverse prognosis; after standardizing for end-systolic volume, the addition to the model of end-diastolic volume or ejection fraction provided no further prognostic information. The importance for prognosis of end-systolic volume is shown in Figure 11-4. As shown in Figure 11-4 (1) ejection fraction and end-systolic volume are inversely related (a mathematical certainty!), (2) patients who die have a higher end-systolic volume for a given ejection fraction than those who survive, and (3) the divergent relationship between those who die and those who survive is readily apparent only when ejection fraction is reduced below about 50% or end-systolic volume is increased above about 100 ml. Figure 11-5 shows the effects of this relationship more clearly. Actuarial survival curves are sharply divergent when ejection fraction is 40 to 49% or less than 40%, according to whether end-systolic volume is, respectively, above or below the median for the group. When ejection frac-

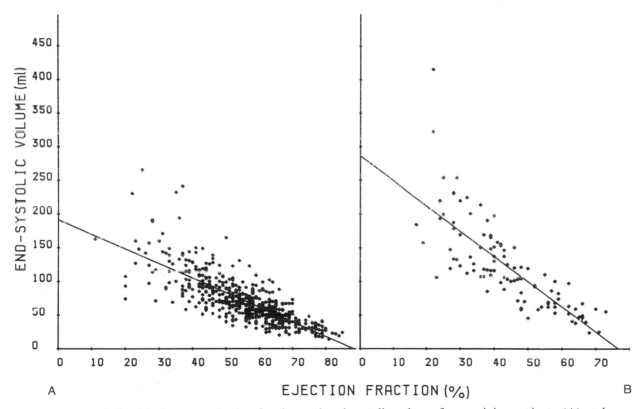

Fig. 11-4. Relationship between ejection fraction and end-systolic volume for surviving patients (**A**) and patients dying of a cardiac cause (**B**). Correlations are similar (r = −0.78) for both groups of patients, but for patients who died the slope of the relationship is significantly steeper than for those who survived (t = 4.6, p <0.001). (From White et al.,[13] with permission.)

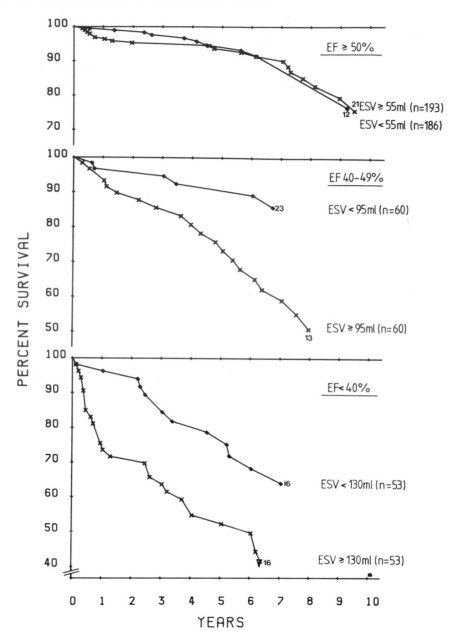

Fig. 11-5. Actuarial curves constructed for three groups of ejection fraction (50% or above, 40% to 49%, and less than 40%). Each group was subdivided according to whether end-systolic volume was above or below the median for that group. Predictive value for end-systolic volume is apparent when ejection fraction is less than 50%, but not when ejection fraction is at least 50%. (From White et al.,[13] with permission.)

tion is 50% or less, however, end-systolic volume carries no further prognostic information.

The idea that cardiac dilation is the single most important predictor of an adverse prognosis has important therapeutic implications. First, cardiac dilation is determined initially by a large infarct size, and infarct size as well as end-systolic volume are limited by thrombolysis.[22] Early thrombolysis to prevent cardiac

dilation should reduce long-term as well as short-term mortality.[35] Second, cardiac dilation is consequent to infarct expansion and remodeling, which occur during healing[44] and can continue for months or years afterward.[45] Recent evidence suggests that cardiac dilation and remodelling can be affected favorably by load reduction by administration of converting enzyme inhibitors[46,47] or nitrates[48] during the recovery phase. It would be predicted from our data that the long-term prognosis should be improved for such patients by administration of these drugs.

It would be expected that end-systolic volume (or ejection fraction) measured after recovery from infarction would be superior as a prognostic indicator to the cruder assessment of the degree of pulmonary venous congestion during the acute phase, a factor that we had introduced as part of the coronary prognostic index during the 1960s and before the widespread use of left ventriculography. However, we found in 1984 that the coronary prognostic index was of approximately equal value to ejection fraction for prediction of prognosis.[12] A very recent report of 1,850 patients followed for a mean period of 2 years showed that the presence of severe pulmonary congestion on admission to the CCU was an independent risk factor for patients with all grades of depression of ejection fraction.[49] In these patients, it appeared that severe pulmonary congestion was measuring something other than systolic dysfunction and is tempting to speculate that diastolic dysfunction during ischemia might be an independent predictor of late mortality. There is no evidence to favor such speculation, but the finding is intriguing and the explanation not immediately obvious.

PROGNOSTIC IMPORTANCE OF ARRHYTHMIAS DURING AND AFTER ACUTE INFARCTION

More than one-half of all patients recovered from an acute infarction die suddenly,[15] and sudden death is more common in patients who have cardiac dilation.[12] Most sudden deaths are caused by ventricular fibrillation.[50] There has been controversy in the literature as to whether arrhythmias detected during Holter monitoring after recovery from infarction constitute an independent adverse prognostic factor for sudden death. There is little doubt that complex ventricular ectopy is a risk factor, but patients with severe cardiac damage tend to have more complex arrhythmias than those who do not.[51] However, it was shown by Bigger et al.,[52] using multivariate analysis of arrhythmias recorded from 24-hour predischarge electrocardiographic (ECG) recordings and ejection fractions recorded by radionuclide ventriculography in 766 patients, that low ejection fraction and runs of ventricular ectopic beats or occurrence of three or more ventricular ectopic beats per hour were independently related to increased cardiac mortality. These results, and those from a similar study,[53] raised the question that suppression of ventricular ectopic beats in asymptomatic patients after recovery from infarction might

reduce the incidence of sudden cardiac death. This hypothesis has been tested, and the unfortunate results of the Cardiac Arrhythmias Suppression Trial (CAST)[54] are well known. The class 1C antiarrhythmic drugs flecainide and encainide significantly increased sudden death and total mortality rate in patients in whom these drugs had been shown to be effective in suppressing ventricular ectopic beats. The increase in mortality was statistically highly significant and led to abandonment of the trial of these drugs on the advice of the Data and Safety Monitoring Board. Trial of a third drug, moricizine (which possesses class 1A and 1B properties) continues, but class 1C agents must now be considered contraindicated for use after MI. Indeed, the only known effective agents for prevention of sudden death after infarction are β-blockers,[55] drugs that, paradoxically and somewhat ironically, do not suppress ventricular ectopic beats in most patients.

Thus, both prevention of sudden death after infarction, and identification of patients at risk of sudden death, remain major challenges. A more promising approach than detection of arrhythmias by Holter monitoring may be by detection of late potentials in signal-averaged ECGs[56] or by inducibility of ventricular tachycardia by programmed stimulation.[57] An important effect of thrombolysis appears to be reduction in the incidence of late potentials[58] and in the inducibility of ventricular arrhythmias by programmed stimulation.[59] Either thrombolysis per se or maintenance of an open infarct-related artery subsequent to thrombolysis may therefore reduce the incidence of late sudden death, although proof of this is not available at present.

PROGNOSIS AND THE SEVERITY OF CORONARY ARTERIAL STENOSES

It was found in three moderately large studies[41–43] that the severity of coronary artery stenoses added prognostic information to the severity of myocardial damage. These studies reported on a total of 667 patients with 41 cardiac deaths, and risk factor analysis was multivariate in one study[41] and univariate in two.[42,43] Using multivariate analysis and the Cox proportional hazards model, we were unable to show an independent effect of coronary stenoses with a long (mean 78 months) follow-up of 605 patients, 101 of whom suffered cardiac death.[13] We used the Brandt scoring system[60] for assessment of stenoses in preference to the conventional system of classification into one, two, and three vessel disease. This system takes into account not only the severity of coronary arterial stenoses but also the volume of myocardium supplied by each stenosed artery; thus, it should be superior as a descriptor of severity to the conventional classification used in the other studies.[41–43] This, and the greater statistical power for our study, cast doubt on the severity of coronary stenoses as an independent prognostic factor.

An alternative method for assessment of the severity of residual coronary stenoses after infarction is by exercise testing with or without thallium imaging. An early report suggested that a positive exercise test carried serious prognostic implications,[61] but we could not confirm this with a larger series of patients.[12] In a small series of 140 patients followed for 15 months, predischarge exercise thallium scintigraphy predicted future cardiac events (mainly severe angina[62]), but as there were only seven deaths, the study had no statistical power for prediction of mortality.

The likely reason for the lack of predictive power of coronary stenoses is that surgical revascularization, and more recently percutaneous transluminal coronary angioplasty (PTCA), is standard treatment for disabling angina after infarction, and surgical treatment for disabling angina prolongs life,[63] even though revascularization for asymptomatic patients may not.[11,64]

PRIMARY RISK FACTORS AFTER MYOCARDIAL INFARCTION

Cigarette smoking has long been recognized as a major risk factor for recurrent events after MI, to the extent that subsequent mortality is approximately doubled in those who continue to smoke after infarction compared with those who renounce the habit.[65,66] Continued cigarette smoking was the only independent risk factor apart from end-systolic volume for late cardiac mortality in our study.[13] We recently found that reinfarction after thrombolysis was predicted not only by smoking status at the time of the index infarct, but also by continued smoking after recovery from the index infarct.[15] Although smoking does accelerate atheroma,[67] there is evidence that, in the coronary circulation, the major risk of smoking is from enhancement of thrombogenesis rather than from exacerbation of atheroma.[68,69] Clearly, a smoker who has had a MI must be advised in the strongest terms to stop smoking, the single most important positive health measure that such a patient can take.

The long-held hypothesis that serum lipis might continue to act as risk factors after recovery from MI and that alteration of lipid levels might improve prognosis is gaining in importance now that powerful methods for controlling lipid metabolism are becoming available. The Coronary Drug Project,[70] which for 10 years was the largest clinical trial ever undertaken, had a negative result, probably because the most pow-

erful lipid-lowering drug (niacin) available at the time lowered cholesterol levels by only 10%. However, a late follow-up evaluation of survivors from this trial at 15 years after entry showed that there had been significantly (12%) fewer cardiac deaths among patients who had taken niacin over the 5-year period of the trial.[71] Among placebo patients, a high serum cholesterol at entry (>250 mg or >280 mg/dl) was a risk factor for 5-year mortality, but the predictive value was not great (total mortality was 3 to 4% higher at 5 years among patients who had a high cholesterol).[72] Mortality risk for patients in the highest quintile for serum cholesterol was 50% higher than for those in the lowest quintile.[73] This increase in risk is clearly a great deal less than the increased risk arising from high end-systolic volume (Fig. 11-3) or, indeed, from indicators of myocardial damage as recorded in the Coronary Drug Project patients.[72]

This modest increase in risk from high cholesterol after infarction does not, however, necessarily mean that lipid levels are not too high for *all* patients with coronary atheroma and that reduction in levels for all patients may not be beneficial. A meta-analysis of the results of the Coronary Drug Project and other much smaller trials[74] suggested that a reduction of cholesterol levels by about 10% would reduce CHD events by about 17% after 2 years of treatment, a result similar to what would be expected from reduction in cholesterol as a primary preventive measure. It should be noted that this prediction applied to coronary events (death plus nonfatal myocardial infarction) and not to coronary deaths alone. A more recent meta-analysis, however, has shown that total cardiovascular mortality was also reduced by cholesterol lowering, but with wider statistical uncertainty (relative risk for treated patients 0.88; 95% confidence limits 0.77 to 0.99).[75]

The introduction of more powerful agents for the treatment of hyperlipidemia, including HMG-Co A reductase inhibitors,[76] has now made it possible to lower cholesterol levels by up to 40%. Very recently, regression of coronary atheroma has been described in men with high levels of apolipoprotein B as a result of 2.5 years treatment with lovastatin and colestipol or niacin and colestipol.[77] Similar regression has been described for partial ileal bypass surgery performed at a mean of 9.7 years previously[78] and by adoption of a vegetarian diet and life-style changes (but no lipid-lowering drugs) over 1 year.[79] Not only did atheroma regress in these trials, but coronary events were also less frequent in treated patients. Death, myocardial infarction, or revascularization occurred in 5 of 94 patients taking the lipid-lowering drug combinations compared with 10 of 52 assigned to conventional therapy (a 72% reduction).[77] Partial ileal bypass reduced coronary events by 35% (p <0.001) and the necessity for coronary artery bypass grafting by 60% (p

<0.0001).[78] Life-style changes were reported to reduce angina to a degree disproportionate to that which would be expected from the regression of atheroma.[79] Reductions in total cholesterol were 28% and 23% from the drug regimens,[77] 23% from partial ileal bypass,[78] and 24% from the vegetarian diet.[79]

Clearly, reduction of serum lipid levels now appears to be the most promising method for secondary prevention of coronary atheroma. As applied in postinfarction patients, however, several caveats are necessary. First, severe myocardial damage remains the most powerful adverse prognostic factor and the severity of coronary stenoses is secondary to this[13]; patients with severe damage are unlikely to benefit from lipid-lowering regimens. Evidence in support of this is already available from the partial ileal bypass trial, in which mortality reduction was confined to patients with an ejection fraction greater than 50%.[78] Second, most patients are not motivated to make drastic changes in life-style, so that the proposed option for lowering lipid levels will in most cases be a lifetime of treatment with expensive drugs. However, other drugs, such as β-blockers,[55] aspirin,[80] and vasodilators,[46–48] might be more cost effective than lipid-lowering drugs for individual patients. Third, indications for lowering lipid levels in the elderly will remain a subject for controversy and value judgment. If, as appears likely, regression of atheroma will become a therapeutic aim, it will likely be the most effective for patients with the most severe atheroma and the least amount of myocardial damage.

CONCLUSION

Mortality rates from AMI continue to decline, with a time course that parallels the decline in community mortality from ischemic heart disease that has occurred since the mid-1960s in the United States, and elsewhere. It is likely that this decline, which is due to better acute treatment (coronary care, thrombolysis) and to the better secondary prevention (stopping smoking, β-blockers, coronary surgery, angioplasty) after infarction, has played a large part in the decline in community mortality from coronary heart disease. The prospect for the 1990s is that secondary prevention by drugs or other measures to cause regression of atheroma may lead to a further decline in coronary mortality so that CHD may cease to be the major killing disease of the Western world.

ACKNOWLEDGMENT

Original work quoted in this chapter has been supported by the Medical Research Council and the National Heart Foundation of New Zealand.

REFERENCES

1. Thom TJ, Maurer J: Time trends for coronary heart disease mortality and morbidity. p. 7. In Higgins MW, Luepker RV (eds): Trends in Coronary Heart Disease Mortality. Oxford University Press, New York, 1988
2. Norris RM, Bensley DF, Caughey DE, Scott PJ: Hospital mortality in acute myocardial infarction. Br Med J 3:143, 1968
3. Norris RM, Brandt PWT, Caughey DE et al: A new coronary prognostic index. Lancet 1:274, 1969
4. Norris RM, Brandt PWT, Lee AJ: Mortality in a coronary-care unit analyzed by a new coronary prognostic index. Lancet 1:278, 1969
5. Norris RM, Caughey DE, Deeming LW et al: Coronary prognostic index for predicting survival after recovery from acute myocardial infarction. Lancet 1:285, 1970
6. Norris RM, Mercer CJ: Long-term prognosis following treatment in a coronary care unit. Aust NZ J Med 1:37, 1973
7. Norris RM, Caughey DE, Mercer CJ, Scott PJ: Prognosis after myocardial infarction. Six year follow-up. Br Heart J 36:786, 1974
8. Merrilees MA, Scott PJ, Norris RM: Prognosis after myocardial infarction; results of 15 year follow-up. Br Med J 288:355, 1984
9. Scott PJ, Norris RM, Merrilees M: Twenty year follow-up of myocardial infarction patients whose data formed the basis of the Norris coronary prognostic index, abstracted. NZ Med J 104:261, 1991
10. Norris RM, Sammel NL: Predictors of late hospital death in acute myocardial infarction. Prog Cardiovasc Dis 23:129, 1980
11. Norris RM, Agnew TM, Brandt PWT et al: Coronary surgery after recurrent myocardial infarction: progress of a trial comparing surgical with nonsurgical management for asymptomatic patients with advanced coronary disease. Circulation 63:785, 1981
12. Norris RM, Barnaby PF, Brandt PWT et al: Prognosis after recovery from first acute myocardial infarction: determinants of reinfarction and sudden death. Am J Cardiol 53:408, 1984
13. White HD, Norris RM, Brown MA et al: Left ventricular end-systolic volume as the major determinant of survival after recovery from myocardial infarction. Circulation 76:44, 1987
14. Stewart AW, Fraser J, Norris RM, Beaglehole R: Changes in severity of myocardial infarction and 3 year survival rates after myocardial infarction in Auckland 1966–67 and 1981–82. Br Med J 297:517, 1988
15. Rivers JT, White HD, Cross DB et al: Reinfarction after thrombolytic therapy followed by conservative management: incidence and effect of smoking. J Am Coll Cardiol 16:340, 1990
16. Norris RM: The changing natural history and prognosis of acute myocardial infarction. p. 87. In Gersh BJ, Rahimtoola SH (eds): Myocardial Infarction. Elsevier, New York, 1990
17. Honey GE, Truelove SC: Prognostic factors in myocardial infarction. Lancet 1:1155, 1957
18. Killip T: In Meltzer LE, Kitchell JR (eds): The Current

Status of Intensive Coronary Care. American College of Cardiology, New York, 1966

19. Norris RM, Barnaby PF, Brown MA et al: Prevention of ventricular fibrillation during acute myocardial infarction by intravenous propranolol. Lancet 2:883, 1984

20. GISSI Trial Group: Effectiveness of intravenous thrombolytic treatment in acute myocardial infarction. Lancet 1:397, 1986

21. ISIS-2 (Second International Study of Infarct Survival) Collaborative Group: Randomised trial of intravenous streptokinase, oral aspirin, both, or neither among 17187 cases of suspected acute myocardial infarction. ISIS 2. Lancet 2:349, 1988

22. White HD, Norris RM, Brown MA et al: Effect of intravenous streptokinase on left ventricular function and early survival after acute myocardial infarction. N Engl J Med 317:850, 1987

23. O'Rourke M, Baron D, Keogh A et al: Limitation of myocardial infarction by early infusion of recombinant tissue-type plasminogen activator. Circulation 77:1311, 1988

24. The TIMI Study Group: Comparison of invasive and conservative strategies after treatment with intravenous tissue plasminogen activator in acute myocardial infarction. N Engl J Med 320:618, 1989

25. Wilcox RG, Olsson CG, Skene AM et al: Trial of tissue plasminogen activator for mortality reduction in acute myocardial infarction. Lancet 2:525, 1988

26. The ISAM Study Group: A prospective trial of intravenous streptokinase in acute myocardial infarction (ISAM). Mortality, morbidity and infarct size at 21 days. N Engl J Med 314:1465, 1986

27. Topol EJ, Califf RM, George BS et al: A randomized trial of immediate versus delayed elective angioplasty after intravenous tissue plasminogen activator in acute myocardial infarction. N Engl J Med 317:581, 1987

28. Topol EJ, Califf RM, George BS et al: Coronary arterial thrombolysis with combined infusion of recombinant tissue-type plasminogen activator and urokinase in patients with acute myocardial infarction. Circulation 77:1100, 1988

29. Topol EJ, George BS, Kereiakes DJ et al: A randomized controlled trial of intravenous tissue plasminogen activator and early intravenous heparin in acute myocardial infarction. Circulation 79:281, 1989

30. Califf R, Topol EJ, Kereiakes DJ et al: Long-term outcome in the thrombolysis and angioplasty in myocardial infarction trial. Circulation. 76:IV-260, 1987

31. Muller DW, Topol EJ, George BS et al: Long-term follow-up in the thrombolysis and angioplasty in acute myocardial infarction (TAMI) trials. Comparison of trials with thrombolysis alone. Circulation, suppl II. 80:II-520, 1989

32. AIMS Trial Study Group: Long-term effects of intraveneous anistreplase in acute myocardial infarction. Lancet 2:427, 1990

33. GISSI Trial Group: Long-term effects of intravenous thrombolysis in acute myocardial infarction: final report of the GISSI study. Lancet 2:871, 1987

34. Van de Werf F, Arnold AE: The European Co-operative rt-PA vs placebo trial: 1 year follow-up. Circulation, suppl II. 80:520, 1989

35. Simoons ML: Long-term benefit of early thrombolytic therapy in patients with acute myocardial infarction: 5 year follow-up of a trial conducted by the Interuniversity Cardiology Institute of the Netherlands. J Am Coll Cardiol 14:1609, 1989

36. Taylor GJ, Sang A, Korsmeyer C et al: Six year survival after thrombolysis for acute myocardial infarction. Circulation, suppl II. 80:520, 1989

37. Norris RM: Letter to the editor. N Engl J Med 323:1704, 1991

38. Goldman L, Cook EF: The decline in ischemic heart disease mortality rates: an analysis of the comparative effects of medical interventions and changes in lifestyle. Ann Intern Med 101:825, 1987

39. Sytkowski PA, Kannel WB, D'Agostino RB: Changes in risk factors and the decline in mortality from cardiovascular disease. N Engl J Med 322:1635, 1990

40. Taylor GJ, Humphries JO, Mellits ED et al: Predictors of clinical course, coronary anatomy and left ventricular function after recovery from acute myocardial infarction. Circulation 62:960, 1980

41. Sanz G, Castaner A, Betriu A et al: Determinants of prognosis in survivors of myocardial infarction. A prospective clinical angiographic study. N Engl J Med 306:1065, 1982

42. De Feyter PJ, van Eenige MJ, Dighton DH et al: Prognostic value of exercise testing, coronary angiography and left ventriculography 6–8 weeks after myocardial infarction. Circulation 66:527, 1982

43. Roubin GS, Harris PJ, Bernstein L, Kelly DT: Coronary anatomy and prognosis after myocardial infarction in patients 60 years of age and younger. Circulation 67:743, 1983

44. McKay RG, Pfeffer MA, Pasternak RC et al: Left ventricular remodelling after myocardial infarction: corollary to infarct expansion. Circulation 74:693, 1986

45. Erlebacher JA, Weiss JL, Eaton LW et al: Late effects of acute infarct dilation on heart size: a two-dimensional echocardiographic study. Am J Cardiol 49:1120, 1982

46. Sharpe DN, Smith H, Murphy J, Hannon S: Treatment of patients with symptomless left ventricular dysfunction after myocardial infarction. Lancet 1:255, 1988

47. Pfeffer MA, Lomas GA, Vaughan DE et al: Effect of captopril on progressive left ventricular dilatation after anterior myocardial infarction. N Engl J Med 319:80, 1988

48. Jugdutt B, Tymchak W, Humen D et al: Prolonged nitroglycerin versus captopril therapy on remodelling after transmural myocardial infarction, abstracted. Circulation, suppl III. 82:442, 1990

49. Gottlieb S, Moss AJ, McDermott M, Eberly S: Prognostic significance and relationship between left ventricular ejection afraction and pulmonary congestion in patients recovering from acute myocardial infarction, abstracted. Circulation, suppl III. 82:204, 1990

50. Liberthson RR, Nagel EL, Hirschman JC et al: Pathophysiologic observations in prehospital ventricular fibrillation and sudden cardiac death. Circulation 49:790, 1974

51. Anderson KP, De Camilla J, Moss AJ: Clinical significance of ventricular tachycardia (3 beats or longer) detected during ambulatory monitoring after myocardial infarction. Circulation 57:890, 1978

52. Bigger JT, Fleiss JL, Kleiger R et al: The relationships among ventricular arrhythmias, left ventricular dysfunction, and mortality in the 2 years after myocardial infarction. Circulation 69:250, 1984

53. Mukharji J, Rude RE, Poole WK et al: Risk factors for sudden death after acute myocardial infarction: two year follow-up. Am J Cardiol 54:31, 1984

54. CAST Investigators: Special Report. Preliminary report: effect of flecainide and encainide on mortality in a randomized trial of arrhythmia suppression after myocardial infarction. N Engl J Med 321:406, 1989

55. Yusuf S, Peto R, Lewis J et al: Beta blockade during and after myocardial infarction: an overview of the randomized trials. Prog Cardiovasc Dis 27:335, 1985

56. Kuchar DL, Thorburn CW, Sammel NL: Late potentials detected after myocardial infarction: natural history and prognostic significance. Circulation 74:1280, 1986

57. Richards DAB, Byth K, Ross DL, Uther JB: What is the best predictor of spontaneous ventricular tachycardia and sudden death after myocardial infarction? Circulation 83:756, 1991

58. Gang ES, Lew AS, Hong M et al: Decreased incidence of ventricular late potentials after successful thrombolytic therapy for acute myocardial infarction. N Engl J Med 321:712, 1989

59. Bourke JP, Young AA, Richards DAB, Uther JB: Reduction in incidence of inducible ventricular tachycardia after myocardial infarction by treatment with streptokinase during infarct evolution. J Am Coll Cardiol 17:229A, 1991

60. Brandt PWT, Partridge JB, Wattie WJ: Coronary arteriography: method of presentation of the arteriogram and a scoring system. Clin Radiol 28:361, 1977

61. Theroux P, Waters DD, Halphen C et al: Prognostic value of exercise testing soon after myocardial infarction. N Engl J Med 301:341, 1979

62. Gibson RS, Watson DD, Craddock GB et al: Prediction of cardiac events after uncomplicated myocardial infarction: a prospective study comparing predischarge exercise thallium-201 scintigraphy and coronary angiography. Circulation 68:321, 1983

63. Rutherford JD, Whitlock RML, McDonald BW et al: Multivariate analysis of the long-term results of coronary artery bypass grafting performed during 1976 and 1977. Am J Cardiol 57:1264, 1986

64. CASS Principal Investigators and Their Associates: Coronary Artery Surgery Study (CASS): a randomized trial of coronary artery bypass surgery. Survival data. Circulation 68:939, 1983

65. Gordon T, Kannel WB, McGee D: Death and coronary attacks in men after giving up smoking. Lancet 2:1345, 1974

66. Wilhelmssohn C, Elmefeldt D, Vedin JA et al: Smoking and myocardial infarction. Lancet 1:415, 1975

67. Auerback O, Carter HW, Garfinkel L, Hammond EC: Cigarette smoking and coronary artery disease. A macroscopic and microscopic study. Chest 70:697, 1976

68. Hartz AJ, Barboriak PN, Anderson AJ et al: Smoking, coronary artery occlusion and non-fatal myocardial infarction. JAMA 246:851, 1985

69. McKenzie WB, McCredie RM, McGilchrist CA, Wilcken DEL: Smoking: a major predictor of left ventricular function after occlusion of the left anterior descending coronary artery. Br Heart J 56:496, 1986

70. The Coronary Drug Project Research Group: Clofibrate and niacin in coronary heart disease. JAMA 231:360, 1975

71. Canner PL, Berge KG, Wenger NK et al: Fifteen year mortality in coronary drug project patients; long term benefit with niacin. J Am Coll Cardiol 8:1245, 1986

72. Schlant RC, Forman S, Stamler J, Canner PL: The natural history of coronary heart disease: prognostic factors after recovery from myocardial infarction in 2789 men. The 5-year findings of the Coronary Drug Project. Circulation 66:401, 1982

73. Coronary Drug Project Research Group: Natural history of myocardial infarction of the Coronary Drug Project: long term prognostic importance of serum lipid levels. Am J Cardiol 42.489, 1978

74. Peto R, Yusuf S, Collins R: Cholesterol lowering trial results in their epidemiological context, abstracted. Circulation 72:III-451, 1985

75. Rossouw JE, Lewis B, Rifkind BM: The value of lowering cholesterol after myocardial infarction. N Engl J Med 323:1112, 1990

76. Grundy SM: HMG-CoA reductase inhibitors for treatment of hypercholesterolemia. N Engl J Med 319:24, 1988

77. Brown G, Allen JJ, Fisher LD et al: Regression of coronary artery disease as a result of intensive lipid-lowering therapy in men with high levels of apolipoprotein B. N Engl J Med 323:1289, 1990

78. Buchwald H, Varco RL, Matts JP et al: Effect of partial ileal bypass surgery on mortality and morbidity from coronary heart disease in patients with hypercholesterolemia. N Engl J MEd 323:946, 1990

79. Ornish D, Brown SE, Scherwitz LW, et al: Can lifestyle changes reverse coronary heart disease? Lancet 1:129, 1990

80. Antiplatelet Triallists' Collaboration: Secondary prevention of vascular disease by prolonged anti-platelet treatment. Br Med J 296:320, 1988

81. American Heart Association: 1991 Heart and Stroke Facts. American Heart Association, NY, 1991, p. 18.

12

Myocardial Infarction: Post-Thrombolytic Risk Assessment and Prognosis

Harvey D. White

Thrombolytic therapy reduces early mortality and preserves left ventricular function.[1-5] Morbidity, including cardiac arrest, the need for pacemakers, and heart failure, is also reduced. The mortality benefit is maintained long term.[6-19]

Thrombolytic therapy saves lives acutely by reperfusing the ischemic myocardium, improving left ventricular (LV) function, and enabling patients who would otherwise die from cardiogenic shock to survive. In our experience, the number of patients dying from cardiogenic shock has decreased from 8% to 2%, and the number of patients with ejection fractions of less than 40% has decreased from about 20% to less than 10%.[5,20]

The frequency of ventricular fibrillation has also been decreased by thrombolytic therapy. In the GISSI trial, ventricular fibrillation was decreased from 3.7% to 2.8%, p < 0.05.[21] In the Second International Study of Infarct Survival (ISIS-2),[2] the incidence of cardiac arrest was reduced with streptokinase therapy from 9.1% to 7.9%, p < 0.01.[2]

Thrombolytic therapy may, however, increase mortality from cardiac rupture or bleeding and cause strokes. The overall risk: benefit ratio needs to be assessed by early mortality trials that also assess disability from stroke. For long-term mortality, LV function appears to be the best prognostic factor.[14,15,17,22,23]

LONG-TERM SURVIVAL

The improvement in long-term survival with thrombolytic therapy has been as impressive as the reduction in early mortality, on the order of 60 to 75% compared with mortality in 1966.[24] One-year mortality for patients leaving the hospital is of the order of 3 to 5% for patients aged less than 70 years and 5-year mortality about 13% (Table 12-1). In GISSI-1[1] and ISIS-2,[2] mortalities have been higher because there was no age limit in these trials. In the trials with age restrictions, there does not seem to be a marked difference between those with high rates of coronary angioplasty and surgery[6,10-17] and those in which intervention rates were more conservative.[1-5,7-9,18,19]

PROGNOSTIC FACTORS

Prior to the thrombolytic era, it was well shown that LV function was the most important prognostic factor after infarction.[25,26] The severity of coronary artery

TABLE 12-1. Late Mortality in the Thrombolytic Era (from the Early Hospital Phase)

Trial	Treatment	No. of Patients	Follow-up	Mortality (%)
ISIS-2[2]	SK + aspirin	3,949	15 mo	10.2
AIMS[3]	APSAC	657	1 yr	4.7
Western Washington[6]	IC SK	129	1 yr	4.6
GISSI-1[7]	SK	5,223	1 yr	7.2
ISAM[8]	SK	805	1.7 yr	8.7
Auckland[9]	SK/rt-PA	430	1 yr	3.5
ECSG I[10]	rt-PA ± PTCA	350	1 yr	3.1
ECSG II[11]	rt-PA	335	1 yr	3.2
TIMI-I[12]	SK/rt-PA	276	1 yr	6.5
TIMI-II[13]	rt-PA ± PTCA ± metoprolol	3,099	1 yr	2.4
TAMI[14]	rt-PA ± PTCA	727	1.5 yr	3.8
Interuniversity[15]	SK	253	5 yr	12.6
PRAIRIE[16]	SK	180	6 yr	11.7
Western Washington[17]	IV rt-PA	109	1 yr	5.4
ASSET[18]	IV rt-PA	2,514	6 mo	3.2
GISSI-2/international[19]	SK	8,685	6 mo	3.4
	rt-PA	8,646	6 mo	3.6

Abbreviations: IC, intracoronary; IV, intravenous; PTCA, percutaneous transluminal coronary angioplasty; rt-PA, tissue plasminogen activator; SK, streptokinase.

disease (CAD)[27–30] and of ventricular arrhythmias[31] was also shown to be important, as was the presence of inducible myocardial ischemia.[32]

Left ventricular function remains a very important prognostic factor following thrombolytic therapy, but there are a paucity of data with respect to additional factors. Patency of the infarct-related artery confers benefits additional to those achieved acutely by reduction of infarct size and preservation of systolic function,[33,34] and has recently been shown to be an independent long-term prognostic factor.[35]

IMPORTANCE OF PATENCY OF THE INFARCT-RELATED ARTERY

Patency of the infarct-related artery may confer benefits by reducing arrhythmias[36] and LV remodeling.[33,37,38] We have shown that end-systolic volume is the most important prognostic factor after recovery from infarction;[26] reperfusion, even if late, may increase the tensile strength of the infarct zone and decrease infarct expansion and dilation of the ventricle.[37,38] Dilation could also be reduced by accelerated infarct healing and salvage of islets of epicardium acting as a splint. Blood in the coronary arteries may also support the infarct zone and reduce infarct expansion, remodeling, and dilation of the noninfarct zone. Sustained patency of an infarct-related artery long-term will also enable collateral blood flow if a subsequent infarct occurs in a different coronary artery territory.

RELATIONSHIP BETWEEN LEFT VENTRICULAR FUNCTION AND PATENCY OF THE INFARCT-RELATED ARTERY

Thrombolytic therapy works by lysing the occluding coronary thrombus and achieving reperfusion of ischemic myocardium. Preservation of LV function is closely related to patency of the infarct-related artery.[39–41] Successful reperfusion results in improved ejection fraction: nonreperfusion results in no change or often deterioration in LV function.[42–44]

A "snapshot in time," such as a 90-minute injection of contrast at angiography, may not reflect the true situation, where the artery may have been closed immediately before or after the contrast injection. Patency of the infarct-related artery is not a static process, and the artery may open and close as reexposure of the endothelium occurs following thrombolysis, with recurring platelet aggregation, spasm, and thrombus formation.[45,46]

Retrospective subgroup analysis of the Western Washington intracoronary streptokinase trial showed that 1-year mortality was improved in the patients who had complete reperfusion (2.5%) compared with the patients in whom the infarct-related artery was either partially reperfused (23.1%) or remained occluded (14.6%), p = 0.008.[6] This study has been widely quoted as showing that patency of the infarct-related artery is an important prognostic factor. However, this analysis evaluated LV function measured acutely when there is both severe stunning of the infarct and

TABLE 12-2. Six-Month Mortality from Hospital Discharge by Hours from Symptom Onset: GISSI-2 and the International Study

Symptom Onset	rt-PA (%)	SK	Risk Ratio (95% CI)	Total (%)
≤1 hr	2.6	2.9	0.89 (0.55–1.45)	2.7
≤3 hr	3.1	3	1.02 (0.82–1.26)	3
>3 hr	4.6	4	1.15 (0.9–1.48)	4.3

Abbreviations: rt-PA, tissue plasminogen activator; SK, streptokinase.

ischemic zones and hyperkinesis of the noninfarct zones. When LV function and patency were measured on day 3, only ejection fraction (p <0.001) and age (p = 0.005) were significant predictors of mortality.[23]

In the Thrombolysis and Angioplasty in Myocardial Infarction (TAMI) trials, ejection fraction was also shown to be the most important predictor of hospital mortality. Analysis of long-term (18-month) follow-up has not shown patency of the infarct-related artery to be a significant prognostic factor, but ejection fraction has been shown to be significantly higher in survivors, 52% versus 46% in nonsurvivors.[14]

In studies such as the TAMI trials, efforts have been made to achieve a patent artery in as many patients as possible before hospital discharge. This makes it very difficult to tease out whether patency is an independent prognostic factor, particularly when the event rate is also low.

Follow-up of the Western Washington intravenous rt-PA trial also shows that LV function is the most important prognostic factor. Cox regression analysis showed that patency of the infarct-related artery at the time of hospital discharge did not give prognostic information.[17]

It is extremely interesting that in the GISSI-2 6-month follow-up, patients treated earlier had the largest reduction in mortality from the hospital period on[19] (Table 12-2). Because of the catch up phenomenon whereby patency of the infarct-related artery becomes similar as time goes on, regardless of which thrombolytic agent is given, patients have the same patency rates after about 3 hr.[47] Differences in patency of the infarct-related artery cannot explain the improved survival with early treatments. It is very likely that this improved survival is due to improved LV function.

ARRHYTHMIAS

The presence of ventricular arrhythmias is an adverse prognostic factor after myocardial infarction, particularly in the presence of LV dysfunction.[31] Re-

perfusion has been shown to reduce the incidence of late potentials on the signal-averaged electrocardiogram (ECG).[48–50] In 55 patients treated with streptokinase, late potentials were present in 16.4% versus 43.3% in 60 control patients. The absence of late potentials also correlated with infarct-related artery patency (sensitivity 80.9%, specificity 89.5%).[50]

Reperfusion may prevent the development of the substrate needed to produce sustained ventricular arrhythmias; perhaps viable islets of myocardium capable of producing microcircuits are killed by reperfusion damage. Several studies have suggested that thrombolysis reduces the incidence of inducible ventricular tachycardia. In a study of 32 patients with anterior infarction and LV aneurysms, Sager et al.[36] showed that thrombolytic therapy reduced ventricular irritability. In patients who did not receive thrombolytic therapy, ventricular tachycardia was induced at electrophysiologic study in 88%, and 50% died suddenly over 11 months of follow-up, whereas ventricular tachycardia at electrophysiologic study occurred in only 8% of patients who received thrombolytic therapy, and there were no deaths at follow-up.

EXERCISE TESTING

Exercise testing after thrombolytic therapy has not been helpful in our experience for predicting patients at risk of reinfarction (Table 12-3). It does not evaluate instability of plaque or propensity of plaque to rupture, but it is very useful for evaluating residual ischemia. Thallium tomography may be more useful in this regard. Jain et al.[51] showed that oral dipyridamole identified more patients with residual ischemia after thrombolytic therapy than did symptom-limited exercise treadmill testing, 74% versus 28%.

OTHER RISK FACTORS

During the first few years postinfarction, the extent of myocardial damage is the prime determinant of prognosis. Long-term, however, the extent of coronary artery disease and risk factors become important. Although aspirin and β-blocker therapy have reduced reinfarction and mortality after infarction, these events still occur frequently,[52] and efforts should be made to modify risk factors associated with the development and progression of coronary artery disease.

Cholesterol

At least 10 trials have shown cholesterol levels to be related to outcome after infarction. Eight secondary prevention trials have involved greater than 3-year fol-

TABLE 12-3. Potential Risk Factors for Reinfarction: Defined 3 Weeks After Index Infarction

Risk Factors	Subsequent Reinfarction (n = 19)	No. of Subsequent Reinfarctions (n = 388)	p
Continued smoking	7 (37%)	28 (8%)	<0.001
Inferior infarction	13 (68%)	212 (55%)	0.35
Non-Q-wave infarction	3 (16%)	93 (24%)	0.59
Female sex	3 (16%)	90 (23%)	0.64
Age (years)	58 ± 10	57 ± 10	0.78
Diabetes	1 (5%)	38 (10%)	0.8
Previous angina	3 (16%)	77 (20%)	0.89
Hypertension	4 (21%)	96 (25%)	0.93
rt-PA therapy	6 (32%)	120 (31%)	1.0
SK therapy	13 (68%)	268 (69%)	1.0
β-Blocker therapy	9 (47%)	175 (45%)	1.0
Catheter data			
n	16	312	
Patent infarct artery	14 (88%)	238 (76%)	0.46
% stenosis in patent infarct artery	84.3 ± 11.7	83.7 ± 17.5	0.9
Exercise test data			
n	16	279	
Exercise duration (minutes)	11.2 ± 3.2	11 ± 3.6	0.81
Angina during test	1 (6%)	45 (16%)	0.48
Peak heart rate (per minute)	131 ± 23	127 ± 24	0.59
Peak systolic blood pressure (mmHg)	168 ± 36	158 ± 28	0.15
ST depression ≥1 mm with exercise	3 (19%)	97 (35%)	0.3

Abbreviations: rt-PA, tissue plasminogen activator; SK, streptokinase.

low-up.[53] These investigations have shown that after about 2 years, cholesterol-lowering therapy results in a decreased incidence of coronary events. Meta-analysis of these trials involving 7.837 patients shows decreased nonfatal (p = 0.001), fatal (p = 0.01) and total (p = 0.001) infarctions with cholesterol-lowering treatment.[53]

Several coronary arteriographic trials have evaluated cholesterol-lowering therapy.[54-59] All of these trials have demonstrated a reduced rate of progression of coronary artery atheroma, and some have shown regression.[56,57,59] The Familial Atherosclerosis Study (FATS) also showed that although the changes in the coronary arteries were small, there were major reductions in clinical events. Death, myocardial infarction, or need for coronary bypass were reduced by 73%:11 events in 52 control patients compared with five events in 94 patients treated.[59] Lipid lowering may have additional important effects on endothelial function, plaque rupture, and thrombus formation.

Smoking

Cigarette smoking is associated with increased risk of myocardial infarction[66]; this risk is increased even when the severity of coronary artery disease is equal.[61,62] Smoking also increases the risk of thrombosis by increasing platelet aggregation,[63-65] and fibrinogen levels[60] and by decreasing the production of prostacyclin.[67]

Our prethrombolytic study of long-term prognosis after myocardial infarction showed that continued cigarette smoking was an independent risk factor for survival.[26] In our study of factors predisposing to reinfarction after thrombolytic therapy, cigarette smoking was the only factor we were able to identify as predictive of reinfarction.[9] Table 12-4 shows the univariate analysis of potential risk factors for reinfarction defined at the time of the initial infarction. Cardiac catheterization and exercise testing were performed 3 weeks postinfarction. Exercise testing and residual stenosis of the patent infarct-related artery were not predictive of subsequent reinfarction (Table 12–3).

TABLE 12-4. Potential Risk Factors for Reinfarction: Defined at Time of Index Infarction

Risk Factors	Reinfarction (n = 43)	No. of Reinfarctions (n = 413)	p
Smoking	29 (67%)	203 (50%)	0.04
Inferior infarction	28 (65%)	221 (54%)	0.2
Female sex	6 (14%)	99 (24%)	0.2
Non-Q-wave infarction	8 (19%)	97 (23%)	0.59
No previous angina	36 (84%)	329 (80%)	0.66
Diabetes	3 (7%)	43 (10%)	0.66
Age (years)	58 ± 9	57 ± 10	0.68
rt-PA therapy	14 (33%)	127 (31%)	0.94
SK therapy	29 (67%)	286 (69%)	0.94
Hypertension	10 (23%)	103 (25%)	0.95

Abbreviations: rt-PA, tissue plasminogen activator; SK, streptokinase.

The only variable associated with reinfarction on multivariate analysis was cigarette smoking on admission. Reinfarction occurred in 12.5% of smokers versus 6.3% of nonsmokers, p = 0.04.

Of the 35 patients who were still smoking at 3 weeks, 20% subsequently reinfarcted versus 5.1% for the 156 previous smokers who had stopped at the time of their infarct, p = 0.01, and 3.4% for the 354 patients who had never smoked. Reinfarction results in significant mortality and worsening of LV function; vigorous efforts should be made to achieve smoking cessation after infarction.

CONCLUSION

The effect of thrombolytic therapy on long-term mortality is as important as the effects on short-term mortality. LV function is the most important long-term prognostic factor, and is closely related to long-term mortality as well as quality of life after infarction. It remains an important and valid objective to try to decrease the amount of LV damage in survivors. Prevention of LV dilation and maintenance of patency of the infarct-related artery may also improve prognosis.

β-Blockers and aspirin should be prescribed. The role of antiarrhythmic drugs is unclear. Angioplasty and coronary surgery should be performed for the relief of important ischemic syndromes.

Vigorous effects should also be made to control primary risk factors by stopping smoking, controlling hypertension, improving the lipid profile, achieving ideal weight, and promoting regular exercise, so as to decrease the progression of CAD in the rest of the coronary arteries.

REFERENCES

1. Gruppo Italiano per lo Studio Della Streptochinasi Nell'Infarto Miocardico (GISSI): Effectiveness of intravenous thrombolytic treatment in acute myocardial infarction. Lancet 1:397, 1986
2. ISIS-2 (Second International Study of Infarct Survival) Collaborative Group: Randomised trial of intravenous streptokinase, oral aspirin, both, or neither among 17,187 cases of suspected acute myocardial infarction: ISIS-2. Lancet 2:349, 1988
3. AIMS Trial Study Group: Effect of intravenous APSAC on mortality after acute myocardial infarction: preliminary report of a placebo-controlled clinical trial. Lancet 1:545, 1988
4. Wilcox RG, von der Lippe G, Ollson CG et al: Trial of tissue plasminogen activation for mortality reduction in acute myocardial infarction. Anglo-Scandinavian study of early thrombolysis (ASSET). Lancet 2:525, 1988
5. White HD, Norris RM, Brown MA et al: Effect of intravenous streptokinase on left ventricular function and early survival after acute myocardial infarction. N Engl J Med 317:850, 1987
6. Kennedy JW, Ritchie JL, Davis KB et al: The western Washington randomized trial of intracoronary streptokinase in acute myocardial infarction: a 12-month follow-up report. N Engl J Med 312:1073, 1985
7. Gruppo Italiano per lo Studio Della Streptochinasi Nell'Infarcto Miocardico: Long-term effects of intravenous thrombolysis in acute myocardial infarction: final report of the GISSI study. Lancet 2:871, 1987
8. Schröder R, Neuhaus KL, Leizorovicz A et al: A prospective placebo-controlled double-blind multicenter trial of streptokinase in acute myocardial infarction (ISAM): long-term mortality and morbidity. J Am Coll Cardiol 9: 197, 1987
9. Rivers JT, White HD, Cross DB et al: Reinfarction after thrombolytic therapy for acute myocardial infarction followed by conservative management: incidence and effect of smoking. J Am Coll Cardiol 16:340, 1990
10. Simoons ML, Arnold A: One year follow-up of rtPA without and with immediate PTCA. Circulation 80:(Suppl II): 520, 1989
11. Van de Werf F, Arnold AE: The European co-operative rt-PA vs placebo trial: 1 year follow-up. Circulation 80: (Suppl II):520, 1989
12. Dalen JE, Gore JM, Braunwald E et al: Six and twelve month follow-up of the phase I thrombolysis in myocardial infarction (TIMI) trial. Am J Cardiol 62:179, 1988
13. Williams DO, Braunwald E and the TIMI investigators. The thrombolysis in myocardial infarction (TIMI) trial: outcome at one year of patients randomized to either invasive or conservative management, abstracted. Circulation 80:II-519, 1989
14. Muller OW, Topol EJ and the Thrombolysis and Angioplasty in Myocardial Infarction Study Group: Long term follow-up in the thrombolysis and angioplasty in myocardial infarction (TAMI) trials: comparison with trials of thrombolysis alone, abstracted. Circulation, suppl II. 80:2068, 1989
15. Simoons ML, Vos J, Tijssen JGP et al: Long-term benefit of early thrombolytic therapy in patients with acute myocardial infarction: 5 year follow-up of a trial conducted by the Interuniversity Cardiology Institute of the Netherlands. J Am Coll Cardiol 14:1609, 1989
16. Taylor GJ, Song A, Korsmeyer C et al: Six year survival after thrombolysis for acute myocardial infarction, abstracted. Circulation 80 (Suppl II): II-520, 1989
17. Flygenring BP, Althouse RG, Sheehan FH et al: Does vessel patency at the time of hospital discharge following thrombolytic therapy predict survival?, abstracted. J Am Coll Cardiol 15:202A, 1990
18. Wilcox RG, von der Lippe G, Olsson CG et al for the Anglo-Scandinavian Study of Early Thrombolysis: Effects of alteplase in acute myocardial infarction: 6-month results from the ASSET study. Lancet 335:1175, 1990
19. GISSI-2/International Study: Follow-up at six months. (in press).
20. White HD, Rivers JT, Maslowski AH et al: Effect of intravenous streptokinase as compared with that of tissue

plasminogen activator on left ventricular function after first myocardial infarction. N Engl J Med 320:817, 1989

21. Volpi A, Cavalli A, Santoro E et al: Incidence and prognosis of secondary ventricular fibrillation in acute myocardial infarction. Evidence for a protective effect of thrombolytic therapy. Circulation 82:1279, 1990

22. White HD: Relation of thrombolysis during acute myocardial infarction to left ventricular function and mortality. Am J Cardiol 66:92, 1990

23. Sheehan FH, Doerr R, Schmidt WG: Early recovery of left ventricular function after thrombolytic therapy for acute myocardial infarction: an important determinant of survival. J Am Coll Cardiol 12:289, 1988

24. Norris RM, Caughey DE, Mercer CJ, Scott PJ: Prognosis after myocardial infarction. Six year follow-up. Br Heart J 36:786, 1974

25. Multicenter Post-infarction Research Group: Risk stratification and survival after myocardial infarction. N Engl J Med 309:321, 1983

26. White HD, Norris RM, Brown MA et al: Left ventricular end-systolic volume as the major determinant of survival after recovery from myocardial infarction. Circulation 76:44, 1987

27. Taylor GJ, Humphries JO, Mellits ED et al: Predictors of clinical course, coronary anatomy and left ventricular function after recovery from acute myocardial infarction. Circulation 62:960, 1980

28. Sanz G, Castaner A, Betriu A et al: Determinants of prognosis in survivors of myocardial infarction: a prospective clinical angiographic study. N Engl J Med 306:1065, 1982

29. De Feyter PJ, van Eenige MJ, Dishton DH et al: Prognostic value of exercise testing, coronary angiography and left ventriculography 6-8 weeks after myocardial infarction. Circulation 66:527, 1982

30. Roubin GS, Harris PJ, Bernstein L, Kelly DT: Coronary anatomy and prognosis after myocardial infarction in patients 60 years of age and younger. Circulation 67:743, 1983

31. Bigger JT, Fleiss JL and the Multicenter Post-infarction Research Group: The relationship among ventricular arrhythmias, left ventricular dysfunction and mortality in the 2 years after myocardial infarction. Circulation 69:250, 1984

32. Gibson RS, Watson DD, Craddock GB et al: Prediction of cardiac events after uncomplicated myocardial infarction: a prospective study comparing predischarge exercise thallium-201 scintigraphy and coronary angiography. Circulation 68:321, 1983

33. White HD: Mechanisms of late benefit in ISIS-2. Lancet 2:914, 1988

34. Braunwald E: Myocardial reperfusion, limitation of infarct size, reduction of left ventricular dysfunction, and improved survival. Should the paradigm be expanded? Circulation 79:441, 1989

35. White HD, Cross DB, Elliott JM et al: Independent long-term prognostic importance of ejection fraction and infarct artery patency after myocardial infarction. J Am Coll Cardiol. 19:237A, 1992

36. Sager PT, Perlmutter RA, Rosenfeld LE et al: Electrophysiologic effects of thrombolytic therapy in patients with a transmural anterior myocardial infarction com-

plicated by left ventricular aneurysm formation. J Am Coll Cardiol 12:19, 1988

37. Hochman JS, Choo H: Limitation of myocardial infarct expansion by reperfusion independent of myocardial salvage. Circulation 75:299, 1987

38. Force T, Kemper A, Leavitt M, Parisi AF: Acute reduction in functional infarct expansion with late coronary reperfusion: assessment with quantitative two dimensional echocardiography. J Am Coll Cardiol 2:192, 1986

39. Spann JF, Sherry S, Carabello BA et al: Coronary thrombolysis by intravenous streptokinase in acute myocardial infarction: acute and follow-up studies. Am J Cardiol 53:655, 1986

40. Schwartz F, Faivre A, Katus H et al: Intracoronary thrombolysis in acute myocardial infarction: an attempt to quantitate its effect by comparison of enzymatic estimate of myocardial necrosis with left ventricular ejection fraction. Am J Cardiol 51:1573, 1983

41. Schröder R, Biamino G, v Leitner E-R et al: Intravenous short-term infusion of streptokinase in acute myocardial infarction. Circulation 67:536, 1983

42. Feyter PJ, Van Eenige ML, Van der Wall EE et al: Effects of spontaneous and streptokinase induced recanalization on left ventricular function in acute myocardial infarction. Circulation 67:1039, 1983

43. Verheugt FWA, Visser FC, Van dur Wall EE et al: Prediction of spontaneous coronary reperfusion in myocardial infarction. Postgrad Med J 62:1007, 1986

44. Jeremy RW, Hackworthy RA, Bautovich G et al: Infarct artery perfusion and changes in left ventricular volume in the month after acute myocardial infarction. J Am Coll Cardiol 9:989, 1987

45. White H: GISSI-2 and the heparin controversy. Lancet 336:297, 1990

46. Kwon KI, Freedman SB, Wilcox I et al: The unstable ST segment early after thrombolysis for acute infarction and its usefulness as a marker of recurrent coronary occlusion. Am J Cardiol 69:109, 1991

47. PRIMI Trial Study Group: Randomised double-blind trial of recombinant pro-urokinase against streptokinase in acute myocardial infarction. Lancet 1:863, 1989

48. Gang ES, Lew AS, Hong M et al: Decreased incidence of ventricular late potentials after successful thrombolytic therapy for acute myocardial infarction. N Engl J Med 321:712, 1989

49. Vatterott PJ, Hammill SC, Bailey VR et al: Reperfusion reduces late potentials independently of left ventricular fucntion, abstracted. Circulation, suppl 2. 80:II-314, 1989

50. Chew EW, Morton P, Murtagh JG et al: Intravenous streptokinase for acute myocardial infarction reduces the occurrence of ventricular late potentials. Br Heart J 64:58, 1990

51. Jain A, Hicks RR, Frantz MM et al: Comparison of early exercise treadmill test and oral dipyridamole thallium-201 tomography for the identificaiton of jeopardized myocardium in patients receiving thrombolytic therapy for acute Q-wave myocardial infarction. Am J Cardiol 66:551, 1990

52. Yusuf S, Wittes J, Friedman L: Overview of results of randomized clinical trials in heart disease. II. Unstable angina, heart failure, primary prevention with aspirin and risk factor modification. JAMA 260:2259–63, 1988

53. Rossouw JE, Lewis B, Rifkind BM: The value of lowering cholesterol after myocardial infarction. N Engl J Med 323:1112, 1990

54. Brensike JF, Levy RI, Kelsey SF et al: Effects of therapy with cholestyramine on progression of coronary arteriosclerosis: results of the NHLBI type II coronary intervention study. Circulation 69:313, 1984

55. Arntzenius AC, Kromhout D, Barth JD et al: Diet, lipoproteins, and the progression of coronary atherosclerosis: the Leiden intervention trial. N Engl J Med 312:805, 1985

56. Blankenhorn DH, Nessim SA, Johnson RL et al: Beneficial effects of combined colestipol-niacin therapy on coronary atherosclerosis and coronary venous bypass grafts. JAMA 257:3233, 1987

57. Ornish D, Brown SE, Scherwitz LW et al: Can lifestyle changes reverse coronary heart disease? Lancet 336:129, 1990

58. Buchwald H, Varco RL, Matts JP et al for the POSCH Group: Effect of partial ileal bypass surgery on mortality and morbidity from coronary heart disease in patients with hypercholesterolemia. N Engl J Med 323:946, 1990

59. Brown G, Albers JJ, Fisher LD, et al: Regression of coronary artery disease as a result of intensive lipid-lowering therapy in men with high levels of apolipoprotein B. N Engl J Med 323:1289, 1990

60. Doyle JT, Dawber TR, Kannel WB et al: The relationship of cigarette smoking to coronary heart disease—the second report of the combined experience of Albany, NY and Framingham Mass studies. JAMA 190:886, 1964

61. Hartz AJ, Barboriak PN, Anderson AJ et al: Smoking, coronary artery occlusion and non-fatal myocardial infarction. JAMA 246:851, 1981

62. McKenzie WB, McCredie RM, McGilchrist CA, Wilcken DEL: Smoking: a major predictor of left ventricular function after occlusion of the left anterior descending coronary artery. Br Heart J 56:496, 1986

63. Fuster V, Chesebro JH, Frye RL, Elveback LR: Platelet survival and the development of coronary artery disease in the young adult: effects of cigarette smoking, strong family history and medical therapy. Circulation 63:546, 1981

64. Mustard JF, Murphy EA: Effect of smoking on blood coagulation and platelet survival in man. Br Med J 1:846, 1963

65. Woolf N, Pittilo RM, Machin SJ: Cigarette smoking and platelet adhesion. Lancet 2:1091, 1983

66. Wilkes HC, Kelleher C, Meade TW: Smoking and plasma fibrinogen. Lancet 1:307, 1988

67. Nadler JL, Velasco JS, Horton R: Cigarette smoking inhibits prostacyclin formation. Lancet 2:1248, 1983

13

Prognostic Significance of Silent Myocardial Ischemia

Bramah N. Singh
Prakash C. Deedwania
Freny Vaghaiwalla Mody

It is estimated that more than six million Americans have chronic coronary heart disease (CHD) and that 1.2 to 1.5 million develop acute myocardial infarction (AMI) each year, resulting in 500,000 patients dying with it annually. The Framingham experience suggested that more than 25% of documented myocardial infarctions (MI) are silent and recognized only during routine electrocardiographic (ECG) examinations,[1] and there is no difference in prognosis between silent and symptomatic infarcts.

Myocardial ischemia is generally accepted as a common expression of coronary artery disease (CAD), and angina has been considered the hallmark symptom of CAD and myocardial ischemia. Recent studies, however, suggest that angina is a relatively insensitive and nonspecific marker of significant CAD. The lack of symptoms does not exclude a severe and potentially lethal degree of coronary arterial stenosis.[2] Even in patients with documented significant CAD, the absence of ischemic symptoms does not necessarily predict a benign prognosis.[3] Furthermore, the severity of anginal symptoms does not necessarily correlate with the extent of CAD or long-term prognosis.[4] Indeed, cardiac ischemia may often occur without associated symptoms. In some cases, sudden cardiac death may be the initial manifestation of CAD.[5] Furthermore, advanced obstructive CAD may exist with minimal or no symptoms and can progress with a rapidly fatal outcome with little or no warning. An estimated 18% of coronary attacks occur with sudden death as the first event.[6] More than 50% of sudden deaths occur without documented history of CAD. Detection of myocardial ischemia during exercise testing in totally asymptomatic patients has also been shown to predict a higher risk of subsequent coronary event and death.[7-10] Although the exact prevalence of asymptomatic CAD in the population at large is not known, it appears that at least 2.5% of middle-aged men in the United States have asymptomatic CAD.[10-12] Therefore, the detection of myocardial ischemia and stratification of its risk potential for adverse prognosis is clearly an important clinical objective. However, it presupposes that therapeutic modalities are available for the effective suppression of ischemia of a sufficient degree that is prognostically meaningful.

Continuous ECG monitoring in patients with various ischemic myocardial syndromes has revealed that most episodes of myocardial ischemia are clinically silent.[13-28] It is also recognized that in patients with asymptomatic CAD; in those with clinically manifest

CAD, incontrovertible evidence of myocardial ischemia may be present *without* symptoms. Such a "discovery" has raised a number of clinically relevant questions. What is the precise incidence of silent myocardial ischemia? Does it differ from symptomatic myocardial ischemia? Does it have the same significance as silent ischemia demonstrated by provocative exercise stress testing with or without the inclusion of radionuclide or ECG parameters of ischemia? Importantly, does silent myocardial ischemia have an independent prognostic significance? For example, does it play a significant role in the development of MI, ventricular dysfunction, arrhythmias, and sudden death? Finally, is it amenable to pharmacologic and nonpharmacologic suppression (e.g., myocardial revascularization with surgery or percutaneous transluminal coronary angioplasty), and what degree of reduction in silent myocardial ischemia might be necessary to favorably alter clinical outcome? The central question is whether silent myocardial ischemia in itself constitutes a marker for sudden death that could be prevented by a measurable reduction in the frequency and duration of asymptomatic ischemic episodes.

Therefore, the purpose of this chapter is to provide the current perspective on the issue of whether silent myocardial ischemia does have an independent prognostic significance that might constitute a clinically valid reason for treating it *independent of symptomatic amelioration*. This is clearly the most crucial issue with respect to the significance of silent myocardial ischemia in clinical therapeutics.

WHAT IS SILENT MYOCARDIAL ISCHEMIA?

Silent myocardial ischemia is thought to be present when unequivocal biochemical, hemodynamic, perfusion, functional, and ECG abnormalities indicative of an imbalance in myocardial oxygen demand and supply develop in the absence of angina or equivalent symptoms. It is clearly desirable to distinguish asymptomatic CAD from silent myocardial ischemia. Asymptomatic CAD provides the substrate for the development of silent myocardial ischemia that may become manifest as the "activity" of the disease changes. Alternatively, the major determinants of oxygen consumption are altered so that the threshold for ischemia is reached. For example, a patient with significant triple vessel CAD may demonstrate no myocardial ischemia during continuous ambulatory ECG monitoring if the disease is not active. On the other hand, under the stress of strenuous exercise treadmill testing, compelling ECG evidence of myocardial ischemia may develop in such a patient *but without angina or its equivalents*. However, in the absence of other confirmatory

evidence of CAD in an individual patient, the significance of the seemingly positive ECG changes on the treadmill test as an isolated phenomenon will be difficult to define.

SILENT MYOCARDIAL ISCHEMIA AS A MEASURABLE CLINICAL ENTITY

In the clinical context, silent myocardial ischemia has been identified by continuous ECG recordings by Holter devices in hospitalized patients and in ambulatory subjects. Ischemia that is silent may also be demonstrated by the performance of exercise treadmill tests combined with radionuclide ventriculography, echocardiography, or perfusion scintigraphy. Irrespective of the method used myocardial ischemia is quantified crudely at best in terms of extent and severity relative to the overall area involved in the ischemic process and its temporal duration when assessed on the basis of the ECG.

The subsets of patients with silent myocardial ischemia are as follows:

Completely asymptomatic subjects
Those with risk factors for CAD
Those without risk factors for CAD
Patients with manifest CAD
Prinzmetal angina
Unstable angina
Chronic stable angina
Postmyocardial infarction
Postmyocardial revascularization

The largest numbers of patients who exhibit the phenomenon of silent ischemia are those who have symptomatic manifestations of CAD. Silent myocardial ischemia should not be confused with silent CAD; the latter represents the state of the susbstrate, the former the manifestations of the degree of abnormality therein. Episodes of silent ischemia simply represent the number of times the imbalance of oxygen supply and demand reaches threshold for manifestation during the course of the day.

SIGNIFICANCE OF SILENT ISCHEMIA DURING ECG MONITORING

The overall data[18,19,21,22,24–29] from studies in patients with rest angina, unstable angina, and chronic stable angina subjected to ambulatory ECG (serial Holter) recordings have revealed a number of significant findings indicative of silent myocardial ischemia:

1. Characteristic pattern of associated heart rate and blood pressure changes

2. Marked variation in duration of individual episodes
3. Considerable temporal variability
4. Exhibits circadian periodicity in chronic stable angina
5. Rarely demonstrable in healthy subjects
6. Most frequently occurs in patients with known and severe coronary artery disease
7. Amenable to reduction by pharmacologic as well as invasive treatment modalities
8. May be of prognostic significance, at least in certain subsets of patients with CAD
9. Prognostic significance probably similar to that with symptomatic ischemia

First, they have shown that more than two-thirds of episodes of myocardial ischemia in all these subsets of patients with CAD are clinically silent. Second, greater than 80 to 90% of episodes of ischemia were not preceded by significant increases in heart rate. These findings are in line with the results of Berndt and co-workers,[30] who reported that the rate-pressure product was significantly lower at the onset of spontaneous ischemia than that at anginal threshold during atrial pacing in patients with CAD and unstable angina. Deanfield and colleagues[24] showed that the peak heart rate is lower in episodes of ischemia that are spontaneous than in episodes induced by exercise in patients with chronic stable angina. Third, the distribution of ischemic episodes over 24-hour periods in chronic stable angina exhibits a circadian rhythm, with very few episodes occurring between midnight and 6 A.M.[31 37] The circadian periodicity coincides with that of heart rate, blood pressure, and the catecholamine surges during the 24 hours. Fourth, increasing data now suggest that the highest incidence of silent myocardial ischemia tends to occur in patients with the most symptomatic and anatomically severe CAD. Of particular interest, in patients with stable CAD, transient ischemic events occur frequently during daily life; the majority (up to 80%) are essentially asymptomatic.[16,34–38] The precise mechanism whereby an episode of ischemia is silent at one time and symptomatic at another time *in the same patient* is unknown. However, whereas the earlier studies suggested the dominant role of myocardial blood flow reduction as the mechanism of silent ischemia even in chronic stable angina,[24] more recent findings emphasize the importance of increases in oxygen demand.[39] In the study conducted by Deedwania et al.,[39] in 25 patients with documented CAD, stable angina, and a positive exercise treadmill test, simultaneous ambulatory ECG and blood pressure monitoring were performed for 24 to 48 hours. The results demonstrated that significant increases in heart rate and systolic blood pressure frequently preceded the onset of silent ischemic events during daily life (Fig. 13-1). They also observed a morning surge in silent ischemic events which was similar to that reported previously and paralleled the morning increases in heart rate and systolic blood pressures[39,40] (Fig. 13-2). These circulatory changes observed prior to the onset of silent ST-segment depression during ambulatory ECG monitoring closely resemble those involved in the pathophysiology of

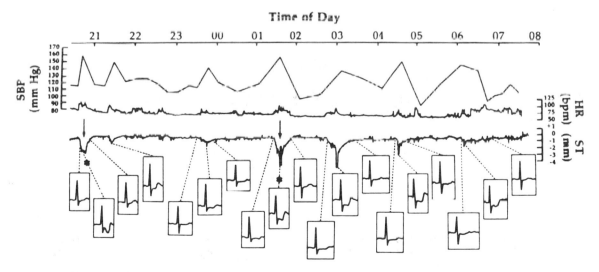

Fig. 13-1. Simultaneous ambulatory ECG and blood pressure monitoring data in a man with CAD. Systolic blood pressure (SBP), heart rate (HR), and ST-segment changes (ST) are plotted against time. The data reveal an increase in HR and SBP preceding and during most time. Asterisk indicates transient ischemic event accompanied by chest pain, requiring use of sublingual nitroglycerin (indicated by arrow). (From Deedwania and Nelson,[39] with permission.)

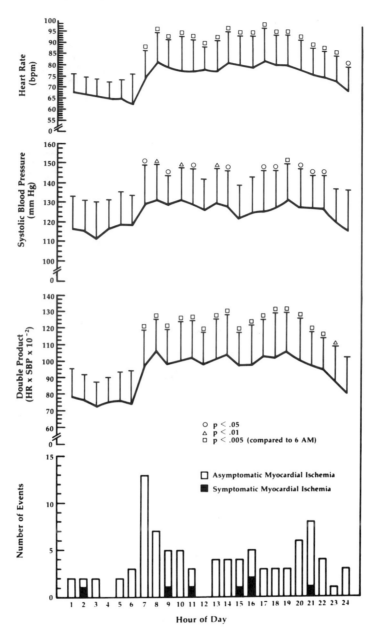

Fig. 13-2. The 24-hour distribution of silent ischemic events during continuous ECG monitoring parallels the circadian pattern of heart rate and systolic blood pressure. Note the simultaneous and significant increases in both the circulatory changes and silent ischemic events between 6:00 and 7:00 A.M. (From Deedwania and Nelson,[39] with permission.)

angina pectoris. Although more data are needed, it seems reasonable to consider that both an increase in myocardial oxygen demand and a decrease in coronary blood supply play a role in the genesis of silent myocardial ischemia. These findings are relevant to the choice of pharmacologic regimens in the suppression of silent ischemia continuously over spans of 24 hours or longer.

SIGNIFICANCE OF SILENT ISCHEMIA DURING TREADMILL EXERCISE TEST

It has long been recognized that the presence of significant CAD can be established with a high degree of sensitivity and specificity by exercise stress testing in an asymptomatic population with a high incidence of the disease.[41] In such patients who test electrocardiographically positive for ischemia, other objective indices such as scintigraphic perfusion defects[42] and segmental wall motion abnormalities[43] are usually present. It is also known that during exercise by patients with CAD, ischemic ST-segment changes may precede the onset of angina, which, in many patients, may fail to develop even at peak levels of stress. For example, in a study involving 92 patients with angiographically documented coronary disease, Amsterdam and associates[44] found ST-segment depression of greater than 1 mm in association with delayed angina in only 39 patients (42%). Lindsey and Cohn[45] studied 122 patients with angiographically documented CAD; they found that in 44 patients no pain developed during exercise stress testing. The data are concordant with the analysis of Rozanski and Berman[46] who, in a review of 13 studies, found that approximately 30% of transient ischemic ST-segment depressions during exercise testing occurred without angina in patients with documented CAD. The extent of CAD evaluated angiographically was similar in the groups with and without pain. The data emphasized that, in patients with known CAD, it is probable that symptomatic as well as silent myocardial ischemia might have the same clinical significance.

Within this context, the data from the Registry (nonrandomized) component of the Coronary Artery Surgery Study (CASS) evaluating 2,982 patients are of particular interest. The 1,583 patients with CAD (70% or greater) were analyzed on the basis of the present of ischemic ST-segment depression (≥1 mm) and oc-currence of anginal symptoms.[47] The cumulative 7-year survival rates for the three groups of patients (with chest pain only, ST-segment depression only, or with both features present) were nearly identical (about 77%). By contrast, in patients without ischemic ST-segment depression or angina, the survival rate was higher (88 percent) (Fig. 13-3). Among patients with silent ischemia during exercise stress testing, survival was related to the severity of CAD as judged by the numbers of coronary arteries with significant stenosis (Fig. 13-4). The findings of the CASS have been supported by those of Falcone and co-workers,[48] who compared the outcomes in 209 patients with silent myocardial ischemia during exercise testing with those of 269 patients with both ischemic ST-segment depression and angina. The mortality rate at 5 years was similar between the two groups, emphasizing that, in patients with known CAD, myocardial ischemia (as demonstrated by exercise stress testing) has the same prognosis whether it is silent or symptomatic.

Numerous studies[17,49–51] have recently attempted to determine the relationship between ischemia demonstrated by exercise treadmill testing and that documented on 24-hour Holter recordings. Emerging data suggest that Holter monitoring as a screening test for CAD has a lower sensitivity and lower predictive accuracy than those of exercise treadmill testing. The occurrence and frequency of silent myocardial ischemia on Holter recordings in totally asymptomatic middle-aged or elderly men with or without risk factors of CAD is not known. It is likely to be low.

As indicated above, the objective evidence of myo-

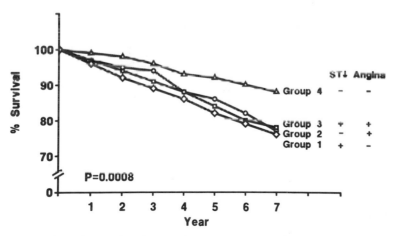

Fig. 13-3. Survival curves in patients with history of chronic stable angina with documented CAD relative to absence (−) or presence (+) of ST-segment depression and angina during exercise treadmill test. Note that when both are absent, the prognosis in terms of survival is the most favorable compared to when one or both the features are present. The data suggest that ischemia, whether symptomatic or silent on treadmill, has the same prognosis in patients with known CAD and stable angina (see text for details). (From Weiner et al.,[47] with permission.)

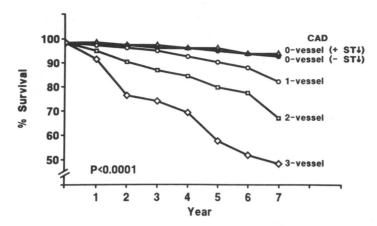

Fig. 13-4. Survival curves in patients with history of chronic stable angina with documented coronary artery disease relative to the number of vessels involved. Note the stepwise increase in attrition rate, over 7 years, as a function of time of vessels significantly stenosed. (Data from Weiner et al.[47])

cardial ischemia can be obtained by stress testing combined with radionuclide techniques in a completely asymptomatic population with CAD.[43] However, without angiographic confirmation and in the absence of pain, it may be difficult to be certain that ECG evidence of a positive test for ischemia is always indicative of significant CAD. The early recognition of ischemia in such patients is nevertheless important, since it might permit identification of asymptomatic subjects with "silent" CAD whose initial presentation of the disease is either AMI or sudden cardiac death. It has been estimated that exercise testing in middle-aged men between the ages of 40 and 60 years suggests a 5% incidence that probably doubles after age 60. Asymptomatic patients with unequivocally positive stress tests may not necessarily have multivessel CAD but, as a group, they have an increased risk of the development of manifestations of ischemic heart disease.[53,54] The important question here is whether among such patients it might be possible to identify by means of Holter monitoring those with silent myocardial ischemia particularly susceptible to a serious morbid coronary event. At present, few systematic and controlled data address this important clinical issue.

PROGNOSTIC SIGNIFICANCE

There is an increasing body of data on the prognostic significance of silent myocardial ischemia in patients with asymptomatic CAD as well as in various subsets of patients with known coronary disease such as those with unstable angina, postinfarct patients, and those with chronic stable angina. Fewer data are available in patients with hypertensive heart disease and in those with hypertrophic or dilated cardiomyopathies.

The available data in well-defined ischemic syndromes are reviewed in brief.

Prevalence and Significance of Silent Myocardial Ischemia in Asymptomatic Subjects

The exact prevalence of silent ischemia in the asymptomatic population is not known. However, results from several screening studies can be used to arrive at an estimate of prevalence of asymptomatic CAD. Data from two large studies in the United States (n = 1,390) and Norway (n = 2,014) in asymptomatic middle-aged men undergoing screening with exercise testing revealed that silent ischemia during exercise with significant angiographic CAD was detected in approximately 2.5% of patients.[10,11] In a smaller study of 129 asymptomatic men (mean age 46) undergoing exercise treadmill testing and fluoroscopy to look for coronary artery calcification, 12 to 129 (10%) patients had evidence of both exercise-induced myocardial ischemia and significant angiographic CAD.[12] The Swedish Study[10] is of particular interest. Patients with a positive stress test without symptoms (i.e., with silent ischemia) were followed for 8 years and then for another 5 years. At the end of the first period, 3 subjects died; 7 had a myocardial infarction, and 16 had developed angina pectoris. Only 17 remained unchanged from the baseline study. At the end of 13 years of follow-up, 11 had died; 8 of the remaining patients had MI, 18 developed angina pectoris and 26 of the remaining men alive had signs of ECG deterioration. The mortality noted correlated well with the extent of angiographic CAD noted at the baseline study. The data document that asymptomatic coronary stenosis is a progressive disease.

Similar prognostic importance of asymptomatic CAD is suggested by other studies. The data from the LRCPPT study of 3,600 men aged 30 to 79 years and without prior evidence of CAD who underwent submaximal exercise treadmill testing showed that men with exercise-induced ischemia had a significantly higher age-adjusted cardiovascular mortality compared with those with a negative test during a mean follow-up period of 8.4 years.[8] In the Multiple Risk Factor Intervention Trial (MRFIT) of asymptomatic middle-aged men with two or more coronary risk factors, the presence of ischemia during exercise testing was highly predictive of cardiac death (relative risk ratio 3.4) compared with those without ST changes.[7] In another prospective study of 135 asymptomatic patients, those with ischemic ST-segment depression during exercise testing had a four- to fivefold increase in the risk of future cardiac events, such as MI, unstable angina, or sudden cardiac death, during a mean follow-up of 6 years.[9]

Unstable Angina and Silent Ischemia

It has long been appreciated that patients with unstable angina are at high risk of morbid coronary events.[57] With the availability of techniques for the quantification of episodes of asymptomatic and symptomatic myocardial ischemia, the question has arisen as to whether the frequency and duration of such episodes might improve prognostic information.

Johnson and associates[58] studied 116 patients with unstable angina who were admitted to the coronary care unit (CCU) and observed them by Holter monitoring for 12 to 50 hours (mean 27 ± 7 hours). Twenty-four patients showed the development of AMI. An analysis of the Holter recordings demonstrated ST segment change in 21 of the 92 remaining patients. Four patients were lost to follow-up. Angiography performed in 43 of the remaining 67 patients indicated that those with triple vessel disease or left mainstem coronary artery stenosis were more likely to have significant ST-segment deviations consistent with ischemic episodes. After a 3-month follow-up, 50 of 63 patients (83%) without ST-segment changes were alive and well on medical therapy. By contrast, only three of 12 (25%) with ST-segment deviations were alive and well, a difference that was highly significant (p < 0.001). Ten (17%) of 60 patients without ST-segment changes had major cardiac events, whereas 58% of patients with ST-segment deviations had major cardiac events. This difference did not reach statistical significance, but the trend of an unfavorable outcome in the group with ST-segment changes on Holter monitoring was striking. However, Johnson and associates[58] did not distinguish between silent and symptomatic episodes.

Two further studies have suggested that silent myocardial ischemia is a marker for an early unfavorable outcome in patients with unstable angina. Gottlieb and co-workers[59] studied Holter recordings in 70 patients admitted to the CCU with unstable angina and treated with triple therapy: β-blockers, calcium-channel blockers, and nitrates. Thirty-seven (group 1) of the patients had at least one episode of silent myocardial ischemia; 33 (group 2) had none. Gottlieb and co-workers examined the differences between the occurrence of MI and the need for myocardial revascularization or percutaneous transluminal coronary angioplasty (PTCA) between the two groups at the end of 1 month of follow-up. Moreover, Kaplan-Meier analysis revealed a significantly higher cumulative probability of infarction or need for revascularization in patients in group 1 (p < 0.002). Of particular interest, 17 of the 37 patients in group 1, whose cumulative silent ischemic episodes after medical therapy exceeded 60 minutes per 24 hours, had a less favorable prognosis than did patients with ischemia (Fig. 13-5). The overall data indicated that 50% of the patients with unstable angina treated with aggressive medical therapy continued to have episodes of silent myocardial ischemia, the duration of which was highly predictive of an unfavorable early clinical outcome.

In the second study reported by Nademanee and colleagues,[60] the data were very similar. These investigators prospectively studied 81 patients with unstable angina admitted to the CCU and treated with conventional therapy. Twenty-nine of these patients (group 1) required emergency coronary angiography. The remaining 52 patients had 24-hour Holter monitoring, the results of which were not used for the purpose of clinical decision-making. Forty-nine patients had Holter data that could be correlated with their short-term prognosis. Twenty of these patients had no myocardial ischemia (group 2A on the Holter recordings; in 11 patients, group 2B), the cumulative duration of ischemia per 24 hours did not exceed 60 minutes; and in the remainder (i.e., 18 patients, group 2C), the cumulative duration of ischemia exceed 60 minutes per 24 hours. It was of interest that the cumulative duration of ischemia also correlated reasonably well with indexes of proximal coronary stenosis scores and with the number of diseased vessels demonstrated on coronary angiography.

Thus, it is clear from these studies that, in patients with unstable angina, *the presence of silent myocardial ischemia persisting after the elimination of symptomatic episodes by medical therapy is of prognostic significance.* What is not clear from these studies, however, is the issue of whether the response to medical therapy in this setting merely identifies a group of patients with inherently better prognosis than for the group in which silent ischemia persists after triple therapy.

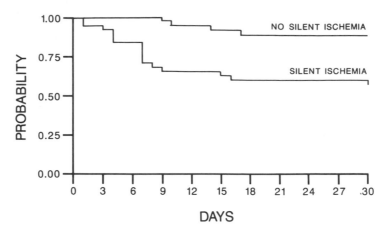

Fig. 13-5. Kaplan-Meier curves comparing the probability of not expecting an unfavorable outcome (myocardial infarction or revascularization for symptoms) over 30 days, for 37 unstable angina patients with silent ischemia and 33 patients without silent ischemia detected by continuous ECG monitoring (p < 0.002). (From Gottlieb et al.,[59] with permission.)

Post-MI Survivors

In a study of 210 survivors of AMI, approximately 18% of patients undergoing a low-level predischarge exercise treadmill test had asymptomatic ischemic ST-segment depression.[61] In another study of 103 high-risk post-MI patients undergoing continuous 24-hour ECG monitoring, approximately 29% demonstrated asymptomatic ischemic ST-segment changes.[62] A review of the available data indicates that 15 to 30% of survivors of AMI may have asymptomatic cardiac ischemia. The prognostic significance of silent myocardial ischemia is also well established in survivors of AMI. The results of predischarge exercise testing in these patients have indicated that the presence of ischemia with or without pain during exercise testing was associated with an increased risk of future cardiac events and death.[61,63] The role of ambulatory ECG monitoring was recently evaluated in 224 low-risk postinfarction patients. There was a fourfold increase in cardiac events in those patients with silent ischemia during ambulatory ECG monitoring compared with those without ischemia during 28-month follow-up.[63]

Prognostic Significance of Silent Myocardial Ischemia in Chronic Stable Angina

In this setting, two types of silent myocardial ischemia should be recognized: those associated with provocative exercise or comparable stress test, and those documented during continuous ambulatory ECG recording. A number of studies in patients with CAD and chronic stable angina have indicated that silent ischemia occurs far more frequently than do symptomatic cases. The pooled data of 1,162 patients from several reports revealed a 27 to 48% incidence of silent ischemia ST-segment changes during exercise ECG.[64,65] In patients with CAD and stable angina undergoing evaluation with Holter monitoring, the prevalence of asymptomatic ST-segment depression ranged from 41 to 56%.[37,38] From these observations, it appears that 2 to 3 million Americans with stable CAD experience silent myocardial ischemia.

A major concern is that in patients with CAD, intensive antianginal drug therapy directed for control of symptoms does not always eliminate silent ischemic episodes.[62,64,65] Recently, in a study of 105 patients with stable angina and CAD who were considered adequately treated with one or more antianginal drugs, Deedwaina and Carbajal[35] found that more than 40% of patients had silent ischemic events (Fig. 13-6) during 24-hour ambulatory ECG monitoring. Most ischemic events occurred during minimal or no physical activity; nearly all were free of symptoms during the monitoring period.

The increased risk of coronary events and cardiac mortality has been well documented in patients with known CAD and evidence of silent ischemia during exercise testing or Holter monitoring.[64,65] The report from the Registry component of the CASS showed that patients with exercise-induced ischemia have a worse prognosis than that of patients with a negative exercise test.[65] In this study in 880 patients with CAD, Weiner and colleagues found that during the 7-year follow-up period, the probability of experiencing MI and sudden death was significantly higher (Fig. 13-3) in pa-

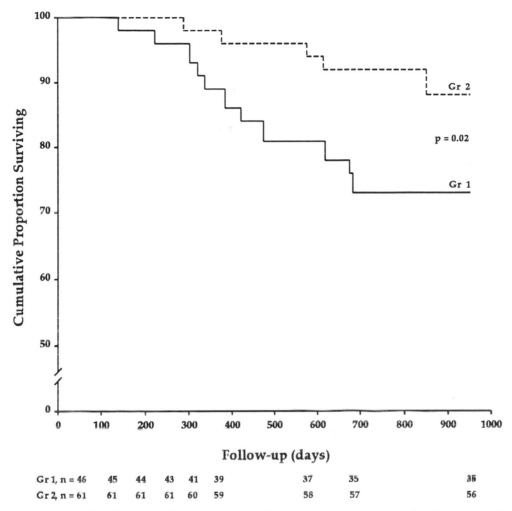

Fig. 13-6. Graph showing Kaplan-Meier curves comparing cumulative proportion of patients surviving without cardiac death during mean follow-up of 2 years for 46 patients with silent ischemia group (Group 1) and 61 patients without ischemia (Group 2) during ambulatory ECG monitoring (p < 0.02). (Adapted from Deedwania and Carabajal,[35] with permission.)

tients with exercise-induced silent (26%) or symptomatic (23%) ischemia compared with patients without exercise-induced ischemia (2%). In another study of 131 asymptomatic or mildly symptomatic patients with CAD undergoing exercise and radionuclide angiography, the presence of exercise-induced silent ischemia and an abnormal left ventricular ejection fraction (LVEF) response during exercise identified a group at high risk of subsequent cardiac death.[64]

A study of 86 patients with chronic exertional angina revealed that silent ischemia during Holter monitoring was associated with a higher risk of unstable angina and revascularization procedures during a 12-month follow-up.[38] In a study of the largest cohort of patients with stable CAD and angina pectoris, Deed-

wania et al.[37] recently reported silent ischemia during ambulatory ECG monitoring (AEM) was the most important predictor of cardiac death. It was found that of 107 patients with known CAD and exertional angina, those with one or more episodes of silent ischemia during Holter monitoring had a threefold (24% mortality) risk of sudden and nonsudden cardiac death compared with those without evidence of ischemia on AEM (8% mortality) during the 2-year follow-up (Fig. 13-6). Multiple regression analysis comparing several established clinical, ECG, and exercise test parameters revealed silent ischemia during AEM as the most powerful and an independent predictor of sudden death. In a recent review of several studies in patients with stable angina, Pepine[66] summarized that presence of ambulatory silent myocardial ischemia is associated with an adverse clinical outcome and increased risk of cardiac mortality. However, the precise reason for an adverse prognosis associated with silent ischemia is not known.

SUPPRESSION OF SILENT MYOCARDIAL ISCHEMIA

Pharmacologic Considerations

There is now growing evidence that various pharmacologic agents, PTCA, or coronary artery bypass surgery are variably effective in suppressing episodes of myocardial ischemia documented on Holter recordings in patients with CAD. However, few comparative studies defining the effects of different classes of antiischemic agents and of invasive interventions have been reported.

Even in the earliest studies, in which silent myocardial ischemic episodes were identified with Holter recordings in patients with CAD, nitrates were found to significantly reduce the number of episodes and their duration.[67] Few systematic studies have been carried out to determine the precise efficacy of these agents in eliminating silent myocardial ischemia. However, studies by Shell[67] indicate that transdermal preparations of nitrates have the propensity for markedly reducing Holter-detected silent myocardial ischemia in patients with chronic stable angina.

In the case of β-adrenergic blocking drugs, the bulk of the pharmacologic effects can ultimately be attributed to the ability of these compounds to competitively antagonize β-adrenoreceptors. Structurally, these compounds are reasonably homogeneous: minor structural differences have produced compounds of variable β-blocking potencies, varied pharmacokinetics, and associated features, such as intrinsic sympathomimetic activity, cardioselectivity, and membrane-depressant propensities. However, while such features may influence the overall profile of side effects of an individual agent, they have little or no effect on their therapeutic efficacy, which results essentially from the blockade of β-adrenoreceptors. The sole exception is the presence of intrinsic sympathomimetic activity that appears to attenuate efficacy. By contrast, calcium antagonists constitute a structurally heterogeneous group of compounds that share two significant properties: (1) the ability to block the slow calcium channel in cardiac muscle, and (2) the capacity to inhibit transmembrane fluxes of calcium in smooth muscle, especially in the coronary and peripheral circulations.[68]

Because of their often striking structural differences, individual calcium-channel blockers may exhibit other pharmacologic actions (e.g., verapamil and diltiazem have noncompetitive sympatholytic actions) that may lead to a complex interplay between their intrinsic properties (demonstrable in isolated tissues) and the reflex changes they may produce as a result of sympathetic activation caused by peripheral vasodilation.[68] Because of the reflex effects and the varying potencies of different calcium antagonists to induce peripheral vasodilatation, the actions of calcium antagonists both in vitro and in vivo may differ markedly. This is particularly striking in the case of atrioventricular (AV) nodal conduction and refractoriness. These electrophysiologic features of the various compounds are of therapeutic significance in the choice of an agent or combination of agents for the control of ischemic syndromes in patients who may have pre-existing conduction system disease. However, from the standpoint of control of ischemia, the comparative cardiocirculatory effects of calcium antagonists and β-antagonists are the most relevant pharmacologic effects.

It is now well-established that most β-antagonists, when administered intravenously or orally, depress heart rate, cardiac output, and indices of ventricular contractility and increase the filling pressures of the ventricle. Thus, the chief mechanism of their antiischemic action is via a reduction in oxygen demand. These drugs may also reduce coronary blood flow commensurate with the reduction in myocardial oxygen demand. From studies using quantitative angiography, it is also known than β-blockers may produce coronary vasoconstriction, an effect that may aggravate the tendency to coronary vasospasm, especially in the setting of Prinzmetal angina in patients with normal coronary vessels. For this reason, β-blockers are unlikely to eliminate episodes of ischemia triggered by coronary vasospasm. On the other hand, in patients whose episodes of ischemia are triggered by vasospasm in the setting of advanced CAD, the increases in heart rate and blood pressure in response to ischemia are likely to augment the overall duration of ischemia. β-Blockers are likely to curtail the duration of such ischemia episodes[69] and perhaps prevent them from reaching the threshold of pain perception. In contrast to the action of β-blockers, the most striking hemodynamic effect of calcium antagonists consists of a predictable and consistent reduction in system vascular resistance accompanied either by no change or by an increase in cardiac output.[69] Furthermore, unlike β-blockers, calcium antagonists reduce coronary vascular resistance, with a tendency for increased coronary sinus flow. Furthermore, these agents have the propensity to dilate resistance as well as capacitance vessels in the coronary circulation,[70,71] while such an effect is modest in extent, lesion dilation even of such a degree is hemodynamically significant.[72] It may be an important component of the anti-ischemic actions of calcium-channel blockers.

The differing pharmacologic effects of β-blockers and calcium-channel blockers therefore provide a rational basis for their combined therapy in the amelioration of transient myocardial ischemia to test the hypothesis that reduction or suppression of silent ischemia improves prognosis.

β-Blockers and Silent Myocardial Ischemia

There appear to be only limited data on this subject, but experience is increasing. However, a recent study[74] has documented that β-blockade exerts a salutary effect on silent myocardial ischemia in patients with chronic stable angina. Imperi and colleagues[74] studied the effects of titrated doses of metoprolol (50 to 100 mg bid) in patients with positive ECG evidence of asymptomatic ischemia but angiographically confirmed CAD. The frequency and duration of silent myocardial ischemia were quantified over 72 hours of Holter monitoring in each patient at baseline and after steady-state therapy at each dose of the β-blocker. A significant reduction was accomplished at each dose with a clear-cut dose-response effect. Imperi et al.[74] reported that metoprolol also reduced the total ischemia time per 24 hours; it attenuated the heart rate at the onset of ischemia while reducing the increases in heart rate associated with individual episodes, the durations of which were also shortened.

The well-known circadian pattern of ischemia distribution[31,32] over 24 hours was markedly attenuated by metoprolol. The blunting of the circadian pattern of silent ischemia in patients with CAD may be one mechanism that reduces the rate of sudden death and reinfarction in survivors of AMI given prophylactic β-blockade.

Suppression of Silent Ischemia by Calcium-Channel Blockers

Again, as in the case of β-blockers, limited data are available on chronic stable angina. The bulk of the reported data deals with the effects of calcium-channel blockers in the setting of vasospastic angina. In this case, the effects of all calcium-channel blockers in silent as well as symptomatic ischemia appear comparable, reflecting their somewhat similar coronary vasodilator propensities. The effects in chronic stable angina undoubtedly stem from a much more complex action of different classes of these agents in relationship to the possibly equally complex mechanisms underlying different episodes of transient ischemia in this setting.

As previously emphasized, there are few systematic data regarding the effects of calcium-channel blockers on silent myocardial ischemic episodes in chronic stable angina. The earliest observations dealt with the effects of bepridil, a calcium antagonist with a complex pharmacologic profile.[74] When 300 mg/day of the compound was given to patients with chronic stable angina and an exercise stress test positive for ischemia, the drug increased the time to angina and to the development of 1-mm ST-segment depression. Twenty-four-hour Holter recordings obtained before and during drug therapy and analyzed by the compact analogue technique indicated that bepridil significantly reduced the cumulative duration of silent myocardial ischemia per 24 hours. Schnellbacher and associates[75] studied the effects of diltiazem (60 mg tid) on silent and symptomatic episodes of myocardial ischemia in 19 patients. Holter monitoring indicated no episodes of ischemia in seven patients. In the remainder, after the first day of therapy with the calcium-channel blockers, the frequency and duration of ischemic episodes (over 90% silent) were reduced by 65 and 77%, respectively, and by 65% and 77%, respectively, and by 69% and 65%, respectively, on the seventh day. Verapamil is likely to exert a similar action on silent myocardial ischemic episodes in chronic stable angina, but systematic data must be obtained in controlled clinical trials.

Combined β-Blockers and Calcium Antagonists

A number of systematic studies dealing with β-blockers and calcium channel-blockers alone or combination have revealed suppressant effects on silent myocardial ischemia.

In the first, Lynch and colleagues[76] objectively evaluated the antianginal and anti-ischemic effects of propranolol, nifedipine, and their combination in 16 patients with severe exertional angina. The study was conducted in a double-blind fashion with multiple endpoints, including parameters of exercise stress tests, subjective features (chest pain, nitroglycerin consumption), and ECG data obtained from 48-hour Holter recordings (the total area and amount of ST-segment depression on the precordial exercise map and the total number of episodes of ST-segment depression). Two doses of each drug were used in the study: nifedipine, 30 and 60 mg/day, and propranolol, 240 and 480 mg/day, each drug given in three divided doses. Both drugs exerted a beneficial effect on the conventional subjective and objective indices of angina and ischemia. The effects of the combination therapy in general were more striking than the effects of either drug given alone at both doses. With respect to the effects and doses of the two drugs and their combination, at both doses, nifedipine and propranolol given along significantly reduced the number of episodes of ST-segment depression per 48 hours (most episodes being silent); propranolol was somewhat more potent in this regard. The combination therapies at both doses were significantly more potent than either drug given alone, with evidence for a synergistic effect. The data (not shown) were also similar for the effects on exercise-induced ST-segment depression during treadmill stress testing.

Another study in chronic stable angina, from our laboratories,[77] was a double-blind study of the antiischemic effects of propranolol and a new dihydropyridine type of calcium antagonist, nicardipine, singly and in combination versus placebo using a protocol with an extended Latin-square design. The goal was to evaluate the relative efficacy of these agents in terms of standard clinical parameters and treadmill variables. The major focus was on the effects of the two classes of drugs and their combination on episodes of silent myocardial ischemia as determined by ST-segment deviations occurring during ambulatory Holter monitoring in patients with chronic stable angina.

Twenty-one men over 21 years of age with at least a 3-month history of classic stable angina were enrolled in the study. They all completed the study. The mean data with respect to the conventional subjective and objective parameters of ischemia were similar to those reported for β-blockers and the dihydropyridine type of calcium antagonists.

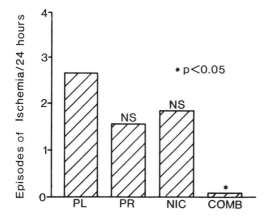

Fig. 13-7. Effects of propranolol (PR), nicardipine (NIC) and combination (COMB) on episodes of myocardial ischemia documented by 24-hour Holter recordings. The design of this study was an extended Latin-square design. Note that the combination was significantly more effective than either regimen alone. (From Khan et al.,[77] with permission.)

The mean data demonstrated the effects of propranolol, nicardipine, and the combination therapy on the number of episodes of ischemia (over 80% being silent) per 24 hours documented on ambulatory ECG recordings. Although both propranolol (-29%) and nicardipine (-18%) given alone reduced the number of episodes of ischemia, the change was not statistically significant. By contrast, combination therapy was effective in significantly ($p < 0.05$) reducing the number of ischemic episodes (-86%) compared with the placebo, the blockers, or the calcium antagonist given alone (Fig. 13-7).

Regarding the effects of these regimens on the maximum duration of ischemia of the longest episode and the total cumulative duration of ischemia per 24 hours, again, neither propranolol nor nicardipine given alone exerted a significant effect on these parameters. The combination regimen reduced the frequency of ischemic episodes by more than 90% ($p < 0.05$), the maximum duration by 90% ($p < 0.05$), and the total duration per 24 hours by 92% ($p < 0.05$). Combination therapy had a significantly greater effect than either propranolol or nicardipine given alone. Deedwania et al.[35] found that patients receiving β-blockers alone or in combination with other drugs had fewer episodes of silent ischemia in the morning hours, and the duration of ischemia per 24 hours was significantly shorter compared with patients not receiving β-blockers. These results are similar to those reported previously in a group of 348 patients with stable angina who were receiving nitrates or a β-blocking agent.[36] In that study, 43% of patients had one or more episodes of transient ischemic St depression (more than 80% silent) during the 48-hour ambulatory ECG monitoring. The high prevalence of residual ischemia reported in these studies suggest that whereas some drugs may be more effective than others, in general, conventional antianginal drug therapy directed for control of angina pectoris does not abolish the silent ischemic events recorded on AEM during routine daily activities.

Recently, in a placebo-controlled double-blind randomized crossover study, Deedwania et al.[78] compared the effects of atenolol and nifedipine in 25 patients with stable CAD, exercise-induced ischemia, and 5 minutes or longer duration of silent ischemia during the 48-hour AEM. The results showed that, although both atenolol and nifedipine treatments reduced the frequency and duration of transient ischemic episodes, atenolol was significantly more effective than nifedipine in reducing the magnitude of ischemic activity as well as total abolition of ischemic episodes (50% versus 25% suppression rate, respectively). During the placebo phase, there was a morning surge in ischemic activity, which was adequately controlled during therapy with atenolol.

Parmley et al.[79] recently investigated the effects of long-acting nifedipine (Nifedipine GITS) alone and in combination with β-blockade on episodes of myocardial ischemia detected by 48-hour ambulatory ECG recordings. A total of 207 patients completed all phases of the study. Overall, nifedipine GITS significantly reduced weekly angina attacks (5.7 to 1.8; p < 0.0001) and the number of ischemic events from 7.28 to 4.0 (mostly silent; p < 0.0001), reported during 48-hour monitoring periods. Nifedipine GITS significantly reduced ischemia during the 48-hour period when administered as monotherapy or in combination with a β-blocker. The morning surge of ischemia was attenuated most effectively by the combination regimen.

THERAPEUTIC IMPLICATIONS

The data outlined in this chapter indicate that both β-blockers and calcium-channel blockers have the potential to reduce silent myocardial ischemic episodes in patients with chronic stable angina. The fact that the suppressant effects of calcium-channel blockers and β-blockers on silent myocardial ischemia in the setting of chronic stable angina are most pronounced when these agents are combined might be of therapeutic significance. Such an effect appears to be synergistic rather than simply additive. It may reflect the complementary effects of two classes of anti-ischemic agents on myocardial oxygen supply and demand relative to their differing hemodynamic effects.

Before embarking on therapy for silent myocardial ischemia in a patient with CAD, one may refer to the currently available data for a number of clinically relevant considerations. As far as Holter monitoring is concerned, if the criteria for the identification of an episode are strictly defined prospectively, rarely is silent myocardial ischemia found in truly normal subjects without risk factors for CAD. However, at present, there are no meaningful studies in completely asymptomatic patients with occult CAD and negative or positive exercise stress tests for myocardial ischemia. Furthermore, there are no data to support or deny the possibility that the presence of ischemia documented on Holter recordings in such patients might provide an incremental prognostic index that allows the clinician to identify a completely asymptomatic subject who is at risk of AMI or sudden cardiac death, the course of which can be altered significantly by aggressive pharmacologic or nonpharmacologic therapy. Thus, the use of Holter monitoring in this group of patients to determine the presence of silent myocardial ischemia for the purposes of instituting therapy currently appears to be neither justified nor warranted.

By contrast, much prognostic data has been obtained with the exercise treadmill in patients with CAD and chronic stable angina. A positive test for myocardial ischemia in these patients is clearly associated with an augmented risk of a morbid coronary event (infarction or sudden death), whether such patients are symptomatic or asymptomatic.[47] It is also well established[47] that in patients whose exercise treadmill test is electrocardiographically positive, the prognosis is identical, whether or not chest pain develops in such patients during the treadmill test. These data indicate that ischemia (as closely correlated with its extent, as reflected in the severity of stenoses and/or the number of the vessels stenosed), rather than its symptomatic manifestations, is prognostically important. Therefore, it is reasonable to assume that a patient with a strongly positive treadmill test should undergo evaluation and treatment of myocardial ischemia, whether it is symptomatic or silent.

As previously indicated, in unstable angina, the persistence of silent myocardial ischemia documented on Holter after elimination of symptomatic episodes by medical therapy appears to be highly predictive of an adverse short-term prognosis.[59,60] Newer data[35-38] provide evidence that the same holds for chronic stable angina. These observations have raised a number of practical questions. For example, does it imply that a concerted effort should be made to further reduce silent myocardial ischemia by intensifying medical therapy? Or are we, with triple drug regimens, already at the upper end of the dose-response curve of medical therapy? The phenomenon of residual ischemia in this setting might simply be an expression of the fact that drug therapy merely distinguishes "responders" from "nonresponders," the latter having an inherently worse prognosis that is unlikely to be influenced significantly by further attempts with more aggressive medical therapy. The implication here might be that the failure of drug therapy to effect a substantive change simply reflects the presence of a substrate not amenable to the influence of pharmacologic regimens. The decisive resolution of this issue is possible only by stringently controlled, adequately designed clinical trials of large sample size. However, such trials are unlikely to be carried out, in the case of unstable angina, because most patients with unstable angina undergo coronary angiography. A strong correlation between the angiographic findings and the frequency and duration of silent myocardial ischemia on Holter recordings has now been demonstrated. Most unstable patients now undergo PTCA or surgical myocardial revascularization. Thus, the use of silent myocardial ischemia as an endpoint to gauge adequacy of therapy in this setting currently appears to have limited practical appeal. The issue of a controlled clinical trial may nevertheless be of fundamental importance in chronic stable angina; however, the difficulties of carrying out meaningful clinical trials of a controlled design in this setting are formidable for a number of reasons. First, patients with chronic stable angina in whom silent ischemia is readily abolished by drug therapy ("responders") may have an inherently good prognosis. Ideally, they need to be randomized in a blinded fashion to placebo versus active therapy. This may not be possible on ethical grounds. In any event, the agents that have the most consistent suppressant effect on silent myocardial ischemia—β-blockers—may exert an effect on mortality independent of their action on ischemia, as suggested by the data in the β-blocker trials in the survivors of AMI. The group with residual ischemia despite aggressive medical therapy ("nonresponders") are those in which the effects of interventions with an endpoint of mortality or recurrent infarction theoretically are the most logical group. Here, the issue of a change in prognosis consequent upon reduction of silent ischemia could be the focus of a trial. On the other hand, as these are subjects in whom drug therapy has essentially failed to produce a satisfactory response, it is clear that the treatment limbs may need to consider PTCA versus surgical revascularization if one were to accept that these two modalities are equally efficacious.

Finally, the issue of whether silent myocardial ischemia documented on Holter recordings should be treated is of particular relevance to patients who have survived cardiac arrest out of the hospital or those who present with sustained symptomatic ventricular tachycardia with the substrate as the CAD. In these patients, myocardial ischemia (presumably silent) may conceivably provide the final trigger for the occurrence of ventricular fibrillation, since more than two-thirds of patients in this category have advanced CAD. This has been established with coronary angiography as well as with exercise stress tests with perfusion scintigraphy. Whether these patients also have episodes of silent myocardial ischemia on Holter monitoring has been conjectural. In recent years, a number of patients had cardiac arrest while wearing Holter recording devices. A careful analysis of the Holter tapes from such patients revealed that fewer than 12% had ST-segment deviations preceding the onset of terminal ventricular tachycardia and fibrillation.[48] These observations indicate that although CAD is the most important factor for sudden cardiac death, in most cases an ischemic episode is not the immediate trigger for the fatal event. However, these findings do not discount the crucial role of ischemia because it is entirely possible that ventricular tachycardia initiated by an early cycle ectopic beat may worsen the imbalance in oxygen supply and demand in a patient with CAD; the resulting ischemia may induce ventricular fibrillation by accelerating the rate of ventricular tachycardia. Clearly, these considerations are relevant to the issue of amelioration of ischemia, silent or symptomatic, as an approach to the prevention of sudden cardiac death in patients with CAD. However, for the present, it appears that the precise link between silent ischemic episodes and the genesis of sudden cardiac death should be defined before therapy to eliminate silent myocardial ischemia can be initiated as a modality to prevent deaths caused by cardiac arrhythmia.

CONCLUSIONS

The sole reason for the treatment of silent myocardial ischemia is to improve prognosis. There is now substantial evidence suggesting that silent myocardial ischemia is a distinct clinical entity and that its presence may be related to adverse clinical outcome, at least in certain subsets of patients. Numerous reports indicate that medical therapy with nitrates, β-blockers, and calcium-channel blockers, as single agents or in combination, is effective in reducing silent myocardial ischemia and its duration. In the case of both unstable as well as chronic stable angina, therapy with single or combination regimens indicate that more than 30% of patients continue to experience silent episodes of ischemia after symptomatic ones have been abolished. However, it remains unclear whether these treatments will influence prognosis when they are effective in suppressing silent ischemia. Nor is it known what degrees of reduction in silent myocardial ischemic episodes or their cumulative durations over a finite period may be necessary in order to effect a favorable change in prognosis. Whether revascularization by PTCA or surgery might be more effective in abolishing silent ischemia is not known. A resolution of these uncertainties by controlled clinical trials will be necessary before the known implications of silent myocardial ischemia can be translated confidently into routine clinical practice.

REFERENCES

1. Kannel WB, Abbot RD: Incidence and prognosis of unrecognized myocardial infarction: an update on the Framingham study. N Engl J Med 311:1144, 1984
2. Reeves T: Relation and independence of angina pectoris and sudden death in persons with coronary atherosclerotic heart disease. J Am Coll Cardiol 5:167B, 1985
3. Cohn PF, Harris P, Barry WH et al: Prognostic importance of anginal symptoms in angiographically defined coronary artery disease. Am J Cardiol 47:233, 1981
4. Hultgren H, Peduzzi P: Participants of the Veterans Administration cooperative study of surgery for coronary arterial occlusive disease. Relation of severity of symp-

toms to prognosis in stable angina pectoris. Am J Cardiol 54:988, 1984

5. Warnes CA, Roberts WC: Sudden coronary death: relation of amount and distribution of coronary narrowing at necropsy to previous symptoms of myocardial ischemia, left ventricular scarring and heart weight. Am J Cardiol 65:6, 1984

6. Kannel W: Prevalence and clinical aspects of unrecognized myocardial infarction and sudden unexpected death. Circulation, suppl II. 75:4, 1987

7. Multiple Risk Factor Interventions Trial Research Group: Exercise electrocardiogram and coronary heart disease mortality in the multiple Risk Factor Intervention Trial. Am J Cardiol 55:16, 1985

8. Gordon D, Ekelund L, Karon J et al: Predictive value of the exercise tolerance test for mortality in North American Men: the lipid research clinics mortality follow-up study. Circulation 74:252, 1986

9. Giagnoni E, Secchi MB, Wu SC et al: Prognostic value of exercise EKG testing in asymptomatic normotensive subjects: a prospective matched study. N Engl J Med 309: 1085, 1983

10. Erikssen J, Thaulow E: Follow-up of patients with asymptomatic myocardial ischemia. p. 156. In Rutishauser W, Roskamm H (eds): Silent Myocardial Ischemia. Springer-Verlag, Berlin, 1984

11. Froelicher V, Yanowitz F, Thompson A, Lancaster MC: The correlation of coronary angiography and the electrocardiographic response to maximal treadmill testing in 76 asymptomatic men. Circulation 48:597, 1973

12. Langou R, Huang E, Kelley M, Cohen LS: Predictive accuracy of coronary artery calcification and abnormal exercise test for coronary artery disease in asymptomatic men. Circulation 62:1196, 1980

13. Stern S, Tzivoni D: Early detection of silent ischemic heart disease by 24-hour electrocardiographic monitoring of active subjects. Br Heart J 36:481, 1974

14. Stern S, Tzivoni D: Early detection of silent ischemic heart disease by 24 hour electrocardiographic monitoring, as validated by coronary arteriography. Circulation 52:1045, 1975

15. Allen RD, Gettes LS, Phalan C et al: Painless ST-segment depression in patients with angina pectoris. Chest 69: 467, 1976

16. Schang SJ, Pepine CJ: Transient asymptomatic ST-segment depression during daily activity. Am J Cardiol 39: 297, 1977

17. Tzivoni D, Gavish A, Benhorin J et al: Myocardial ischemia during daily activities and stress. Am J Cardiol 58:47B, 1982

18. Nademanee K, Intarachot V, Singh BN et al: Characteristics and clinical significance of silent myocardial ischemia in unstable angina. Am J Cardiol 58:26B, 1986

19. Singh BN, Nademanee K, Figueras J et al: Hemodynamic and electrocardiographic correlates of symptomatic and silent myocardial ischemia: pathophysiologic and therapeutic implications. Am J Cardiol 38:3B, 1986

20. Figueras J, Singh BN, Ganz W et al: Mechanism of rest and nocturnal angina: Observations during continuous hemodynamic and electrocardiographic monitoring. Circulation 59:955, 1979

21. Nademanee K, Singh BN, Guerrero J et al: Accurate rapid compact analog method for the quantification of frequency and duration of myocardial ischemia by semiautomated analysis of 24-hour Holter ECG recordings. Am Heart J 103:802, 1982

22. Wolf E, Tzivoni D, Stern S: Comparison of exercise stress tests and 24-hour ambulatory electrocardiographic monitoring of St-T changes. Br Heart J 86:501, 1980

23. Biagini A, Antonelli R, Michelassi C et al: Analisi di tracuati Holter in forma analogica compattata per il riconoscionento di episodi ischemia miocardica transitoria. G Ital Cardiol 10:668, 1980

24. Deanfield JE, Maseri A, Selwyn AP et al: Myocardial ischemia during daily life in patients with stable angina. Its relation to symptoms and heart rate changes. Lancet 2:753, 1983

25. Cecchi A, Dovellini EV, Morchi F et al: Silent myocardial ischemia during ambulatory electrocardiographic monitoring in patients with effort angina. J Am Coll Cardiol 1:934, 1983

26. Cocco G, Brown G, Strozzi C et al: Asymptomatic myocardial ischemia in patients with stable and typical angina pectoris. Clin Cardiol 5:403, 1982

27. Chierchia S, Brunelli C, Simonetti I et al: Sequence of events in angina at rest: primary reduction in coronary flow. Circulation 61:759, 1980

28. Biagini A, Mazzei MG, Carpeggiani C et al: Vasospastic ischemic mechanism of frequent asymptomatic transient ST-T changes during continuous electrocardiographic monitoring in selected unstable angina patients. Am Heart J 103:13, 1980

29. Nesto RW, Kowalchut GJ: The ischemic cascade: temporal sequence of hemodynamic, electrocardiographic and symptomatic expressions of ischemia. Am J Cardiol 57:23C, 1987

30. Berndt TB, Fitzgerald J, Harrison DC et al: Hemodynamic changes at the onset of spontaneous versus pacing-induced angina. Am J Cardiol 39:784, 1977

31. Nademanee K, Intarachot V, Josephson MA et al: Circadian variation in occurrence of transient overt and silent myocardial ischemia in chronic stable angina and comparison with Prinzmetal angina in men. Am J Cardiol 60: 494, 1987

32. Rocco MB, Nabel EG, Selwyn AP: Circadian rhythms and coronary artery disease. Am J Cardiol 59:13C, 1987

33. Rocco MB, Barry J, Campbell S et al: Circadian variation of transient myocardial ischemia in patients with coronary artery disease. Circulation 75:395, 1987

34. Mulcahy D, Keegan J, Crean P et al: Silent myocardial ischemia in chronic stable angina: a study of its frequency and characteristics in 150 patients. Br Heart J 60: 417, 1988

35. Deedwania P, Carbajal E: Prevalence and patterns of silent myocardial ischemia during daily life in stable angina patients receiving conventional antianginal drug therapy. Am J Cardiol 65:1090, 1990

36. Cohn P, Vetrovec G, Nesto R, Gerber F: The Nifedipine-total ischemia awareness program: A national survey of painful and painless myocardial ischemia including results of antiischemic therapy. Am J Cardiol 63:534, 1989

37. Deedwania P, Carbajal E: Silent ischemia during daily

life is an independent predictor of mortality in stable angina. Circulation 81:748, 1990

38. Rocco M, Nabel E, Campbell S et al: Prognostic importance of myocardial ischemia detected by ambulatory monitoring in patients with stable coronary artery disease. Circulation 78:877, 1988

39. Deedwania P, Nelson J: Pathophysiology of silent myocardial ischemia during daily life: hemodynamic evaluation by simultaneous electrocardiographic and blood pressure monitoring. Circulation 82:1296, 1990

40. Rocco M, Barry J, Campbell S et al: Circadian variation of transient myocardial ischemia in patients with coronary artery disease. Circulation 75:395, 1987

41. Ellestad MH, Allen W, Wan MCK et al: Maximal stress testing for cardiovascular evaluation. Circulation 39:517, 1969

42. Gibson RS, Beller GA, Keiser DL: Prevalence and clinical significance of painless ST-segment depression during early post infarction exercise testing. Circulation 75:1136, 1987

43. Bonow RD, Kent KM, Rosing DR et al: Exercise-induced ischemia in mildly symptomatic patients with coronary artery disease and preserved left ventricular function: identification of subgroups at risk of death during medical therapy. N Engl J Med 331:1339, 1984

44. Amsterdam EA, Martschinske R, Laslett LJ et al: Symptomatic and silent myocardial ischemia during exercise testing in coronary artery disease. Am J Cardiol 58:43B, 1986

45. Lindsey HE, Cohn PF: "Silent" myocardial ischemia during and after exercise testing in patients with coronary artery disease. Am Heart J 95:441, 1978

46. Rozanski A, Berman DS: Silent myocardial ischemia: pathophysiology, frequency of occurrence and approaches toward detection. Am Heart J 114:615, 1987

47. Weiner DA, Ryan TJ, McCabe CH et al: Significance of silent myocardial ischemia during exercise testing in coronary artery disease. Am J Cardiol 59:725, 1987

48. Falcone C, DeSevi S, Porna E et al: Clinical significance of exercise-induced silent myocardial ischemia in patients with coronary artery disease. J Am Coll Cardiol 9:295, 1987

49. Campbell S, Barry J, Rocco MB et al: Features of the exercise test that reflect ischemic heart disease activity out of hospital. Circulation 74:72, 1986

50. Nademanee K, Intrachot V, Piontek M et al: Relationship of myocardial ischemia detected by compact Holter analog technique to that induced by ETT. Circulation, suppl II. 70:451, 1984

51. Mody FV, Nademanee K, Intarachot V et al: Severity of silent myocardial ischemia on ambulatory ECG monitoring in patients with stable angina pectoris: relation to prognostic determinants during exercise stress testing and coronary angiography. J Am Coll Cardiol 12:1169, 1988

52. Parmley W: Prevalence and clinical significance of myocardial ischemia. Circulation, suppl IV. 80:68, 1989

53. Epstein SE: Implications of probability analysis of the strategy used for the non-invasive detection of coronary artery disease. Am J Cardiol 46:491, 1980

54. Froelicher VF, Maron D: Exercise testing and ancillary techniques to screen for coronary heart disease. Prog Cardiovasc Dis 14:261, 1981

55. Sharma B, Asinger R, Francis G: Demonstration of exercise-induced painless myocardial ischemia in survivors of out-of-hospital ventricular fibrillation. Am J Cardiol 59:740, 1987

56. Diamond GA, Forrester JS: Analysis of probability as an aid in the clinical diagnosis of coronary-artery disease. N Engl J Med 300:1350, 1979

57. Heng MK, Norris RM, Singh BN, Partridge JP: Prognosis in unstable angina. Br Heart J 38:921, 1976

58. Johnson SM, Mauritson DR, Winniford MD et al: Continuous electrocardiographic monitoring in patients with unstable angina pectoris: identification of high-risk subgroup with severe coronary disease, variant angina, and/or impaired early prognosis. Am Heart J 103:4, 1982

59. Gottlieb SO, Weisfeldt ML, Ouyang P et al: Silent ischemia as a marker for early unfavorable outcomes in patients with unstable angina. N Engl J Med 314:1214, 1986

60. Nademanee K, Intarachot V, Josephson MA et al: Prognostic significance of silent myocardial ischemia in patients with unstable angina. J Am Coll Cardiol 10:1, 1987

61. Theroux P, Waters DD, Halphen C et al: Prognostic value of exercise testing soon after myocardial infarction. N Engl J Med 301:341, 1979

62. Gottlieb SO, Gottlieb SH, Achuff SC et al: Silent ischemia on Holter monitoring predicts mortality in high-risk postinfarction patients. JAMA 249:1030, 1988

63. Tzivoni D, Gavish A, Zin D et al: Prognostic significance of ischemic episodes in patients with previous myocardial infarction. Am J Cardiol 62:661, 1988

64. Bonow R, Bacharach S, Green M et al: Prognostic implications of symptomatic versus asymptomatic (silent) myocardial ischemia induced by exercise in mildly symptomatic and in asymptomatic patients with angiographically documented coronary artery disease. Am J Cardiol 60:778, 1987

65. Weiner D, Ryan T, McCade C et al: Risk of developing an acute myocardial infarction or sudden coronary death in patients with exercise-induced silent myocardial ischemia. A report from the Coronary Artery Surgery Study (CASS) Registry. Am J Cardiol 62:1155, 1988

66. Pepine CJ: Is silent ischemia a treatable risk factor in patients with angina pectoris? Circulation, suppl II. 82:II–135, 1990

67. Shell WE: Mechanisms and therapy of silent myocardial ischemia and the effect of transdermal nitroglycerin. Am J Cardiol 56:231, 1985

68. Singh BN, Hecht HS, Nademanee K et al: Electrophysiologic and hemodynamic effects of slow channel blocking drugs. Prog Cardiovasc Dis 23:103, 1982

69. Singh BN, Nademanee K: Beta-adrenergic blockade and unstable angina. Am J Cardiol 57:992, 1986

70. Hossack KF, Brown BG, Stewart DK et al: Diltiazem-induced effects on sympathetically medicated constriction of normal and diseased coronary arteries: lack of epicardial coronary dilatory effect in humans. Circulation 70:465, 1984

71. Brown BG, Bolson EL, Dodge HT: Dynamic mechanisms in human coronary stenosis. Circulation 70:917, 1984

72. Singh BN, Chew CYC, Josephson MA: Pharmacologic and hemodynamic mechanisms underlying the antianginal actions of verapamil. Am J Cardiol 50:886, 1982

73. Imperi GA, Lambert CR, Coy K et al: Effects of titrated beta-blockade (metoprolol) on silent myocardial ischemia in ambulatory patients with coronary artery disease. Am J Cardiol 60:519, 1987

74. Nademanee K, Singh BN, Piontek M et al: Antianginal efficacy of bepridil, a novel calcium antagonist: double blind evaluation by quantitating myocardial ischemia by compact Holter analog technique in chronic stable angina. J Am Coll Cardiol 3:551, 1984

75. Schnellbacher K, Droste C, Roskamm H: Medical and surgical therapy of patients with asymptomatic ischemia. p. 154. In Arnim TV, Maseri A (eds): Silent Ischemia. Springer-Verlag, New York, 1987

76. Lynch P, Dargie H, Krikler S et al: Objective assessment of anti-anginal treatment: a double-blind comparison of propranolol, nifedipine and their combination. Br Med J 281:184, 1980

77. Khan S, Nademanee K, Intarachot V, Singh BN: Effects of nicardipine and propranolol, alone and in combination, on silent myocardial ischemia in patients with chronic stable angina. Submitted Am Heart J 1992

78. Deedwania PC, Carbajal EV, Nelson JR, Hait H: Antiischemic effects of atenolol versus nifedipine in patients with coronary artery disease and ambulatory silent ischemia. J Am Coll Cardiol 17:963, 1990

79. Parmley W, Deanfield J, Gottlieb S et al: Attenuation of the circadian patterns of myocardial ischemia with nifedipine GITS in chronic stable angina patients. J Am Coll Cardiol 19:380, 1992

14

Risk Assessment, Stratification, and Prognosis of Young Patients After Myocardial Infarction

Amar S. Kapoor

Myocardial infarction (MI) is a common occurrence in hospitalized patients. In the United States alone, 1.5 million patients experience an MI each year. For a North American man, there is a 20% chance of suffering either MI or sudden cardiac death before the age of 65.[1] Coronary artery disease (CAD) is generally thought to be a disease that occurs in middle-aged or advanced-aged persons, but CAD is a common finding in young adults. Autopsy studies from the Korean War demonstrated that 77% of 300 soldiers (average age, 22 years) had evidence of significant CAD, and 10% showed total or nearly total occlusion of a major artery.[2] Approximately 1% of men aged 30 to 62 years have manifest CAD each year.[3] Of these patients, about 40% present with MI as their initial manifestation.

There has been a focus of attention on the subject of MI in young patients in several reports.[4,5] Epidemiologic and pathologic data[6–9] indicate that about 3 to 6% of MIs occur in adults under 40 years of age. Evidence suggests that CAD patterns in young adults differ from those in older patients.[10,11] In a previous report,[11] young postinfarct patients were categorized into four different subsets. The spectrum of coronary artery anatomy includes congenital coronary anomalies, normal coronary arteries with large infarcts, and coronary atherosclerosis, as is commonly seen in older patients. For the purpose of this review, young age group are arbitrarily defined as those no more than 40 years of age.

EPIDEMIOLOGIC STUDIES

The epidemiology of CAD is well established for rates of occurrence in different population groups, but there is a scarcity of data on the epidemiology of MI in young age groups, making it difficult to estimate whether the incidence of MI in this age group in the United States is decreasing or increasing. Using a common strategy of comparison of CAD rates and associated characteristics of large population groups, such as between countries, there is a steep increase in CAD rates in young age groups in Northern Ireland, Denmark, and Poland.[6] The data from the World Register Study shows a relatively high incidence of coronary morbidity in the 20- to 64-year age group in Helsinki (8/1,000/year).[6]

There is a definite declining trend of mortality attributable to CAD in the United States. Epidemiologic data are lacking in corroborating the prevalence of CAD and occurrence of MI in young patients, especially when looking at the declining trend of coronary epidemic. The mortality from CAD shows a striking relationship with age. The disease is a major cause of death for men aged 35 to 44 years. The mortality from CAD rapidly increases, so that by age 55 to 64 years, 40% of all deaths among men are due to this single cause. According to data from Lamm's[6] study, there is a steep gradient of MI when comparing the 20- to 39-year age group with the 50- to 54-year age group. In men in the older age group, MI is 25 times more prevalent than in the young age group. However, in selected studies in some communities there has been a decline in mortality from CAD in the younger age group. In the Allegheny County Coronary Heart Disease Mortality Study in white men (aged 35 to 44 years), the CAD mortality rate fell from 90.6/100,000/year during 1970 to 1972 to 40.3/100,000/year during 1985 to 1986.[12] Two-thirds of the decline was related to a decline in sudden deaths. On the other hand, the CAD deaths in young diabetics increased dramatically from 6.5% during 1970 to 1972 to 23.0% during 1985 to 1986.[12]

RISK FACTOR SURVEY IN YOUNG PATIENTS

There is general consensus of a multifactorial etiology for CAD and for increased incidence with age. Four risk factors appear most significant in terms of linking CAD and onset of clinical coronary atherosclerotic heart disease. The cardinal risk factors in the older population are diabetes mellitus, hypertension, hypercholesterolemia, and cigarette smoking. However, some variations in risk factors affect the younger populations. Smoking has been the most common risk factor in this age group (70 to 90%).[13] According to the Heidelberg Myocardial Infarction Registry area, 74% were smokers,[13,14] and 6% had no risk factors. A family history of significant atherosclerosis or death from MI in first-degree relatives is a major risk factor in the younger population than the older patients.[15] This may represent a genetic predisposition to atherosclerosis and is probably interrelated to familial hyperlipidemia and other metabolic risk factors. The strong familial component in the younger patients needs to be emphasized and can be used as a predictor of risk and for screening persons at high risk.[16]

Obesity has been suggested as a minor risk factor, and its independent effect has been questioned, as several studies have shown that the relationship of CAD

TABLE 14-1. Comparative Risk Factor Significance in Different Age Groups With Coronary Artery Disease

	Young Patients Aged <40 Yr	Older Patients Aged <55 Yr
Hypertension	+	+ + +
Diabetes mellitus	+	+ + +
Hypercholesterolemia	+ + +	+ + +
Cigarette smoking	+ + + +	+ + +
Obesity	+ + +	+
Family history	+ +	+
No risk factors	+ +	+
Multiple risk factors	+ + +	+ +

+, small percentages + + + +, very high percentage of patients having that risk factor.

to obesity is virtually entirely accounted for by the relationship of obesity to hypertension, hyperlipidemia, and glucose intolerance. The role of obesity as an independent contributor in young adults with low levels of other risk factors has been observed in more than 50% of younger patients.[14] In large-scale studies of Japanese men in Hawaii and in a cohort of young American men after a 26-year observation period, obesity has been found to be an independent contributor.[17,18]

Intensive physical exertion before MI has been observed in many young patients. Coronary atherosclerosis is found in the exercise MI group. The period after intense exercise is regarded as one of vulnerability. It is a time when perfusion of the myocardium is still unstable. Arrhythmias, biochemical alterations, and coronary spasm may be causative factors.

The mosaic of risk-factor pattern in the young age group may be helpful in identifying and screening persons with clinical or advanced disease. In short, the most common risk factors in young patients are cigarette smoking (70 to 90%), followed by obesity (53%), hypercholesterolemia (41%), and a family history of MI or cerebrovascular accident (CVA) (38%).[19–22] Comparison of risk factors in the young and older age groups is shown in Table 14-1. The presence of several risk factors appears to be common in the younger MI patients.[13,14] This appears to contradict that most patients have no risk factors.

PATHOANATOMY OF MYOCARDIAL INFARCTION IN YOUNG PATIENTS

Coronary artery anatomy in young postinfarction patients is heterogeneous, and there are four distinctly different subsets[10]:

TABLE 14-2. Angiographic Studies in Young Post-MI Patients

	Series			
Status	Roskamm (1973–1978) (n = 500)	Hamby (1974–1978) (n = 51)	Sheldon (1971–1978) (n = 236)	Kapoor (1980–1982) (n = 54)
Normal coronaries	6.6%	0%	—	8%
One vessel	50.2%	50%	63.5%	46%
Two vessel	21.6%	28%	27.7%	24%
Three vessel	18.2%	21%	8.4%	22%
Left main	(Included)	NS	0.5%	1.5%

Congenital coronary anomalies
   Anomalous origin of coronary artery from the pulmonary artery
   Coronary arteriovenous fistulas
Normal coronary arteries with large or medium infarcts
   Young women taking oral contraceptives and smoking heavily
   Young men after strenuous physical exercise
   Spontaneous dissection of coronary artery
One vessel coronary artery disease
Multivessel coronary artery disease
   Patients without diffuse disease
   Patients with diffuse distal disease

Hence, the pathologic mechanisms for each subset are different but may overlap. Each of the four subsets will be described in some detail in order to clarify the pathophysiologic mechanisms responsible for the underlying pathology. In older patients, almost all MIs result from atherosclerosis and thrombosis of the coronary arteries. However, in younger patients, atherosclerosis may not be present in 15 to 20% of patients. The size and location of a particular infarction depend on the severity of the coronary artery lesion, the presence and severity of coronary arterial spasm, the size of the vascular bed perfused by the stenotic artery, and the extent of collateral blood vessels. Results of angiographic studies from different series are shown in Table 14-2.

CONGENITAL CORONARY ANOMALY

Congenital coronary anomaly is a rare but correctable disorder that may manifest in adolescence. Anomalous origin of the coronary artery from the pulmonary artery is a rare malformation that occurs in 0.4% of patients with congenital cardiac anomalies.[23,24] In more than 90% of cases, the left coronary artery has an anomalous origin from the posterior sinus of the pulmonary trunk. The common clinical presentations are those of infants who suffer an MI and in whom congestive heart failure (CHF) develops. The infant

syndrome usually becomes manifest at 2 to 4 months of age with angina-like symptoms. In 10 to 15% of patients, myocardial ischemia never occurs because an extensive coronary collateral vessel system permits a survival to adolescence. Young adults usually present with a continuous murmur or mitral regurgitation resulting from papillary muscle dysfunction. These young adults may also present with angina or heart failure, or experience sudden death. Patients having congenital coronary arteriovenous fistulas survive to adulthood when they may have signs and symptoms of left ventricular failure secondary to significant left-to-right shunt.

NORMAL CORONARY ARTERIES WITH INFARCTION

The occurrence of MI with normal coronary arteries has been well documented. The true incidence of this pathophysiologic entity is not known, since postmortem examinations confirming the myocardial lesion and the patency of the coronary arteries are infrequent. The incidence of normal coronary arteriograms in patients with MI ranges from 1 to 15%.[25,26] However, in younger patients with MI, more than 15% may have normal coronary arteriograms; some are women taking oral contraceptives in addition to smoking heavily.[27,28] Most of these patients exhibit a regional wall-motion abnormality corresponding to the electrocardiographic (ECG) site of infarction.

The mechanism responsible for such incidence of acute MI remains speculative. Spontaneous lysis of an occlusive thrombus as a possible mechanism has been postulated.[29] The known effects of oral contraceptives on blood clotting factors and on the microstructure of the vessel wall combined with the synergistic effects of nicotine on platelet aggregation[30] suggests that thromboembolic mechanisms may be active in such cases, although coronary spasm and immunologic phenomena have also been implicated. There is a small subset of patients who present with MI and spontaneous dissection of coronary artery.

Myocardial infarctions have been documented in

young men with normal coronary angiograms after intensive physical activity. Coronary vasospasm has been implicated as a causative factor; the role of coronary vasospasm in the genesis of angina and MI has been well documented in both young and old patients. Maseri and others[31,32] have carried out elegant studies and demonstrated that changes in coronary vasomotor tone play a dominant role in the genesis of transient coronary ischemic attacks in these patients. Furthermore, they performed angiograms during an ischemic attack and demonstrated vasospastic ischemia and later MI in the same myocardial region showing ECG ST-segment changes during ischemia. The causes of coronary spasm and the irreversibility of the spasm remain elusive. It is possible that other factors, such as platelet aggregation and thromboxane A_2 (TxA_2) release, could play a modulating role in maintaining vascular contraction and producing lumen occlusion while favoring the onset of thrombus formation that could subsequently be lysed.

There is no single cause for MI in this group of patients. It is also possible to speculate that cigarette smoking leads to a change in the vascular endothelium. Young men with CAD have shortened platelet survival.[33,34] Abnormal platelet activity could be an initiating factor for an imbalance or thrombosis resulting in MI and subsequent spontaneous lysis.

ONE VESSEL CORONARY ARTERY DISEASE

One vessel CAD is the most common lesion in young patients with MI. In autopsy studies, 60% of patients had evidence of prior MI.[35] The artery most commonly involved with atherosclerosis in the left anterior descending (LAD) vessel, followed by the right coronary, left circumflex (CX), and left main coronary arteries. Several autopsy series on young patients after sudden death or MI report a high incidence of LAD involvement with associated anterior wall infarction.[36] Depending on the location of the stenosis, the size of the MI may be very large; for example, in patients with major occlusion of the proximal LAD there may be massive infarction. In spite of only having one vessel involved, the extent of left ventricular (LV) dysfunction equals that of older patients with extensive CAD. These findings suggest that the development of coronary occlusion in young patients occurs rather rapidly, without leaving time for coronary collateral vessels to become established, and hence an extensive MI occurs. It is possible that LAD disease may occur earlier in the natural course of coronary atherosclerotic heart disease. The prevalence of one vessel disease is more than 50% in younger patients, in contrast with older

patients after MI where multivessel disease predominates.[37–39]

MULTIVESSEL CORONARY ARTERY DISEASE

Three vessel CAD is seen in less than 20% of younger patients with MI. Two vessel CAD is seen in 30 to 40% of this younger population. There is also a subset of this group who have a very aggressive and progressive disease pattern. In patients with one vessel disease, regression is frequently seen and progression is rare but can be present if patients share multiple risk factors. There is little tendency for deterioration of LV function. By contrast, patients with multivessel involvement have two different patterns. In the first, the progression is common.[13] This is the disease pattern commonly seen in older patients. In the second subset, patients have multivessel disease with diffuse and extensive involvement. In these patients, there is positive history of familial hyperlipidemia and precocious atherosclerosis. The disease is progressive and unrelenting. Prognosis in this subgroup is less favorable compared with other CAD patterns. Young patients with multivessel involvement have more risk factors, compared with similarly affected older patients.[40,41]

ASSESSMENT OF RISK IN YOUNG POSTINFARCTION PATIENTS

The natural history has been defined for the postinfarct patient. A very substantial risk of death exists during the first 6 months after hospital discharge. Clinical outcome and profile of risk categorization have been assembled by various clinical markers of risk in the postinfarct patients. During the phase of acute MI, the principal determinant of mortality is infarct size since 10% of LV damage results in decreased ejection fraction; the mortality is 5 to 10% in this case. In patients with greater than 40% LV damage, cardiogenic shock usually results, and mortality is in excess of 80%.

Prognosis has been related to multiple variables: (1) extent of myocardial damage as reflected by global pump dysfunction, (2) the extent of viable myocardium at risk of ischemia or the extent and severity of CAD, and (3) the degree of electrical instability. A host of noninvasive and invasive tests have been employed to properly identify and stratify these patients in the hope that outcome can be improved by appropriate treatment of the physiologic and functional abnormality. Physiologic and functional derangements are different in the young post-MI patients, and some of the

TABLE 14-3. Killip Classification

Class	Definition	Patients (%)	Mortality (%)
1	No rales or gallop	30–40	6–8
2	Rales	30–50	17–30
3	Rales in 50% of lung fields	5–10	38–44
4	Cardiogenic shock	10	80–95

laboratory methods for evaluating young post-MI subjects are not predictive as in older patients.

ASSESSMENT DURING THE ACUTE PHASES

For a definitive diagnosis of acute MI, two of the following three must be evident: a typical history, ECG abnormalities, or abnormal elevations of cardiac enzyme levels. The hemodynamic changes that occur with acute myocardial infarction (AMI) are diverse and numerous, resulting from reduced contractile mass and alterations in LV compliance. In addition, mechanical dysfunction, altered contractility, and the peripheral circulation interact to produce wide divergence among clinical and hemodynamic features from case to case, as well as during the course of the disease.

The prognosis of patients with AMI can be based on clinical presentations and hemodynamic abnormalities.[42] The clinical indexes of Killip and Kimball,[43] Peel and associates,[44] and Norris and co-workers[45] estimated prognosis based on classification and numeric scoring of salient features of the history, physical examination, and laboratory data. The Killip index is frequently used; it classifies patients into four clinical subsets (Table 14-3).

The clinical applications of Swan-Ganz catheter have provided physiologic measurements of LV filling pressure and cardiac index in patients with AMI, which can further characterize LV function. Abnormally elevated LV filling pressure and a reduced cardiac index are the mechanical expressions of LV failure. However, the hemodynamic measurements do not closely correlate with the physical findings in terms of the development of pulmonary rales and ventricular gallop in the early stage of AMI.

Forrester and colleagues[46,47] devised a system based on hemodynamic data. Using the Forrester classification system, patients can be placed into one of four hemodynamic subsets, based on measurements of pulmonary capillary wedge pressure and cardiac index (Table 14-4).

The use of these hemodynamic subsets is helpful for prognostication and is critical for therapeutic decisions. The hemodynamic defects could be employed for triaging the patients who may need acute medical or surgical interventions. Patients with AMI are a heterogeneous group, both hemodynamically and prognostically. Increased pulmonary capillary pressure and diminishing cardiac output are the final common pathways for the production of heart failure, cardiogenic shock, and circulatory collapse. Generally, pulmonary capillary wedge pressure greater than 18 mmHg and a cardiac index of less than 2.2 is prognostically a poor sign. In the Forrester classification, patients belonging to subset 4 with cardiogenic shock have a mortality of 56%, which is much lower than Killip's class 4 (80 to 95%). This may be due to differences within subset 4.

ASSESSMENT DURING EARLY CONVALESCENCE

A stepwise risk stratification procedure combining historic and clinical characteristics, and treadmill exercise variables provide important prognostic information.[48] Postinfarction patients at very high risk of subsequent morbidity and mortality can be identified on the basis of clinical presentation of congestive heart failure (CHF) and unstable angina. These high-risk patients would not be suitable for treadmill testing and might benefit from invasive laboratory methods. A whole array of diagnostic technologies can be used in the stratification and prognostication of young post-MI patients:

Clinical
  Early postinfarction angina
  Congestive heart failure
  ECG predictors
  ECG ischemia
  Arrhythmia detection by Holter monitoring

TABLE 14-4. Forrester Classification

Hemodynamic Subset	Cardiac Index	Pulmonary Wedge Pressure (mmHg)	Clinical Class	Mortality (%)
1	2.7 ± 0.5	12 ± 7	Normal	3
2	2.3 ± 0.4	23 ± 5	LV failure	9
3	1.9 ± 0.4	12 ± 5	Hypovolemia	23
4	1.6 ± 0.6	27 ± 8	Cardiogenic shock	56

Noninvasive laboratory techniques
  Low-level treadmill testing predischarge
  Treadmill exercise test 3–8 weeks postdischarge
  Exercise thallium 201 perfusion scintigraphy
  Resting and exercise radionuclide ventriculography
  Two-dimensional echocardiography
Cardiac catheterization
  Left ventriculography
  Coronary angiography

The information content of the various tests is different, and we get different probability estimates. When so many tests are available and each one gives a certain magnitude of abnormality, one is obliged to use multiple diagnostic or predictive tests to assess functional impairment and estimate survivability. This discussion attempts to present all facts of different issues and establish the interrelations among the various diagnostic modalities with respect to quantifying the extent of ischemia and damage.

EARLY POSTINFARCTION ANGINA

Angina is apparent after infarction in nearly 50% of patients. The development of angina following MI has important prognostic and therapeutic implications. The 5-year mortality in survivors of an AMI was 18% if patients were asymptomatic, but 60% if they had angina.[49] Two types of early postinfarction angina have been described,[50] ischemia at a distance from the infarcted area and ischemia in the infarct zone. The former is angina with new ECG changes distant from the acute infarct, and the latter angina with new ECG changes indicated in the area initially involved by the acute infarct. Patients with ischemia at a distance represent an especially high-risk subset of patients with large areas of ischemic myocardium; their mortality is 72%. Anginal chest pain after MI suggests, but does not prove, that the patient has multivessel disease. Chest pain is absent in many patients with extensive CAD.

The prognosis of patients with silent ischemia caused by exercise is not different from that of patients with symptomatic ischemia. There are no long term studies to suggest whether there is any prognostic difference between silent and painful myocardial ischemia postinfarct at rest.

ELECTROCARDIOGRAPHIC PREDICTORS OF MULTIVESSEL DISEASE

After a patient survives an inferior infarction, the likelihood of multivessel disease is greater than after an anterior infarction,[51,52] and inferior wall necrosis appears to be an independent predictor of more extensive arterial involvement. The large incidence of multivessel disease in patients with a previous inferior infarction has been noted by Miller and associates[53] in an older patient population with a mean age of 53 years. Multivessel disease is found in 85% of the patients with ECG evidence of ischemia distant from the site of MI.

PREDISCHARGE HOLTER MONITORING

Twenty-four-hour Holter monitoring has proved far superior to the standard ECG and clinical examination in identifying patients with complex arrhythmias. Twenty-four-hour Holter monitoring has demonstrated that complicated premature ventricular contractions (PVCs) are significant, whereas simple PVCs are not. Patients with complex PVCs run a significantly higher risk of sudden death following discharge from the hospital. Holter monitoring provides valuable insight into ventricular arrhythmias, conduction disorders, ischemic ST-segment changes, heart rate trends during activity and sleep, and supraventricular arrhythmias.

Several studies have confirmed an association between ventricular arrhythmias and left ventricular failure in patients in the convalescent phase of AMI. The association holds good for different indexes of LV failure, including third heart gallop, decreased exercise duration, low ejection fraction, and cardiomegaly with pulmonary vascular congestion. Ventricular arrhythmias and LV dysfunction contribute independently to mortality risk in the year after the AMI.

PREDISCHARGE TREADMILL EXERCISE TESTING

The feasibility and safety of predischarge treadmill exercise testing after an uncomplicated MI has been established. In addition, the development of certain abnormalities during low-level treadmill exercise testing has been reported to predict future cardiac events. The following exercise parameters are important for prognostic purposes: duration of treadmill exercise, exercise-induced ST-segment depression, ST-segment depression with angina, and inadequate blood pressure response to exercise.

Patients with evidence of myocardial ischemia or an inadequate blood pressure response to exercise, at low levels of workload, have a greater incidence of future cardiac events, specifically unstable angina and cardiac death. When subjects with ischemic treadmill abnormalities are combined with the patients exhibiting an inadequate blood pressure response, they have statistically greater incidence of cardiac death than that of a patient without treadmill abnormalities.[54]

A treadmill exercise test, however, does not always identify a high-risk patient, so a symptom-limited treadmill exercise test should be carried out 6 to 8 weeks after the MI. The usefulness of exercise ECG in the presence of MI may be limited by the MI itself.[55]

TREADMILL EXERCISE ELECTROCARDIOGRAPHY AND MYOCARDIAL STRESS PERFUSION SCINTIGRAPHY

Risk can be classified using a different set of determinants, especially those that encompass cardiovascular functional components, namely ischemic potential, hemodynamic dysfunction, and arrhythmic potential. Exercise testing yields information on different parameters of cardiovascular function that appear to be related to the various determinants of prognosis after MI:

Extent of coronary artery disease
    Presence of ST-segment depression
    Depth of ST-segment depression
    Ischemic chest pain
LV function
    Exercise tolerance level
    Blood pressure response
    Heart rate response
Arrhythmia potential
    Premature ventricular contractions

Weld and co-workers[56] studied a series of 250 patients who underwent a 9-minute treadmill test before hospital discharge and found that exercise limitation of less than 6 minutes was one of the most powerful independent predictors of a poor prognosis; much more so than the presence of ST-segment depression.

Most of the reported series show an association between ST-segment changes during an exercise test and late mortality; in fact, the risk of late mortality appears to be doubled. In the series reported by Schwartz and co-workers,[57] the 2-year mortality in 48 patients was 19% in the presence of ST-segment depression, compared with 10% in its absence; Weld and associates[56] reported a 1-year mortality of 16% versus 8% in patients with or without exercise-induced ST changes, respectively.

The problems in interpreting the results of exercise stress testing in the presence of an abnormal postinfarct ECG are now well recognized. Routinely performed stress tests predischarge and 8 weeks postdis-

charge in young postinfarct military patients were of little value in predicting multivessel disease.[58] There was one patient with significant left main coronary artery stenosis who had a negative ischemic response. The presence of chest pain and the total workload performed did not improve the predictive accuracy. In another study, by DeBusk et al.,[59] patients with a negative symptom-limited exercise stress test after an uncomplicated MI have a 1-year cardiovascular mortality of less than 2%. However, these data do not pertain to younger patients.

In older patients, the history, clinical characteristics, and treadmill testing were useful in discriminating high-risk patients, whereas negative response was nonspecific.[53] ST-segment depression or chest pain during exercise testing are unreliable predictors of the extent of CAD.[60] Although the presence of exercise-induced ST-segment depression identifies older patients with multivessel CAD, it is not certain whether a positive exercise ECG identifies patients with a poor prognosis due to large infarcts or extensive CAD. The many false-negative and false-positive results obtained with exercise ECG after a first MI[60] lend support to the proposal that coronary angiography should be recommended to every young patient after a first MI.[60,61]

Exercise thallium 201 imaging can identify jeopardized myocardium after AMI and can assess perfusion of specific coronary vascular distribution. There is not much information available on the prognostic capability of stress thallium imaging in the younger patients. In older patients, exercise thallium imaging was useful in discriminating between high-risk and low-risk groups after MI. According to Patterson and colleagues,[61] patients with thallium perfusion defects outside the region of the infarct, decreasing blood pressure during exercise, or failure to achieve 85% of age predicted heart rate have a high probability of having left main coronary artery or three vessel CAD. However, another study[62] found that exercise thallium imaging is less sensitive in predicting three vessel or left main CAD even in older patients. Myocardial perfusion scintigraphy has a low sensitivity for the accurate detection of left main disease. However, by using maximal stress testing in conjunction with myocardial perfusion imaging, one can identify approximately two-thirds of symptomatic patients with left main or three vessel CAD before coronary angiography.[63] The criteria for evaluating cardiovascular status are used to identify high-risk patients (see above).

PROGNOSTIC INDICATORS FROM RADIONUCLIDE ANGIOGRAPHY

Functional alternations during exercise after AMI may be a better prognostic indicator than mere knowledge of coronary artery anatomy or residual left ventricular function. The exercise ejection fraction is most accurately predictive of future cardiac events, followed by ejection fraction at rest, wall motion abnormalities, and exercise time. Although more studies need to be conducted, the exercise ejection fraction may turn out to be a better prognostic predictor than resting ventricular function, coronary artery anatomy, exercise-induced ST-segment changes, or exercise duration.

Ventricular function in patients with CAD may improve, remain unchanged, or worsen with exercise. The exercise ejection fraction describes the change in ventricular function that occurs with exercise. For example, for a patient with a resting ejection fraction of 55%, a decrease to 40% with exercise is associated with a worse prognosis than is an increase to 60% with exercise. The addition of radionuclide studies to the exercise test has not increased the predictive and screening power to the latter.

PROGNOSTIC INDEX BY CORONARY ANGIOGRAPHY

The angiographic assessment of coronary pathology is closely related to the overall prognosis of CAD and represents an important predictor of survival potential (Table 14-5). The two prognostic indicators are the degree and the extent of coronary artery obstruction and the degree of LV dysfunction. More quantitative information from the coronary angiogram can be derived if a scoring system is used, taking into account the degree of narrowing, the localization and extension of coronary artery obstructions, and predominance of the right or left coronary artery.

Our noninvasive technology does not permit determination of the extent and severity of CAD with acceptable accuracy and precision. Even with thallium 201 exercise testing, it is not possible to quantitate the severity of coronary artery obstruction, the number of

vessels involved, the proximal or distal nature of the obstructive lesions, and the overall pathologic picture for making sound therapeutic decisions and prognostic implications.

Until better diagnostic methods become available that can quantitate either ischemia or the severity of coronary artery lesions, coronary angiography should be recommended for young patients who have survived their first MI. It seems that with the present-day trend of treating AMI with either thrombolytic therapy or other acute pharmacologic intervention, all patients may undergo coronary angiography sooner than later.

Coronary angiography has established that long-term survival of patients with CAD varies inversely with the number of significantly diseased major vessel.[64] A low ejection fraction (less than 30%) and the presence of three vessel disease are the best catheterization variables for prediction of cardiac death. Left ventricular end-diastolic pressure (LVEDP) alone or in combination with these variables does not add to the predictive accuracy. Abnormalities of wall motion after infarction are not as useful as global abnormalities in predicting prognosis.

It is practical to identify high-risk and low-risk groups. Exercise test variables may be useful in identifying low-risk patients only; the high efficiency of catheterization variables makes high-risk detection more reliable. For example, an exercise tolerance criterion of 10 minutes or more using the Bruce protocol results in the identification of a very low-risk group for future cardiac events, whereas an ejection fraction of less than 30% or the presence of critical three vessel disease identifies a high-risk group for predicting cardiac death or recurrent MI.

OUTCOME OF REVASCULARIZATION PROCEDURES IN YOUNG PATIENTS

It is extremely important to select the best treatment strategy for a young patient in whom coronary revascularization is deemed necessary. In considering revascularization, one must take into account perioperative mortality, short-term and long-term outcome, quality of life, and prolongation of survival.

Coronary angioplasty has emerged as an attractive alternative to coronary bypass surgery. There are no randomized trials to compare directly the results of medical, surgical, and angioplasty treatment modalities in young patients. Medical treatment of young adults is associated with 17 to 30% mortality rate during the 5 years post-MI.[65,66] In another study, a 5-year mortality rate of 33% was documented,[67] suggesting

TABLE 14-5. Risk Predictors of Cardiac Death

	Annual Mortality (%)
Vessel involvement	
1 vessel	1.8
2 vessels	2.1
3 vessels	6.2
Left ventricular (LV) dysfunction	
Mild LV dysfunction	1.5
Moderate LV dysfunction	2.5
Severe LV dysfunction	8.9
Arrhythmias	
Without significant arrhythmias	1.6
With significant arrhythmias	3.6

poor long-term outcome with medical therapy. The poor outcome was related to prior infarction, decreased LV function, multivessel disease, and progression of atherosclerosis. A more recent 3-year follow-up study[68] is indicative of a better outcome with a 3-year mortality rate of only 1.2% in 85 young adults treated medically, surgically, or with angioplasty. The better outcome in this study is attributable to the fact that a large number of patients had single vessel disease, and only 35% required revascularization.

Coronary bypass surgery in young patients is performed in higher-risk patients with extensive CAD, high prevalence of risk factors, and LV dysfunction. In this group of young patients, the perioperative mortality from coronary bypass surgery ranged from 0 to 4.9%.[68–73] There is also a 1.6 to 8.4% rate of MI. Actuarial 5-year survival after coronary bypass surgery ranged from 80 to 94%.[69,71–73] (Fig. 14-1) Lytle and associates[73] at Cleveland Clinic demonstrated actuar-

ial survival free of early or late clinical events was 77% at 5 years and 53% at 10 postoperative years.[73] Late clinical events were 15 late deaths, 23 nonfatal MI, 13 reoperations, and return of severe angina in a study group of 107 patients aged 35 years or younger. In their study, bypass vein graft patency at 24 months of 47 vein grafts 21 (43%) were patent, 20 grafts were totally occluded, and 6 had hemodynamically significant stenoses. For mammary artery grafts, 14 of 14 were patent at less than 24 months, and 11 of 13 were patent at 24 months or more. The mammary grafts exhibited much better patency even at 10 years.

In another study[75] of 38 subjects aged 39 years and younger, bypass graft patency significantly declined from 91% early after operation to 55% at 10 years, and only 29% of the grafts were free of disease at 7.5 years. No mammary grafts were performed in this study.

Most of the studies were performed during the late 1970s and early 1980s and, since that time, many im-

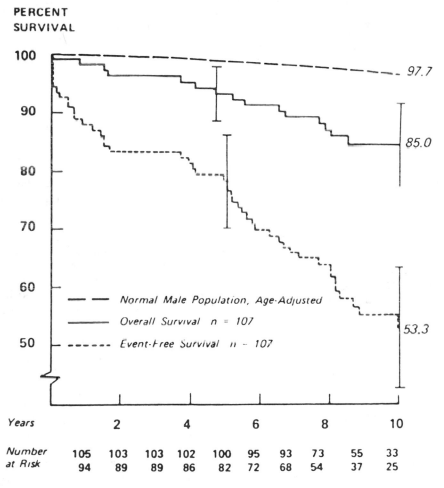

Fig. 14-1. Survival (Kaplan-Meier) and event-free survival of patients undergoing bypass surgery compared with the expected survival of an age-matched sample of men from the United States population. (From Cohen et al.,[74] with permission.)

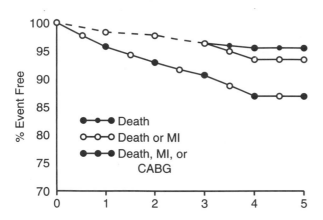

Fig. 14-2. Outcome after coronary angioplasty in 130 patients under 40 years of age. Life-table analysis depicts freedom from death, or myocardial infarction (MI) and death, infarction or coronary artery bypass surgery (CABG). (From Simpfendorfer et al.,[77] with permission.)

provements in myocardial protection and surgical techniques have taken place. Poor late outcome after bypass surgery is due to a high rate of vein graft failure. Internal mammary artery bypass graft has excellent patency rate and it should be the bypass graft of choice for these patients.

Coronary angioplasty in young patients has provided initial gratifying results. Webb and associates[76] performed coronary angioplasty on 148 patients under 40 years of age. Angioplasty was performed on a single vessel in 70% of patients and on multiple vessels in 30%. Angioplasty was successful in 90.5% of patients, complicated by MI in 0.7%, emergency bypass surgery in 0.7%, and death in 0.7%. There was high rate of restenosis ranging from 19 to 41%. The actuarial 5-year survival rate was 95% (Figs. 14-2 and 14-3). Hypertension, diabetes, and LV dysfunction were markers of poor prognosis after angioplasty in their study. Late bypass surgery was required in 8.5% of patients.

In two other angioplasty studies[77,78] of young patients, survival was 94 and 98.6% at a mean follow-up of 2.5 and 2.7 years, respectively. Early and 5-year results after coronary angioplasty in selected young patients are favorable. Late revascularization procedures for restenosis or disease progression are common. There are no randomized studies to compare the outcome in medical, surgical, or angioplasty treatment in young patients.

CONCLUSION

Myocardial infarction at young age is an important cause of long-term disability and has a great impact on the future job activity and productivity of the indi-

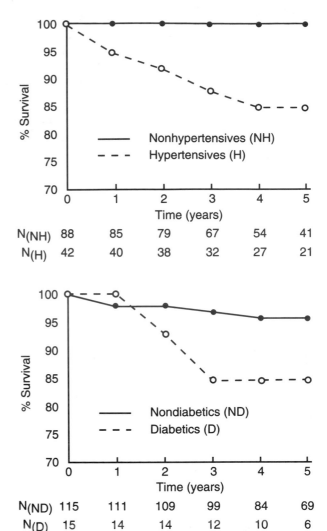

Fig. 14-3. Late outcome in 130 patients with and without hypertension and diabetes. 42 Hypertensive patients (H) and 15 diabetic (D) patients were at increased risk of death. ND, no diabetes; NH, no hypertension. (From Simpfendorfer et al.,[77] with permission.)

vidual patient. It is important to know the extent and severity of CAD in young people in order to better advise them of their future activity and prognosis.

Patients with MI and normal coronary angiograms have a favorable 5-year prognosis. They are not susceptible to recurrent MI, especially if they stop smoking and discontinue using oral contraceptives (women). Coronary angiography will help allay long-term anxiety, reassuring both the patient and the physician.

In patients with one vessel disease and other vessels showing only minimal narrowing disease, progression is rare and slow, and prognosis is generally good if the risk factors are controlled.

In patients with multivessel CAD, progression is common and rapid. Prognosis is less favorable when compared with patients having one vessel disease. In young patients with diffuse, extensive coronary atherosclerosis, progression of the disease is more rapid in comparison with older age groups. These patients will need careful and aggressive medical and/or surgical management to have any significant long-term impact on their survival. Coronary angioplasty is a promising therapeutic modality in young patients.

REFERENCES

1. Stamler J: The primary prevention of coronary heart disease. p. 219. In Braunwald E (ed): The Myocardium: Failure and Infarction. HP Publishing, New York, 1974
2. Blackburn H: Progress in the epidemiology and prevention of coronary heart disease. p. 1. In Yu PN, Goodwin JF (eds): Progress in Cardiology. Lea & Febiger, Philadelphia, 1974
3. Oberman A, Kouchoukos NI, Holt JH et al: Long term results of the medical treatment of coronary artery disease. Angiology 28:160, 1977
4. Nixon JV, Lewis HR, Smitherman TC et al: Myocardial infarction in men in the third decade of life. Ann Intern Med 85:759, 1976
5. Dolder MA, Oliver MF: Myocardial infarction in young men; study of risk factors in nine countries. Br Heart J 37:493, 1975
6. Lamm G: The epidemiology of acute myocardial infarction in young age groups. p. 5. In Roskamm H (ed): Myocardial Infarction at Young Age. Springer-Verlag, Heidelberg, 1981
7. Bergsrand R, Vedin A, Wilhelmsson C et al: Myocardial infarction among men below age 40. Br Heart J 40:783, 1978
8. Simonson E, Berman R: Myocardial infarction in young people: experience in USSR. Am Heart J 84:814, 1972
9. Silver M, Baroldi G, Mariani F: The relationship between acute occlusive coronary thrombus and myocardial infarction studied in 100 consecutive patients. Circulation 61:219, 1980
10. Kapoor AS: Assessment, risk stratification and prognosis of young patients after myocardial infarction. Cardiovasc Rev Rep 1(7):14, 1986
11. Burkart F, Salzmann C: Angiographic findings in postinfarction patients under age of 35. p. 56. In Roskamm H (ed): Myocardial Infarction in Young Age. Springer-Verlag, Heidelberg, 1981
12. Kuller H, Traven ND, Rutan GH et al: Marked decline in coronary heart disease mortality in 35-45 year old white men in men in Alleghency County, Pennsylvania. Circulation 80:261, 1989
13. Gohlke H, Golkhe-Barwolf C, Sturzenhofecke P et al: Myocardial infarction at young age: Correlation of angiographic findings with risk factors and history in 619 patients. Circulation, suppl 3. 62:39, 1980
14. Uhl GS, Farrel PW: Myocardial infarction at young age: risk factors and natural history. p. 29. In Roskamm H
(ed): Myocardial Infarction at Young Age. Springer-Verlag, Heidelberg, 1981
15. Kannel WB, Sorlie P, McNamara PM: Prognosis after initial myocardial infarction: The Framingham study. Am J Cardiol 44:53, 1979
16. Rissanen A, Nikkila: Coronary artery disease and its risk factors in families of young men with angina pectoris and in controls. Br Heart J 39:875, 1977
17. Kagan A, Gordon T, Rhoads GG et al: Some factors related to coronary heart disease incidence in Honolulu Japanese men: the Honolulu Heart study. Int J Epidemiol 4:271, 1975
18. Rabkin SW, Mathewson FAL, Hsu P: Relation of body weight to development of ischemic heart disease in a cohort of young North American men after a 26 year observation period: the Mannitoba study. Am J Cardiol 39:452, 1971
19. Heinle RA, Leng RI, Fredrickson DS: Lipid and cardohydrate abnormalities in patients with angiographically documented coronary artery disease. Am J Cardiol 24:178, 1969
20. Ostrander LD, Neff BJ, Block WD et al: Hyperglycemia and hypertriglyceridemia among persons with coronary heart disease. Ann Intern Med 67:34, 1967
21. Truett T, Cornfield J, Kannel W: A multivariate analysis of the risk of coronary heart disease in Framingham. Chronic Dis 20:511, 1967
22. Keen H, Reese G, Pkye DA et al: Blood sugar and arterial disease. Lancet 2:505, 1965
23. Schwartz RP, Robicsek F: An unusual anamoly of coronary system—origin of the anterior descending interventricular artery from the pulmonary trunk. J Pediatr 78:123, 1971
24. Wesselhoeft H, Fawcett JS, Johnson AL: Anomalous origin of the left coronary artery from the pulmonary trunk. Its clinical spectrum, pathology and pathophysiology based on a review of 140 cases with seven further cases. Circulation 38:403, 1968
25. Thompson SL, Vieweg WVR, Alpert JS et al: Evidence and age distribution of patients with myocardial infarction with normal coronary arteriograms. Cathet Cardiovasc Diagn 3:1, 1977
26. Arnett EN, Roberts WC: Acute myocardial infarction and angiographically normal coronary arteries. An unproven combination. Circulation 53:395, 1976
27. Engel HJ, Page HL, Campbell WB: Coronary artery disease in young women. JAMA 230:1531, 1974
28. Engel HJ, Hundeshagen H, Lichtlen P: Transmural myocardial infarctions in young women taking oral contraceptives: evidence of reduced flow in spite of normal coronary arteries. Br Heart J 39:477, 1977
29. Engel HJ, Lichtlen P: Evidence of spontaneous thrombolysis in the human coronary system. p. 127. In Kaltenbach M, Lichtlen P, Balcom R et al (eds): Coronary Heart Disease. Thieme, Stuttgart, 1979
30. Mann JI, Vessey MP, Thorogood M et al: Myocardial infarction in young women with special reference to oral contraceptive practice. Br Med J 11:241, 1975
31. Maseri A, L'Abbate A, Baroldi G et al: Coronary vasospasm as a possible cause of myocardial infarction. N Engl J Med 299:1271, 1978

32. Maseri A, Chiechia S, L'Abbate A: Pathogenetic mechanism underlying clinical events associated with atherosclerotic heart disease. Circulation, suppl 5. 62:3, 1980

33. Steel P, Battock D, Genton E: Effects of clofibrate and sulfinpyrazone on platelet survival time in coronary artery disease. Circulation 52:473, 1975

34. Gold F, Steele P: Relationship of age and serum cholesterol to platelet survival time in men with coronary artery disease. p. 143. In Roskamm H (ed): Myocardial Infarction at Young Age. Springer-Verlag, Heidelberg, 1981

35. Roberts WC, Buja IM: The frequency and significance of coronary arterial thrombi and other observations in fatal acute myocardial infarction. A study of 107 necropsy patients. Am J Cardiol 52:425, 1971

36. Waller BF, Roberts WC: Comparison of luminal narrowing by atherosclerotic plaques in young and very old necropsy patients with fatal coronary events. p. 162. In Roskamm H (ed): Myocardial Infarction at Young Age. Springer-Verlag, Heidelberg, 1981

37. Savran SV, Bryson L, Welch TG et al: Clinical correlates of coronary angiography in young males with myocardial infarction. Am Heart J 91:551, 1976

38. Davia JE, Hallal FF, Cheitlin MD et al: Coronary artery disease in young patients: arteriographic and clinical review of 40 cases aged 35 and under. Am Heart J 87:689, 1974

39. Proudfit WL, Shirey EL, Sones MF: Selective cinecoronary arteriography: correlation with clinical findings in 1000 patients. Circulation 33:901, 1966

40. Sanmarco ME, Selvester RH, Brooks SH et al: Risk factors reduction and changes in coronary arteriography. Circulation, suppl 2. 56:140, 1976

41. Selvester RH, Camp J, Sanmarco ME: Effects of exercise training on progression of documented coronary arteriosclerosis in men. p. 495. In Milvy P (ed): The Marathon: Physiological, Medical, Epidemiological and Psychological Studies. New York Academy of Sciences, New York, 1977

42. Kapoor AS, Dang NS: Reliance on physical signs in acute myocardial infarction and its complications. Heart Lung 7:1020, 1978

43. Killip T III, Kimball JT: Treatment of myocardial infarction in coronary care unit: a two year experience with 250 patients. Am J Cardiol 20:457, 1967

44. Peel AAF, Semple T, Wang I et al: A coronary prognostic index grading the severity of infarction. Br Heart J 24: 745, 1962

45. Norris RM, Brandt PWT, Caughey DE et al: A new coronary prognostic index. Lancet 1:274, 1969

46. Forrester JS, Diamond G, Chatterjee K et al: Medical therapy of acute myocardial infarction by application of hemodynamic subsets. Part I. N Engl J Med 295:1356, 1976

47. Forrester JS, Diamond G, Chatterjee K et al: Medical therapy of acute myocardial infarction by application of hemodynamic subsets. Part II. N Engl J Med 295:1404, 1976

48. DeBusk RF, Kraemer HC, Nash E et al: Stepwise risk stratification soon after acute myocardial infarction. Am J Cardiol 52:1161, 1983

49. Matthews E, Amsterdam EA, Lee G et al: Occurrence of angina pectoris in relation to history of myocardial infarction: lack of abolition of angina by infarction, abstracted. Circulation, suppl 3. 55:5, 1977

50. Schuster EH, Bulky BH: Early post-infarction angina: ischemia at a distance and ischemia in the infarct zone. N Engl J Med 305:1101, 1981

51. Harris PJ, Harrell FE, Jr, Lee KL et al: Survival in medically treated coronary artery disease. Circulation 60: 1259, 1979

52. Vanhaecke J, Piessens J, Willens JL et al: Coronary arterial lesions in young men who survived a first myocardial infarction: clinical and electrocardiographic predictors of multivessel disease. Am J Cardiol 47:810, 1981

53. Miller RR, De Maria AN, Vismara et al: Chronic stable inferior myocardial infarction: unsuspected harbinger of high-risk proximal left coronary arterial obstruction amenable to surgical revascularization. Am J Cardiol 39: 954, 1977

54. Starling MR, Crawford MH, O'Rourke RA: Exercise testing early after myocardial infarction: predictive value for subsequent unstable angina and death. Am J Cardiol 46: 909, 1980

55. Cohn PF, Vokonas PS, Herman MV et al: Post-exercise EKG in patients with abnormal resting EKG. Circulation 43:648, 1971

56. Weld FM, Chu KL, Bigger JT et al: Risk stratification with low level exercise testing 2 weeks after acute myocardial infarction. Circulation 64:306, 1981

57. Schwartz KM, Turner JD, Shefield LT et al: Limited exercise testing soon after myocardial infarction. Correlation with early coronary and left ventricular angiography. Ann Intern Med 94:724, 1981

58. Kapoor AS, Dassah H, Synder M et al: The prognostic spectrum of coronary artery disease 8 weeks after myocardial anfarction. Chest 84:312, 1983

59. DeBusk RF, Blomqvist CG, Kouchoukos NT et al: Identification and treatment of low-risk patients after acute myocardial infarction and coronary-artery bypass graft surgery. N Engl J Med 314:161, 1986

60. Pichard AD: Coronary arteriography—for everyone? Am J Cardiol 38:533, 1976

61. Patterson RE, Horowitz SF, Calvin E et al: Can noninvasive exercise test criteria identify patients with left main or 3-vessel coronary disease after a first MI? Am J Cardiol 51:361, 1983

62. Webster JS, Moberg C, Rincon G: Natural history of severe proximal coronary artery disease as documented by coronary cineangiography. Am J Cardiol 33:195, 1974

63. Dash H, Massie BM, Botvinick EH et al: The noninvasive identification of left main and three-vessel coronary artery disease by myocardial stress perfusion scintigraphy and treadmill exercise electrocardiography. Circulation 60:276, 1979

64. Humphries JO, Kuller L, Ross RS et al: Natural history of ischemic heart disease in relation to arteriographic findings. Circulation 49:489, 1974

65. Gertler MM, White PD, Simon R et al: Long-term follow-up of young coronary patients. Am J Med Sci 247:145, 1964

66. Roth O, Berki A, Wolff GD: Long range observations in fifty-three young patients with myocardial infarction. Am J Cardiolo 19:331, 1967

67. Klein LW, Agarwal JB, Herlich MB et al: Prognosis of symptomatic coronary artery disease in young adults aged 40 years or less. Am J Cardiol 60:1269, 1987

68. Lim JS, Proudfit WL, Sones FM, Jr et al: Selective coronary arteriography in young men: a follow-up of 449 patients. Circulation 49:1122, 1974

69. De Oliveria SA, Santana GP, Barchi CA et al: Direct myocardial revascularization in young patients: analysis of 100 consecutive cases without operative mortality. J Cardiovasc Surg 18:9, 1977

70. Laks H, Kaiser GC, Barner HB et al: Coronary revascularization under age 40: risk factors and resutls of surgery. Am J Cardiol 41:584, 1978

71. Kelly TF, Craver JM, Jones EL et al: Coronary revascularization in patients 40 years and younger: surgical experience and long term follow-up. Am Surg 44:675, 1978

72. Jones JW, Ochsner JL, Mills NL et al: Long term results of myocardial revascularization in early-onset arteriosclerosis. Surgery 88:760, 1980

73. Lytle BW, Kramer J R, Golding LAR et al: Young adults with coronary atherosclerosis. 10 year results of surgerical myocardial revascularization. J Am Coll Cardiol 4:445, 1984

74. Cohen DJ, Basamania C, Graeber GM et al: Coronary artery bypass grafting in young patients under 36 years of age. Chest 89:811, 1986

75. Fitzgibbon GM, Hamilton MG, Leach AJ et al: Coronary artery disease and coronary artery bypass in young men. J Am Coll Cardiol 9:977, 1987

76. Webb JG, Myler RK, Shaw RE et al: Coronary angioplasty in young adults: Initial results and late outcome. J Am Coll Cardiol 16:1569, 1990

77. Simpfendorfer C, Tuzcu EM, Badhwar K et al: Percutaneous transluminal coronary angioplasty in the young adult. Cleve Clin J Med 56:569, 1989

78. Stone GW, Ligon RW, Rutherford BD et al: Short-term outcome and long-term follow-up following coronary angioplasty in the young patients: an 8-year experience. Am Heart J 118:873, 1989

15

Assessment of Prognosis in Patients With Suspected Coronary Artery Disease Using Planar Thallium 201 Imaging

Sanjiv Kaul

Planar thallium 201 imaging has now been used for more than 15 years in clinical cardiology. Abundant data have accumulated regarding the role of this technique for determining prognosis in patients with suspected coronary artery disease (CAD). Although single photon emission computed tomography (SPECT) is now being used increasingly in lieu of planar imaging in the clinical setting, all prognostic data thus far have been accumulated from planar images. Furthermore, certain prognostically important information, such as the lung-heart thallium 201 ratio, can only be obtained from planar images. Consequently, until prognostic data using SPECT imaging have been collated, planar thallium 201 imaging remains the thallium 201 procedure of choice for determining prognosis. Planar thallium 201 imaging has been demonstrated to provide useful prognostic information in the following clinical conditions:

A. Resting thallium 201 imaging
   1. Known or suspected acute myocardial infarction (AMI)
   2. Where left ventricular (LV) dysfunction exceeds measured infarct size
   3. In patients receiving reperfusion therapy for AMI
B. Exercise thallium 201 imaging
   1. Ambulatory patients with stable angina pectoris
   2. Patients with uncomplicated infarctions who did not receive thrombolytic therapy
   3. Patients with uncomplicated infarctions who received thrombolytic therapy
C. Dipyridamole thallium 201 imaging

213

1. In patients who cannot exercise but are suspected to have CAD
2. In patients referred for major vascular surgery
3. In patients with AMI

To understand its value in determining prognosis in patients with suspected CAD, certain aspects of thallium 201 kinetics must be understood. The uptake of thallium 201 by myocytes involves an active process using the Na^+,K^+ pump. If there is loss of cell membrane integrity, thallium 201 uptake will be reduced despite adequate blood flow. Irreversibly damaged myocardial tissue cannot concentrate thallium 201 intracellularly.[1]

After initial uptake, there is a continuous exchange of thallium 201 between the intracellular compartment and the blood pool that recirculates through the myocardium.[2-9] A region of the myocardium that has received less thallium 201 initially because of reduced blood flow will therefore continue to accumulate thallium 201 over time, as long as the myocardial cells are viable. By contrast, a region that has received adequate thallium 201 initially will show a net loss of thallium 201 over time in proportion to the decrease in blood thallium 201 levels. The disparity noted in the thallium 201 activity on the initial image between regions of normal and decreased flow will, consequently tend to become less over time. This phenomenon is known as *redistribution;* it can be seen when a delayed image (taken 2 to 4 hours after injection of thallium 201) is compared with the initial image (taken 5 minutes after the injection of thallium 201) (Fig. 15-1). This reversal of the initial disparity can either be *complete* (indicating that the entire region of the myocardium showing the initial defect is viable) or *partial* (implying that some viable tissue is present within the region of the initial defect). Redistribution is best assessed using quantitative techniques.[10]

When thallium 201 uptake is reduced in the initial image with no redistribution noted in the delayed image, a *persistent defect* is said to be present.[3] Persistent defects can be of several grades depending on the initial uptake of thallium 201 in that region. When the uptake is very reduced, such that there is virtual absence of thallium 201 activity in that region both in the initial and in the delayed images (Fig. 15-2), a *severe defect* is said to be present. Presence of severe defects has been correlated with previous myocardial infarction, Q waves on the electrocardiogram (ECG), and akinetic or dyskinetic left ventricular regions on angiography.[11,12]

Because redistribution implies the presence of hypoperfused viable myocardium, the absence of redistribution has, unfortunately, been interpreted as the lack of viability.[13,14] The lack of redistribution in an image

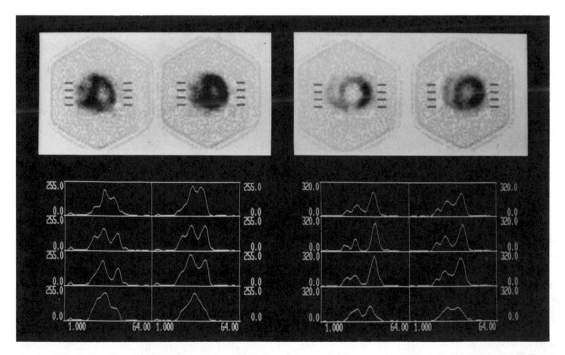

Fig. 15-1. "Complete" redistribution in the anterolateral wall (anterior projection) and "partial" redistribution in the interventricular septum (45-degree left anterior oblique projection). The initial defect noted in the interventricular septum shows less "fill-in" in the 2-hour image compared with that noted in the anterior wall. (From Kaul,[67] with permission.)

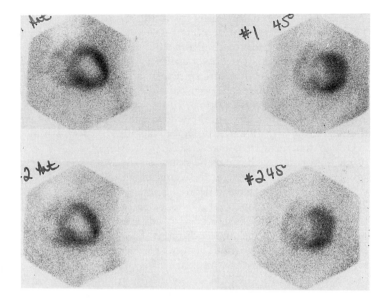

Fig. 15-2. Severe "persistent" defect in the interventricular septum in the 45-degree left anterior oblique projection. The initial defect is severe with hardly any counts seen, and there is no "fill-in" noted in this region, even at 2 hours. (From Kaul,[67] with permission.)

showing a severe initial defect as illustrated in Figure 15-2 probably does imply the absence of viable tissue in that region. When initial defects are *mild*, however (there is reduced but definite uptake of thallium), and thallium 201 activity is present in the delayed image without any evidence of redistribution (Fig. 15-3), they

probably represent a mixture of viable and nonviable tissue. If there is only nonviable tissue in these regions, there should be no uptake of thallium 201 in the first place, and certainly there should be no reason for the myocardium to retain thallium several hours later. This contention is supported by normal uptake of thal-

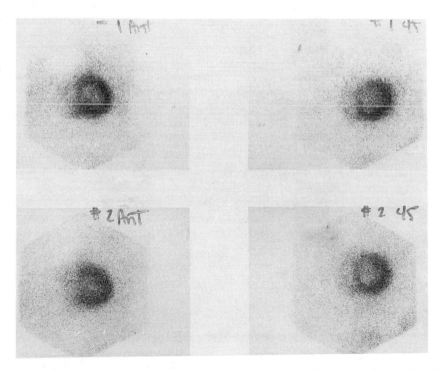

Fig. 15-3. Mild "persistent" defect in the interventricular septum in the 45-degree left anterior oblique projection with no "fill-in" noted in this region in the delayed image. The thallium 201 counts within the defect are not as low as those noted in Fig. 15-2. Despite a "fixed defect," this region of hypoperfusion denoted viable myocardium. (From Kaul,[67] with permission.)

lium 201 in such regions after revascularization.[15,16] These fixed defects also demonstrate oxygen utilization.[14] On reinjection of thallium 201, most of these defects also demonstrate reversibilty.[17] Put together, these data indicate that unless severe, a fixed defect showing some thallium 201 uptake indicates the presence of viable myocardium. Data regarding the amount of thallium 201 uptake within a defect versus the degree of viability are, however, lacking.

Other than *persistent defect* and *redistribution*, another abnormality that can be noted on thallium 201 images is *reverse redistribution*. This phenomenon is said to occur when there is normal uptake of thallium 201 in the initial image, but a defect occurs in the delayed image[18] (Fig. 15-4). Reverse redistribution has different implications under different conditions. In patients with CAD without a recent infarction, this phenomenon implies the presence of a severely stenotic vessel. In this situation, myocardium supplied by a less stenotic artery will demonstrate a faster

wash-out of thallium 201 compared with that supplied by a more stenotic vessel. The region supplied by the less stenotic vessel will therefore demonstrate reverse redistribution, whereas it is actually the myocardium remote from this region that is supplied by the more stenotic vessel.

In patients who have been imaged after a recent myocardial infarction, reverse redistribution implies successful reperfusion (either spontaneous or related to thrombolytic therapy).[19,20] The precise mechanism of reverse redistribution in such patients is not known. Some have postulated that hyperemic blood flow in the noninfarcted epicardial tissue of the reperfused zone results in increased initial thallium 201 uptake in that region. During the interval between the initial and delayed images, there is faster wash-out of thallium 201 from this region compared with normal areas, resulting in appearance of a defect in the delayed images (reverse redistribution).[19] In the canine model, regional hyperemia following coronary reper-

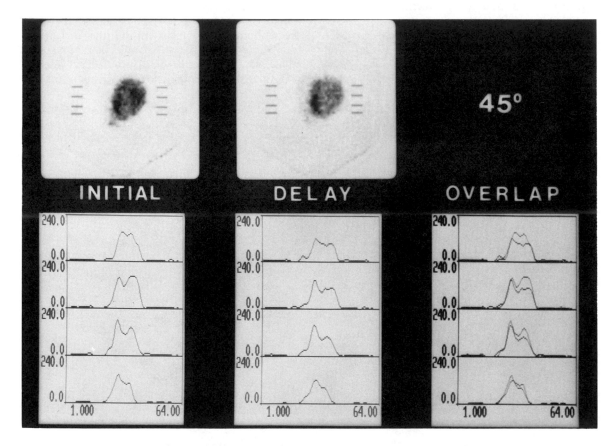

Fig. 15-4. Phenomenon of "reverse redistribution." In the initial image, the counts in both the postero-lateral wall and the interventricular septum appear to be equal, although a defect is noted in the inferoapical region. In the 2-hour image, however, the counts in the posterolateral wall are significantly lower than those in the interventricular septum, resulting in a defect in the posterolateral wall in the delayed images. (From Kaul,[67] with permission.)

fusion has been reported to result in accelerated thallium 201 clearance[21] and may be related to initial accumulation of thallium in the interstitial space. Although the precise mechanism of reverse redistribution post-thrombolysis remains unclear, it is associated with improvement in regional function, hence viable myocardium.[19,20]

Lung-heart thallium 201 ratio also provides important information. This ratio is best assessed using quantitative techniques.[10] Increased lung uptake of thallium 201 during exercise implies exercise-induced pulmonary edema and has been correlated with the presence of multivessel disease, number of myocardial segments demonstrating redistribution and abnormal wall motion, presence of large infarcts, and heart failure.[22–25] Abnormally high lung uptake has also been correlated with larger infarct size and lower ejection fractions in patients with AMI who have undergone a submaximal exercise test.[26] In addition, lung thallium 201 activity at rest in patients with AMI has been correlated with the presence of heart failure and large areas of hypoperfusion on thallium 201 images.[27] Lung thallium 201 activity after intravenous infusion of dipyridamole has been correlated with the presence of redistribution and transient LV dilation on thallium 201 images and ST-segment depression on the ECG.[28] The correlates of the increased lung-heart thallium 201 ratio are as follows:

A. At rest
1. Congestive heart failure
2. Number of segments with initial defects
3. Resting left ventricular ejection fraction (LVEF)
B. During exercise
1. Congestive heart failure
2. Resting LVEF
3. Prior MI
4. Poor exercise double product
5. Number of segments with redistribution
6. Number of segments with initial defects
C. During dipyridamole imaging
1. Number of segments with redistribution
2. ST-segment depression
3. LV dilation

The discussion relating to the value of planar thallium 201 imaging in determining prognosis is divided into three components: (1) thallium 201 imaging at rest, (2) exercise thallium 201 imaging, and (3) dipyridamole thallium 201 imaging.

THALLIUM 201 IMAGING AT REST

Known or Suspected Acute Myocardial Infarction. There are several clinical situations in which thallium 201 imaging can provide useful prognostic information. As would be expected, the size of the perfusion defect after AMI on thallium 201 imaging provides important prognostic information.[29] Figure 15-5 illustrates acturial survival curves from patients experiencing a myocardial infarction based on the thallium 201 defect size. Patients with high-risk scans did much worse than those with low-risk scans. Thallium 201 imaging

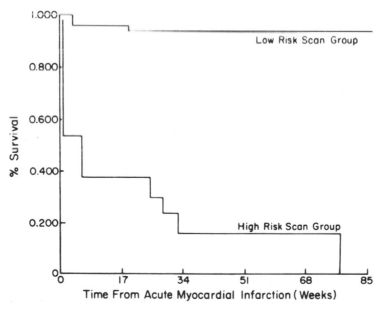

Fig. 15-5. Actuarial survival in patients after acute myocardial infarction who have a high-risk versus a low-risk thallium scan. (From Silverman et al,[29] with permission.)

is also useful for determining disposition in patients admitted to the hospital with nondiagnostic clinical and ECG features.[30,31] In such patients, thallium 201 imaging can identify those likely to have suffered an infarction. Figure 15-6 depicts thallium 201 findings in patients referred to the coronary care unit (CCU) with chest pain in whom the diagnosis of AMI was uncertain. On thallium 201 imaging, only those with acute ischemic syndromes (specifically, AMI) demonstrated definite abnormalities.[30] On the basis of these findings, it has been suggested that patients suspected to have acute ischemic syndromes but having nondiagnostic ECGs should undergo rest thallium 201 imaging. Patients with abnormal thallium 201 findings should be transferred to the CCU for further care.[30,31] From these data one can extrapolate that thallium 201 imaging at rest would also have a high sensitivity for the detection of AMI in patients presenting to the emergency department with chest pain and nondiagnostic ECGs.

Left Ventricular Dysfunction That Exceeds Infarct Size During Acute Myocardial Infarction. There are several instances in which patients with no evidence of prior infarction present with AMI and who have left ventricular dysfunction far in excess of the ongoing infarction judged from creatine kinase levels or ECG. Such patients might have ischemia in myocardial beds remote

from the infarct zone and tend to have a grave prognosis.[32,33] Rest thallium 201 images have been shown to be useful in determining the extent of ischemia in such patients.[34] The presence of redistribution in regions beyond the ongoing infarction can help determine whether immediate revascularization is needed. Figure 15-7 illustrates initial and delayed rest thallium 201 images in such a patient at time of hospital admission. This patient had ECG evidence of anterior infarction with a peak creatine kinase-MB of 284 IU/dl. The resting left ventricular ejection fraction (LVEF) was 0.30. The thallium 201 images demonstrated ischemia in the entire anterolateral wall, interventricular septum and anterior wall. Figure 15-8 illustrates exercise thallium 201 images in the same patient after revascularization. Only a small infarct is noted in the anteroapical and distal interventricular septal regions in the exercise image; all other areas that showed redistribution on the rest images prior to surgery now show normal perfusion. The resting LVEF in this patient improved to 0.45.

Patients Undergoing Reperfusion Therapy for Acute Myocardial Infarction. A patient in whom chest pain develops after reperfusion therapy might have ischemia within the infarct zone or in a remote myocardial bed. Because regional wall-motion abnormality can persist for 5 to 10 days after successful reperfusion,[35] its pres-

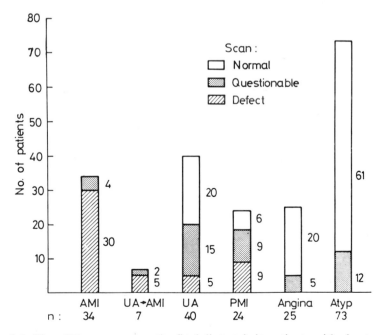

Fig. 15-6. Results of thallium 201 scans versus the final diagnosis in patients with chest pain syndromes and equivocal electrocardiograms admitted to the hospital. Definite defects were noted in most of the patients with acute myocardial infarction (AMI) and those with unstable angina progressing to acute infarction (UA→AMI). Patients with angina and those with atypical chest pain had either questionable or normal scans. (From Wackers et al.,[30] with permission.)

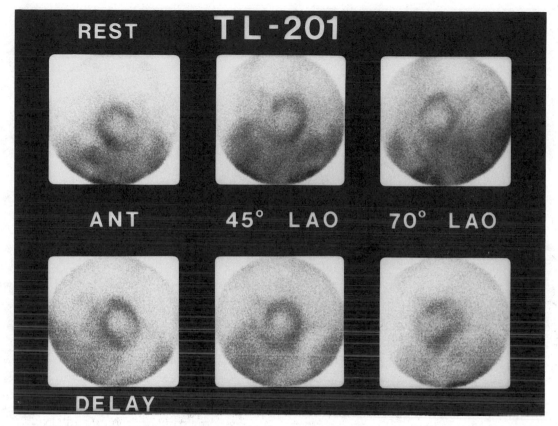

Fig. 15-7. Resting thallium images in a patient with Q waves in V1 to V4 and a peak creatine kinase-MB level of 284 IU/dl whose left ventricular (LV) dysfunction was far in excess of infarct size (LV ejection fraction of 0.30). This patient showed a mild persistent defect in the lower interventricular septum and anterior wall with partial redistribution to these regions as well as redistribution to other beds. (From Smucker et al.,[34] with permission.)

ence does not indicate the absence of viable myocardium. Uptake of thallium 201 in the infarct zone that persists in the delayed image can be said to indicate viable myocardium. Similarly, rest redistribution in remote beds indicates ischemia in those beds. In either case, thallium 201 imaging will help in determining the therapeutic strategy. There is controversy regarding the optimal timing of thallium 201 imaging after reperfusion therapy. It has been suggested that because of hyperemia or tissue edema, or both, after reperfusion, if injected immediately after reperfusion therapy, thallium 201 might accumulate in areas that are not viable.[36,37] This does not occur if thallium 201 is injected approximately 48 hours after reperfusion.[36]

EXERCISE THALLIUM 201 IMAGING

Ambulatory Patients With Stable Angina Pectoris. The following thallium 201 imaging variables have been shown to predict adverse prognosis in ambulatory patients with chest pain:

1. Lung-heart thallium 201 ratio
2. Number of segments with redistribution
3. Number of segments with initial defects
4. LV dilation
5. Reverse redistribution

The number of myocardial segments showing redistribution on delayed thallium 201 images has been shown to be a strong predictor of prognosis in several studies (Fig. 15-9).[38–43] The cardiac event rate has been exponentially related to the number of segments with redistribution[41] (Fig. 15-10). Patients without evidence of redistribution on delayed images have a much better event-free survival rate than do those who demonstrate redistribution. In several studies comparing both angiographic and catheterization variables, only the presence of redistribution predicted the occurrence of future nonfatal MI.[39–41] Coronary anatomy and rest and exercise LV ejection fraction were not as useful in this regard. These latter variables are, however, important as predictors of mortality.[38]

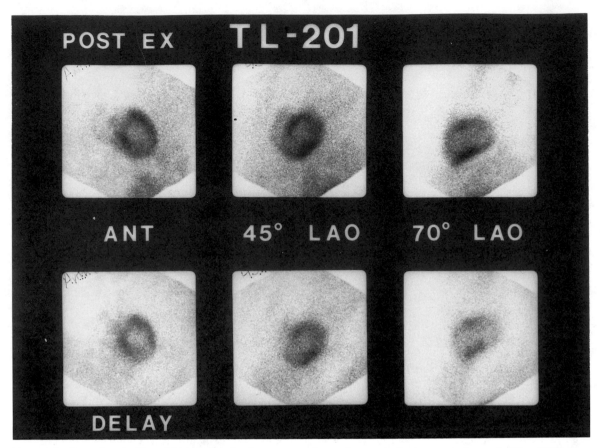

Fig. 15-8. Exercise thallium 201 imaging in the same patient whose rest images are shown in Fig. 15-7 after the patient underwent bypass surgery to all three major coronary arteries. The resting left ventricular ejection fraction improved to 0.45. There is only a mild persistent apical and lower septal defect. Perfusion to all other regions is normal. (From Smucker et al.,[34] with permission.)

The lung-heart ratio of thallium 201 has also been shown to be a strong predictor of future events.[39,42] In these studies, this ratio was a better predictor of events than the presence of redistribution. In two studies in which angiographic and thallium 201 data were compared, the lung-heart ratio of thallium 201 was better than the number of diseased vessels. Figure 15-11 illustrates the event-free rate in 204 patients with stable symptoms who were followed for a period of 4 to 9 years. The presence of multivessel disease (Fig. 15-11A) had a slightly lower predictive power for cardiac events than the presence of increased lung-heart ratio of thallium 201 (Fig. 15-11B). In comparison, the presence of redistribution on delayed thallium 201 images (Fig. 15-11C) was not as powerful a predictor of future events as either the lung-heart thallium 201 ratio or coronary anatomy, and the presence of ST-segment depression on the ECG was the least powerful of these four predictors[39] (Fig. 15-11D). The superiority of the lung-heart ratio of thallium 201 for predicting future events (especially mortality) should not be surprising. Increased lung uptake of thallium 201 during exercise indicates the presence of pulmonary edema and thus, in the setting of CAD, the presence of LV dysfunction. The presence of increased lung uptake of thallium 201 should therefore provide the same information as a decrease in the LV ejection fraction during exercise.

More importantly, thallium 201 imaging added incremental prognostic information in the presence of known clinical and exercise stress test variables[44] (Fig. 15-12). When the lung-heart thallium 201 ratio was excluded from analysis, coronary angiography provided further additional prognostic information to that available from clinical and exercise thallium 201 data. When lung-heart thallium 201 ratio was included in the analysis, coronary angiography did not add any prognostic information to known clinical and exercise thallium 201 data. These data are of great practical significance. It is one thing to demonstrate that a certain variable has great prognostic merit; it

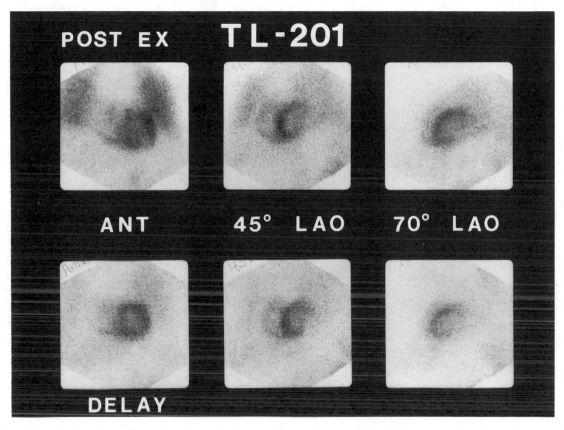

Fig. 15-9. High-risk thallium 201 study with increased lung-heart thallium 201 ratio and multiple defects with and without redistribution. (From Kaul,[68] with permission.)

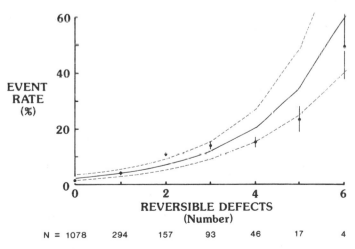

Fig. 15-10. Relationship of cardiac event rate (y-axis) to number of segments with redistribution on exercise thallium 201 images. An exponential relation is noted. (From Ladenheim et al.,[41] with permission.)

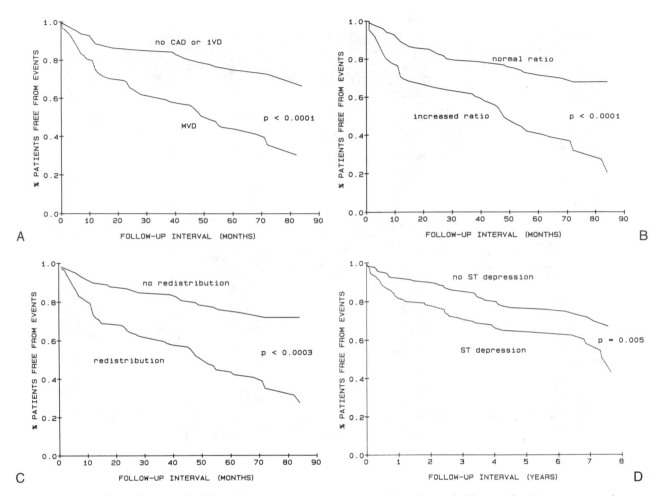

Fig. 15-11. Event-free survival based on coronary anatomy (**A**), lung-heart thallium ratio (**B**), presence of redistribution (**C**), and presence of ST-segment depression (**D**). The lung-heart ratio of thallium is the best predictor of future events followed closely by the number of diseased vessels. (From Kaul et al.,[39] with permission.)

is another to show that it adds prognostic information when examined in light of known and easily available clinical data.

Not only have predictors such as the number of segments with redistribution and the lung-heart thallium 201 ratio found to be of importance in determining prognosis in individual studies but, when models have been derived based on these variables in one study population, they have been found to be powerful predictors of events in an unrelated patient population.[44] Testing the validity of these models in unrelated populations has not been attempted for any other test and provides a unique and powerful insight into the prognostic value of exercise thallium 201 imaging. Other thallium 201 predictors found to correlate with the

occurrence of future events include the number of defects on the initial images and the degree of initial defect (mild or severe).[45,46]

Several studies have indicated that patients with chest pain and normal exercise thallium 201 images have an excellent prognosis, even if underlying CAD has been demonstrated angiographically. Figure 15-13 is an example of a normal thallium 201 study. One study reported a 0.1% event rate in 500 patients with normal thallium 201 images,[46] while another reported a yearly cardiac mortality of 0.5% in 345 patients with chest pain and normal thallium 201 images.[47] Similarly, no deaths and two nonfatal infarctions were reported during a 2-year follow-up evaluation of 95 patients with normal exercise thallium 201 images.[48]

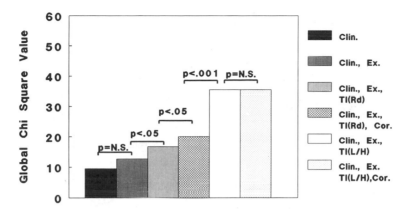

Fig. 15-12. Incremental prognostic value of tests done in succession in patients with suspected coronary artery disease (see text for details). Clin, clinical; Ex, exercise; Tl(Rd), thallium-201 redistribution; Cor, coronary angiography; Tl(L/H), thallium 201 lung-heart ratio. (From Pollock et al.,[44] with permission.)

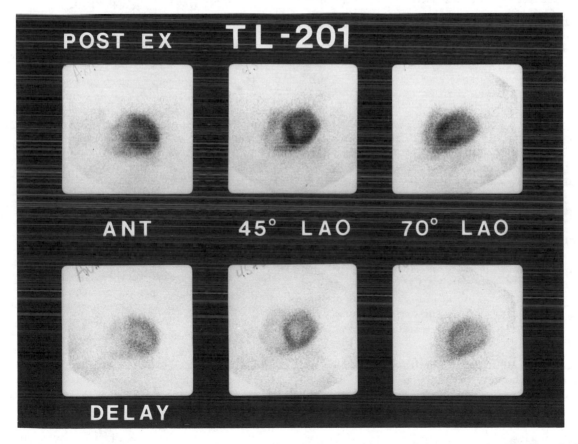

Fig. 15-13. Normal exercise thallium 201 images. A patient with such a result has a very low likelihood of suffering an adverse cardiac event. (From Kaul,[68] with permission.)

Patients with chest pain and insignificant CAD on angiography who had normal exercise thallium 201 images had no events in a 4- to 8-year follow-up in one study compared with 4 of 24 patients with insignificant CAD but abnormal thallium 201 images who had nonfatal cardiac events.[49]

High-risk exercise thallium 201 findings are more prevalent than high-risk exercise ECG findings in patients with left main coronary artery and three vessel disease.[50,51] In one study, high-risk thallium 201 images were seen in 38 of 40 patients with three vessel CAD. In these same patients, only 15 (38%) had greater than 2 mm ST-segment depression on the ECG within 6 minutes of exercise.[50] In another study, 70% of patients with greater than 50% left main coronary artery stenosis and 50% of patients with proximal three vessel disease had high-risk thallium 201 images that were more prevalent than high-risk ECG findings during exercise stress testing.[51] Thallium 201 variables may be more predictive of future cardiac events in comparison with the exercise ECG alone because of better detection of multivessel ischemia by the former.

Uncomplicated Infarction in Patients Who Did Not Receive Thrombolytic Therapy. Patients at high risk of subsequent cardiac events after an uncomplicated AMI can be identified using thallium imaging in conjunction with low-level treadmill exercise testing.[26,52–54] A prospective study in which such patients were followed for a mean interval of 15 months found that while 49% of patients with future events had ST-segment depression and 60% had angina during exercise, 86% had high-risk thallium 201 images[52] (Fig. 15-14). The high-risk thallium 201 findings are listed on page 219. Coronary angiography did not add to the prognostic power of the test. Future nonfatal ischemic events were predicted better by thallium 201 imaging than by coronary angiography. In another study, a combination of thallium 201 imaging and hemodynamic and ECG findings complemented each other in identifying three vessel and left main coronary artery disease in patients who had recently suffered an MI.[53] In a more recent study, lung-heart ratio of thallium 201 during predischarge exercise testing was found to relate closely with the extent and severity of CAD, residual ischemia, and resting LV systolic function.[26]

Uncomplicated Infarction in Patients Who Received Thrombolytic Therapy. In addition to the findings listed above, patients who receive thrombolytic therapy during their infarction can show another thallium 201 imaging finding postinfarction, which reflects the presence of viable myocardium.[19,20] This finding is "reverse redistribution" and has been alluded to earlier (Fig. 15-4).

The incidence of reverse redistribution in patients receiving thrombolytic therapy depends on the defini-

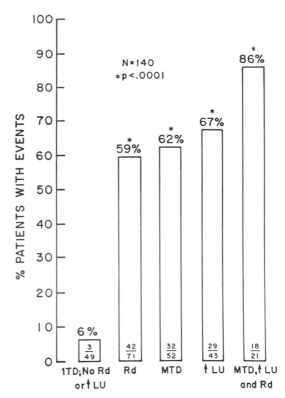

Fig. 15-14. Relationship between cardiac event rate and thallium 201 abnormalities during submaximal exercise stress test in patients who were discharged from the hospital following an uncomplicated myocardial infarction. (From Gibson et al.,[52] with permission.)

tion of the term. If reverse redistribution is said to occur in a segment showing decreased counts in the delayed image, even if there is a partial defect in the initial image, the incidence can be as high as 75%.[19] If, however, it is said to be present when there is no numerically significant defect in the initial image, but a significant defect in the delayed images, the incidence is about 25%.[30] Reverse redistribution on planar thallium 201 images is usually seen only in the inferoapical and low posterolateral regions. One possible explanation is that these regions are thin, and there is also less tissue overlay. By contrast, the interventricular septum in the thallium 201 images represents a summation image of the right ventricle and both the anterior and posterior interventricular septum. Heterogeneity of blood flow between the epicardium and endocardium is therefore less likely to be detected in this region. It has also been suggested that reverse redistribution could be an artifact of background subtraction.[55] It is readily observed, however, in the analogue non-background subtracted images.

Recent data suggest that, unlike postinfarction patients who have not received thrombolytic therapy, the detection rate of multivessel disease is low on pre-discharge exercise thallium 201 imaging in patients who have received thrombolytic therapy.[56] Although thallium 201 imaging continues to be superior to exercise ECG in detecting multivessel disease in such cases, the overall predictive power for detecting multivessel disease is significantly lower by both tests in such patients. The reason for this phenomenon is not known, and its prognostic implications are undefined.

DIPYRIDAMOLE THALLIUM 201 IMAGING

Dipyridamole, recently approved by the Food and Drug Administration (FDA) for intravenous use in humans, is a phosphodiesterase inhibitor that causes vascular smooth muscle dilation. It causes a severalfold increase in blood flow through normal coronary arteries without changing flow to a similar extent in arteries with critical stenosis. This disparity in flow results in mismatch of thallium 201 uptake in different regions of the myocardium. In this regard, dipyridamole achieves the same objective as exercise. Dipyridamole thallium 201 imaging has been suggested as an alternate approach to exercise imaging,[11,57] especially in patients who are unable to exercise. The specific situations in which dipyridamole thallium 201 imaging has provided important prognostic information are discussed.

Patients Who Cannot Exercise But Suspected of Having Coronary Artery Disease. Patients with physical limitations such as severe peripheral vascular disease, amputation, arthritis, or limiting respiratory disease are candidates for dipyridamole thallium 201 imaging. In such patients, the presence of initial defects and redistribution offer a high sensitivity for the detection of CAD.[57,58] Although no studies have been done so far to demonstrate long-term outcome in patients who have undergone dipyridamole thallium 201 imaging for routine detection of CAD, variables such as increased lung-heart ratio have been correlated with the extent of ischemia in a manner similar to patients undergoing exercise thallium 201 imaging.[28]

Patients Referred for Major Vascular Surgery. Because most patients with peripheral vascular disease have CAD, the risk of intraoperative cardiac events is high if these patients undergo major vascular surgery, especially that requiring aortic cross-clamping.[59,60] The latter procedure increases afterload to the heart, resulting in greater myocardial oxygen demand. In the presence of critical coronary stenoses, this increase in demand could result in myocardial ischemia and infarction.[60] As a result, several institutions routinely perform coronary angiography in these patients and, if significant CAD is present, perform bypass surgery either before or during the vascular procedure.[61]

Because these patients cannot exercise on a treadmill, dipyridamole thallium 201 imaging has been attempted and found to be successful in identifying patients who are at increased risk of a cardiac event either in the operating room or shortly thereafter.[62] The presence of redistribution is particularly useful in this regard and, when combined with other clinical

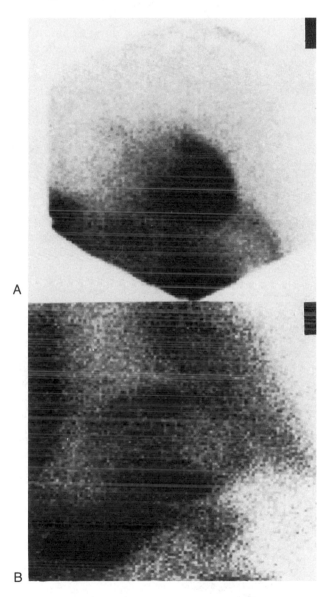

Fig. 15-15. Rest dipyridamole images. **(A)** Patient with normal coronary arteries. **(B)** Patient with multivessel coronary artery disease. Note the increased splanchnic and lung activity, as well as multiple defects. (From Villanueva et al.,[28] with permission.)

variables, can offer a high degree of certainty in identifying high-risk patients.[63] Figure 15-15 includes examples of both normal high-risk dipyridamole thallium 201 images. On the basis of these results, dipyridamole thallium 201 imaging is now being performed routinely in such patients in several institutions.

Patients With Acute Myocardial Infarction. Dipyridamole thallium 201 imaging has been safely performed in patients who have suffered an MI, in an effort to identify those who are at increased risk of a subsequent cardiac event following discharge. In an earlier study, the presence of redistribution was found to be a strong predictor of events (e.g., mortality, unstable angina, and death) in such patients.[64] In this study, dipyridamole was given 10 to 16 days after the infarction. This method of risk stratification after AMI may be particularly suited in patients who are unable to undergo submaximal symptom-limited exercise testing. A more recent study reported no adverse effects using dipyridamole thallium 201 imaging as early as 1 to 4 days after infarction.[65] The best predictor of in-hospital events in this study was the presence of redistribution within the infarct zone. Similar results have been reported by others.[66] Early risk stratification after AMI may therefore become feasible in the future, allowing shortening of the hospital course in those with low-risk studies and aggressive intervention in those with high-risk studies.

SUMMARY

Planar thallium 201 imaging at rest, during exercise, and during pharmacologic intervention with dipyridamole has been shown to provide valuable prognostic information in patients with suspected CAD. The information provided with this technique equals or exceeds that provided by any other noninvasive technique as well as coronary angiography, particularly when the lung-heart thallium 201 ratio is also analyzed. This technique is far superior to exercise ECG in determining prognosis. Because of the superior diagnostic and prognostic information provided by this test, it should be considered for routine use in assessing patients with suspected CAD.

REFERENCES

1. Goldhaber SZ, Newell JB, Ingwall JS et al: Effects of reduced coronary flow on thallium-201 accumulation and release in an in vitro rat heart preparation. Am J Cardiol 51:891, 1983
2. Grunwald AM, Watson DD, Holzgrefe HH et al: Myocardial thallium-201 kinetics in normal and ischemic myocardium. Circulation 64:610, 1981
3. Pohost GM, Zir LM, Moore RH et al: Differentiation of transiently ischemic from infarcted myocardium by serial imaging after a single dose of thallium-201. Circulation 55:294, 1977
4. Beller GA, Watson DD, Ackell P et al: Time course of thallium-201 redistribution after transient myocardial ischemia. Circulation 61:791, 1980
5. Gerry JL, Becker LC, Flaherty JT et al: Evidence for a flow-independent contribution to the phenomenon of thallium redistribution. Am J Cardiol 45:58, 1980
6. Okada RD, Jacobs ML, Daggett WM et al: Thallium-201 kinetics in nonischemic myocardium. Circulation 65:70, 1982
7. Nishiyama H, Adolph R, Gabel M et al: Effect of coronary blood flow on thallium-201 uptake and washout. Circulation 65:534, 1982
8. Pohost GM, Okada RD, O'Keefe DB et al: Thallium redistribution in dogs with severe coronary artery stenosis of fixed caliber. Circ Res 48:439, 1981
9. Okada RD, Leppo JA, Strauss HW et al: Mechanisms and time course for the disappearance of thallium-201 defects at rest in dogs: relation of time to peak activity to myocardial blood flow. Am J Cardiol 49:699, 1982
10. Kaul S, Chesler DA, Okada RD, Boucher CA: Computer versus visual analysis of exercise thallium-201 images: a critical appraisal in 325 patients with chest pain. Am Heart J 114:1129, 1987
11. Leppo J, Boucher CA, Okada RD et al: Serial thallium-201 myocardial imaging after dipyridamole infusion: diagnostic utility in detecting coronary stenoses and relationship to regional wall motion. Circulation 66:649, 1982
12. Bodenheimer MM, Banka VS, Fooshee C et al: Relationship between regional myocardial perfusion and the presence, severity and reversibility of asynergy in patients with coronary heart disease. Circulation 58:789, 1978
13. Kiess MC, Fung AY, Thompson CR et al: Can thallium scan alone determine viability post thrombolytic therapy?, abstracted. Circulation, (suppl II.) 78:91, 1988
14. Brunken RC, Kottori S, Nienaber CA et al: PET detection of viable tissue in myocardial segments with persistent defects at Tl-201 SPECT. Radiology 172:65, 1989
15. Gibson RS, Watson DD, Taylor GJ et al: Prospective assessment of regional myocardial perfusion after coronary revascularization surgery by quantitative thallium-201 scintigraphy. J Am Coll Cardiol 1:804, 1983
16. Liu P, Kiess MC, Okada RD et al: The persistent defect on exercise thallium imaging and its fate after myocardial revascularization: does it represent scar or ischemia? Am Heart J 110:996, 1985
17. Dilsizian V, Rocco TP, Freedman NMT et al: Enhanced detection of ischemic but viable myocardium by the reinjection of thallium after stress redistribution. N Engl J Med 323:141, 1990
18. Hecht HS, Hopkins JM, Rose JG et al: Reverse redistribution: Worsening of thallium-201 myocardial images from exercise to redistribution. Radiology 140:177, 1981
19. Weiss AT, Maddahi J, Lew AS et al: Reverse redistribution of thallium-201: a sign of nontransmural myocardial infarction with patency of the infarct related coronary artery. J Am Coll Cardiol 7:61, 1986

20. Touchstone DA, Beller GA, Nygaard TW et al: Functional significance of predischarge exercise thallium-201 findings following intravenous streptokinase therapy during acute myocardial infarction. Am Heart J 116:1500, 1988

21. Okada RD: Kinetics of thallium-201 reperfused canine myocardium after coronary artery occlusion. J Am Coll Cardiol 3:1245, 1984

22. Boucher CA, Zir LM, Beller GA et al: Increased lung uptake of thallium-201 during exercise myocardial imaging: clinical, hemodynamic and angiographic implications in patients with coronary artery disease. Am J Cardiol 46:189, 1980

23. Homma S, Kaul S, Boucher CA: Correlates of lung/heart ratio of thallium-201 in coronary artery disease. J Nucl Med 28:1531, 1987

24. Kushner FG, Okada RD, Kirshenbaum HD et al: Lung thallium-201 uptake after stress testing in patients with coronary artery disease. Circulation 63:341, 1981

25. Bingham JB, McKusick KA, Strauss HW et al: Influence of coronary artery disease on pulmonary uptake of thallium-201. Am J Cardiol 46:821, 1980

26. Al-Khwaja I, Lahiri A, Rodrigues EA et al: Clinical significance of exercise-induced pulmonary uptake of thallium-201 in uncomplicated myocardial infarction. Am J Cardiol Imag 2:135, 1988

27. Jain D, Lahiri A, Raftery EB: Clinical and prognostic significance of lung thallium uptake on rest imaging in acute myocardial infarction. Am J Cardiol 65:154, 1990

28. Villanueva F, Kaul S, Smith WH et al: Prevalence and correlates of increased lung/heart thallium-201 during dipyridamole stress imaging for suspected coronary artery disease. Am J Cardiol 66:1324, 1990

29. Silverman KJ, Becker LC, Bulkley BH et al: Value of early thallium-201 scintigraphy for predicting mortality in patients with acute myocardial infarction. Circulation 61:996, 1980

30. Wackers FJT, Lie KI, Liene KL et al: Potential value of thallium-201 scintigraphy as a means of selecting patients for the coronary care unit. Br Heart J 41:111, 1979

31. Van der Wieken LR, Kan G, Belfer AJ et al: Thallium-201 scanning to decide CCU admissions in patients with nondiagnostic electrocardiograms. Int J Cardiol 4:285, 1983

32. Touchstone DA, Nygaard TW, Kaul S: Correlation between left ventricular risk area and clinical, electrocardiographic, hemodynamic, and angiographic variables during acute myocardial infarction. J Am Soc Echo 3:106, 1990

33. Jaarsma W, Visser CA, Eenige VMJ et al: Prognostic implications of regional hyperkinesia and remote asynergy of noninfarcted myocardium. Am J Cardiol 58:394, 1986

34. Smucker ML, Beller GA, Watson DD, Kaul S: Left ventricular dysfunction in excess of the size of infarction: a possible management strategy. Am Heart J 115:749, 1988

35. Touchstone DA, Beller GA, Nygaard TW et al: Effects of successful intravenous reperfusion therapy on regional myocardial function and geometry in humans: a tomographic assessment using two-dimensional echocardiography. J Am Coll Cardiol 13:1506, 1989

36. Okada RD, Pohost GM: The use of pre-intervention and post-intervention thallium imaging for assessing the early and late effects of experimental coronary arterial reperfusion in dogs. Circulation 69:1153, 1986

37. Forman R, Kirk ES: Thallium-201 accumulation during reperfusion of ischemic myocardium: dependence on regional blood flow rather than viability. Am J Cardiol 54:659, 1984

38. Brown KA, Boucher CA, Okada RD et al: Prognostic value of exercise thallium-201 imaging in patients presenting for evaluation of chest pain. J Am Coll Cardiol 1:994, 1983

39. Kaul S, Finkelstein DM, Homma S et al: Superiority of quantitative exercise thallium-201 variables in determining long-term prognosis in ambulatory patients with chest pain: a comparison with cardiac catheterization. J Am Coll Cardiol 12:25, 1988

40. Kaul S, Lilly DR, Gascho GA et al: Prognostic utility of the exercise thallium-201 test in ambulatory patients with chest pain: comparison with cardiac catheterization. Circulation 77:745, 1988

41. Ladenheim MC, Pollock BH, Rozanski A et al: Extent and severity of myocardial hypoperfusion as predictors of prognosis in patients with suspected coronary artery disease. J Am Coll Cardiol 7:464, 1986

42. Miller DD, Kaul S, Strauss HW et al: Increased exercise thallium-201 lung uptake: a noninvasive prognostic index in two-vessel coronary artery disease. Can J Cardiol 4:270, 1988

43. Gill JB, Ruddy TD, Newell JB et al: Prognostic importance of thallium uptake by the lungs during exercise in coronary artery disease. N Engl J Med 317:1485, 1987

44. Pollock SG, Abbott RD, Boucher CA et al: Independent and incremental prognostic value of tests performed in hierarchical order to evaluate patients with suspected coronary artery disease and validation of models based on these tests. Circulation 85:237, 1992

45. Iskandrian AS, Hakki AH, Kane-Marsch S: Prognostic implications of exercise thallium-201 scintigraphy in patients with suspected or known coronary artery disease. Am Heart J 110:135, 1985

46. Staniloff HM, Forrester JS, Berman DS, Swan HJC: Prediction of death, myocardial infarction, and worsening chest pain using thallium scintigraphy and exercise electrocardiography. J Nucl Med 27:1842, 1986

47. Pamelia FX, Gibson RS, Watson DD et al: Prognosis with chest pain and normal thallium-201 exercise scintigrams. Am J Cardiol 55:920, 1985

48. Wackers FJ, Russo DS, Russo D, Clements JP: Prognostic significance of normal qualitative planar thallium-201 stress scintigraphy in patients with chest pain. J Am Coll Cardiol 6:27, 1985

49. Kaul S, Okada RD, Pohost GM, Boucher CA: How valid is it to classify coronary artery disease based on the number of diseased vessels?, abstracted. Circulation, (suppl II. 74:473, 1986

50. Canhasi B, Dae M, Botvinick E et al: Interaction of "supplementary" scintigraphic indicators of ischemia and stress electrocardiography in the diagnosis of multivessel coronary disease. J Am Coll Cardiol 6:581, 1985

51. Nygaard TW, Gibson RS, Ryan JM et al: Prevalence of high-risk thallium-201 scintigraphic findings in left main coronary artery stenosis: comparison with patients with multi- and single-vessel coronary artery disease. Am J Cardiol 53:462, 1984

52. Gibson RS, Watson DD, Craddock GB et al: Prediction of cardiac events after uncomplicated myocardial infarction: A prospective study comparing predischarge exercise thallium-201 scintigraphy and coronary arteriography. Circulation 68:321, 1983
53. Patterson RE, Horowitz SF, Eng C et al: Can noninvasive exercise test criteria identify patients with left main or three-vessel coronary disease after a first myocardial infarction? Am J Cardiol 51:361, 1983
54. Hung J, Goris ML, Nash E et al: Comparative value of maximal treadmill testing, exercise thallium myocardial perfusion scintigraphy, and exercise radionuclide ventriculography for distinguishing high- or low-risk patients soon after acute myocardial infarction. Am J Cardiol 53:1221, 1984
55. Brown KA, Benoit L, Clements JP, Wackers FJT: Fast washout of thallium-201 from area of myocardial infarction: possible artifact of background subtraction. J Nucl Med 28:945, 1987
56. Haber HL, Gimple LW, Watson DD, Beller GA: Value and limitations of thallium-201 scintigraphy in myocardial infarction patients after thrombolytic therapy, abstracted. J Am Coll Cardiol 17:182A, 1991
57. Josephson MA, Brown BG, Hecht HS et al: Noninvasive detection and localization of coronary stenoses in patients: comparison of resting dipyridamole and exercise thallium-201 myocardial perfusion imaging. Am Heart J 103:1008, 1982
58. Ruddy TD, Dighero HR, Newell JB et al: Quantitative analysis of dipyridamole-thallium images for the detection of coronary artery disease. J Am Coll Cardiol 10:142, 1987
59. Thompson JE, Garrett WV: Peripheral-arterial surgery. N Engl J Med 302:491, 1980
60. Attia RR, Murphy JD, Snider M et al: Myocardial ischemia due to infrarenal aortic cross-clamping during aortic surgery in patients with coronary artery disease. Circulation 53:961, 1976
61. DeBakey ME, Lawrie GM: Combined coronary artery and peripheral vascular disease: recognition and treatment. J Vasc Surg 1:605, 1984
62. Boucher CA, Brewster DG, Darling RC et al: Determination of cardiac risk by dipyridamole-thallium imaging before peripheral vascular surgery. N Engl J Med 312:389, 1985
63. Eagle K, Coley CM, Newell JB et al: Combining clinical and thallium data optimizes preoperative assessment of cardiac risk before major vascular surgery. Ann Intern Med 110:859, 1989
64. Leppo JA, O'Brien J, Rothendler JA et al: Dipyridamole-thallium-201 scintigraphy in the prediction of future cardiac event after acute myocardial infarction. N Engl Med J 310:1014, 1984
65. Brown KA, O'Meara J, Chambers CE, Plante DA: Ability of dipyridamole thallium-201 imaging 1 to 4 days after acute myocardial infarction to predict in-hospital and late recurring myocardial ischemic events. Am J Cardiol 65:160, 1990
66. Bosch X, March R, Magrina J et al: Prediction of in-hospital cardiac events using dipyridamole perfusion scintigraphy after myocardial infarction, abstracted. Circulation, (suppl II. 80:II–307, 1989
67. Kaul S: A look at 15 years of planar thallium-201 imaging. Am Heart J 118:581, 1989
68. Kaul S: Identification of high risk patients with coronary artery disease: an overview. p. 275. In Miller DD, Burns RJ, Gill JB, Ruddy TD (eds): Clinical Cardiac Imaging. McGraw-Hill Book Company, New York, 1987

16

Risk Assessment of Patients Undergoing Coronary Artery Bypass Surgery

Bradford P. Blakeman
Roque Pifarré

Defining the risk of coronary artery bypass surgery for patients is imperative. Not only is it necessary to answer the questions of patients and fellow medical personnel, but to assess which mode of therapy—medical, angioplasty, or surgery—is in the patient's best interest. Although the efficacy of any treatment for coronary artery disease (CAD) can best be judged by how well it relieves a patient's symptoms and prolongs life expectancy, the intent of this chapter is to look specifically at the perioperative risk factors for coronary artery surgery.

The capability of pinpointing risk factors for morbidity and mortality is hindered by changes in patient population over a period of years, as well as differences in medical institutions. Also, definitions of elective, urgent, and emergent patients vary from center to center. Despite these differences, this chapter evaluates the general trends in patient population, perioperative morbidity, and mortality of the past two decades and provides a more detailed discussion of the risk factors.

CHANGE IN POPULATION

Understanding the risks of coronary artery surgery requires tracing the evolution of patient population undergoing bypass surgery over the past 20 years. In general, there has been an increase in the age of patients operated on.[1-5] Oldham et al. reported the average age to be 50 in 1972 for patients presenting to surgery.[3] By 1980, the average age reported was 54.6 at the Emory University[4] Medical Center and 58.1 at the Cleveland Clinic.[1] And in 1985, the reported mean age was 61.1.[5] Similarly, patients over the age of 70 undergoing revascularization composed 0.6% of the group in 1973, but 9.1% by 1982.[1] This trend toward an older population continues into the 1990s.

The next significant change is the larger proportion of patients that are female. During the 1970s, the increase was nearly twofold at most institutions.[2,4,6] In a recent publication, Naunheim et al.,[5] noted that 23% of the patient population was female.

Associated medical problems also represent an area

of change over the past two decades. Although there is a decline in patients with a recent smoking history, more patients with chronic obstructive pulmonary disease are presenting to surgery.[1,5] A gradual increase in patients with insulin-dependent diabetes mellitus (IDDM) has been reported for the decades of the 1970s and 1980s.[1,5] Other peripheral vascular problems, including hypertension, cerebrovascular disease, peripheral vascular disease, and renal disease associated with coronary disease, although not consistent in all institutions, are more prevalent.[1,2,5]

Coronary catheterization data concerning patients presenting to surgery have undergone change as well. Left ventricular dysfunction, whether calculated by the complex equation of the Coronary Artery Surgery Study (CASS) or by a much simpler ejection fraction, has diminished in quality.[1,2,4,5] In three large series, severe ventricular impairment is now seen in 33.3 to 44% of patients.[1,2,4] The extent of coronary disease likewise has increased over this same time period in most institutions with three vessel disease, now making up more than 50% of the patients.[1,2,5] As a result, there has been an increase in patients presenting with congestive heart failure (CHF). Whether there is an increase in unstable angina or in emergent cases, or both, varies among institutions. Although the Cleveland Clinic has noted a decrease in both subgroups, other institutions have reported an increase.[1,2,5] A history of previous myocardial injury has remained relatively constant over the past 20 years.[1,2,5] Finally, more patients are presenting for redo revascularization and with concomitant cardiac problems such as valvular disease, ventricular aneurysm, or arrhythmias requiring surgical intervention.

In summary, the patient of the 1990s is more likely to be older, increasingly female, with more associated medical problems, more extreme CAD, and poorer ventricular function than the patient operated on 20 years ago.

CHANGES IN TECHNIQUE

Fortunately for the cardiac surgeon, there are many improvements in technique and better equipment with which to facilitate the procedure. Cardioplegia as a means to protect the myocardium was introduced in 1973 by Gay and Ebert.[5] Ventricular fibrillation with intermittent cross-clamping for cardiac protection was phased out at most medical centers. By 1979, nearly all patients were done by cardioplegic arrest using crystalloid or blood cardioplegia.[1,2] Topical hypothermia was also used during the early 1970s and continues as a mainstay in our practice to provide better protection of the myocardium during periods of ischemia.

Better lighting and magnification to visualize proximal and distal anastomoses were introduced during the late 1970s; by 1981, most surgeons employed ×2.5 or ×3.5 lenses for coronary work. Thanks to these advances, more complete revascularization has been performed and has resulted in decreased perioperative infarction rates and improved overall prognosis.[1,2,4] Even the addition of the internal mammary artery, with its greater technical demands, has not increased overall mortality.[1]

MORBIDITY

Changes both in the types and in the numbers of complications have occurred as well. Perioperative myocardial infarction (PMI) as defined by a new Q wave seen on the electrocardiogram (ECG) postoperatively has decreased in incidence. Rates of PMI ranged from 4.2 to 14.1% in 1973; however, rates now are more commonly seen in the range of 1.0 to 4.5% for nonredo revascularization.[1,2,4–6] No doubt improvement in protection and completeness of revascularization are responsible for this improvement. Mortality associated with perioperative myocardial infarction has remained significant, however, over these two decades and ranges from 8 to 28% in several studies.[5–7]

A decrease in the number of reoperations for bleeding is seen today with an expected rate of 2.5 to 6.0%.[1,6] And this problem does not increase significantly with age.[1,8,9] Although the incidence of cerebrovascular accident (CVA) has not changed significantly (1.4%), the subgroup of patients over age 60 and certainly over age 70 demonstrates an increase in perioperative strokes.[1,8,9] Rates in patients over 70 years of age range from 2.4 to 9%.[1,8,9]

Pulmonary complications have remained stable in the population as a whole but, as the group ages, it becomes a more significant problem.[1,5,9] A recent study on septagenarians showed significantly pulmonary complications, including pleural effusion, adult respiratory distress syndrome (ARDS), pulmonary embolus, pneumonia, and atelectasis, in 18%.[9] Other complications, such as wounds and renal failure, have demonstrated no change over time.[1,6]

MORTALITY

When tracking mortality over two decades in multiple institutions, several trends become apparent. There has been a general decline in operative mortalities for elective surgery.[1–17] Mortality published from three large centers during the late 1970s and early 1980s approached 0.8%.[1,2,4] Rates published from Coronary Artery Surgery Study (CASS) showed a mortality of 2.3%, including data gathered from 15 centers with 6,176 total patients.[16] More recent data published from four medical institutions begins to demonstrate a slight increase in mortality: 3.1 to 8%.[5,6,12–14] The explanation provided has been a higher number of complex cases and volume of emergent surgery performed. Edwards et al.[12] noted that 40% of their cases were emergent, and this group of patients accounted for 81% of their deaths. Elective mortalities at these respective centers range from 0.6 to 2.5%.[5,6,12,14] This recent trend needs to be examined further in the 1990s.

Several changes have also occurred in the way in which patients die. While cardiac death remains the leading cause, the percentage of deaths directly related to cardiac dysfunction has decreased. At the Cleveland Clinic, cardiac death accounted for 74.7% during the early 1970s, but for only 58.8% during the early 1980s.[1] Also, as patients get older, in terms of decades, cardiac death as a percentage of total deaths decreases.[1,8,9] Two causes of death have become more prevalent: neurologic and subsystem failure. Cosgrove et al.[1] reported a gradual increase over 13 years of neurologic death from 7.2 to 19.6% of total deaths. Miller et al.[2] noted a similar incidence of neurologic death. Subsystem failure coupled with a longer interval of time from surgery until death has also been noted.[1,6] Both neurologic and subsystem death have an increased prevalence as the patient population ages.

RISK FACTORS

This section examines the specific causes of morbidity and mortality. No importance is necessarily attached to the order of each section. Also, no attempt is made to look at a detailed statistical analysis, but rather a picture of the trends is provided. The following risk factors continue to predict an increased morbidity or mortality well into the 1990s:

Emergent revascularization
Congestive heart failure
Age above 70 years
Female gender
Incomplete revascularization
Recent myocardial infarction
Perioperative myocardial infarction
Redo revascularization

Often, patients have many of these factors, which affect their prognosis, to varying degrees.

AGE AND SEX

As noted in an earlier section, the average age and percentage of patients who are female has increased over the past two decades. Older age and female gen-

der both lead to a higher mortality for coronary revascularization.[1,2,5,6,8–11,15,16] The age at which operative mortality significantly increases has changed. Oldham et al. in 1972 noted a higher mortality in patients over age 50; the CASS noted an increased mortality over age 60, and more recent publications demonstrate the higher mortality occurs over the age of 70.[1,3,5,8,9,10,16] The chance of operative mortality over 70 years of age ranges from 1.2 to 10.5%.[1,9,14] This compares with operative mortalities of 0.6 to 3.5% in the same institutions under 70 years of age.[1,9,14] The primary cause of death in this older age group continues to be cardiac (myocardial infarction, arrhythmias, heart failure), although neurologic, subsystem failure, and respiratory causes are more prevalent than the under-age 70 subset.[1–17]

Female gender as an increased risk factor for mortality was present through the decade of the 1970s, reaching statistical significance during the 1980s in one large study.[1] This finding has been consistent at all institutions, except Stanford, which noted, in a well-matched group of men, that no difference could be found.[2] The CASS demonstrated the likelihood of mortality for women to be twice that for men and for persons over age 60; the ratio achieved proportions of 3:1.[16] Similar findings were seen in other studies.[1,3–17] In fact, one paper showed the operative mortality of women over age 70 to be 28.6%, while the mortality for women under age 70 was 5.5%.[9] Even the Stanford group agreed that women over age 70 achieved a statistically higher mortality.[2] Again, the most deaths are due to cardiac problem.[1,17] The most commonly offered theory as to why women have an increased risk is their smaller physical stature and the smaller size of their coronary arteries.[15] With further improvements in microvascular technique and more extensive use of the internal mammary artery with its better size proportion and patency, this difference should be greatly reduced or eliminated. Morbidity, when compared by gender, does not differ greatly.[1]

OTHER MEDICAL CONDITIONS

There has been an increase in the percentage of patients with hypertension, diabetes mellitus, cerebrovascular disease, peripheral vascular disease, and chronic obstructive pulmonary disease.[5] The only associated medical risk factor that has decreased is smoking.[1,5] Despite this general increase in the severity of medical problems, no statistically significant trend can be seen for increased perioperative morbidity or mortality. The Stanford group suggested that hypertension might be a predictor of risk, but it should be noted that this study dates back to the late 1970s. Methods of blood pressure control have markedly improved and have decreased the likelihood that this would be a consistent predictive factor of increased risk.[2]

PREOPERATIVE MYOCARDIAL INFARCTION AND PERIOPERATIVE INFARCTION

The number of patients with a history of preoperative myocardial infarction (MI) has not changed over a period of time and has remained in the range of 30 to 50%.[1–5,7–9] Remote myocardial injury (defined as 30 days before surgery) has no significant effect on prognosis.[1–3,5–17] The Emory experience demonstrated an operative mortality of 1% for patients with no MI, 1.8% for one MI, and 2.2% for more than one MI.[4] However, remote myocardial injury reported in most articles is not a predictive factor.[1–3,5–17]

Recent myocardial injury (occurring in less than 30 days), including hyperacute injury and postinfarction angina, shows a different trend.[5] The primary indication for surgery in this group is persistent angina with compelling anatomy that demonstrates areas of reversible ischemia.[18] Cooley and co-workers[26] published a mortality of 38.1% if operated within 7 days and 16.% if operated 16 to 30 days post-MI. More recent data would suggest that this mortality is in the range of 0 to 16% no matter which period within the 30 days the patient is operated.[18–25] If the patient is operated for postinfarct angina only, the mortality is clearly less. However, if the patient is operated on with any evidence of power failure, the mortality increases markedly.[18–26] This problem was clearly magnified in our group of 107 patients operated on during 1983 to 1984. Of the nine mortalities, six of the patients were in heart failure.[18] No other factors in this subset were predictive of an increased mortality. As expected, this group of patients has a significantly increased need for intra-aortic balloon pump, inotropic support, and intravenous use of nitroglycerin both pre- and postoperatively.[18–26]

PMI has clearly seen a decrease as a risk factor surrounding coronary artery revascularization in all studies. The only definition of infarction agreed on in the literature is occurrence of a new Q wave in the postoperative electrocardiogram. Enzyme released MI infarctions have a varied definition in the literature. The incidence of PMI has decreased from a range of 4.2 to 14.6% during the 1970s to a range of 1 to 7% during the 1980s.[1–17] The one fact that remains disturbingly high is the mortality associated with a new Q-wave infarct. Pelletier et al.[7] published a mortality of 28%; 90% of the infarcts occurred in the distribution of a patent graft as proved by autopsy. Recent papers published during the late 1980s continue to show a mortality resulting from perioperative MI of 8 to 11%.[5,6] There are some soft indications that PMIs may be related to New York Heart Association (NYHA) groups 3 and 4 and prolonged periods of cardiopulmonary bypass at revascularization.[6] In conclusion, remote MIs do not significantly affect prognosis; however, recent MIs do affect prognosis particularly if heart failure persists. Although PMIs have decreased in incidence, their occurrence continues to have an ominous prognosis.

EXTENT OF CORONARY ARTERY DISEASE AND COMPLETENESS OF REVASCULARIZATION

Mortality was linked to severity of CAD during the past two decades.[1–17] This has best been measured by degree of left main coronary artery disease and by the number of patients presenting with single, double, triple, or multivessel disease. Mortality at the Cleveland Clinic increased with number of vessels diseased until the mid-1970s when this risk factor was neutralized primarily by better methods of myocardial protection and complete revascularization.[1] Left main coronary artery disease also carried an increased mortality until the 1980s. Mortalities decreased from 10.7% during the early 1970s to essentially none for left main coronary artery disease in the elective situation.[1] Elimination of left main coronary artery disease as an ominous predictor too was echoed by other centers.[2,7,10] Likewise, the number of grafts performed does not affect surgical outcome.[1]

One factor that has emerged as a predictor of increased risk of morbidity and mortality is incomplete revascularization.[1,10] Mortalities during 1980 to 1982 were doubled if incomplete revascularization was performed (1.3 versus 0.6%). A paper from the Emory University Medical Center demonstrated a trend toward better prognosis with complete revascularization, but this did not achieve statistical significance.[4] A more recent paper from St. Louis University also showed a trend toward better prognosis with complete revascularization.[5] The degree of CAD cannot be linked to increased morbidity and mortality; however, a lack of complete revascularization is related.

VENTRICULAR DYSFUNCTION

The discussion of ventricular dysfunction as a potential risk factor is clouded by several issues.

Method of Assessment

The first issue is the method by which ventricular function is assessed. The CASS devised a complicated formula that divided the ventricle angiographically into five segments. Each segment was then evaluated as to whether it was normal (score of 1) and ranged to aneurysmal (score of 6). The sum of the five segments then yielded a number called a wall motion score, 5 being normal ventricular function ranging up to 30, which theoretically would be an aneurysmal ventricle.[16] Another common method is to evaluate the right anterior oblique view of the ventricle angiographically and determine a number called left ventricular ejection fraction (LVEF). At least one investigator has shown reasonable evidence for similar prognostic ability for these two numbers.[13] The third method that has gained some popularity recently is a nuclear medicine method called a multigated acquisition analysis (MUGA).

Definition of Moderate to Severe Dysfunction

The second factor is the precise definition of moderate to severe dysfunction. Passamani et al.[28] defined an ejection fraction below 50% as the separation point. Another center quoted 40% and still another defined 30% as the separation point.[11,27] Hochberg et al.[27] evaluated 5% intervals of LVEF down to 10%. It is clear that no number exists in the literature as a definitive cutoff point for moderate to severe LV dysfunction.

Differentiation from Cardiac Heart Failure

The last issue that is reasonably well clarified is the differentiation of ventricular dysfunction from cardiac heart failure as a risk factor. Most institutions have made a definite separation of these two variables.[1,2,4,16]

Severe Ventricular Dysfunction—Not a Risk Factor

Severe ventricular dysfunction has been eliminated as a risk factor for increased operative mortality in recent years,[1] with the realization that throughout the 1970s it was an important determinant of poor prognosis.[1,2,3,4,11] The one exception may be extremely poor ventricular dysfunction (LVEF <20%). In a small group of patients, Hochberg et al.[27] demonstrated an operative survival of only 63 percent for patients with LVEF below 20 percent. The fairest statement would be that ventricular dysfunction, in well-compensated heart failure and with clinical symptoms of reversible ischemia is not a predictor of increased risk.

CONGESTIVE HEART FAILURE

Congestive heart failure (CHF), as defined by clinical symptoms (dyspnea, rales, cardiomegaly, and pulmonary edema), increased LV end-diastolic pressure, and elevated pulmonary artery wedge pressures, has consistently remained a predictor of perioperative mortality.[1-17,27-29] During the early 1970s, both Sabiston and Loop noted that CHF was the leading predictor of perioperative death.[1,3] The CASS data too demonstrated CHF as a predictor of increased morbidity and mortality through the late 1970s.[16] Publications during the past decade have demonstrated that CHF increased the likelihood of perioperative mortality by two to ten times over patients not in heart failure.[1,2,4–7] The fact that CHF remains a risk factor during the 1990s reflects that, despite major advances in medical management, this subgroup of patients must be operated on with great concern. Patients with CHF caused by reversible ischemia or correctable valvular disease, or both conditions, have the best prognosis.

EMERGENT SURGERY

Emergent surgery as defined by the need for coronary revascularization immediately after cardiac catheterization or due to a deteriorating condition within 24 hours of cardiac catheterization has been a consistent predictor of mortality associated with coronary bypass surgery.[1-17,27-32] The indications included for this condition vary but generally include unstable angina despite maximal medical management, cardiogenic shock, evolving MI, CHF, and urgent revascularization resulting from angioplasty failure.

The mortality associated with emergent surgery overall was 13% during the late 1970s but has decreased to 4.9%, with better medical management.[1] This number remains a sevenfold increase over elective revascularization. Miller et al.[2] noted a 6.7% mortality for emergent revascularization (13-fold increase over elective surgery), and a threefold greater probability of perioperative myocardial infarction. The CASS experience demonstrated an urgent/emergent mortality of 4.4% versus 1.7% for elective revascularization.[16] As stated previously, emergent surgery at one center accounted for 40% of the coronary bypasses but was responsible for 81% of mortality.[12]

In order to investigate this risk factor further, individual problems leading to the emergent surgery may be broken down.

Unstable Angina

First, unstable angina has not been a consistent predictor of increased mortality. Both the Stanford and Emory studies noted the same mortality for stable and unstable angina.[2,4] Miller et al.[2] noted a slight increase in PMI. This finding reflects the fact that in some patients a PMI was evolving at surgery. The Cleveland

Clinic does not separate unstable angina as a risk factor from the emergent group.[1] The statement is made that better medical management has reduced the mortality of the emergent group. Data from the CASS experience demonstrated an increased risk factor: 3.9% mortality for unstable versus 2.3% overall.[30] Four recent publications from the late 1980s have shown a definite increase in perioperative mortality with unstable angina.[5,6,31,32] Perioperative morbidity was not affected, however.[6] Further data on unstable angina from more centers are needed to clarify this discrepancy.

Cardiogenic Shock

There is no question that cardiogenic shock with evolving MI carries an ominous prognosis. Medical management has a predicted mortality that is uniformly fatal.[33] This grim outcome justifies an operative mortality that approximates 50%.[5]

Urgent Revascularization for Failed Angioplasty

The subset of urgent revascularization for angioplasty represents patients going directly to the operating room from the catheterization laboratory or within hours for an obvious infarct in progress. Angioplasty is established as a method of treatment for single vessel disease and, at many centers, for multivessel disease. The incidence of failure for angioplasty and the need for urgent surgery ranges from 2.7 to 16%.[34–41] Bredlau et al.[38] identified five risk factors predictive of a major complication at angioplasty: multivessel coronary disease, lesion eccentricity, presence of calcium, female gender, and lesion length. The primary pathologic indication of a procedural problem was the occurrence of a dissection with or without occlusion of the coronary artery.[34–36,38,40] The clinical indicator for urgent revascularization with the worst prognosis was hemodynamic instability. Preoperative cardiogenic shock or cardiac arrest carries a mortality ranging from 34 to 80%.[38,41,42] Insertion of an intra-aortic balloon pump and timely operative revascularization are imperative to reduce these mortalities.

Morbidity associated with urgent revascularization after failed angioplasty ranges from 10 to 54%.[36,38,43] The most common perioperative complication cited was progression to a transmural MI in the distribution of the failed angioplasty. Criteria used to differentiate a new infarct include a new Q wave seen on electrocardiogram (ECG) and cardiac enzyme elevation more than three times the expected normal values. Using these criteria, the rate of MI in this emergent group will be 8.6 to 60%.[34–44] Again, hemodynamic instability caused a significantly increased risk of transmural

infarct. Other complications noted to be increased were low cardiac output, postoperative hemorrhage, ventricular arrhythmias, and sternal wound problems. At all centers, the complications cited—especially perioperative myocardial infarction—were significantly higher than their elective surgical population.[34–44]

Mortality for failed angioplasty with emergent need for revascularization ranges from 0 to 12%.[34–44] Again, the strongest predictor of death is hemodynamic instability resulting from angioplasty. The most common cause of death is cardiac failure attributable to MI. Other causes cited include organ failure and irreversible neurologic injury. It should be noted, however, that the overall risk of death resulting from angioplasty at two large volume centers (including our own) approaches 0.1%.[38,44] Angioplasty has a reasonable success rate, but the group of patients needing urgent revascularization after angioplasty carries a significant risk of increased morbidity and mortality.

REDO REVASCULARIZATION

Data from several institutions demonstrate the clinical efficacy and safety of reoperative coronary revascularization, even if two or more previous attempts have been made.[45–48] As the population of revascularized patients from the two previous decades advances in age, large numbers can be expected to return for reoperative coronary bypass surgery (CABS).[49,50] The most current information on the morbidity and mortality of reoperative coronary surgery from the CASS shows no significant difference in the incidence of PMI, ventricular arrhythmias, cardiogenic shock, CHF, neurologic events, respiratory failure, significant bleeding requiring reexploration, renal failure, or wound infection in the reoperative versus the primary revascularization group.[47] Although the CASS demonstrated a slight increase in operative mortality on the day of surgery, this difference was lost after postoperative day 1.[47] Furthermore, the most recent data from the Cleveland Clinic have shown a reduction of operative mortality from 3.1% (31/1,000) to only 2% (5/250)—a figure nearer that for primary revascularization surgery.[50]

Using multivariate analysis, Cosgrove and Loop and co-workers[50] showed that the absence of an internal mammary artery graft and incomplete revascularization are the surgical variables that predict the requirement for subsequent reoperative bypass surgery. This association with the lack of an internal mammary artery graft is so strong that medical risk factors such as hypertension, hypercholesterolemia, and smoking were actually neutralized as predictors of reoperative surgery.[51] The use of the internal mammary graft as well as complete revascularization will continue to be important during the 1990s or complex reoperative cases.[45,52]

Another group of redo coronary bypass patients has emerged during the 1980s; these are candidates for a third revascularization. Two studies—those conducted by Brenowitz et al.[45] our group[48]—have not shown the mortality to differ significantly from the figures previously noted for first redo revascularization. In our group of patients, there was, however, a slight increase in reexploration for bleeding (8%) and perioperative infarcts (12%) over the CASS data.[48] However, our series and that of Brenowitz and co-workers demonstrate that a third revascularization can be performed with a reasonable morbidity and mortality.

CONCOMITANT SURGERY

When considering concomitant surgery with coronary revascularization, differences in morbidity and mortality can be found. The specific procedures examined in this section are aortic valve replacement (AVR), mitral valve replacement, and resection of ventricular aneurysm.

The overall mortality when CABS is added to AVR does not significantly increase the mortality for aortic valve replacement alone.[5,53–59] The mortality associated with this combined procedure in recent years ranges from 3 to 5%.[5,54–59] This finding shows a definite improvement in mortality, which was 15.6% during the 1970s.[54] A similar decline has been seen in the number of PMIs from a rate of 14.2% during the early 1970s to 2% during the 1980s.[54] Again, this is attributed to improved methods of myocardial protection. At least one paper compared two groups of patients with aortic stenosis and significant CAD. One group received appropriate revascularization, and one did not. The respective mortalities were 3.6% with CAB and 17.9% without indicated CABS.[56] Thus, coronary revascularization in appropriate patients with aortic valvular diseases actually decreases morbidity and mortality.

When considering coronary revascularization in conjunction with mitral valve replacement it is important to remember that two groups of patients exist: (1) those with mitral valve disease and CAD with different etiologies, and (2) those with mitral valvular insufficiency secondary to CAD.[58] Overall, mortalities, no matter the mitral valve pathology, for this combined procedure range from 3.5 to 18%.[58,60–63] The rate of survival generally does not depend directly on the degree of CAD.[58] Risk was significantly increased under the following conditions: (1) the case was done as an emergency, (2) LV dysfunction was severe, (3) the pa-

tient was in NYHA class 4 for failure, (4) mitral regurgitation was severe, and (5) the ventricular dysfunction was secondary to CAD.[58,60,63] Mortalities for emergency procedures approached 45 to 60% at certain institutions.[60,61] If the emergency procedures were removed from the formula, the mortality for mitral valve replacement in combination with revascularization dropped down to 5.8%—a figure not too different from mortality for isolated mitral stenosis or mitral regurgitation.[61] In conclusion, CAD probably does not increase the perioperative mortality of patients with mitral valve disease; however, if the mitral valve disease is secondary to CAD, the perioperative mortality is markedly increased.[58,60,61,63]

When evaluating patients with ventricular aneurysm and CAD, the operative mortality is probably increased by the severity of CAD.[64] Mortalities ranged from 6.5% for aneurysm resection with single vessel disease to 19.4% with triple vessel disease.[64] Other factors that increased mortality in this subset were severe CHF and an increased NYHA classification. Other complications, including postoperative bleeding, wound healing, renal failure, stroke, and septicemia, did not differ significantly in the groups of patients for revascularization with or without an aneurysm.[6]

CONCLUSION

The data presented are extrapolated from multiple centers, some from high-volume centers and some from low-volume centers. Because of differences in patient populations at these institutions, it is impossible to apply all risk factors directly to each and every center. The intent of this discussion is to provide general insight into the many risks that persist with coronary revascularization. Cardiac centers and surgeons would be well advised to evaluate their own surgical results, using this summary as a guideline.

REFERENCES

1. Cosgrove DM, Loop FD, Lytle BW et al: Primary myocardial revascularization: trends in surgical mortality. J Thorac Cardiovasc Surg 88:673, 1984
2. Miller DC, Stinson EB, Oyer PE et al: Discriminant analysis of the changing risks of coronary artery operations: 1971–1979. J Thorac Cardiovasc Surg 85:197, 1983
3. Oldham HN, Kong Y, Bartel AG et al: Risk factors in coronary artery bypass surgery. Arch Surg 105:918, 1972
4. Jones EL, Craver JM, King SB et al: Clinical, anatomic and functional descriptors influencing morbidity, survival and adequacy of revascularization following coronary bypass. Ann Surg 192:390, 1980
5. Naunheim KS, Fiore AC, Wadley JJ et al: The changing

profile of the patient undergoing coronary artery bypass surgery. J Am Coll Cardiol 11:494, 1988

6. Stahle E, Bergstrom R, Nystrom SO, Hansson HE: Predictive value of factors affecting early results and complications in eight years of coronary artery bypass surgery. Thorac Cardiovasc Surg 37:355, 1989

7. Pelletier C, Cossette R, Dontigny L et al: Determinants of mortality following coronary bypass surgery. Can J Surg 23:199, 1980

8. Hochberg MS, Levine FH, Daggett WM et al: Isolated coronary artery bypass grafting in patients seventy years of age and older. J Thorac Cardiovasc 84:219, 1982

9. Faro RS, Golden MD, Javid H et al: Coronary revascularization in septuagenarians. J Thorac Cardiovasc 86:616, 1983

10. Chaitman BR, Rogers WJ, Davis K et al: Operative risk factors in patients with left main coronary-artery disease. N Engl J Med 303:953, 1980

11. Hammermeister KE, Kennedy JW: Predictors of surgical mortality in patients undergoing direct myocardial revascularization. Circulation, suppl. 49:II-112, 1974

12. Edwards FH, Albus RA, Zajtchuk R et al: Use of a bayesian statistical model for risk assessment in coronary artery surgery. Ann Thorac Surg 45:437, 1988

13. Pierpont GL, Kruse M, Ewald S, Weir EK: Practical problems in assessing risk for coronary artery bypass grafting. J Thorac Cardiovasc Surg 89:673, 1985

14. Junod FL, Harlan BJ, Payne J et al: Preoperative risk assessment in cardiac surgery: comparison of predicted and obsrved results. Ann Thorac Surg 43:59, 1987

15. Fisher LD, Kennedy JW, Davis KB et al: Association of sex, physical size, and operative mortality after coronary artery bypass in the Coronary Artery Surgery Study (CASS). J Thorac Cardiovasc Surg 84:334, 1982

16. Kennedy JW, Kaiser GC, Fisher LD et al: Multivariate discriminant analysis of the clinical and angiographic predictors of operative mortality from the collaborative study in coronary artery surgery (CASS). J Thorac Cardiovasc Surg 80:876, 1980

17. Loop FD, Berrettoni JN, Pichard A et al: Selection of the candidate for myocardial revascularization: a profile of high risk based on multivariate analysis. J Thorac Cardiovasc Surg 69:40, 1975

18. Jones RN, Pifarre R, Sullivan HJ et al: Early myocardial revascularization for postinfarction angina. Ann Thorac Surg 44:159, 1987

19. Jones EL, Waites TF, Craver JM et al: Coronary bypass for relief of persistent pain following acute myocardial infarction. Ann Thorac Surg 32:33, 1981

20. Singh AK, Rivera R, Cooper GN, Karlson KE: Early myocardial revascularization for postinfarction angina: results and long-term follow-up. J Am Coll Cardiol 6:1121, 1985

21. Molina JE, Dorsey JS, Emanuel DA, Reyes J: Coronary bypass operation for early postinfarction angina. Surg Gynecol Obstet 157:455, 1983

22. Hartz RS, Hoyne WP, LoCicero J et al: Risk assessment of coronary artery bypass grafting within one month of acute myocardial infarction. Am J Cardiol 62:964, 1988

23. Breyer RH, Engleman RM, Rousou JA, Lemeshow S: Postinfarction angina: an expanding subset of patients undergoing coronary artery bypass. J Thorac Cardiovasc Surg 90:532, 1985

24. Hochberg MS, Parsonnet V, Gielchinsky I et al: Timing of coronary revascularization after acute myocardial infarction: early and late results in patients revascularized within seven weeks. J Thorac Cardiovasc Surg 88:914, 1984

25. Nunley DL, Grunkemeier GL, Teply JF et al: Coronary bypass operation following acute complicated myocardial infarction. J Thorac Cardiovasc Surg 85:485, 1983

26. Dawson JT, Hall RJ, Hallman GL, Cooley DA: Mortality in patients undergoing coronary artery bypass surgery after myocardial infarction. Am J Cardiol 33:483, 1974

27. Hochberg MS, Parsonnet V, Gielchinsky I, Hussain SM: Coronary artery bypass grafting in patients with ejection fractions below forty percent: early and late results in 466 patients. J Thorac Cardiovasc Surg 86:519, 1983

28. Passamani E, Davis KB, Gillespie MJ, Killip T: A randomized trial of coronary artery bypass surgery: survival of patients with a low ejection fraction. N Engl J Med 312:1665, 1985

29. Jones EL, Craver JM, Kaplan JA et al: Criteria for operability and reduction of surgical mortality in patients with severe left ventricular ischemia and dysfunction. Ann Thorac Surg 25:413, 1978

30. McCormick JR, Schick EC, McCabe CH et al: Determinants of operative mortality and long-term survival in patients with unstable angina: the CASS experience. J Thorac Cardiovasc Surg 89:683, 1985

31. Edwards FH, Cohen AJ, Bellamy RF et al: Risk assessment in urgent/emergent coronary artery surgery. Chest 97:1125, 1980

32. Teoh KH, Christakis GT, Weisel RD: Increased risk of urgent revascularization. J Thorac Cardiovasc Surg 93:291, 1987

33. Vlietstra RE, Assad-Morrell JL, Frye RL et al: Survival predictors in coronary artery disease: medical and surgical comparisons. Mayo Clin Proc 52:85, 1977

34. Reul GJ, Cooley DA, Hallman GL et al: Coronary artery bypass for unsuccessful percutaneous transluminal coronary angioplasty. J Thorac Cardiovasc Surg 88:685, 1984

35. Pelletier LC, Pardini A, Renkin J et al: Myocardial revascularization after failure of percutaneous transluminal coronary angioplasty. J Thorac Cardiovasc Surg 90:265, 1985

36. Cowley MJ, Dorros G, Kelsey SF et al: Emergency coronary bypass surgery after coronary angioplasty: the National Heart, Lung, and Blood Institute's percutaneous transluminal coronary angioplasty registry experience. Am J Cardiol 53:22C, 1984

37. Golding LAR, Loop FD, Hollman JD et al: Early results of emergency surgery after coronary angioplasty. Circulation, suppl. 74:III-26, 1986

38. Bredlau CE, Roubin GS, Leimgruber PP: In-hospital morbidity and mortality in patients undergoing elective coronary angioplasty. Circulation 72:1044, 1985

39. Smith CW, Hornung CA, Sutton JP et al: Coronary bypass for failed angioplasty. Circulation, suppl. 70:II-254, 1984

40. Connor AR, Vlietstra RE, Schaff HV et al: Early and late results of coronary artery bypass after failed angioplasty. J Thorac Cardiovasc Surg 96:191, 1988

41. Parsonnet V, Fisch D, Gielchinsky I et al: Emergency operation after failed angioplasty. J Thorac Cardiovasc Surg 96:1988, 1988

42. Killen DA, Hamaker WR, Reed WA: Coronary artery bypass following percutaneous transluminal coronary angioplasty. Ann Thorac Surg 40:133, 1985

43. Brahos GJ, Baker NH, Ewy G et al: Aortocoronary bypass following unsuccessful PTCA: experience in 100 consecutive patients. Ann Thorac Surg 40:7, 1985

44. Doud DN, Killian DM, Johnson SA et al: Emergency myocardial revascularization after failed angioplasty. Chest, suppl. 98:455, 1990

45. Brenowitz JB, Johnson WD, Kayser KL et al: Coronary artery bypass grafting for the third time or more—results of 150 consecutive cases. Circulation, suppl. 78:I-166, 1988

46. Schaff HV, Orszulak TA, Gersh BJ et al: The morbidity and mortality of reoperation of coronary artery disease and analysis of late results with use of actuarial estimate of event-free interval. J Thorac Cardiovasc Surg 85:508, 1983

47. Foster ED: Reoperation for coronary artery disease. Circulation, suppl. 72:V-59, 1985

48. Blakeman BP, Thomas NJ, Sullivan HJ et al: Myocardial revascularization for the third time: clinical characteristics and follow-up. Chest 98:1099, 1990

49. Foster ED, Fisher LD, Kaiser GC, Myers WO: Comparison of operative mortality and morbidity for initial and repeat coronary artery bypass grafting: the Coronary Artery Surgery Study (CASS) registry experience. Ann Thorac Surg 38:563, 1984

50. Loop FD, Lytle BW, Gill CC et al: Trends in selection and results of coronary artery reoperations. Ann Thorac Surg 36:380, 1983

51. Cosgrove DM, Loop FD, Lytle BW et al: Determinants of 10-year survival after primary myocardial revascularization. Ann Surg 202:480, 1985

52. Baillot RG, Loop FD, Cosgrove DM, Lytle BW: Reoperation after previous grafting with the internal mammary artery: technique and early results. Ann Thorac Surg 40:271, 1985

53. Takaro T, Ankeney JL, Laning RC, Peduzzi PN: Quality control for cardiac surgery in the Veterans Administration. Ann Thorac Surg 42:37, 1986

54. Nunley DL, Grunkemeier GL, Starr A: Aortic valve replacement with coronary bypass grafting: significant determinants of ten-year survival. J Thorac Cardiovasc Surg 85:705, 1983

55. Miller DC, Stinson EB, Oyer PE et al: Surgical implications and results of combined aortic valve replacement and myocardial revascularization. Am J Cardiol 43:494, 1979

56. Lund O, Nielsen TT, Pilegaard HK et al: The influence of coronary artery disease and bypass grafting on early and late survival after valve replacement for aortic stenosis. J Thorac Cardiovasc Surg 100:327, 1990

57. Lytle BW, Cosgrove DM, Loop FD et al: Replacement of aortic valve combined with myocardial revascularization: determinants of early and late risk for 500 patients, 1967–1981. Circulation 68:1149, 1983

58. Karp RB, Mills N, Edmunds LH: Coronary artery bypass grafting in the presence of valvular disease. Circulation, suppl. 79:I-182, 1989

59. Reed GE, Sanoudos GM, Pooley RW et al: Results of combined valvular and myocardial revascularization operations. J Thorac Cardiovasc Surg 85:422, 1983

60. DiSesa VJ, Cohn LH, Collins JJ et al: Determinants of operative survival following combined mitral valve replacement and coronary revascularization. Ann Thorac Surg 34:482, 1982

61. Magovern JA, Pennock JL, Campbell DB et al: Risks of mitral valve replacement and mitral valve replacement with coronary artery bypass. Ann Thorac Surg 39:346, 1985

62. Lytle BW: Combined surgery for valve and coronary artery disease. Cleve Clin J Med 55:79, 1988

63. Connolly MW, Gelbfish JS, Jacobwitz IJ et al: Surgical results for mitral regurgitation from coronary artery disease. J Thorac Cardiovasc Surg 91:379, 1986

64. Barratt-Boyes BG, White HD, Agnew TM et al: The results of surgical treatment of left ventricular aneurysms. J Thorac Cardiovasc Surg 87:87, 1984

Section III

RISK ASSESSMENT AND PROGNOSIS OF VALVULAR HEART DISEASE

17

Natural History, Risk Assessment, and Prognosis of Patients With Mitral Stenosis

Sarana Boonbaichaiyapruck
Amar S. Kapoor

Mitral valve stenosis is an important entity in many countries around the world. The incidence of rheumatic fever and rheumatic heart disease has declined markedly in the United States.[1] Mortality rates for rheumatic fever and rheumatic heart disease have significantly decreased as well.[2] There are intermittent outbreaks of rheumatic fever throughout the United States,[3,4] and certain subgroups are still at high risk of development of the disease. These include the poor, American Indians, inner city and rural blacks, and Hispanics. Refugees and immigrants from areas of high prevalence also contribute to the existence of this disease in the United States.

PATHOPHYSIOLOGY

Rheumatic fever is believed to be the initiating event for the development of mitral stenosis.[5] About one-half of patients with this disease recall such previous illness of rheumatic fever. The peak incidence is at 5 to 25 years of age. The disease rarely involves the heart, if it occurs in age groups above 20 years.[6] With acute rheumatic fever, carditis mitral and/or aortic insufficiency can be detected early. In fact, evidence of valvulitis discovered by either diastolic murmur or systolic murmur is a good predictor of subsequent sequelae. Mitral stenosis usually becomes evident 2 or 3 years after the initial insult and is the most frequent chronic sequelae of rheumatic carditis.[7,8]

Rheumatic mitral stenosis involves the contact edge of the leaflets, the valve cusps, and the chordae tendineae. The rheumatic process results in fusion of the commissures, thickening of the leaflets, as well as fusion and shortening of the chordae. These lead to both valvular and subvalvular obstruction of blood flow from the left atrium into left ventricle during diastole. This obstruction leads to subsequent clinical events in patients with this disease. When the valve area is reduced from the normal diameter of 4 to 6 cm² to the level of about 1 cm², severe mitral stenosis occurs. Resistance to flow across the mitral valve raises the pressure in the left atrium, passively increases the pressure in the pulmonic vein and pulmonary capillaries, and eventually increases total pulmonary vascular resistance. Passive elevation of the pressure in the pulmonary capillaries increases total lung water and lung compliance is reduced. These hemodynamic derangements mark the development of symptoms of dyspnea and reduced functional ability. When the capacity of lymphatic compensation is stretched by pulmonary capillary pressure, pulmonary edema ensues. Elevated pulmonary vascular resistance causes right side heart failure in some patients. Chronic elevation of pressure in the left atrium causes dilation of the chamber that can lead to atrial arrhythmias. Thrombus formation in the atrium is likely to occur with a dilated atrium and arrhythmias coexist. The thromboembolic phenomenon is believed to be secondary to clot formation in the atrium. Life span is shortened in patients with this disease, secondary to congestive heart failure (CHF) and thromboembolic phenomenon.

NATURAL HISTORY: CARDIOVASCULAR RISKS

Mitral stenosis is a progressive disease in most patients. As depicted in Figure 17-1, an average of 19 years elapses before the onset of dyspnea. Recognition of the disease in the asymptomatic group occurs within this time frame. The development of symptomatic disease is accelerated in underdeveloped countries. It takes approximately 7 years for the development of total disability. Cardiovascular events that occur as part of the natural history in patients with mitral stenosis are reduced functional ability, thromboembolic phenomenon, development of atrial arrhythmias, ineffective endocarditis, severe CHF, and early death. Medical therapy and valve intervention are currently included in the natural history.

Before the surgical era, the outlook for patients with this disease was unfavorable. From 1925, Rowe et al.[9] followed 250 patients with mitral stenosis for 10 years and 150 patients for 20 years. The diagnosis was made purely on the basis of clinical examination. The patient population was heterogeneous in terms of age and functional class; 33% of the patients were younger than 20 years and one-half were asymptomatic. The asymptomatic group was confined to the younger population. By 10 years, 39% of patients had died, 22% had become more dyspnic, and 16% had developed at least one thromboembolic phenomenon. By 20 years, 79% had died, 8% had become more symptomatic, and 26% had developed at least one thromboembolic event.

Olesen[10] published his experience with 271 patients in 1962. The cohort of patients in this group had more advanced symptoms than those in the series conducted by Rowe et al.[9] The mean age of patients in this series was 41.5 years, and all had at least functional class 2, with most in functional class 4, according to the American Heart Association (AHA) classification. By 11 years, 70% had died, and by 18 years 83% had died. Only 3% remained unchanged in terms of functional class. The major causes of death were complications of mitral stenosis.

Progression of the disease is the rule, especially in the symptomatic group.[11,12] There is a variation in the rate of progression, with rapid progression in one group and a steady course in another. Worsening of symptoms tends to parallel the process of valve narrowing; in a small subgroup, the deterioration was induced by arrhythmias or by a transient decrease in cardiac output. Selzer and colleagues studied 42 patients with mitral stenosis and followed these patients by repeat cardiac catheterization for hemodynamic parameters.[11,13] Twenty-seven patients demonstrated progressive disease of mitral valve area and worsening of their clinical condition. Fifteen patients had stable valve area. However, 50% of these patients with a stable valve area deteriorated in terms of functional class, which was virtually caused by the development of atrial fibrillation. In the group with progression of the disease, it is not known whether continued rheumatic activity causes further damage or the turbulence caused by commissural fusion promotes further fibrosis and calcification. It is also not known whether the process of stenosis progresses steadily or is episodic and periodic.[14]

Pathologically, the disease process is progressive.

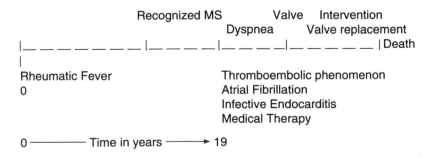

Fig. 17-1. Natural history of patient with rheumatic mitral stenosis.

The younger patients seem to have a more benign picture than that of their older counterparts. Calcification and fibrosis of the mitral valve become worse with age and result in valvular immobility.[15] In addition, subvalvular apparatus involvement becomes part of the picture in the older population. These pathologic processes and the status of the left atrium determine the risk in the natural history and the response to certain treatment modalities. Symptomatic and hemodynamic parameters do not correlate with pathologic findings. In certain parts of the world (e.g., India), the malignant picture of pathology can occur in the younger age group. There are inadequate data to explain this phenomenon in the younger age group. However, it is believed that the recurrent attacks of rheumatic fever with cardiac involvement cause more valvular damage. Of interest, follow-up evaluation of these patients with an erythrocyte sedimentation rate (ESR) and serology did not reveal evidence of recurrent infections with streptococci.

CONGESTIVE HEART FAILURE

Development of dyspnea or deterioration of functional ability is secondary to two mechanisms: progressive narrowing of the valve, and occurrence of other precipitating factors in a stable narrowed valve. The major precipitating factors are atrial fibrillation, pregnancy, and anemia. With atrial fibrillation, there is a loss of atrial contribution; along with tachycardia, there is significant reduction of cardiac output. In pregnancy and anemia, increased flow per minute as well as increased heart rate are responsible for the development of a high gradient across the mitral valve. These hemodynamic alterations increase the pressure in the left atrium and mark the development of dyspnea.

Tables 17-1 and 17-2 are derived from follow-up studies conducted by 250 patients by Rowe et al.[9] At the beginning of the study, 47% had dyspnea, 8% had pulmonary edema, and 9% had right-sided heart failure. At 10-year follow-up of 250 patients, 65% had dyspnea, 15% had pulmonary edema, and 24% had developed right-sided heart failure; of 115 patients who

TABLE 17-1. Progression of CHF in Mitral Stenosis

Major Symptom	Prior to 1st Visit (%)	After 10 Yr (%)	After 20 Yr (%)
Dyspnea	47	65	69
Pulmonary edema	8	15	21
Right-sided failure	9	24	36

(From Rowe et al.,[9] with permission.)

TABLE 17-2. Rate of Progression of CHF in Mitral Stenosis at the End of 1st 10 Years

Grade[a]	Same (%)	Worse (%)	Dead (%)
1	59	25	16
2	21	21	58
3	4	11	85
4	0	0	100
All patients	39	22	39

[a] Grade 1, auscultatory signs of mitral stenosis without symptom; grade 2, mild symptoms with normal rhythm or atrial fibrillation with or without symptoms; grade 3, moderate to moderately severe symptoms or a major complication; grade 4, chronic heart failure. (From Rowe et al.,[9] with permission.)

were followed for as long as 20 years, 69% had developed dyspnea and 36% had developed heart failure. Table 17-2 demonstrates the rate of progression of CHF among different functional classes. The likelihood of progression parallels the severity of the symptom. In the asymptomatic group at 10 years of follow-up, 59% were asymptomatic, 25% had become symptomatic, and 16% had died. In the mildly symptomatic group, 21% remained mildly symptomatic, 21% had become more symptomatic, and 58% had died. In the moderately symptomatic and chronic heart failure groups, most had died by 10 years, and only 4% had remained in the same status. The number at 20 years follow-up confirms the grave prognosis in the symptomatic group.

However, these studies were performed during the earlier era, when several medical therapeutic agents were not yet available. Diuretics and digoxin were the mainstay of treatment. Diuretics improve the congestive symptoms through reduction of the preload. Digoxin works well in the setting of atrial fibrillation predominantly by slowing the ventricular response, as left ventricular (LV) function is normal in most patients with mitral stenosis.[16] β Blockers also proved effective in increasing exercise tolerance in patients with mild to moderate symptoms even those with sinus rhythm.[17] Calcium-channel blockers with the same atrioventricular (AV) node suppressant ability as β-blocker also slow ventricular response and improve exercise tolerance. The progressive nature of the disease process has changed somewhat with currently available therapeutic modalities. Surgical palliative correction of the valve-narrowing process has a significant beneficial effect in patients with this disease. Medical treatment has a place mainly in mildly symptomatic patients and in patients with a temporary change in cardiac output (e.g., pregnancy and anemia). Timing of valvular replacement in patients with advanced disease and not suitable for valvotomy can be delayed with the judicious use of medical treatment, including anticoagulation.

Valvotomy has been demonstrated to improve the hemodynamic profile of heart failure in mitral stenosis and has become part of the natural history. Several alternatives exist to relieve the narrowing of the valve. Transthoracic commissurotomy (either closed or open) and valve replacement have been the standard therapy for patients with symptomatic mitral stenosis. Transvenous catheter balloon commissurotomy is currently an attractive alternative. These modes of commissurotomy are not curative, but palliative, and place the patient back in the early phase of the natural history. Recurrence of symptoms is the rule with repeat interventions or valve replacement performed with the return of symptoms.

THROMBOEMBOLIC PHENOMENON IN MITRAL STENOSIS

Enlargement of the left atrium and the development of atrial fibrillation encourage thrombus formation in that chamber. The thrombogenic potential of an enlarged atrium is exacerbated by enhanced platelet adhesion/aggregation and increased coagulant capacity.[18] Increased level of von Willebrand factor (vWf) and α_2-antiplasmin as well as decreased level of antithrombin III were noted in patients with mitral stenosis.[19] It is generally agreed that visualization of thrombus will correlate well with the history of thromboembolism and is a good predictor of subsequent embolism. Dislodgement of this clot is believed to be the major mechanism of this complication after valve intervention. The thromboembolic phenomenon can be the first clinical presentation of patients with this disease. It can occur in three different states of mitral stenosis: in virgin stenotic mitral valves, in the peri-interventional phase, and in the postinterventional phase.

In the virgin mitral valve, the chance of thromboembolic insult ranges from 13 to 25% during a lifetime. The risk increases with age and atrial fibrillation. Coulshed et al.[20] reported the data for 839 patients with rheumatic mitral valve disease followed from 1952 to 1965, 737 of whom had predominant mitral stenosis. Systemic embolization occurred in 140 patients with mitral stenosis who had never undergone any valve intervention. Strong predictors of systemic emboli are age and the presence of atrial fibrillation. The incidence ranges from 4.5% in the patients under 35 of age and in sinus rhythm to 32.3% in the group above 35 years of age who had atrial fibrillation. The interval from the onset was extrapolated from the data. Of interest, 31 of 140 (20%) patients were in sinus rhythm at presentation with systemic emboli. However, most of these patients had a previous history of paroxysmal arrhythmia. There is no correlation between functional status and the incidence of thromboembolic complications.

Other predictors of thromboembolic phenomenon are previous episodes of systemic emboli and large left atrium. Patients with more than two episodes of embolization are at high risk of another episode. This risk seems to persist through life, even after valvular intervention and resumption of sinus rhythm. Presence of left atrial enlargement was considered the major risk of thromboembolism. In fact, the development of atrial fibrillation and left atrial enlargement may be due to the same process: chronic elevation of left atrial pressure. Several noninvasive methods has been used to evaluate left atrium size and risk of thromboembolic phenomenon. Conventional chest radiography is sensitive enough to evaluate the size of the left atrium.[20]

Echocardiography has emerged as a very useful tool in detecting left atrium size and has practically replaced conventional the chest radiograph as the mode of evaluation of this cardiac chamber. Transthoracic M-mode and two-dimensional echocardiography were the standard method of measuring the size of left atrium thrombus found in the left atrium by two-dimensional echocardiography correlates well with a history of thromboembolic phenomenon.[21] The transesophageal route provides a new window in visualizing the left atrium, especially its appendage. Spontaneous echo contrast characterized by dynamic clouds of echoes curling up slowly in a circular or spiral shape within the atrial cavity may be helpful in identifying the patient at risk of this complication.[22] However, the presence of thrombus or of spontaneous echos is prevalent in the left atrium and may merely represent abnormal flow in the enlarged chamber, by itself a strong predictor of thromboembolic phenomenon.

Anticoagulation has been the method of choice in lowering the risk of thromboembolic phenomenon. Valvular intervention (either closed or open commissurotomy) in the pliable noncalcific mitral valve may prevent the risk of this complication.[23] Data from the 1960s suggest that the incidence of systemic emboli in patients who were receiving coumadin was about 2% per patient year.[20] Follow-up data from the study[20] also noted a lower incidence of systemic emboli in patients who underwent surgical valvotomy compared with the group treated with medical therapy. However, this medical therapy group were not on anticoagulants during the study. A much lower incidence was noted in patients under 35 years of age and in sinus rhythm.

During mitral valve surgery, especially closed mitral commissurotomy, the increased incidence of thromboembolic complication was attributed to the presence of a clot found during surgery, as well as atrial fibrillation and a heavily calcified valve. This increased incidence was reduced, to a certain extent, by the use of prophylactic preoperative anticoagulation but was not totally eliminated. The possibility of calcific debris dislodgement with the embolic phenomenon may explain the continued number of thromboembolic complication with mitral valve surgery. In another study,[24] the incidence of postoperative embolism was 0.4% in 256 patients who had atrial fibrillation and placed on anticoagulation 3 weeks before surgery. The incidence in 204 patients with atrial fibrillation but no anticoagulation was 6.25%. Patients with sinus rhythm had a 0.95% incidence of this complication.[24]

Thromboembolic complication is quite rare after tranvenous balloon mitral valvuloplasty. This may be attributable to better case selection with noninvasive techniques before the procedure and the use of anticoagulation as a routine prophylactic measure. Two-dimensional echocardiography has been used as a standard to evaluate the mitral valve, mitral apparatus, left atrium size, and the possibility of thrombus in this chamber. At some institutions, transesophageal echocardiography is used to evaluate these parameters before valvuloplasty. An early report from Inoue's group, using two-dimensional echocardiography as a screening method before transvenous mitral balloon valvuloplasty had shown 0% for thromboembolic complication.[25] Of course, anticoagulation was used before the procedure and heavily calcified valves were not considered suitable for this intervention.

The postintervention probability of a thromboembolic complication is again related to the state of atrial rhythm, atrial size, and mitral valve prosthesis. Because of the continuation of thromboembolic risk, patients with atrial fibrillation or an enlarged left atrium should not be treated with a tissue valve. The risk of this complication postoperatively has to be weighed against the risk of anticoagulation itself. The risk of the thromboembolic phenomenon in patients with mitral valve prosthesis depends on the type of prosthesis used and is 1 to 2% per patient-year.

Anticoagulation could be started prophylactically in patients with mitral stenosis at high risk of thromboembolic complication and who do not have any contraindications for anticoagulation. The high-risk group includes the following:

1. All age groups with atrial fibrillation documented anytime in their lifetime
2. Patients above 35 of age with enlarged left atrium detected by noninvasive test, regardless of the cardiac rhythm
3. Patients with a history of unexplained transient ischemic attacks (TIAs) or documented stroke

A new catheter balloon valvuloplasty technique may prove effective in preventing progression of disease and in preventing the complication of thromboembolism.

INEFFECTIVE ENDOCARDITIS

Bacterial infection of stenotic mitral valve has not been a major problem. During the pre-antibiotic era, 5 of 250 patients (2% incidence) with mitral stenosis followed over 10 years showed the development of bacterial endocarditis.[9] However, its incidence is significant in the patients who also have aortic or mitral regurgitation. It is standard practice to administer prophylactic antibiotics to all patients with this valvular disease. This complication, however, is still a problem following artificial heart valve surgery and seems to play a major role in morbidity and mortality after mechanical valve replacement.

MITRAL VALVE INTERVENTIONS

There are currently four major procedures for the treatment of mitral stenosis. As the disease is progressive in nature, these intervention are part of natural history of mitral stenosis. The timing of intervention varies from one individual to another. Generally, the indication for mitral valve intervention is at least functional class 2. The following list compares the different interventions:

1. Surgical closed mitral commissurotomy
2. Surgical open mitral commissurotomy
3. Surgical valve replacement
4. Percutaneous balloon mitral commissurotomy

Surgical closed commissurotomy was first reported in England in 1925. The procedure was replaced in the United States by the open direct visualized method in mid-1970. Mitral valve replacement was initiated after the development of cardiac valve prosthesis with the first artificial mechanical valve being Starr-Edward valve in late 1960. The selection of either valve replacement or open commissurotomy was made at the time of surgery and has been dictated by valve pathology and the degree of valve incompetency. Catheter balloon valvuloplasty of the mitral valve was introduced as a effective alternative in patients who would have had a surgical commissurotomy.[25]

Selection of these methods of intervention depends mostly on valve pathology. Availability and skill of the interventional cardiologist and cardiac surgery also play a part in the choice of intervention. These procedures have proved to alter the life history of patients with symptomatic mitral stenosis. Prolonged survival has been noted by all surgical methods, as well as with catheter balloon technique.[15,24,26–28] Hemodynamic improvement occurs in more than 90% of patients after the intervention and usually parallels with the symptomatic improvement. It remains to be seen whether early commissurotomy, either by catheter or

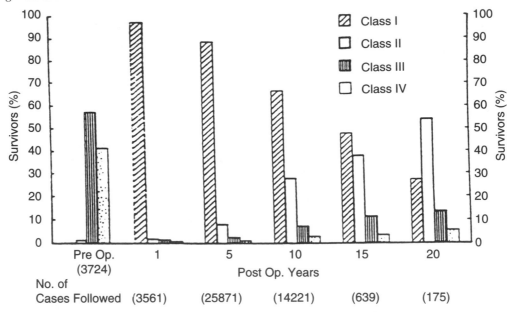

Fig. 17-2. Functional status of patients at different stages of follow-up. (From John et al.,[24] with permission.)

surgically, would prevent thromboembolic complication in patient with benign pathology and sinus rhythm.

Morbidity and mortality after surgical commissurotomy was statistically lower than surgical valve replacement. The intraoperative mortality rate was 2 to 3% in the commissurotomy group, in contrast to 10 to 15% after surgical valve replacement. Functional class and age are the predictors of postoperative mortality for commissurotomy surgery. With regard to the two types of surgical commissurotomies, open or direct visual surgical commissurotomy has been claimed to have a better outcome than the closed technique.[29–31] Data from one institution at which the two procedures were done by the same group of surgeons have shown the two techniques to be quite comparable.[28]

Catheter balloon commissurotomy became an important alternative to surgical commissurotomy.[25] The procedure has proved safe and effective, even in the group considered to be poor surgical candidates.[32] The postprocedure complication rate has been slightly lower than in those with surgical commissurotomy. This may represent a better case selection. A lower rate of thromboembolic complication is probably secondary to the use of echocardiography in case selection.[27,33] Severe mitral regurgitation and subsequent mitral valve replacement are not common. However, iatrogenic atrial septum defect is a potential problem, although shunt size is not believed to be significant in most cases. Follow-up for as long as 3 years has shown that the hemodynamic as well as symptomatic improvement were sustained in the majority of patients.[34,35]

In the vast majority of cases, life expectancy has improved after the intervention, but a good number of patients remain at risk after the procedure.[36,37] Because of the progressive nature of the disease, recurrence of symptoms is part of natural history after the intervention requiring a second intervention at a later date. Figure 17-2 shows the trend of functional class after commissurotomy of the mitral valve. Immediately after the procedure, most of the patients were in class 1 and 2. The percentage of patients with a class 3 increases with longer follow-up. The major causes of recurrent symptoms and reoperation are residual stenosis, restenosis, and mitral regurgitation. However, repeat intervention has been proved practical and improves the quality of life in these recurrent symptomatic patients.[37] Figure 17-3 demonstrates a reduction in the number of patients with class 3, purely the result of an increased number of interventions, either repeat commissurotomy or valve replacement.

MITRAL VALVE REPLACEMENT

Mitral valve replacement is an important part of the history of many patients with mitral stenosis. An estimated 20% of patients after commissurotomy would have to undergo mitral valve replacement in 10 years.[36] The number goes up to more than 50% in 20 years. Indications for mitral valve replacement in mitral stenosis are severely damaged valve and heavy calcification to begin with and residual stenosis or restenosis not suitable for recommissurotomy. Patients

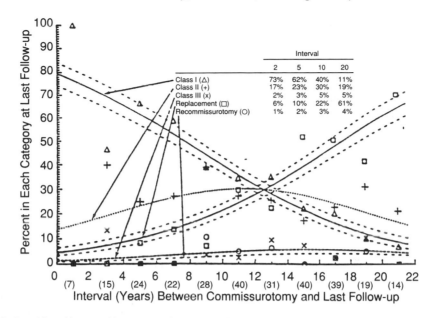

Fig. 17-3. Relationship of interval between mitral commissurotomy and last follow-up study to the functional status (prevalence of functional class) in the 213 patients at last follow-up evaluation and to the prevalence of a repeat commissurotomy and mitral valve replacement. Symbols represent the actual proportions at the odd-year intervals. Continuous curves (—, ---) are nomograms of the parametric predictions or the prevalences of the outcome events; (– – –), around class I and (mitral valve) replacement enclose the 70% confidence intervals. Percentages in each category total 100% at each time interval. Numbers in parentheses on the X axis are numbers of patients at each follow-up interval. (From Hickey et al.,[28] with permission.)

with mitral regurgitation tend to have mitral prosthesis placed early after the commissurotomy usually within 1 year. Morbidity and mortality after valve replacement are higher than commissurotomy. The operative mortality is about 10%. The postoperative thromboembolic phenomenon is about 2.2% per year, about twice that after commissurotomy. In any event, mitral valve replacement is beneficial in improving functional status. The survival rate after mitral valve replacement was 95% at 5 years and 73% at 10 years by the same study.

TIMING OF INTERVENTION

Clinical class as well as valve pathology plays an important part in the timing of intervention. Generally, functional class 2 warrants intervention if the valve is pliable. Early mitral intervention may slow the progressive nature of the disease and may lower the incidence of thromboembolic complications. However, higher threshold of intervention should be set if one is dealing with a heavily diseased valve, if valve replacement is the more appropriate intervention. In this case, time can be bought and functional status improved by the judicious use of medical therapy, including anticoagulation. Although effective surgical

commissurotomy lowers the incidence of thromboembolism, it has not been used as an indication for valvular intervention.

RISK ASSESSMENT IN PATIENTS WITH MITRAL STENOSIS

History

The history is probably the most important predictor of complication in mitral stenosis. Dyspnea suggests significant narrowing of the valve and in most cases predicts the progression of disease and mortality. Dyspnea can be recipitated by arrhythmias, pregnancy, and anemia. Symptoms of thromboemboli (e.g., TIA) suggest thrombogenic atrium and further embolization. By contrast, asymptomatic patients can remain asymptomatic for quite some time.

Clinical Examination

Clinical examination is a useful tool for diagnosis but may not be sensitive enough to predict cardiovascular events. Most young patients with this disease are asymptomatic but their condition can be detected by clinical examination. However, a loud first heart

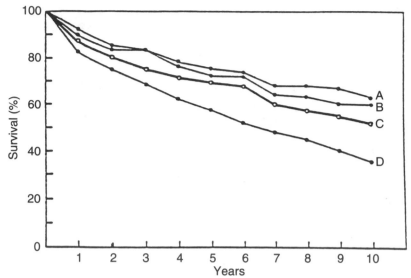

Fig. 17-4. Life expectancy in patients with mitral stenosis before surgical era. (*A & B*, data from Rowe et al.,[9] *C & D*, data from Olesen.[10])

sound and open snap suggest a pliable valve. Chest radiography and electrocardiography (ECG) are part of the routine laboratory workup and may give some clue about the status of left atrium and right ventricle, indirectly identifying the patient with pulmonary hypertension. Pulmonary hypertension is an ominous sign of this disease. These parameters are not sensitive but are quite specific. Atrial fibrillation is a predictor of subsequent thromboembolism. Mitral stenosis may lead to any of the following events:

Congestive heart failure
Thromboembolism
Infective endocarditis
Mitral valve intervention
Death
Recurrent rheumatic fever

Noninvasive Diagnostic Tools

In the practice of the current era, noninvasive cardiology has a prominent part in evaluating patients. Treadmill ECG is usually not useful in assessing the risk but may be helpful in identifying patients who have poor exercise reserve. It may also be beneficial in evaluating medical treatment in terms of slowing the ventricular response. Ambulatory ECG may be useful in identifying those with intermittent atrial fibrillation and who are unaware of it. Although there is no proof that using this method aids in predicting the risk, starting anticoagulation once this dysrythmia was noted may be indicated. Doppler-enhanced echocardiography has become the most widely used tool in establishing diagnosis and evaluating the mitral valve status. Information in regard to valve mobility, thick-

ness, calcification, subvalvular involvement, and degree of mitral regurgitation as well as the status of the left atrium can be obtained. These criteria are crucial for selecting an intervention and for estimating its risk. The transesophageal route has provided an excellent window of visualizing the mitral valve and left atrium.

Cardiac Catheterization

Cardiac catheterization have been used as the gold standard for establishing the degree of stenosis. The hemodynamic data, however, do not correlate with the pathology of the valve and do not predict any response of the disease. In addition, hemodynamics at any given time do not predict the rate of progression of the disease. Current noninvasive methods, especially echocardiography, have been as effective as cardiac catheterization in establishing diagnosis and severity. Some centers will operate on patients with pure mitral stenosis on the basis of echocardiography, without cardiac catheterization.

LIFE EXPECTANCY

During the presurgical era, the cause of death was CHF and systemic embolization in most the cases, while pulmonary emboli and bacterial endocarditis were minor causes. Figure 17-4 demonstrates survival during the presurgical era, derived from several studies. The mortality rate has declined over the past three decades. This improvement in the death rate is probably secondary to the decline in the rate of rheumatic

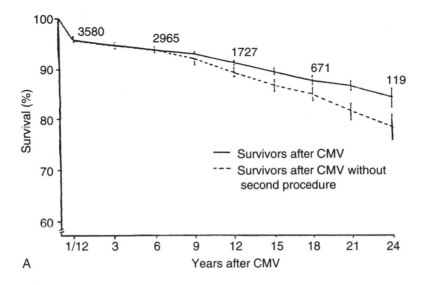

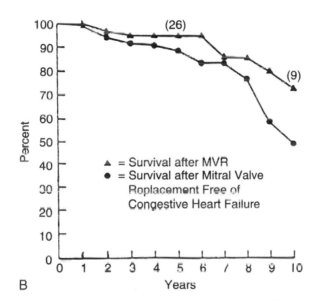

Fig. 17-5. Survival curve of patients with mitral stenosis following surgical interventions. **(A)** Actuarial survival curve after closed mitral commissurotomy. (From John et al.,[24] with permission.) **(B)** Actuarial analysis of survival and survival free of congestive heart failure after mitral valve replacement. (From Rutledge et al.,[38] with permission.)

fever, advancement of medical therapy, and the development of mitral valve intervention. The survival of patients with this disease after surgical commissurotomy is shown is Figure 17-5. Life expectancy has dramatically improved as compared with the presurgical era. However, some of the deaths during the current era with valve intervention are due to CHF. The risks of dying from this disease and from valve intervention are directly related to the age and functional class of the patient, as well as to valve pathology and the de-

gree of mitral regurgitation. The increased risk in the sicker group should alert us to earlier diagnosis and timely treatment.

REFERENCES

1. Gillum RF: Trends in acute rheumatic fever and chronic rheumatic heart disease: a national perspective. Am Heart J 111:430, 1986

2. Masseli BF, Chute CG, Walker AW, Kurland GS: Penicillin and the marked decrease in Morbidity and mortality from rheumatic fever in the United States. N Engl J Med 318:280, 1988
3. Bisno AL: Acute rheumatic fever: forgotten but not gone. (Editorial.) N Engl J Med 316:476, 1987
4. Wallace MR, Garst PD, Papadimos TJ, Oldfield EC: The return of acute rheumatic fever in young adults. JAMA 262:2557, 1989
5. Feinstein AR, Di Massa R: Prognostic significance of valvular involvement in acute rheumatic fever. N Engl J Med 260:1001, 1959
6. Feinstein AR, Spagnuolo M: The clinical patterns of acute rheumatic fever: a reappraisal. Medicine (Baltimore) 41:381, 1962
7. Cheitlin MD, Byrd RC: Mitral Valve Disease. Valvular Heart Disease. 1st Ed. PSG, 1987
8. Braunwald E: Valvular Heart Disease. Heart Disease, A Textbook of Cardiovascular Medicine. 3rd Ed. WB Saunders, Philadelphia, 1988, p. 1023
9. Rowe JC, Bland EF, Sprague HB, White PD: The course of mitral stenosis without surgery: ten- and twenty-year perspectives. Ann Intern Med 52:741, 1960
10. Olesen KH: The natural history of 271 patients with mitral stenosis under medical treatment. Br Heart J 24:349, 1962
11. Selzer A, Cohn KE: Natural history of mitral stenosis. A review. Circulation 45:878, 1972
12. Rapaport E: Natural history of aortic and mitral valve disease. Am J Cardiol 35:221, 1975
13. Dubin AA, March HW, Cohn K, Selzer A: Longitudinal hemodynamic and clinical study of mitral stenosis. Circulation 44:381, 1971
14. Hugenholtz PG, Ryan TJ, Stein SW, Abelmann WH: The spectrum of pure mitral stenosis. Hemodynamics studies in relation to clinical studies. Am J Cardiol 10:773, 1962
15. Ellis LB, Benson H, Harken DE: The effect of age and other factors on the early and late results following closed mitral valvuloplasty. Am Heart J 75:743, 1968
16. Heller SJ, Carleton RA: Abnormal left ventricular contraction in patients with mitral stenosis. Circulation 42:1099, 1970
17. Meister SG, Engel TR, Feitosa GS et al: Propranolol in mitral stenosis during sinus rhythm. Am Heart J 94:685, 1977
18. Steele PP, Weily HS, Davies H, Genton E: Platelet survival in patients with rheumatic heart disease. N Engl J Med 290:537, 1974
19. Penny WF, Weinstein M, Salzman EW, Ware JA: Correlation of Circulating von Willebrand factor levels with cardiovascular hemodynamics. Circulation 83:1630, 1991
20. Coulshed N, Epstein EJ, Mckendrick CS et al: Systemic embolism in mitral valve disease. Br Heart J 32:26, 1970
21. Bansal RC, Heywood T, Applegate PM, Jutzy KR: Detection of left atrial thrombi by two-dimensional echocardiography and surgical correlation in 148 patients with mitral valve disease. Am J Cardiol 64:243, 1989
22. Daniel WG, Nellessen U, Schroder E et al: Left atrial spontaneous echo contrast in mitral valve disease: An indicator for an increased thromboembolic risk. J Am Coll Cardiol 11:1204, 1988
23. Kirklin JW, Barratt-Boyes BG: Acquired Valvular Heart Disease. Textbook of Cardiac Surgery. 1st Ed. John Wiley & Sons, New York, 1986
24. John S, Bashi VV, Jairaj PS et al: Closed mitral valvotomy: early results and long-term follow-up of 3724 consecutive patients. Circulation 68:891, 1983
25. Noboyoshi M, Hamasaki N, Kimura T et al: Indications, Complications, and Short-term clinical outcome of Percutaneous transvenous mitral commissurotomy. Circulation 80:782, 1989
26. Commerford PJ, Hastie T, Beck W: Closed mitral valvotomy: actuarial of results in 654 patients over 12 years and analysis of preoperative predictors of long term survival. Ann Thorac Surg 33:473, 1982
27. Matorras R, Reque JA, Minguez JA et al: Commissurotomy and pregnancy. A study of 245 cases. Acta Obstet Gynecol Scand 65:847, 1986
28. Hickey MS, Blackstone EH, Kirklin JW, Dean LS: Outcome probabilities and life history after surgical mitral commissurotomy: implications for balloon commissurotomy. J Am Coll Cardiol 17:29, 1991
29. Smith WM, Neutze JM, Barret-Boyes BG, Lowe JB: Open mitral valvotomy. Effect of preoperative factors on result. J Thor Cardiol Surg 82:738, 1981
30. Housman LB, Bonchek L, Lambert L et al: Prognosis of patients after open mitral commissurotomy. Actuarial analysis for late results in 100 patients. J Thorac Cardiol Surg 73:742, 1977
31. Gross RI, Cunningham JN, Snively SL et al: Long-term results of open radical mitral commissurotomy: ten years follow-up study of 202 patients. Am J Card 47:821, 1981
32. Mckay CR, Kawanishi DT, Kotlewski A et al: Improvement in exercise capacity and exercise hemodynamics 3 months after double-balloon, catheter balloon valvuloplasty treatment of patients with symptomatic mitral stenosis. Circulation 77:1013, 1988
33. Herrmann HC, Wilkins GT, Abascal VM et al: Percutaneous balloon mitral valvotomy for patients with mitral stenosis. Analysis of factors influencing early results. J Thor Cardiol Surg 96:33, 1988
34. Reid CL, Chandraratna PAN, Kawanishi DT et al: Influence of Mitral valve morphology on double-balloon catheter balloon valvuloplasty in patients with mitral stenosis. Analysis of factors predicting immediate and 3-month results. Circulation 80:515, 1989
35. Kawanishi D, Reid CL, Stellar WA, Rahimtoola SH: Long-term follow-up of patients undergoing balloon catheter balloon commissurotomy for mitral stenosis. J Am Coll Cardiol 17:253A, 1991
36. Higgs LM, Glancy DL, O'Brien KP et al: Mitral restenosis: an uncommon cause of recurrent symptoms following mitral commissurotomy. Am J Cardiol 26:34, 1970
37. Peper WA, Lytle BW, Cosgrove DM et al: Repeat mitral commissurotomy: long-term results. Circulation 76:III-97, 1987
38. Rutledge R, McIntosh CL, Morrow AG et al: Mitral valve replacement after closed mitral commissurotomy. Circulation 66:I-162, 1982

18
Mitral Regurgitation

Larry A. Osborn
Michael H. Crawford

Prognosis in mitral valvular regurgitation is affected by acuity, etiology, left ventricular (LV) function, and the age and medical condition of the patient. This chapter discusses prognostic factors in patients with chronic mitral regurgitation. The etiology of mitral valvular regurgitation, pathophysiology of chronic mitral insufficiency, natural history of acute and chronic mitral regurgitation, and the impact of operative intervention are addressed. In addition, the predictors of poor versus good surgical outcome and the optimal timing of surgery are elucidated.

ETIOLOGIES OF MITRAL REGURGITATION

The clinical presentation of mitral regurgitation may be classified as acute or chronic. The pathologic processes that can disrupt the mitral valve include degenerative, inflammatory, congenital and traumatic injury. Regurgitation can be caused by disruption of any component of the mitral apparatus (i.e., mitral leaflets, annulus, or subvalvular structures).

Acute Mitral Regurgitation

The causes of acute mitral regurgitation (AMI) are as follows[1,3]:

1. Chordal rupture
   a. Infective endocarditis
   b. Trauma
   c. Degenerative disease
   d. Hypertension
2. Papillary muscle pathology, dysfunction, or rupture
   a. Ischemic
   b. Myocardial infarction
   c. Trauma
   d. LV enlargement
3. Disruption of mitral valve leaflets
   a. Infective endocarditis
   b. Trauma
   c. Complication of cardiac surgery
   d. Myxoma of the left atrium
4. Prosthetic valve dysfunction

As summarized by Rapaport,[1] acute mitral regurgitation may result from chordal rupture, diseases of the papillary muscles, or primary valvular damage. In addition, mechanical prosthetic valve malfunction often causes acute regurgitation.

Chronic Mitral Regurgitation

There are a number of causes of chronic mitral regurgitation[1,3]:

1. Rheumatic heart disease
2. Rheumatologic diseases
3. Hereditary connective tissue diseases
4. Myxomatous changes (mitral valve prolapse)
5. Calcification of the mitral annulus
6. Infective endocarditis
7. Subvalvular apparatus rupture or dysfunction
8. Congenital
9. Hypertrophic cardiomyopathy

Included are inflammatory, infective, connective tissue, degenerative, structural, and hereditary disorders.

As can be seen above, the etiologies of acute and chronic mitral regurgitation are often the same, but the resulting structural abnormality is usually more severe in acute regurgitation. Consequently, acuity of mitral regurgitation is an operational classification based on the need for urgent intervention in acute cases.

PATHOPHYSIOLOGY OF CHRONIC MITRAL REGURGITATION

Chronic mitral insufficiency may be well tolerated for years. The volume load imposed on the left atrium and left ventricle results in enlargement of these chambers. Because of increased compliance, the volume excess may be accommodated with minimal to no change in left ventricular (LV) diastolic pressure.[2,3] The increased LV volume results in the development of eccentric hypertrophy, which tends to normalize LV wall stress. In time, LV afterload begins to rise as the left ventricle continues to dilate without an adequate increase in LV wall thickness. Furthermore, the severity of mitral regurgitation increases because the progressive LV enlargement causes increasing mitral annular dilation. Eventually, pulmonary hypertension and subsequent right heart heart failure may ensue. Death ultimately occurs from biventricular backward failure.

Chronic Compensated Mitral Regurgitation

The volume overload of chronic mitral insufficiency results in myocellular changes which include the loss of z-line register and the development of new sarcomeres (eccentric hypertrophy).[4] Increased sarcomere length (preload) coupled with the addition of new sarcomers provides improved contractile performance.[5]

A major adaptive response to the volume overload of mitral regurgitation is the development of increased LV and left atrial size and compliance. With increased diastolic compliance, the LV filling pressure may remain normal or only mildly increased despite a large increase in end-diastolic volume.[1,2] In the study conducted by Wong and Spotnitz,[6] analysis of the diastolic pressure-volume relationship in chronic mitral insufficiency indicated that compliance was increased.

Recently, there has been a change in our understanding of afterload in chronic mitral regurgitation. The prevailing hypothesis had been that regurgitation into the left atrium provides reduced LV afterload secondary to the mitral valvular leak. More recent data, however, indicate that mean systolic afterload is normal in chronic compensated mitral regurgitation. Wall stress (afterload) can be estimated by the law of Laplace:

$$\text{Stress} = \frac{p \times r}{2h}$$

where p is systolic pressure, r is ventricular radius, and h is ventricular wall thickness. In mitral regurgitation, r increases as the left ventricle dilates, yet h, or the ventricular wall thickness, usually remains constant.[2] Corin et al.[7] determined that mean systolic wall stress is essentially the same in normal subjects as in patients with chronic compensated mitral regurgitation. However, this was due to a counterbalance between elevated ejection phase stress related to increased ventricular volume and reduced pre-ejection stress caused by decreased ventricular pressure during regurgitation into the left atrium.

Because of loading alterations in chronic mitral regurgitation, special techniques must be employed to determine intrinsic myocardial contractility. Wisenbaugh[8] studied contractile function in chronic severe mitral regurgitation using load-independent measurements. Four of 13 patients with ejection fractions >0.60 and 10 of 14 with ejection fractions of <0.60 had muscle dysfunction. Thus, most patients with compensated mitral regurgitation and an ejection fraction >0.60 have normal contractile function.

Decompensated Chronic Mitral Regurgitation

Measured afterload (wall stress) is normal in compensated mitral regurgitation. However, Corin et al.[7] demonstrated that patients with mitral regurgitation and depressed ejection phase indices had elevated mean systolic wall stress. This increased afterload likely accelerates the deterioration of LV function.[2]

Muscle function decline in chronic decompensated mitral incompetence is related to the declining mass to volume ratio, as increases in ventricular volume are not matched by increases in wall thickness. Each unit of myocardium is therefore subjected to greater demand. The failure of wall thickness to increase in response to greater afterload is similar to the pathophysiology of dilated cardiomyopathy.[2]

ASSESSMENT OF SEVERITY OF MITRAL REGURGITATION

Clinical

In general, the diastolic volume of the left ventricle reflects the severity of mitral regurgitation.[9] Chronic severe mitral regurgitation is characterized by radiographic cardiomegaly with LV and left atrial enlargement. Physical examination in severe chronic mitral insufficiency may reveal (1) wide splitting of the second heart sound secondary to an earlier aortic component, (2) an accentuated pulmonic component when pulmonary hypertension is present, and (3) palpable evidence of enlarged left heart chambers. However, the loudness of the systolic murmur does not correlate well with the severity of regurgitation.[3] Symptoms of fatigue and exhaustion suggest an advanced degree of regurgitation with low forward cardiac output.[3]

Cardiac Catheterization

The angiographic grading of mitral regurgitation is generally classified from 1+ to 4+. With 1+ mitral regurgitation, the contrast clears the left atrium with each diastole; in 2+ mitral regurgitation, there is opacification of the left atrium after several beats, which is less than LV dye density; in 3+ mitral regurgitation, there is equal opacification of the left atrium with the left ventricle; and in 4+ mitral insufficiency, opacification of the left atrium is noted within one beat, progresses with each beat, and dye is noted in the pulmonary veins.[10] However, in a study by Croft et al.[11] the 1 to 4+ angiographic severity of mitral insufficiency did not correlate well with regurgitant flow; the regurgitant flow had wide variation within each angiographic grade, and there was considerable regurgitant volume index overlap between the grades.

The regurgitant fraction is determined as follows: angiographic flow (angiographic stroke volume × heart rate) minus the measured forward flow by Fick or indicator dilution technique divided by angiographic flow. Less than 20% is considered mild, 20 to 40% moderate, 40 to 60% moderately severe, and greater than 60% severe regurgitation.[10]

There have been attempts to correlate the magnitude of left atrial V waves with the severity of mitral regurgitation, but the V-wave amplitude is dependent on left atrial size and compliance and cardiac output. Severe mitral regurgitation may therefore exist in the absence of prominent V waves.[10]

Doppler Echocardiography

Early Doppler evaluations of mitral regurgitation used localized pulsed Doppler sampling in the left atrium to map the extent of detected regurgitant flow velocities. This tedious analysis was shown to correlate fairly well with angiographic severity ratings in the same patients.[12] More recently, color Doppler encoding has permitted the visualization of regurgitant jets in the left atrium. Spain and colleagues[13] recently demonstrated that Doppler color flow mapping of the regurgitant jet correlates with angiographic grades of mitral regurgitation with an r value of 0.76; but, similar to the cardiac catheterization study of Croft et al.,[11] Doppler grading of severity correlated poorly with the regurgitant volume and did not predict hemodynamic dysfunction.

Radionuclide Angiography

The regurgitant volume may be calculated noninvasively using radionuclide angiographic techniques. In these studies, the difference in stroke counts per beat between the left and right ventricles is measured. The stroke count difference is proportional to the regurgitant stroke volume. When divided by the LV end-diastolic counts, it becomes the regurgitant fraction, a unitless measure of the severity of regurgitation. However, values of ±20% can be measured in patients without mitral regurgitation.[14]

Cine Magnetic Resonance Imaging

Aurigemma et al.[15] performed a study that compared cine MRI with Doppler. These investigators found the cine MRI classification of mitral regurgitation severity to be the same as pulsed Doppler echocardiography in 87% of patients and color flow Doppler in 80%. However, as previously discussed, these gradings would not be expected to correlate with the regurgitant flow volume.

Summary

Accurate quantitation of the severity of mitral regurgitation is not achievable by current invasive or noninvasive techniques. However, the extent of LV dilation, LV dysfunction, and pulmonary hypertension can be accurately assessed by invasive and noninvasive techniques. Fortunately, these latter parameters are useful for estimating prognosis and planning therapy in patients with mitral regurgitation. As long as the severity of mitral regurgitation is at least moderate, assessment of LV function and pulmonary pressures are warranted. Whether current invasive and noninvasive techniques can accurately separate mild from moderate cases has not been proved but seems to be a reasonable expectation.

NATURAL HISTORY

Appropriate management, medical versus surgical, of a patient with mitral regurgitation must entail consideration of the expected natural history versus the anticipated short-term and long-term outcome of surgery. Therefore, it is extremely important to have an understanding of the natural history of mitral regurgitation, both acute and chronic.

Acute Mitral Regurgitation

The hallmark of acute mitral insufficiency is severe LV failure, with associated pulmonary edema or peripheral hypoperfusion, or both. Death may occur within a matter of days, and decisions about surgery are usually urgent to emergent.[1,3] However, acute mitral regurgitation may be mild to moderate in some patients. Patients with a mild degree of acute mitral regurgitation may be managed without surgery. The clinical course in patients with moderate acute mitral regurgitation will determine whether mitral valve operation is required. Patients with acute mitral insufficiency who do not require surgery will need to be followed in a manner similar to patients with chronic mitral regurgitation.

Chronic Mitral Regurgitation

The course of chronic mitral regurgitation depends on the stage of the disease at the time of patient evaluation. Furthermore, the natural history is significantly influenced by the intrinsic contractile state of the left ventricle. Acknowledging that a spectrum of risk exists among medically treated patients with chronic mitral regurgitation, Rapaport[1] cites an overall 5-year survival rate of 80% and 10-year survival rate of 60% in unoperated patients with isolated mitral insufficiency. Munoz et al.[16] reported that medically treated patients with severe mitral regurgitation have a 45% 5-year survival rate. The major prognostic factors in chronic mitral regurgitation include the following:

1. LV ejection fraction.[45,46]
2. RV ejection fraction (poor prognosis when ≤0.30).[46]
3. NYHA functional class (in predicting morbidity).[45]
4. Stage of disease at the time of patient encounter.[1]
5. Etiology.[9]

Summary

Acute moderately severe to severe mitral regurgitation usually requires urgent or emergent operative intervention. Patients with mild acute mitral regurgitation or moderate acute mitral regurgitation not requiring surgery should be managed and followed like other patients with chronic mitral insufficiency.

Chronic mitral insufficiency is usually an insidious disorder which may be well tolerated for years.[1,17] Impairment of LV contractile performance may develop and progress with little or no symptomatology.[1,3] It is important in chronic mitral regurgitation to assess ventricular function serially and understand the associated expected natural history. In this fashion, follow-up and management, including appropriately timed operative intervention when indicated (vide infra), may be better planned.

CHRONIC MITRAL REGURGITATION: PROGNOSTIC FACTORS

Etiology

Concomitant coronary artery disease (CAD) with mitral regurgitation confers a worse prognosis than that of isolated mitral insufficiency.[18,19] Also, operative mortality is increased in patients with ischemic mitral valve apparatus dysfunction compared with those patients in whom CAD and mitral regurgitation coexist but are not causally related.[18,20]

Influence of Mitral Valve Surgery

Hammermeister et al.[21] found that surgically treated patients with mitral insufficiency had a marginally improved (p = 0.07) 10-year survival compared with those treated medically. The influence of CAD was not studied. These investigators emphasized that valve replacement superimposes new outcome variables due to prosthetic valve related complications.

Myocardial Function

Many studies have demonstrated that prognosis in mitral regurgitation, either operated or unoperated, is related to the intrinsic function of the left ventricle.[1,22–25] Significant impairment of load-independent LV performance is clearly associated with decreased long-term medical survival, reduced postoperative survival, and higher operative mortality.[1,22,26] These concepts and the related criteria for optimal timing of mitral valve surgery are further discussed below.

VASODILATOR THERAPY

Acute Mitral Regurgitation

The treatment of acute moderate to severe mitral regurgitation encompasses conventional heart failure and pulmonary edema therapies, including diuretic treatment, appropriate oxygen administration, and afterload reduction.[3] In severely compromised patients, intravenous nitroprusside may be required; in addition, placement of an intra-aortic balloon for counterpulsation may assist in the management of selected patients.[3]

Chronic Mitral Regurgitation

In chronic mitral regurgitation, short-term hemodynamic benefits have been achieved with both venodilator and arterial dilator therapy. However, currently there is no established role for long-term vasodilator therapy in patients with chronic mitral regurgitation,[27] and further studies are needed.

IMPACT OF SURGICAL TREATMENT ON PATIENTS WITH CHRONIC MITRAL REGURGITATION

Factors Affecting Surgical Results

Rahimtoola[28] has summarized the essential elements of operative outcome as survival, valve function, surgical complications, functional class, and cardiac performance. These major outcome variables are influenced by the preoperative clinical condition of the patient; the etiology of mitral regurgitation; intraoperative management; whether mitral valve replacement or repair is performed; and, if replacement is undertaken, which type of prosthesis is selected. In addition, long-term postoperative results are influenced by patient follow-up and treatment, including surveillance for prosthetic valve dysfunction and appropriate management of anticoagulant therapy when indicated.

Left Ventricular Function and Volume

Multiple studies have demonstrated a significant reduction in ejection fraction following mitral valve replacement for chronic mitral regurgitation. Examples include a decline in average ejection fraction from 0.55 to 0.43 in the study by Kennedy et al.[29] from 0.56 to 0.45 in the report by Crawford et al.,[23] and from 0.66 to 0.48 in the study by Boucher and colleagues.[30] Since mortality is increased postoperatively with an ejection fraction ≤0.50,[23] it is important to time mitral valve replacement with the expectation that the postoperative ejection fraction will be >0.50.

Mitral Valve Repair

Mitral valve repair in eligible patients results in preservation of ejection fraction.[31,32] In the study by Goldman et al.,[31] the intraoperative echocardiographic ejection fraction was maintained after mitral valve repair. This and other studies[33] support the concept that preservation of the papillary muscles by performing mitral valve reconstruction contributes to maintaining ejection fraction. The technique of mitral valve repair is most applicable to degenerative mitral regurgitation, as compared with rheumatic fibrosis and calcification.[32]

Mitral Valve Replacement

The decrease in ejection fraction with mitral valve replacement reflects the loss of diastolic volume with relatively little change in end-systolic volume. In the study by Crawford et al.,[23] the average LV end-diastolic volume index declined from 117 to 89 ml/m², but the LV end-systolic volume index decreased minimally, from a mean of 54 to 50 ml/m². Boucher and colleagues[30] also reported essentially no change in end-systolic volume after mitral valve replacement. However, after mitral valve repair, Lessana et al.[34] and Bonchek et al.[35] found that end-systolic volume decreased, preserving ejection fraction.

Afterload

Left ventricular wall stress has been demonstrated to increase immediately after discontinuation of cardiopulmonary bypass in patients undergoing mitral valve replacement.[6] However, Schuler et al.,[5] Boucher et al.,[30] and Crawford et al.[23] did not observe changes in end-systolic volume after mitral valve replacement, suggesting little change in afterload. In mitral valve repair, however, the fall in end-systolic volume indicates that afterload probably lessens after this procedure.

Operative Mortality

Christakis and colleagues[24] reported an 8.7% operative mortality in their mitral regurgitation patients. Mitral valve operative mortality ranges from 4% to 10% in the absence of symptomatic CAD.[18,19]

Symptomatic CAD significantly increases the operative mortality for mitral regurgitation. In patients with symptomatic ischemic heart disease the operative mortality of mitral valve replacement without coronary artery bypass surgery is 29%.[19] The combined operation of mitral valve replacement and coronary artery bypass surgery carries a 3 to 20% mortality.[18,20] When the mitral insufficiency is ischemic, the operative mortality is 11 to 38%.[18–20,36,37]

Postoperative Survival

Phillips et al.[25] reported an 82% 5-year survival rate for mitral valve replacement for isolated mitral regurgitation. However, age over 60 decreased the 5-year survival rate to 72%. With a preoperative ejection fraction of <0.40, the 5-year survival rate fell dramatically to 38%.

The coexistence of significant CAD with mitral insufficiency influences 5-year survival following operation. Mitral valve replacement plus coronary artery bypass surgery for rheumatic or degenerative mitral valve disease carries a 60 to 70% 5-year survival rate,[18] whereas 5-year survival ranges from 30 to 40% after mitral valve replacement and coronary artery bypass surgery for ischemic mitral insufficiency.[18,19]

Mitral valve repair, with preservation of the subvalvular components of the mitral valve apparatus, appears to improve postoperative survival. In the study by Galloway et al.,[32] the 30-day hospital mortality for isolated mitral reconstruction was 1.2%. Sand et al.[38] reported a 5-year survival rate of 76% after mitral valve repair, compared with 56% after replacement (p=0.005); however, by multivariate analysis, valve replacement was not found to be a significant risk factor. These data suggest, but do not prove, reduced mortality risk with valve repair.

Functional Status

Mitral valve repair or replacement provides significant improvement in symptoms in most patients. In the report by Phillips and colleagues,[25] 78% of patients preoperatively were in New York Heart Association (NYHA) functional class 3 or 4; after mitral valve replacement, 98% of patients were in functional class 1 or 2, with most in the former. Likewise, in the study by Breisblatt et al.,[39] 90% of patients were in functional class 3 or 4 preoperatively, and postoperatively 28% were in either of these classes. It is evident from these and other studies that most symptomatic patients with mitral insufficiency experience a significant reduction in their symptomatology following operation.

Mitral Valve Repair Versus Replacement

Two additional well-substantiated advantages of mitral valve reconstruction are freedom from thromboemboli and reduced rates of endocarditis.[32] Approximately 95% of patients remain free from thromboemboli for 5 to 10 years after mitral valve repair, contrasted with 65 to 90% of patients with a mechanical prosthesis. The reported incidence of late endocarditis after mitral valve replacement is 3 to 6%, but this complication is quite rate after mitral valve reconstruction.

Since mitral valve reconstruction has the following advantages:

1. Preservation of LV ejection fraction
2. Reduced risk of thromboembolism
3. Trend toward improved mortality
4. Reduced risk of infective endocarditis

it should be considered in patients with mitral insufficiency who have indications for operation. However, as discussed by Kulick and Rahimtoola,[17] although mitral valve reconstruction may appear possible preoperatively, it may be discovered during the operation that replacement is required. Therefore, patients who are referred for mitral valve surgery must be considered candidates for mitral valve replacement, although mitral valve repair is desired. If mitral valve replacement is necessary, every attempt should be made to preserve the annular-chordal structures.

TIMING OF MITRAL VALVE OPERATION

To time mitral valve repair or replacement optimally in patients with mitral regurgitation, it is important to (1) appreciate the expected natural history of the disease in individual patients, (2) be aware of the operative and postoperative mortality and morbidity statistics at one's institution, (3) grade the patient's symptoms by functional class, and (4) assess one or more of the objective parameters that predict good versus poor operative outcome.

Functional Class

Mitral valve repair or replacement is indicated in patients with mitral regurgitation who are in NYHA functional class 3 or 4. In addition, operation should be considered in functional class 2 patients with hemodynamic predictors of poor outcome despite vigorous medical therapy.[3]

Objective Variables That Predict Operative Outcome

There has been considerable interest in the predictive value of load-independent measures of myocardial contractility. Carabello et al.[22] found the ratio of end-systolic wall stress (ESWS) to end-systolic volume index (ESVI) significantly predicted surgical outcome. Patients with a ratio of <2.5 had an unsatisfactory outcome, either remaining in functional class 3 or 4 or dying during the perioperative period. However, only 21 patients were studied, and simultaneous pressure and volume measurements were not performed.

An even more elaborate parameter was analyzed by Breisblatt et al.,[39] the tension-volume ejection fraction (TVEF). To calculate the TVEF, end-systolic wall stress is divided by the product of the end-systolic volume index and ejection fraction. In their study, the TVEF index accurately predicted the operative results in all 40 patients. A TVEF index of <1.47 dynes/cm²/m² predicted a poor operative outcome with 100% accuracy. Likewise, a TVEF index of >1.47 had a 100% positive predictive value, accurately identifying all patients in

NYHA functional class 1 or 2 after mitral valve replacement. The TVEF index, as used in their study, requires invasive measurements and is not appropriate for the long-term follow-up of mitral regurgitation patients. However, the authors suggest that noninvasive determination of the TVEF index should be feasible. Higher patient number studies of the predictive value of the ESWS-ESVI ratio and TVEF in mitral regurgitation are needed.

Several studies have addressed the prognostic value of LV end-systolic volume. In the study by Borow et al.,[40] a left ventricular end-systolic volume index of 60 ml/m² differentiated good (<60) versus poor (>60) postoperative ventricular function. Crawford et al.[23] found that a preoperative end-systolic volume index <50 ml/m² generally predicted a postoperative end-diastolic volume index of ≤101 ml/m² in patients undergoing mitral valve replacement. Similarly, in the echocardiographic study by Zile and colleagues,[41] a LV end-systolic dimension index >2.6 cm/m² predicted an unfavorable outcome for mitral valve replacement in chronic mitral insufficiency.

Since ejection fraction may be easily measured and serially compared using noninvasive techniques, multiple studies have evaluated its prognostic role in chronic mitral regurgitation. Phillips and colleagues[25] studied 105 patients undergoing mitral valve replacement and found that a preoperative ejection fraction of >0.50 was associated with a 5-year survival of 89%, but patients with an EF of <0.40 had a 38% 5-year survival rate. Boucher et al.[30] noted that the postoperative ejection fraction will likely be normal only when the preoperative resting EF is >0.60. Crawford et al.[23] found that the best predictor of postoperative ejection fraction is the preoperative ejection fraction. They observed increased mortality in patients having a postoperative ejection fraction of <0.50. Of 17 patients with an ejection fraction of <0.60 preoperatively, 15 had a postoperative ejection fraction of <0.50. Of 21 patients with an ejection fraction of <0.50 postoperatively, 15 had a preoperative ejection fraction of <0.60. On the basis of these data, mitral valve replacement should be considered before the ejection fraction is <0.60 and strongly considered before the ejection fraction is <0.50.

The predictors of suboptimal to poor results from mitral valve replacement in chronic mitral insufficiency include the following:

1. LV ejection fraction <0.60[23,30]
2. LV ejection fraction <0.50[17,23,25]
3. End-systolic wall stress to end-systolic volume index ratio <2.5[22]
4. Tension-volume ejection fraction <1.47 dynes/cm²/m²[39]
5. LV end-systolic volume index >50 ml/m²[23] to 60 ml/m²[40]
6. LV end-systolic dimension index >2.6 cm/m²[41]

Comparable criteria for mitral valve repair are not available at this time; however, as stated above, patients who are candidates for mitral valve repair may find themselves undergoing mitral valve replacement based upon intraoperative findings; therefore, it is prudent to evaluate patients as potential candidates for mitral valve replacement.[17] Surgical intervention should ideally be performed while predictors of good operative outcome are still in effect, but even if preoperative predictors of poor long-term results are present, many patients will experience significant symptomatic improvement after valve replacement or repair.

PERIOPERATIVE AND POSTOPERATIVE PROGNOSTIC DETERMINANTS

Intraoperative and Perioperative Factors

Postoperative prognosis is influenced by the type of surgery for mitral regurgitation (repair versus replacement); the operative and perioperative management expertise; the level of patient education during the perioperative period, including information about endocarditis prophylaxis and anticoagulation therapy; and the quality of long-term care.[28]

Type of Prosthesis

Two studies[42,43] have demonstrated similar up to 7-year outcomes with mechanical prosthetic and bioprosthetic valves. However, in patients under the age of 35, the risk of bioprosthetic valve failure is high. Over the age of 50, the risk of bioprosthetic valve failure is reduced.[28,44] Whether a bioprosthetic or a mechanical valve is selected involves consideration of patient age, compliance, and anticoagulation risk-benefit issues. Rahimtoola[28] emphasizes that valve-related problems are more significantly influenced by patient-related issues than the type of prosthesis.

CONCLUSIONS

Major compensatory mechanisms in chronic mitral insufficiency include (1) increased LV and left atrial size with increased compliance, and (2) eccentric hypertrophy. Eventually, without operative intervention, decompensation occurs as (1) LV afterload increases, (2) the LV mass-to-volume ratio decreases, and (3) because the annular dilation resulting from LV enlargement results in worsening of the mitral regurgitation.

Careful analysis of natural history versus postoperative outcomes indicate that mitral valve surgery provides marginally significant long-term survival benefits but significant symptomatic improvement in most patients.

Surgery for moderate to severe chronic mitral insufficiency is advised for patients with functional class 3 to class 4 symptoms and selected patients in NYHA functional class 2. Mitral valve surgery should be carefully considered before reaching the objective parameters listed in the section on Chronic Mitral Regurgitation: Prognostic Factors.

Mitral valve repair provides several advantages over mitral valve replacement, including preservation of LV function and reduced postoperative rates of infective endocarditis and thromboembolic complications. However, since the final decision about mitral valve repair versus replacement is necessarily made intraoperatively, patients who are candidates for mitral valve surgery must be assessed as potential candidates for mitral valve replacement.

ACKNOWLEDGMENT

We wish to acknowledge Ms. Sharon Binyon for her excellent preparation of the manuscript.

REFERENCES

1. Rapaport E: Natural history of aortic and mitral valve disease. Am J Cardiol 35:221, 1975
2. Carabello BA: Mitral regurgitation. Part 1. Basic pathophysiological principles. Mod Concepts Cardiovasc Dis 57:53, 1988
3. Braunwald E: Valvular heart disease. p. 1023. In Braunwald E (ed): Heart Disease. 3rd Ed. WB Saunders, Philadelphia, 1988
4. Ross J, Sonnenblick EH, Taylor RR et al: Diastolic geometry and sarcomere lengths in the chronically dilated canine left ventricle. Circ Res 28:49, 1971
5. Schuler G, Peterson KL, Johnson A et al: Temporal response of left ventricular performance to mitral valve surgery. Circulation 59:1218, 1979
6. Wong CYH, Spotnitz HM: Systolic and diastolic properties of the human left ventricle during valve replacement for chronic mitral regurgitation. Am J Cardiol 47:40, 1981
7. Corin WJ, Monrad ES, Murakami T et al: The relationship of afterload to ejection performance in chronic mitral regurgitation. Circulation 76:59, 1987
8. Wisenbaugh T: Does normal pump function belie muscle dysfunction in patients with chronic severe mitral regurgitation? Circulation 77:515, 1988
9. Cheitlin MD, Bonow RO, Parmley WW et al: Task force II: acquired valvular heart disease. J Am Coll Cardiol 6: 1209, 1985
10. Grossman W: Profiles in valvular heart disease. p. 359. In Grossman W (ed): Cardiac Catheterization and Angiography. 3rd Ed. Lea & Febiger, Philadelphia, 1986
11. Croft CH, Lipscomb K, Mathis K et al: Limitations of qualitative angiographic grading in aortic or mitral regurgitation. Am J Cardiol 53:1593, 1984
12. Abbasi AS, Allen MW, DeCristofaro D, Ungar I: Detection and estimation of the degree of mitral regurgitation by range-gated pulsed Doppler echocardiography. Circulation 61:143, 1980
13. Spain MG, Smith MD, Grayburn PA et al: Quantitative assessment of mitral regurgitation by Doppler color flow imaging: angiographic and hemodynamic correlations. J Am Coll Cardiol 13:585, 1989
14. Sorenson SG, O'Rourke RA, Chaudhuri TK: Noninvasive quantitation of valvular regurgitation by gated equilibrium radionuclide angiography. Circulation 62:1089, 1980
15. Aurigemma G, Reichek N, Schiebler M et al: Evaluation of mitral regurgitation by cine magnetic resonance imaging. Am J Cardiol 66:621, 1990
16. Munoz S, Gallardo J, Diaz-Gorrin JR, Medina O: Influence of surgery on the natural history of rheumatic mitral and aortic valve disease. Am J Cardiol 35:234, 1975
17. Kulick DL, Rahimtoola SH: Selection of patients for cardiac valve replacement: p. 257. In Braunwald E (ed): Heart Disease—Update. 3rd Ed. WB Saunders, Philadelphia, 1990
18. Karp RB, Mills N, Edmunds LH: Coronary artery bypass grafting in the presence of valvular disease. Circulation, suppl I. 79:I–182, 1989
19. Czer LSC, Gray RJ, DeRobertis MA et al: Mitral valve replacement: impact of coronary artery disease and determinants of prognosis after revascularization. Circulation, suppl. I. 70:I–198, 1984.
20. Karp RB: Mitral valve replacement and coronary artery bypass grafting. Ann Thorac Surg 34:480, 1982
21. Hammermeister KE, Fisher L, Kennedy JW et al: Prediction of late survival in patients with mitral valve disease from clinical, hemodynamic and quantitative angiographic variables. Circulation 57:341, 1978
22. Carabello BA, Nolan SP, McGuire LB: Assessment of preoperative left ventricular function in patients with mitral regurgitation: value of the end-systolic wall stress—end-systolic volume ratio. Circulation 64:1212, 1981
23. Crawford MH, Souchek J, Oprian CA et al: Determinants of survival and left ventricular performance after mitral valve replacement. Circulation 81:1173, 1990
24. Christakis GT, Weisel RD, David TE et al: Predictors of operative survival after valve replacement. Circulation, suppl I. 78:I–25, 1988
25. Phillips HR, Levine FH, Carter JE et al: Mitral valve replacement for isolated mitral regurgitation: analysis of clinical course and late postoperative left ventricular ejection fraction. Am J Cardiol 48:647, 1981
26. Ross J: Afterload mismatch in aortic and mitral valve disease: implications for surgical therapy. J Am Coll Cardiol 5:811, 1985
27. Greenberg B: Use of vasodilators for valvular insufficiency. Choices Cardiol 3:315, 1989
28. Rahimtoola SH: Perspective on valvular heart disease: an update. J Am Coll Cardiol 14:1, 1989

29. Kennedy JW, Doces JG, Stewart DK: Left ventricular function before and following surgical treatment of mitral valve disease. Am Heart J 97:592, 1979

30. Boucher CA, Bingham JB, Osbakken MD et al: Early changes in left ventricular size and function after correction of left ventricular volume overload. Am J Cardiol 47:991, 1981

31. Goldman ME, Mora F, Guarino T et al: Mitral valvuloplasty is superior to valve replacement for preservation of left ventricular function: an intraoperative two-dimensional echocardiographic study. J Am Coll Cardiol 10:568, 1987

32. Galloway AC, Colvin SB, Baumann FG et al: Current concepts of mitral valve reconstruction for mitral insufficiency. Circulation 78:1087, 1988

33. David TE, Uden DE, Strauss HD: The importance of the mitral apparatus in left ventricular function after correction of mitral regurgitation. Circulation, suppl II. 68:II–76, 1983

34. Lessana A, Herreman F, Boffety C et al: Hemodynamic and cineangiographic study before and after mitral valvuloplasty (Carpentier's technique). Circulation, suppl II. 64:II–195, 1981

35. Bonchek LI, Olinger GN, Siegal R et al: Left ventricular performance after mitral reconstruction for mitral regurgitation. J Thorac Cardiovasc Surg 88:122, 1984

36. DiSesa VJ, Cohn LH, Collins JJ et al: Determinants of operative survival following combined mitral valve replacement and coronary revascularization. Ann Thorac Surg 34:482, 1982

37. Magovern JA, Pennock JL, Campbell DB et al: Risks of mitral valve replacement and mitral valve replacement with coronary artery bypass. Ann Thorac Surg 39:346, 1985

38. Sand ME, Naftel DC, Blackstone EH et al: A comparison of repair and replacement for mitral valve incompetence. J Thorac Cardiovasc Surg 94:208, 1987

39. Breisblatt W, Goodyer AVN, Zaret BL, Francis CK: An improved index of left ventricular function in chronic mitral regurgitation. Am J Cardiol 57:1105, 1986

40. Borow KM, Green LH, Mann T et al: End-systolic volume as a predictor of postoperative left ventricular performance and volume overload from valvular regurgitation. Am J Med 68:655, 1980

41. Zile MR, Gaasch WH, Carroll JD, Levine HJ: Chronic mitral regurgitation: predictive value of preoperative echocardiographic indexes of left ventricular function and wall stress. J Am Coll Cardiol 3:235, 1984

42. Hammermeister KE, Henderson WG, Burchfiel CM et al: Comparison of outcome after valve replacement with a bioprosthesis versus a mechanical prosthesis: initial 5 year results of a randomized trial. J Am Coll Cardiol 10:719, 1987

43. Bloomfield P, Kitchen AH, Wheatley DJ et al: A prospective evaluation of the Björk-Shiley, Hancock and Carpentier-Edwards heart valve prostheses. Circulation 73:1213, 1986

44. Jamieson WRE, Rosado LJ, Muniro AI et al: Carpentier-Edwards standard porcine bioprosthesis: primary tissue failure (structural valve deterioration) by age groups. Ann Thorac Surg 46:155, 1988

45. Ramanathan KB, Knowles J, Connor MJ et al: Natural history of chronic mitral insufficiency: relation of peak systolic pressure/end-systolic volume ratio of morbidity and mortality. J Am Coll Cardiol 3:1412, 1984

46. Hochreiter C, Niles N, Devereux RB et al: Mitral regurgitation: relationship of noninvasive descriptors of right and left ventricular performance to clinical and hemodynamic findings and to prognosis in medically and surgically treated patients. Circulation 73:900, 1986

19
Aortic Valve Stenosis

Arthur Selzer

Aortic stenosis represents a deformity of the aortic valve that narrows the outflow orifice from the left ventricle to the point of offering resistance to flow, manifested by higher pressure in the ventricle than the aorta and producing a pressure gradient. The valve is either completely competent during diastole, or it may be associated with trivial aortic regurgitation. The term *valvular aortic stenosis* is frequently used, as distinguished from *subvalvular stenosis (subaortic stenosis)* and *supravalvular aortic stenosis.*

ETIOLOGY AND PATHOLOGY

The aortic valve may be deformed at birth or may be altered during life by various pathologic processes. Consequently, three types of aortic stenosis are recognized[1-5]:

Congenital aortic stenosis. In this type of aortic stenosis, there may be a fusion of the commissures, leaving a central small opening or a "unicommissural valve" in which the fused valve tissue has a horseshoe appearance. The term congenital aortic stenosis should not be applied to a bicuspid aortic valve that usually functions normally for decades but that may be a site of secondary changes causing stenosis or incompetence later in life.

Inflammatory aortic stenosis: The cause of inflammatory aortic stenosis is rheumatic fever. Once widely prevalent throughout the world, rheumatic fever has almost disappeared from most developed countries but still represents a major health problem in many third world countries. Valvular stenosis produced by rheumatic fever represents a late result of scarring of the initial rheumatic lesions on the valve leaflets.[6] The prime target of rheumatic fever is the mitral valve. The time interval from the acute stage to the development of significant mitral stenosis ranges from one to five decades; aortic stenosis develops more slowly and is seldom found less than two decades after the attack. Aortic stenosis is a less common consequence of rheumatic fever, present in less than one-half of cases of chronic rheumatic heart disease. It is usually present in combination with mitral valve disease; pure aortic stenosis occurs in only 5% cases of rheumatic heart disease.[1]

Degenerative aortic stenosis: This is a disease of old age, found as one of two subsets: calcific aortic stenosis developing in patients with congenital bicuspid aortic valve, in which the degenerative process is secondary, and senile calcification of a normal tricuspid aortic valve. Thus, significant aortic stenosis of congenital etiology occurs in infants or children; inflammatory aortic stenosis is a disease of middle age. Degenerative aortic stenosis occurs in the sixth or seventh decade in its secondary form (bicuspid aortic stenosis) and in the eighth or ninth decade in its primary form.

The pathology of stenotic aortic valves differs in the congenital and inflammatory varieties from that in the degenerative etiology (Fig. 19-1). In the former, there is a fixed reduced opening during systole produced by fusion of the commissures. Patients surviving beyond middle age may show superimposed calcification of aortic cusps. Degenerative aortic stenosis does not affect valvular commissures that remain free. Stenosis

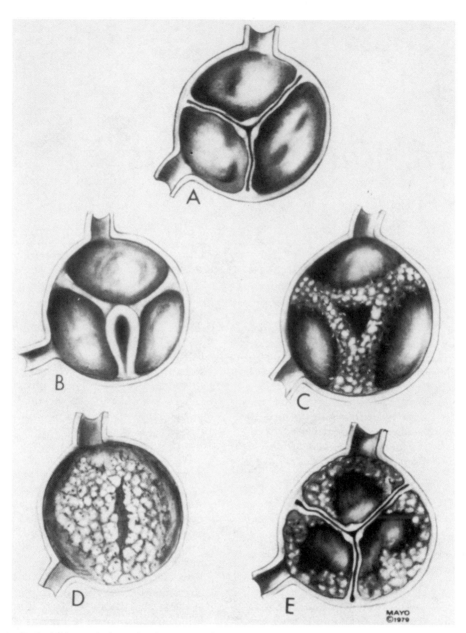

Fig. 19-1. Pathologic varieties of valvular aortic stenosis. **(A)** Normal aortic valve. **(B)** Congenital aortic stenosis. **(C)** Inflammatory (rheumatic) aortic stenosis. **(D)** Degenerative (calcific) aortic stenosis of the secondary variety, based on congenital bicuspid valve. **(E)** Primary degenerative (calcific) aortic stenosis. (From Edwards,[2] by permission of Mayo Foundation.)

is caused by an inability of the stiff, heavy calcified cusps to be lifted open under physiologic pressure generated by the left ventricle.

In the United States and other Western countries, aortic stenosis is predominantly a disease of old age. Degenerative varieties of aortic stenosis, often referred to as *calcific aortic stenosis*, represent the bulk of cases requiring surgical treatment. Cardiovascular surgeons report that the commonest variety of aortic stenosis requiring valve replacement is calcific infiltration of congenital bicuspid aortic valve. Although no good statistics are available, it may be assumed that, in the third world, a high proportion of cases are of rheumatic etiology.

PATHOPHYSIOLOGY

With the exception of congenital aortic stenosis, the disease process narrowing the aortic orifice involves a slow, chronic progression. The size of the aortic orifice during systole has to be reduced to less than one-half its original size in order to interfere with left ventricular (LV) systolic outflow. The earliest effect of reduction of aortic outflow orifice is a change from laminar to turbulent flow, manifesting as a murmur, at which point no transvalvular gradient is present. A low gradient of some 20 mmHg develops when the aortic orifice is reduced to about 1.5 cm^2 for an average adult heart. Moderately severe aortic stenosis is present when the size of the orifice falls below 1.0 cm^2; severe aortic stenosis is present when the valve area is less than 0.7 cm^2.

Estimation of the area of the orifice size is based on a hydraulic formula using data obtained during cardiac catheterization. The two critical measurements determining the area are transvalvular pressure gradient and the magnitude of blood flow through the orifice. However, there is no straight line relationship between the two: the flow through the orifice is related to the square root of the pressure gradient, which means that for each orifice size, changes in flow (i.e., cardiac output) are associated with changes in pressure gradient of much higher magnitude. For example, if the cardiac output were reduced to one-half its original size, the pressure gradients would fall to one-fourth its previous level.[7]

The transvalvular pressure gradient is frequently used as an index of the severity of aortic stenosis. This index reflects the extent of stenosis only in patients in whom a normal or near-normal cardiac output is expected. Thus, in late-stage aortic stenosis, when heart failure may lead to a fall in cardiac output, transvalvular pressure gradient is often misleadingly low and, if relied on, may grossly underestimate aortic stenosis.

The consequence of significant aortic stenosis is increased workload on the left ventricle.[8] Inasmuch as the systolic pressure in the aorta is determined by systemic peripheral resistance, thus independent of aortic ejection of LV function, the systolic pressure in the left ventricle is the sum of systolic pressure in the aorta and the transvalvular pressure gradient. As an example, in an average case of moderately severe to severe aortic stenosis, ventricular pressure may be 220/10 and aortic pressure 110/80.

The response of the LV myocardium to pressure overload is the development of concentric hypertrophy, that is, increase thickness of the LV wall without an increase in the volume of the LV cavity. By contrast, volume overload (e.g., in aortic regurgitation) produces excentric hypertrophy, that is, increased wall thickness with an enlarged ventricular cavity.

LV hypertrophy increases the strength of contraction of that chamber, thereby fulfilling a compensatory role, that is, maintenance of circulation capable of satisfying all metabolic demand despite the increased workload. With increased severity of aortic stenosis, there is a progressive increase in LV muscle mass. However, at a certain point, the negative effect of hypertrophy may become apparent: cellular hypoxia or other metabolic abnormalities may develop producing fibrotic changes and eventually leading to a mismatch between metabolic demands and available perfusion. These changes precipitate the development of heart failure.

Aortic stenosis with resulting concentric hypertrophy is capable of producing two types of cardiac failure: systolic LV malfunction and diastolic LV malfunction. The former is in line with cardiac failure resulting from most cardiac disease (primary myocardial diseases or end effect of overload). It is characterized by an increased LV cavity, as shown by lowered ejection fraction, increased left-sided filling pressure with its secondary effects on the pulmonary circulation, and, often, a drop in cardiac output. Diastolic malfunction consists of the inability of the stiff and noncompliant left ventricle to fill adequately.[9,10] Here the systolic function of the left ventricle remains normal, as is the ejection fraction. Yet, inadequate ventricular filling in diastole may elevate LV filling pressure and may even produce pulmonary edema.

It is important to recognize the basic difference between concentric hypertrophy produced by pressure overload (aortic stenosis) and excentric hypertrophy produced by volume overload (aortic regurgitation). The latter is characterized by early dilation of the LV cavity. Systolic malfunction appears relatively early and may be associated with irreversible changes in the hypertrophic myocardium; namely, relief of the overload can no longer restore normal function; often, even improvement of LV function is no longer possible.

The consequences of aortic stenosis are more benign than those of aortic regurgitation; given comparable degrees of hypertrophy, the prognosis of aortic stenosis is much more favorable in its response to surgical treatment than that of aortic regurgitation.

In calcific aortic stenosis of the elderly, there is a major prognostic difference between systolic LV failure and diastolic LV failure. The former may present an ominous situation and may call for emergency surgical treatment; the reduced ejection fraction often associated with fall in cardiac output may cause an inordinate reduction of LV pressure, thereby reducing the force opening the aortic cusps (see above).

The mode of ejection of blood through a stenotic aortic valve produces certain consequences unique to this lesion. Reflexes originating in the left ventricle may affect baroreceptor control of the peripheral circulation during exercise, which may lead to a precipitous fall in systemic pressure, resulting in syncope.[11] Furthermore, the discrepancy between the high intraventricular pressure and the low perfusion pressure of the coronary arteries (perfused under aortic pressure) often produces myocardial ischemia in the form of effort angina—in the absence of coronary disease.[11,12]

NATURAL HISTORY

Aortic stenosis represents a purely mechanical lesion that produces pressure overload (systolic overload) on the left ventricle. It is most often a progressive disease, with its course extending over decades. The natural history and prognosis of aortic stenosis depend on the severity of the lesion and the capacity of the ventricle to adapt to the overload by means of compensatory hypertrophy.[13] There is a straight relationship between these two factors and the course of aortic stenosis is a given case. Complications that could abruptly alter the prognosis at any stage of the disease are rare, in contrast to other valve lesions. The risk of infective endocarditis is much rarer in aortic stenosis than in aortic regurgitation; proneness to atrial flutter or fibrillation (as is present in mitral stenosis) does not exist.

Progression of aortic stenosis depends on the etiologic variety of this lesion. In congenital aortic stenosis, narrowing of the outflow orifice is there since birth; further changes are variable. Wagner et al.[14] reported that in 294 medically treated cases of congenital aortic stenosis, one-third showed an increased transvalvular gradient in longitudinal observation, 12 patients showed a decrease, and the remainder showed no change in the severity of the lesion. The inflammatory variety of aortic stenosis is characterized by postrheumatic scarring, which fuses the valve commissures. This is a finite process, however, that at a certain point becomes complete in determining the severity of aortic stenosis. From this point on, further progression is very slow and depends on secondary deposition of calcium in the cusps later in life. Degenerative aortic stenosis, which depends entirely on calcification of the cusps, progresses at variable rate, but often very rapidly.

Inasmuch as calcific aortic stenosis accounts for the greatest majority of cases, its natural history is best known. Early deposition of calcium, as stated, first narrows the orifice mildly, producing a systolic murmur without a pressure gradient. This phenomenon, a precursor of degenerative aortic stenosis, is often referred to as *aortic sclerosis*. Further progression of calcification produces mild aortic stenosis, which may have no significant effect on circulatory dynamics. Eventually the calcification produces increasing degrees of stenosis up to "critical" aortic stenosis, with a valve area of less than 0.5 cm^2. The development of symptoms varies a great deal. It is not unusual to reach this stage without any symptoms, as the patient is capable of unrestricted physical activity.

Looking at the natural history from the clinician's standpoint, the following stages can be recognized[1]:

Stage 1: Asymptomatic. The clinical diagnosis when the patient is asymptomatic, in most cases, recognized on the basis of routine examination or as an accidental finding in patients with other medical problems.
Stage 2: Prefailure symptoms. The presence of prefailure symptoms is found when cardiac performance by clinical and laboratory criteria is still normal, but the patient begins to suffer from symptoms related to aortic stenosis, still fully compensated (e.g., angina-like chest pain on exertion and/or attacks of exertional syncope).
Stage 3: LV failure. The patient is in this stage when effort tolerance is reduced by dyspnea; the patient may suffer from paroxysmal dyspnea.
Stage 4: Congestive heart failure. CHF encompasses fully developed biventricular failure.
Stage 5: Postoperative. At this stage, the patient has problems related to prosthetic valves or those following other interventional therapy.

As already emphasized, there are large individual variations regarding the timing of the development of cardiac symptoms. In general, symptomatic stages of aortic stenosis are progressively more ominous. Prefailure symptoms (e.g., angina and syncope) appear generally in the presence of severe aortic stenosis but are not present in all cases.[7] They are, as a rule, self-limited and reversible and least significant from the prognostic standpoint, largely because LV function tends to be normal and the overload fully compensated.

The development of LV failure represents a major

turning point in the natural history of LV failure. As explained, the two varieties of LV failure have different prognostic significance; therefore, appropriate identification of the type of failure is of considerable practical importance. Diastolic malfunction, the more benign of the two, may be subjected to medical therapy; systolic malfunction has to be considered an ominous prognostic sign and calls for evaluation of the patient from the standpoint of surgical treatment.

The stage of congestive heart failure (CHF) is almost always related to systolic malfunction, representing emergent consideration of surgical removal of the LV overload; it is probably the principal background condition responsible for sudden cardiac death, which is traditionally associated with aortic stenosis and which is rare in patients with well functioning left ventricles. Fully developed CHF is now relatively rare, as patients are usually operated on before its onset. It is primarily seen in patients in whom the underlying aortic stenosis has been missed or in patients in whom surgical treatment is contraindicated or refused.

THERAPEUTIC OPTIONS

Medical therapy for aortic stenosis plays a lesser role than in other valvular diseases and has to be always considered in its relationship to surgical treatment. During the long asymptomatic stage of aortic stenosis, standard prophylactic treatment for endocarditis is the only obligatory therapeutic step. When the patient enters the symptomatic stage, the type and severity of symptoms determine the choice between medical and interventional therapy. The symptomatic stages of aortic stenosis fall into two prognostic phases: (1) the benign phase, which has a favorable prognosis, in which individual decisions regarding timing of interventional therapy are indicated; and (2) the precarious phase, which carries a poor prognosis, requiring relief of overload as promptly as possible. The first phase includes asymptomatic patients and those with pre-failure symptoms (e.g., angina, syncope) and those with LV failure demonstrated to have diastolic malfunction. The second phase includes patients with systolic LV malfunction and those with CHF. A special category of patients includes those in whom interventional therapy is contraindicated or those who refuse surgical treatment. In these cases, medical therapy is the only option.

Aortic stenosis represents a single mechanical defect affecting the function of the heart: malfunction of the aortic valve. Theoretically, if the faulty valve could be replaced by one functioning flawlessly or could be repaired by successful restoration of normal function, this disease could be cured. Thus, it is not surprising that attempts to restore aortic valve function were among the earliest approaches to cardiac surgery. More than five decades ago,[15] encouraged by successful dilation of stenotic mitral valves and stenotic congenital pulmonary valves, procedures aimed at dilating aortic valves in the beating heart were performed. However, poor results, caused mostly by unacceptable aortic regurgitation, led to abandonment of this procedure. Since the development of cardiopulmonary bypass opened the field of surgery performed under direct vision in an open heart, two types of operations have been developed: aortic valvotomy applicable to congenital aortic stenosis, and valvuloplasty, consisting of mobilization of calcified stiff valve by removal of calcium ("debridement") from the cusps. Both procedures showed considerable immediate success: aortic valvotomy is still the standard method of treatment for congenital aortic stenosis in children and adults. Debridement has been abandoned, however, because redeposition of calcium on aortic valves has occurred in most cases, leading to restenosis of the valve.

The major breakthrough came around 1960, when a successful prosthetic valve was developed—the Starr-Edwards valve consisting of the plastic or metal ball in a cage.[15] During systole, the ball was ejected to the top of the cage with blood freely flowing around it; in diastole, the ball fell back into the ring inserted at the aortic orifice, preventing regurgitation. Despite many problems arising from the use of this prosthetic valve, in many patients spectacular successes could be observed with total reversal of heart failure.

During the past three decades, a great many models of prosthetic cardiac valves have been developed—a point indicating that no ideal valve is yet available. The most important problem related to prosthetic valves is thrombosis, which could be a source of systemic embolization or could develop in situ, eventually interfering with motion of the prosthesis. Other problems with ball valves include infection, mechanical failure, and appearance of aortic regurgitation. The function of ball valves is related to its size, which, in turn depends on the size of the patient's aortic annulus. There is some resistance to outflow produced by the blood encircling the ball, rather than flowing out straight. Later models of mechanical valves attempted to overcome some of the problems. Less thrombogenic material was used, and the ball was replaced by tilting disks. Parallel to the development of mechanical prosthetic valves, a variety of biologic prostheses have been tried; these include cadaver homograft; autograft (the use of patient's own pulmonary valve sutured into the aortic orifice); animal heterograft; and valves molded from human tissue, including some taken from the patient's own, such as pericardium, and fascia lata. Biologic valves were very much less thrombogenic, yet less durable than mechanical valves. The biologic valve prosthesis that has stood the test of time and that continues to be popular is commercially prepared porcine heterograft. These valves have an excellent record of low thrombogenesis (90% freedom from thromboembolism in 10 years, as reported in Magilligan's series).[16] The median lifetime of porcine valves is estimated at 13 years if "high-risk" patients are excluded.[17] The highest risk of early degeneration of porcine heterograft is young age. The use of this valve in children and adolescents has been abandoned, and the recommended use is above the age 35. Another high-risk factor is low cardiac output. It has also been suggested that female patients have more problems with this valve than are found among males patients.

The most important consideration regarding aortic valve prosthesis is the fact that, in the great majority of patients, a transvalvular gradient is still present occasionally at rest, but most often during exercise. This finding indicates that prosthetic valves have mild aortic stenosis rather than reestablishment of an entirely normal valve function. The presence or absence of a pressure gradient depends on the size of the prosthesis (i.e., the size of the aortic annulus). Only the largest valve approaches the normal flow into the aorta.

The most recent method of relief of aortic stenosis was developed approximately a decade ago in the form of balloon valvuloplasty.[16] Using the principle of successful dilation of stenotic lesions in arteries, percutaneous introduction of one or two balloons may permit considerable dilation of a stenotic valve orifice. Of the valves submitted for balloon valvuloplasty, the aortic valve probably has the poorest long-range success. Balloon separation of fused valve commissures, as is possible in mitral stenosis or congenital pulmonary stenosis, may produce lasting dilation of valve orifice, although seldom complete restoration of a free valve orifice. In the vast majority of cases of aortic stenosis, however, where the stenosis is produced by inability to move heavily calcified valve, the immediate success of balloon valvuloplasty may depend on the fracture of calcified valves. The high incidence of restenosis within months of the procedure has suggested that this method is suitable primarily for patients who are disqualified from open heart surgery or as a temporary palliative procedure to be followed by surgery.

TIMING OF INTERVENTIONAL THERAPY

There are two ways of approaching the selection of patients with aortic stenosis for interventional treatment: (1) accepting the hypothesis that aortic stenosis is a purely mechanical problem that can be eliminated by surgical intervention (i.e., making aortic stenosis a surgical disease that can be corrected as soon as the severity of aortic stenosis reaches a significant hemodynamic level); and (2) carefully evaluating the prognosis of each patient medically treated, matching it with estimated prognosis of surgically treated patient. The first approach would be justifiable if an ideal prosthetic valve were available. The second approach is a realistic appraisal of the limitations of the available interventional therapy.

It has been mentioned in a preceding section that the natural history of aortic stenosis can be divided into two prognostic phases: the benign phase and the precarious phase. In reviewing data from the presurgical era, Ross and Braunwald[18] found that the survival curve of aortic stenosis shows a gentle downward course (representing the benign phase), which abruptly changes into a precipitous fall of survival. According to today's concepts, the sharp angle is reached when systolic left ventricular (LV) malfunction becomes apparent. The "precarious" phase represents an absolute indication for interventional therapy as the prognosis of unoperated patients at this stage is far worse than can be expected with a postsurgical course.

Selection of patients for interventional therapy during the benign phase often presents considerable difficulties and is subject to controversy. In order to consider the principal factors in decision-making, it is necessary to review briefly some of the factors needed to appraise individual prognosis of a patient.

The asymptomatic stage of aortic stenosis extends for many years or decades and, as a rule, involves progression of the degree of stenosis, ranging from minimal to rapid development of critical stenosis. It has been pointed out that symptoms are likely to develop in the presence of advanced stenosis but, even in critical stenosis, the patient may remain asymptomatic and fully active. The progressive nature of aortic stenosis brought about for consideration the question of whether prophylactic operation could forestall the late effects of aortic stenosis. Operating on patients with significant aortic stenosis before symptoms appear would provide an attractive possibility, considering the early removal of the mechanical barrier in the aortic orifice, provided that treatment could be performed with minimal risk and the relief could be permanent. Inasmuch as symptoms guide the prognosis and timing of the interventional treatment, surgical treatment of asymptomatic patients would be particularly valuable, if (1) sudden cardiac death could be prevented, or (2) irreversible LV malfunction could be obviated. The prophylactic approach to interventional therapy has stirred considerable controversy. In recent years, a consensus evolved opposing surgery in asymptomatic patients—a consensus accepted by most but not all experts.[19–21] The compelling arguments involve the observation that sudden cardiac death, although occurring more often in aortic stenosis than in other valve lesions, is very rare in the absence of severe symptoms. Furthermore, irreversible damage to the function of the left ventricle seldom develops in aortic stenosis and is easily preventable if surgery is planned during the precarious phase of aortic stenosis. Another cogent argument against early operations is the fact that, in many patients, progression of aortic stenosis is so slow that many years of asymptomatic stage may elapse until the warning symptoms appear.

In the stage of what one may call "benign symptoms" (i.e., angina, syncope, diastolic LV malfunction), individual appraisal is made, on the basis of the severity of aortic stenosis and the degree of clinical disability produced by symptoms. Medical treatment consisting of antianginal drugs or the use of calcium channel blocking agents or β-adrenergic agents for diastolic ventricular malfunction represents an acceptable option. Obviously, asymptomatic or mildly symptomatic patients provided medical therapy must be carefully followed, particularly in regard to the progression of the severity of aortic stenosis (which can now be noninvasively evaluated by echo-Doppler studies). Another important factor in evaluation of the patient is the relationship of symptoms to aortic stenosis. The principal variety of aortic stenosis—degenerative calcific stenosis, affects primarily older patients. Syncope caused by factors other than aortic stenosis, angina due to coexisting coronary artery disease (CAD), or dyspnea caused by obstructive pulmonary disease may provide an alternative explanation of the patient's symptoms. The presence of symptoms in patients with only moderate degree of aortic stenosis should be considered with great caution as an indication for surgery.

In evaluating patients for interventional therapy, one has to consider the other side of the equation: the risk of operation and the postoperative course. The usual mortality figures for aortic valve replacement are quoted as at 2 to 10% during the perioperative period. It is important, however, to recognize that these are the best figures obtained from tertiary high-volume cardiac referral centers and cannot be considered overall averages, particularly in the United States, where there are 793 open-heart surgical units, many located in community hospitals. Furthermore, risk of interventional treatment includes the course and complications of prosthetic valves. Considering the fact that the great majority of patients with prosthetic aortic valves show significant relief of symptoms and reduction in LV overload, indications in patients with the precarious phase of aortic stenosis are clear cut. However, in the "benign" phase of aortic stenosis, careful individual analysis, perhaps combined with a period of observation regarding progress of disease, is justified.

PROSTHETIC AORTIC VALVE DISEASE

As stated, the size of the aortic prosthetic valve depends on the size of the aortic ring to which the prosthesis is to be attached. Large valve prostheses that permit aortic ejection without any gradient are in the minority. As a rule, some transvalvular gradient is present, indicating residual mild aortic stenosis. Perhaps the most important aspects of the valve size is whether the relief of LV overload is complete enough to induce *regression* of LV hypertrophy (as determined by ECG or echocardiography). Regression of LV hypertrophy represents the best overall prognostic sign.

The second prognostic aspect of aortic valve prosthesis is its durability. Determination of durability of prosthetic valves requires years of observation. Tragic consequences have been observed with some prostheses that showed considerable short-term advantages but that later developed serious malfunctions. The widely used porcine heterograft has many advantages and fair durability but is limited to older patients. Deterioration of this graft consists of calcification of the leaflets, which can produce aortic stenosis or regurgitation. While it maintains its function on the average of a decade (median life 13 years), early degeneration may develop in some patients. It is noteworthy that reoperation for replacement of malfunctioning prosthetic valve carries a considerably higher operative risk than does the original operation.

Among complications altering the course of prognosis of patients with prosthetic aortic valves, the most important is thromboembolism. Thrombus formation on prosthetic material occurs with great frequency; therefore, an anticoagulant regimen has been introduced as a routine treatment in all patients, except in the presence of specific contraindications, soon after the introduction of mechanical valve prostheses. The enthusiasm concerning bioprosthetic valves was largely due to the greatly reduced risk of thromboembolism. Bioprosthetic valves are being used without anticoagulant regimen, often with platelet antiaggregant aspirin. Nevertheless, protection from thrombus formation is not complete in either group of patients. The risks of thromboembolism include systemic embolization or thrombus formation on the valve, or both, eventually interfering with its function.

Infective endocarditis represents another complication, which though rare (probably less than 5%), may have a devastating effect on the course. Endocarditis developing within 4 to 8 weeks after the operation ("early endocarditis") is often caused by difficult-to-treat organisms, such as staphylococci or fungi, and is assumed to represent contamination during the perioperative period. Late endocarditis resembles infection on unoperated valves and can be cured by anti-biotic therapy in most cases. Early endocarditis almost always requires reoperation and replacement of the infected prosthesis at a high operative risk. Other complications include perivalvular leaks producing aortic regurgitation and, rarely, valve dehiscence may develop, requiring prompt surgery.

SUMMARY

Aortic stenosis is a mechanical lesion producing reduced aortic orifice in systole. There are three etiologies of aortic stenosis: congenital, inflammatory (rheumatic), and degenerative ("calcific aortic stenosis"). In the Western world, the great majority of cases of aortic stenosis involve the degenerative variety; aortic stenosis is thus a disease of the seventh, eight, and ninth decades of life. Stenosis of the valve is usually progressive; however, the rate of progression varies widely, ranging from a nonprogressive form over a few decades to a rapidly progressive form, particularly in calcific stenosis.

The natural history of aortic stenosis involves two principal phases: the benign phase, which includes the long asymptomatic stage and the presence of some early, nondisabling symptoms; and the precarious stage, which is present when systolic malfunction of the hypertrophied LV develops, characterized by high mortality and a tendency to sudden cardiac death.

The LV overload producing hypertrophy of that chamber can be relieved by the removal of stenotic valve and replacement with a valve prosthesis or, in rare cases, by repair of the valve. Interventional therapy is the only effective treatment for aortic stenosis. Such treatment is mandatory in patients in the precarious phase of the disease. Those in the benign phase are considered candidates for interventional therapy only after careful evaluation of all factors and estimation of the prognosis of unoperated patients against the risk and consequences of surgical therapy.

REFERENCES

1. Selzer A: Changing aspects of the natural history of valvular aortic stenosis. N Engl J Med 317:91, 1987
2. Edwards JE: Calcific aortic stenosis: pathologic features. Mayo Clin Proc 36:44, 1961
3. Pomerance A: Pathogenesis of aortic stenosis and its relation to age. Br Heart J 34:569, 1972
4. Pomerance A: Pathology and valvular heart disease. Br Heart J 34:347, 1972
5. Davis MJ: Pathology of Cardiac Valves. Butterworth, London, 1980, p. 18
6. Tweedy PS. The pathogenesis of valvular thickening in rheumatic heart disease. Br Heart J 18:173, 1956
7. Wagner S, Selzer A: Patterns of progression of aortic stenosis: a longitudinal hemodynamic study, Circulation 65:709, 1982
8. Sasayama S, Ross J, Jr, Franklin D et al: Adaptation of the left ventricle to chronic pressure overload. Circ Res 38:172, 1976
9. Peterson KL, Tsuji J, Johnson A et al: Diastolic left ventricular pressure-volume and stress-strain relations in patients with aortic stenosis and left ventricular hypertrophy. Circulation 58:77, 1978
10. Dineen E, Brent BN: Aortic valve stenosis: comparison of patients with to those without chronic congestive failure. Am J Cardiol 57:419, 1986
11. Mark AL, Kioschos JM, Abboud FM et al: Abnormal vascular responses to exercise in patients with aortic stenosis. J Clin Invest 52:1138, 1973
12. Marcus ML, Doty DB, Hiratzka LF et al: Decreased coronary reserve: a mechanism for angina pectoris in patients with aortic stenosis and normal coronary arteries. N Engl J Med 307:1362, 1982
13. Lombard JT, Selzer A: Valvular aortic stenosis: clinical and hemodynamic profile of patients. Ann Intern Med 106:292, 1984
14. Wagner JR, Ellison RC, Keane JF et al: Clinical course in aortic stenosis. Circulation, suppl I. 56:47, 1977
15. Selzer A: Fifty years in cardiology: a personal perspective. Circulation 77:955, 1988
16. Magilligan DJ, Jr, Lewis JW, Jr, Stein P, Adams A: The porcine bioprosthetic heart valve experience at 15 years. Ann Thorac Surg 48:324, 1989
17. Starr A, Grunbenmeier GL: The expected life time of porcine valves. Ann Thorac Surg 48:317, 1989
18. Ross J, Jr, Braunwald E: Aortic stenosis. Circulation, suppl 5. 38:61, 1974
19. Pellikka PA, Nishimura RA, Bailey KR, Tajik AJ: The natural history of adults with asymptomatic hemodynamically significant aortic stenosis. J Am Coll Cardiol 15: 1012, 1991
20. Braunwald E: On the natural history of severe aortic stenosis. J Am Coll Cardiol 15:1018, 1990
21. Rackley CE, Edward JE, Wallace RB, Katz NM: Aortic valve disease. p. 795. In Hurst JW, Schlant RC (eds): The Heart, Arteries, Veins. 7th Ed. McGraw-Hill, New York, 1990

20

Risk Assessment, Timing of Surgery, and Prognosis of Patients With Aortic Regurgitation

Robert Stauffer
Amar S. Kapoor

The critical question in assessing the risk of aortic regurgitation is the timing of aortic valve replacement. The examiner must weigh the risks of operative mortality and the long-term complications of aortic valve replacement versus the risk of irreversible left ventricular (LV) dysfunction and the inherent associated increases in morbidity and mortality. In light of the fact that the operative mortality is approximately 3 to 5% and the long-term complication rate can be as high as 30 to 50% at 6 years,[1] the decision to replace the aortic valve must be made on firm clinical grounds. One must therefore, have a solid understanding of both the natural history of aortic regurgitation and the effect of aortic valve replacement.

The algorithm shown in Figure 20-1 is a simplified attempt at classifying patients with aortic regurgitation on the basis of clinical status. The first division is between acute and chronic aortic regurgitation. Because of the inability of the left ventricle to tolerate a sudden increase in volume, numerous studies have shown that the outcome associated with surgical correction is superior to that with medical treatment.[2-7] The decision as when to intervene in chronic aortic regurgitation is much more complex and is the primary focus of this chapter.

RISK ASSESSMENT OF CHRONIC AORTIC REGURGITATION

As Figure 20-1 depicts, the first assessment in chronic aortic regurgitation involves determining whether the patient is asymptomatic or symptomatic. Thus, the most important step in the initial assessment is a good history. Many patients may not complain of symptoms initially but, on further questioning, they may realize that they have been limiting their activities compared with their previous abilities. Furthermore, an objective test such as the treadmill may help quantify a patient's symptoms. The differentiation between asymptomatic and symptomatic patients is cru-

269

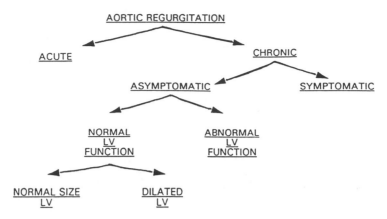

Fig. 20-1. Simplified approach to assessing the risk of patients with aortic regurgitation.

cial because they have vastly different natural histories. We will begin by discussing the symptomatic patient.

RISK ASSESSMENT OF SYMPTOMATIC PATIENTS

The symptomatic patient with aortic regurgitation presents with dyspnea on exertion and with signs of increased pulmonary pressures. Other symptoms include, rarely, angina with or without underlying coronary artery disease (CAD) and occasionally syncope or presyncope. The natural history of symptomatic patients without surgical intervention is poor. The 1-year survival rate after an episode of congestive heart failure (CHF) is approximately 30 to 50 percent[8] with a 5-year survival rate of 15%.[9] In symptomatic patients without CHF, the 5-year survival was 68 to 78% and at 10 years 34 to 66%. The major cause of death is progressive CHF or infective endocarditis. Figure 20-2 shows the natural history data from Rappaport[10] and

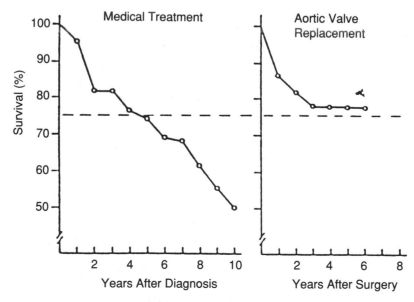

Fig. 20-2. Mortality data comparing a group of patients treated medically (Rappaport[10]) versus a group that had aortic valve replacement (Greeves et al.[11]) showing the benefit of surgical intervention.

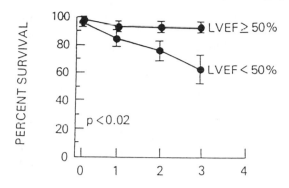

Fig. 20-3. Forman's study depicting the prognostic significance of preoperative left ventricular ejection fraction (LVEF) on survival after aortic valve replacement in symptomatic patients with chronic aortic regurgitation. (From Forman et al.,[12] with permission.)

compares them with data from patients who underwent aortic valve replacement.[11] These figures show that, without surgical intervention, the long-term prognosis of symptomatic patients is poor, forming the basis for the recommendation valves be replaced in symptomatic patients, both for symptomatic improvement and for increased longevity.

The next step in assessing the patient's risk once the patient has been determined to be symptomatic and in need of an aortic valve replacement should be the preoperative risk evaluation of the patient's long-term prognosis after aortic valve replacement. The most important predictor of outcome after aortic valve replacement is LV function. Figure 20-3 depicts a study by Forman et al.,[12] illustrating that patients with an ejection fraction of less than 50% had a 3-year survival of only 65% compared with 93% if the ejection fraction was greater than 50%. In addition, Greeves et al.[11] showed that patients with class 3 and class 4 symptoms of CHF had a substantially better outcome if LV function was normal, with a difference in survival of 63% versus 90% at 3 years. Thus, even patients with severe symptoms do well postoperatively if they have good LV function. Fractional shortening using echocardiography has also been evaluated as a modality in assessing LV function. A National Institutes of Health (NIH) study showed a significant reduction in survival among patients whose fractional shortening was less than 29% (62% versus 91%).[13] Figure 20-4 depicts this study. These studies suggest that aortic valve replacement can be delayed until symptoms develop in patients with normal LV function, since it has been determined that these patients do well even if symptomatic. However, once symptoms do develop in a patient with decreased LV function, surgery is then undertaken at a much greater risk.

The LV end-systolic size has also been found to be a strong predictor of postoperative outcome. Studies done at both the Mayo Clinic[14] and the NIH[15] have

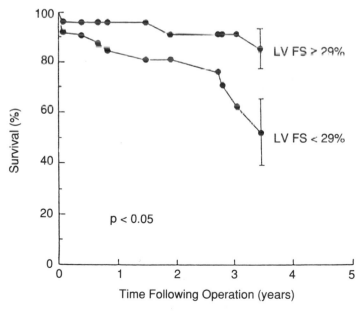

Fig. 20-4. National Institutes of Health study depicting the prognostic significance of preoperative left ventricular (LV) fractional shortening on postoperative survival for symptomatic patients with chronic aortic regurgitation.

shown that an LV end-systolic dimension greater than 55 mm on M-mode echocardiography predicts significantly lower long-term survival. Figure 20-5 shows the results of Bonow's group at the NIH. Furthermore, Borow et al.[16] used contrast angiography and Boucher et al.[17] used radionuclliotide angiography to show that LV end-systolic volume was the strongest preoperative predictor of postoperative end-diastolic volume and postoperative contractility. Furthermore, Borow's study showed that LV systolic volume was the strongest predictor of perioperative death, particularly if the systolic volume was greater than 90 ml/m². In these studies, the left ventricular end-diastolic volume was found to be less accurate at predicting postoperative outcome. It should be noted that persistent LV dilation after surgery is strongly associated with increased risk of progressive CHF and greatly increased mortality.[14,18–21] Looking at both fractional shortening and the LV end-systolic dimension, Henry et al.[13] found that out of 13 patients with both a fractional shortening of less than 29% and a LV dimension greater than 55 mm, nine died and two of the remaining patients had CHF postoperatively. In a study by Roman et al.[22] at New York Hospital, 86% of patients with an LV end-systolic dimension of less than 55 mm had a normal LV size after surgery, while 81% of patients with persistent LV dilation postoperatively had an LV end-systolic dimension of greater than 55 mm preoperatively. Thus, patients with increased an LV end-systolic dimension of have an increased likelihood of persistent

LV dilation and an inherent increased risk of progressive CHF and death.

The response of the left ventricle to exercise has also been looked at as a prognostic indicator. Most symptomatic patients will have a decrease in ejection fraction with exercise, even with a normal resting ejection fraction. However, no level of exercise response has been associated with decreased survival or irreversible dysfunction. Instead, there is growing evidence that the LV dysfunction is reversible after aortic valve replacement. Furthermore, there is a strong correlation between LV end-systolic dimension and the response to exercise.[23] Therefore, the response of the left ventricle to exercise has not been a useful prognostic indicator and does not offer additional information beyond that of the much-simpler-to-assess echocardiographic estimate of LV end-systolic dimension.

The exercise capacity and the degree of symptoms, however, have been shown to be a strong predictor of postoperative outcome. The Mayo Clinic[11] and the University of Oregon[15] have demonstrated that patients in New York Heart Association (NYHA) class 1 and class 2 have a much better outcome than do the more symptomatic patients in class 3 and class 4. Figure 20-6 shows the improved survival of the less symptomatic patients. Furthermore, Bonow at the NIH looked objectively at exercise capacity, using a special treadmill protocol to assess exercise capacity. Figure 20-7 shows that patients able to exercise more than 22 minutes or at about 8 METS had 100% survival at 4

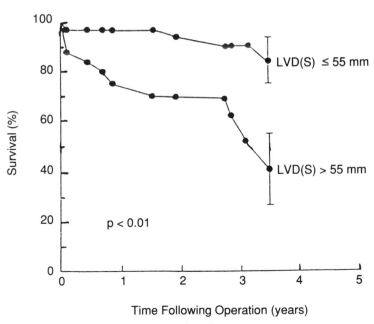

Fig. 20-5. Prognostic significance of preoperative left ventricular (LV) end-systolic dimension in symptomatic patients with chronic aortic regurgitation. (From Bonow et al.,[15] with permission.)

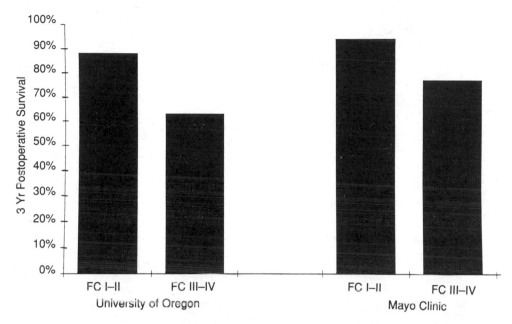

Fig. 20-6. Survival data comparing postoperative outcome versus New York Heart Association (NYHA) functional preoperative class, showing the superior outcome of the less symptomatic patients. (Data from Bonow et al.,[15] and Greeves et al.[11])

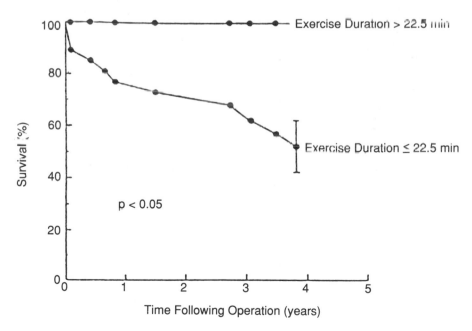

Fig. 20-7. Postoperative survival curve for patient's with aortic valve replacement based on their preoperative exercise capacity and ability to complete stage 1 of the National Institutes of Health (NIH) exercise protocol without symptoms. (From Bonow et al.,[21] with permission.)

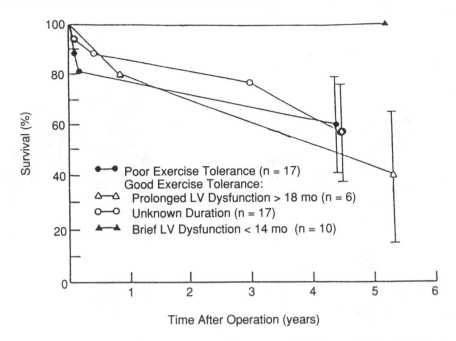

Fig. 20-8. Postoperative survival data from patients with preoperative left ventricular (LV) dysfunction showing the poor outcome of patients with prolonged left ventricular dysfunction. (From Bonow et al.,[24] with permission.)

years, while those who failed had significant mortality.[21]

The duration of LV function also dictates postoperative survival. Bonow et al.[24] looked at 37 patients and compared LV dysfunction lasting less than 14 months with LV dysfunction lasting more than 18 months. Figure 20-8 shows that patients with a short duration of LV dysfunction had excellent postoperative survival as compared with those with long-term LV dysfunction, even if the exercise capacity was preserved. Furthermore, reversal of LV dysfunction was also dependent on duration. Thus, in patients with aortic regurgitation and decreased LV function, reversibility of the ventricular function is dependent on both the severity of symptoms and the duration of the LV dysfunction.

Another modality used to assess whether LV dysfunction is reversible is the use of wall stress, the concept being that cardiac decompensation occurs when the ventricle can no longer enlarge to normalize wall stress. Gaasch et al.[20] looked at the end-diastolic radius-to-wall-thickness ratio and found that it may be

TABLE 20-1. Natural History Studies Illustrating the Long Duration of Symptom-Free Intervals in Patients With Aortic Regurgitation

Reference	No. of Pts.	% of Pts. Symptom Free at Specified Year			Groups Studied
		5	7	10	
Spagnuolo et al.[25]	174	98		95	Low risks (normal BP/ECG/CXR)
		25		5	High risk (SBP >140, DBP <40, LVH on ECG, cardiomegaly on CXR)
Goldschlager et al.[26]	126			100	11–20 years of age
				76	21–30 years of age, % of patients
				65	31–40 years of age, symptom free
				29	41–50 years of age, grouped by age
				23	51–60 years of age
				11	61–70 years of age
Bonow et al.[23]	77	81%	75%		

a strong predictor of LV regression after valve replacement. Further work assessing the clinical usefulness of wall stress may prove helpful in the future.

RISK ASSESSMENT OF ASYMPTOMATIC PATIENTS

In assessing the risk of the asymptomatic patient, one must understand the natural history both of asymptomatic patients with normal LV function and of those with abnormal LV function. The critical question to be asked is whether these patients have long periods of clinical stability that would permit delaying aortic valve replacement. Multiple natural history studies of patients with aortic regurgitation have shown that patients with a normal left ventricle have long periods of clinical stability without deterioration of LV function. Table 20-1 shows several of the natural history studies done in the past illustrating the long symptom-free intervals. Bonow et al.[23] followed 77 patients with normal LV function and aortic regurgitation for a mean period of 49 months. The patients had 3–4 plus aortic regurgitation (64/77) or a wide pulse pressure of greater than 70 (14/77). Patients were followed for the need for aortic valve replacement, which was performed either for symptoms or for decreased LV function. Of the 77 patients, 12 patients required an aortic valve replacement. A breakdown of these 12 patients revealed that six patients had symptoms with a normal left ventricle, five patients had both an abnormal left ventricle and symptoms, and one patient had an abnormal left ventricle and was asymptomatic. Figure 20-9 shows the clinical course of these patients. At 3 years, 90% of patients were asymptomatic, at 5 years 81% were asymptomatic, and at 7 years 75% were asymptomatic. The aortic valve replacement rate was approximately 4% per year.

A breakdown of these data shows a strong correlation between left ventricular end-systolic dimension and progression to aortic valve replacement. Patients with an left ventricular end-systolic dimension of less than 41 mm had no progression to aortic valve replacement, while only 31% of patients with an left ventricular end-systolic dimension greater than 50 mm were asymptomatic at follow-up. Figure 20-10 depicts these findings. Most importantly, of the 12 patients who eventually had aortic valve replacement, there was no mortality, LV dilation was reversed, and the left ventricular ejection fraction (LVEF) normalized in all patients. Another study done by the Oregon Health Sciences University and the University of California at San Francisco looked at 50 patients with normal LV function and a dilated left ventricle.[27] Approximately 10 patients needed an aortic valve replacement at 5 years (4%/year). The rate of progression to aortic valve replacement correlated to an end-systolic volume of greater than 60 mm/ml^2, end-systolic volume greater than 50 mm, increased wall stress greater than 86 dynes, and an ejection fraction of less than 50% with

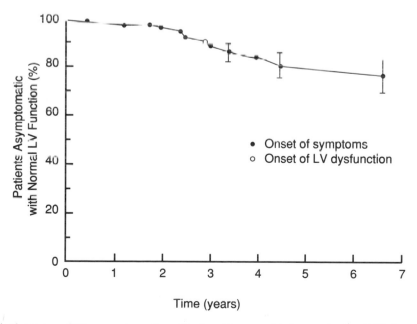

Fig. 20-9. Clinical course of 77 asymptomatic patients with normal left ventricular (LV) function illustrating the clinical stability of this group of patients. (From Bonow et al.,[23] with permission.)

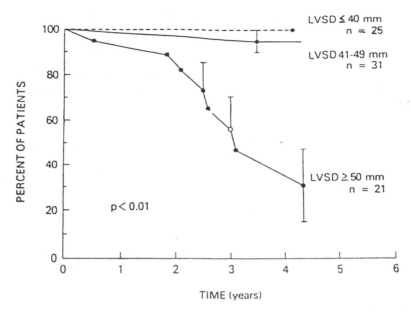

Fig. 20-10. Influence of left ventricular (LV) end-systolic dimension in asymptomatic patients showing an increased rate or progression to valve replacement in patients with an LV systolic dimension of greater than 50 mm. (From Bonow et al.,[23] with permission.)

maximum exercise. In conclusion, asymptomatic patients with normal LV function can be safely watched, with aortic valve replacement delayed, until the development of symptoms or LV dysfunction. In particular, patients with an increased LV end-systolic dimension should be watched very carefully, as their rate of progression to LV dysfunction is much quicker. However, these patients have a good outcome if operated on before the development of LV dysfunction.

Asymptomatic patients with decreased LV function form a different subset. If indeed these patients were noted to have long periods of clinical stability, observation might be indicated and aortic valve replacement delayed, sparing the patient the associated morbidity and mortality of an aortic valve replacement. However, the natural history of these patients is that most will become symptomatic within 3 years.[28–30] Thus, patients with decreased LV function and who are asymptomatic will become symptomatic within 3 years; they will now be operated on with a higher mortality, since they are now symptomatic patients with decreased LV function. Clearly, these patients should be operated on before symptoms develop.

MANAGEMENT STRATEGY: TIMING OF SURGERY

The application of the results and information from the studies cited in this chapter can lead to a management strategy. Figure 20-11 is a management strategy for patients with aortic regurgitation based on a review of this literature. In review, the initial step is to determine the length of duration of the aortic regurgitation. If the aortic regurgitation is acute, early surgical intervention is warranted. However, if the aortic regurgitation is chronic, further evaluation is necessary to determine the approach to management. The first step is to assess the patient for symptoms, both by subjective means such as NYHA class and by a good comprehensive history, as well as objectively, by means of the treadmill stress test. Patients who are clearly symptomatic or who have poor exercise tolerance should undergo aortic valve replacement as soon as possible. Preoperative assessment of LV function and size will be helpful in determining postoperative prognosis and regression of LV size. Recent studies have suggested that even patients with markedly decreased LV function have a good outcome if operated on.[31–33] Asymptomatic patients should have LV function assessed by echocardiography or radionucliotide angiography. Patients with decreased LV function with ejection fractions of less than 50% or fractional shortening of less than 29% on multiple studies with good correlation should also undergo aortic valve replacement. Asymptomatic patients with normal LV function may have a long period of clinical stability and thus should be observed for symptoms and deterioration of LV function. Patients with a normal-size ventricle should undergo annual echocardiograms and biannual multiple gated acquisition analysis (MUGA) scans to assess LV function. Patients with a dilated

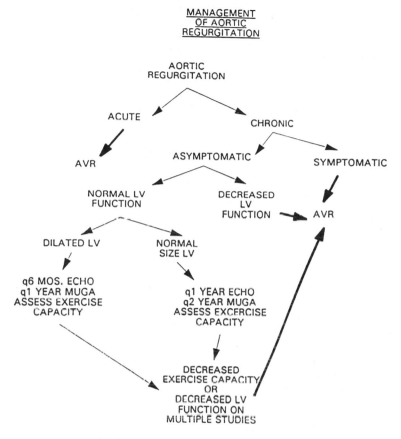

Fig. 20-11. Management strategy for following and treating patients with aortic regurgitation. See text for further explanation.

left ventricle should be watched more carefully with echocardiograms every 6 months and a MUGA scan every year secondary to a tendency to more rapid progression to LV dysfunction. Any patient with either new onset of symptoms, significant decrease in exercise capacity, or LV dysfunction should be operated on. Finally, it is important to keep in mind that LV deterioration is a dynamic process and that no defined setpoints can be used in the individual patient. Rather, decisions for intervention must be made not only on that patient's condition at a specific time, but how that patient's LV function has changed over time. Furthermore, the limitations of the tests used to assess LV function must be entered into the equation; decisions regarding operating should be based on a series of tests and not on any single specific test.

The role of vasodilators remains controversial. Numerous studies have shown impressive hemodynamic improvement with afterload reduction in the short term in patients with aortic regurgitation.[34–37] Several

recent studies have also looked at long term afterload reduction with nifedipine (Procardia) and hydralazine.[38–40] These studies have all shown reduced LV end-diastolic volume, improved LVEF, and decreased wall stress. However, presently what is not known is whether afterload reduction prevents the progression of irreversible LV dysfunction in asymptomatic patients with normal LV function and thereby delay the need for aortic valve replacement. Furthermore, afterload reduction should not be used in place of aortic valve replacement in symptomatic patients.

The role of vasodilators is not clearly defined. Patients who are symptomatic but who are either not surgical candidates or who refuse surgery should have a trial of afterload reduction to see whether there is improvement in symptoms, and possibly to prevent further LV deterioration. Furthermore, patients with severe LV dysfunction who not considered surgical candidates secondary to increased perioperative mortality also can be placed on vasodilators. The other

TABLE 20-2. Determinants of Outcome by Cox Regression Analysis

Variable	Univariate Analysis		Age-Corrected	
	t	p	t	p
Age	2.24	<0.005	—	—
Echocardiogram				
LV diastolic dimension	4.29	<0.001	4.69	<0.001
LV systolic dimension	4.93	<0.001	5.35	<0.001
LV fractional shortening	−2.95	<0.001	−2.96	<0.001
LV wall thickness	1.12	NS	1.19	NS
Radionuclide angiogram				
LVEF at rest	−1.99	<0.05	−1.61	NS
LVEF during exercise	−4.17	<0.001	−4.57	<0.001
LVEF exercise response	−3.92	<0.001	−3.78	<0.001

Abbreviations: LV, left ventricular; LVEF, left ventricular ejection fraction; NS, not significant.
(From Bonow et al.,[23] with permission.)

group of patients that may benefit are symptomatic elderly patients with a short expected life span. Whether vasodilators should be used in asymptomatic patients with normal LV function is not known. The use of vasodilators in patients with increased LV size or increased wall stress should be considered, since these patients have an increased rate of progression to LV deterioration. However, it should be done with the understanding that this concept has not been proved and could mask the progression of LV deterioration.

PROGNOSIS OF PATIENTS WITH AORTIC REGURGITATION

In patients with chronic symptomatic aortic regurgitation, the prognosis is dependent on the state of the left ventricle. Critical LV dilation and measures of LV end-systolic volume and end-systolic dimension clearly identify patients who are at risk of persistent LV dysfunction and death over the long term after aortic valve replacement. Two important LV crite-

ria—end-systolic dimension greater than 55 mm and LV end-systolic volume greater than 90 ml/m²—are associated with persistent LV dilation following valve replacement and also increased risk of progressive heart failure and greatly increased mortality.[14,17–21]

However, the data on asymptomatic patients with chronic aortic regurgitation are less clear. Bonow and associates at the NIH have studied 104 asymptomatic patients with a mean follow-up period of 8 years (range 2 to 16 years).[23] They used the same indexes with serial echocardiographic and radionuclide angiographic studies, using Kaplan–Meir life-table analysis; 58 + 9% of patients remained asymptomatic with no change in ejection fraction at 11 years, 2 patients died suddenly, 4 developed asymptomatic LV dysfunction, and 19 underwent become symptomatic and required valve replacement (Fig. 20-12).

The two deaths in their series give a mortality rate of 0.4%/year. By univariate Cox regression analysis, Bonow et al. found that several variables were significantly associated with subsequent clinical outcome: LV dimensions at end-diastole, at end-systole, and

TABLE 20-3. Multivariate Cox Regression Analysis of Variables on Serial Studies Associated With Dead or Symptoms

Variable	Initial Value (p)	Rate of Change (p)
Age	<0.05	—
Echocardiogram		
LV end-diastolic dimension	NS	NS
LV end-systolic dimension	<0.001	<0.05
LV fractional shortening	NS	NS
Radionuclide angiogram		
LVEF at rest	NS	<0.05
LVEF during exercise	NS	NS
LVEF response to exercise	NS	NS

Abbreviations: LV, left ventricular; LVEF, left ventricular ejection fraction; NS, not significant.
(From Bonow et al.,[23] with permission.)

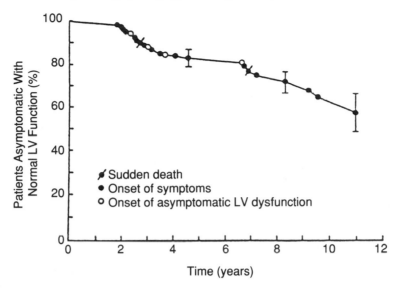

Fig. 20-12. Life-table analysis depicting the clinical course of 104 patients. At 11 years, 58 + 9% of patients were alive and asymptomatic with normal left ventricular (LV) function. (From Bonow et al.,[23] with permission.)

fractional shortening by echocardiography and the LVEF by radionuclide angiography (Table 20-2). They used these data to subgroup the patients for risk stratification. Using multivariate Cox regression analysis of the initial variables, LV end-systolic dimension and age were significantly associated with clinical outcome (Table 20-3). The LVEF during exercise or the change in LVEF during exercise did not provide independent prognostic information. When all variables were included in a multivariate Cox analysis, only age (p <0.05), initial end-systolic dimension (p < 0.001), and the rate of change in end-systolic dimension and resting LVEF during serial studies predicted outcome. In conclusion, according to Bonow and associates, the end-systolic dimension provided the greatest discrimination. In patients with an initial end-systolic dimension of less than 40 mm, the outcome was excellent, whereas patients with an end-systolic dimension of 50 mm or greater had a 19% likelihood per year of incurring cardiac events. Noninvasive studies can be safely used to follow the course of asymptomatic patients and to identify those patients who are at risk.

REFERENCES

1. Clark DG, McAnulty JH, Rahimtoola SH: Valve replacement in aortic insufficiency with LV dysfunction. Circulation 61:411, 1980
2. Wise JR, Cleland WP, Hallidie-Smith KA et al: Urgent aortic valve replacement for acute aortic regurgitation due to infective endocarditis. Lancet 2:115, 1971
3. Braniff BA, Shumway NE, Harrison DC: Valve replacement in active bacterial endocarditis. N Engl J Med 276:1464, 1967
4. Levine RJ, Roberts WC, Morrow AG: Traumatic aortic regurgitation. Am J Cardiol 10:752, 1962
5. Marcus FI, Ronan J, Masanik LF, Ewy GA: Aortic insufficiency secondary to spontaneous rupture of a fenestrated leaflet. Am Heart J 66:675, 1983
6. Hutter AM, Jr, DeSanctis RW, Nathan MJ et al: Aortic valve surgery as an emergency procedure. Circulation 41:623, 1970
7. Wiggle ED, LaBrosse CJ: Sudden, severe aortic insufficiency. Circulation 32:708, 1965
8. Scott RW: Symptoms and clinical course of syphilitic aortic insufficiency. Am Heart J 6:86, 1930
9. Padget P, Moore JE: Results of treatment of cardiovascular syphilis. Am Heart J 10:1017, 1935
10. Rappaport E: Natural history of aortic and mitral valve. Am J Cardiol 35:221, 1975
11. Greeves J, Ramintoola SH, McAnulty JH et al: Preoperative criteria predictive of late survival following valve replacement for severe AR. Am Heart J 101:300, 1981
12. Forman R, Firth BG, Barnard MS: Prognostic significance of preoperative left ventricular ejection fraction and valve lesion in patients with aortic valve replacement. Am J Cardiol 45:1120, 1980
13. Henry WL, Bonow RO, Borer JS et al: Observations on the optimum time for operative intervention for aortic regurgitation. I. Evaluation of the results of aortic valve replacement in symptomatic patients. Circulation 61:471, 1980
14. Cunha CL, Giuliani ER, Fuster V et al: Preoperative M-mode echocardiography as a predictor of surgical results in chronic aortic insufficiency. J Thorac Cardiovasc Surg 79:256, 1980
15. Bonow RO, Rosing DR, Kent KM, Epstein SE: Timing of

operation for chronic aortic regurgitation. Am J Cardiol 50:325, 1982

16. Borow KM, Green LH, Mann T et al: End systolic volume as a predictor of postoperative left ventricular performance in volume overload from valvular regurgitation. Am J Med 47:991, 1981

17. Boucher GA, Bingham JB, Osbakken MD et al: Early changes in left ventricular size and function after correction of left ventricular volume overload. Am J Cardiol 47: 991, 1981

18. Clark RD, Korcuska KL, Cohn K: Serial echocardiographic evaluation of left ventricular function in valvular disease, including guideline for serial studies. Circulation 62:564, 1980

19. Gaasch WH, Carroll JD, Levine HJ, Criscitiello MG: Chronic aortic regurgitation: prognostic value of left ventricular end-systolic dimension and end-diastolic radius/thickness ratio. J Am Coll Cardiol 1:775, 1983

20. Gaasch WH, Andrias CW, Levine HJ: Chronic aortic regurgitation: the effect of aortic valve replacement on left ventricular volume, mass, and function. Circulation 58: 825, 1978

21. Bonow RO, Borer DR, Rosing DR et al: Preoperative exercise capacity in symptomatic patients with aortic regurgitation as a predictor of postoperative left ventricular function and long term prognosis. Circulation 62: 1280, 1980

22. Roman MJ, Klein L, Devereux et al: Reveral of left ventricular dilatation, hypertrophy, and dysfunction by valve replacement in aortic regurgitation. Am Heart J 118:553, 1989

23. Bonow RO, Rosing DR, McIntosh CL et al: The natural history of asymptomatic patients with aortic regurgitation and normal left ventricular function. Circulation 68: 509, 1983

24. Bonow RO, Rosing DR, Maron BJ et al: Reversal of left ventricular dysfunction after aortic valve replacement for chronic aortic regurgitation: influence of duration of preoperative left ventricular dysfunction. Circulation 70: 570, 1984

25. Spagnuolo M, Kloth H, Taranta A et al: Natural history of rheumatic aortic regurgitation: criteria predictive of death, congestive heart failure, and angina in young patients. Circulation 44:368, 1971

26. Goldschlager N, Pfeifer J, Cohn K et al: Natural history of aortic regurgitation: a clinical and hemodynamic study. Am J Med 54:577, 1973

27. Siemienczuk D, Greenberg B, Morris C et al: Chronic aortic insufficiency: factors associated with progression to aortic valve replacement. Ann Intern Med 110:587, 1989

28. Bonow RO: Aortic Regurgitation: Medical and Surgical Management. Marcel Decker, New York, 1986, p. 67

29. Henry WL, Bonow RO, Rosing DR, Epstein SE: Observation on the optimum time for operative intervention for aortic regurgitation. II. Serial echocardiographic evaluation of asymptomatic patients. Circulation 61:484, 492, 1980

30. McDonald IG, Jelinek VM: Serial M-mode echocardiography in severe chronic aortic regurgitation. Circulation 62:1291, 1980

31. Fioretti P, Roelandt J, Bos RJ et al: Echocardiography in chronic aortic insufficiency: is valve replacement too late when left ventricular end-systolic dimension reaches 55mm? Circulation 67:216, 1983

32. Fioretti P, Roelandt J, Sclavo M et al: Postoperative regression of left ventricular dimensions in aortic insufficiency: a long term echocardiography study. J Am Coll Cardiol 5:856, 1985

33. Daniel WG, Hood WP, Siart A et al: Chronic aortic regurgitation: reassessment of the prognostic value of preoperative left ventricular end-systolic dimension and fractional shortening. Circulation 71:669, 1985

34. Bolen JL, Alderman EL: Hemodynamic consequences of afterload reduction in patients with chronic aortic regurgitation. Circulation 53:879, 1976

35. Miller RR, Vismara LA, DeMarta AN, Mason DT: Afterload reduction with nitroprusside in severe aortic regurgitation: improved cardiac performance and reduced regurgitant volume. Am J Med 38:564, 1976

36. Greenberg BH, Demots H, Murphy E, Rahimtoola S: Beneficial effect of hydralazine on rest and exercise hemodynamics in patients with chronic aortic insufficiency. Circulation 62:49, 1980

37. Greenberg BH, Demots H, Murphy E, Rahimtoola SH: Mechanism for improved cardiac performance with arteriolar dilators in aortic insufficiency. Circulation 63:263, 1981

38. Dumesnil J, Tran K, Dazenais G: Beneficial long term effects of hydralazine in aortic regurgitation. Arch Intern Med 150:757, 1990

39. Greenberg B, Massie B, Bristow D et al: Long term vasodilator therapy of chronic aortic insufficiency: a randomized double-blinded, placebo controlled clinical trail. Circulation 78:92, 1988

40. Scognamiglio R, Giuseppe F, Ponchia A, Dalla-Volta S: Long-term Nifedipine unloading therapy in asymptomatic patients with chronic severe aortic regurgitation. J Am Coll Cardiol 16:424, 1990

41. Bonow RO, Lakatos E, Maron BJ et al: Serial long-term assessment of the natural history of asymptomatic patients with chronic aortic regurgitation and normal left ventricular systolic function. Circulation 84:1625, 1991

Section IV

PROGNOSIS WITH CARDIOMYOPATHIES AND PERICARDIAL DISEASES

21

Chronic Heart Failure: Incidence, Prognosis, and the Effects of Medical Interventions

Thomas S. Rector
Jay N. Cohn

Many pathologic processes can cause cardiac dysfunction that can progress to the clinical syndrome of heart failure and premature death. The criteria used to establish the onset and progression of heart failure have not been standardized. The diagnosis in practice is often based on subjective signs and symptoms, such as an S_3 gallop, rales, pedal edema, jugular venous distention, dyspnea on exertion, orthopnea, and cardiomegaly.[1,2] These clinical signs and symptoms are not necessarily sensitive or specific indicators of abnormal physiologic measurements such as left ventricular ejection fraction (LVEF), cardiac index, pulmonary capillary wedge pressure, and exercise tolerance time or peak oxygen consumption.[2–5] Nevertheless, the symptoms and functional limitations imposed on a patient's life-style along with the high mortality rate are the primary concerns in the syndrome of chronic heart failure. Although asymptomatic ventricular dysfunction could be appropriately classified as heart failure, this overview pertains to the symptomatic syndrome associated with ventricular dysfunction.

INCIDENCE OF HEART FAILURE

Given the relatively poor prognosis, once heart failure becomes symptomatic, consideration of its development and prevention is warranted. The incidence of symptomatic heart failure secondary to the multitude of pathologies that can lead to this condition has not been the focus of many reports. Selected data from different populations at risk are summarized in Table 21-1. The Framingham cohort of 5,192 patients had annual incidence rates of less than 1 per 1,000 for persons under 50 years of age, increasing to more than 4 per 1,000 among those aged 60 or older.[6] Overall, symptomatic heart failure developed in 2.7% of this cohort during the 16 years of follow-up, which began in 1949. Heart failure was diagnosed in this study, using only clinical signs and symptoms. This Framingham sample had a substantial 21% prevalence of rheumatic heart disease prior to the onset of heart failure. Another 35% of this cohort had hypertension (>160/95

TABLE 21-1. Incidence of Heart Failure

Study	Year of Initiation	No.	Age (yr)	Incidence Estimates
Framingham[6] (general population)	1949	5,192	30–62	<1/1,000/yr if <50 yr >4/1,000/yr if >60 yr 2.7% over 16 yr
Gothenburg[9] (general male population)	1963	855	50	1.5/1,000/yr of 50–54 10.2/1,000/yr if 61–67
LRC-CPPT[10] (hyperlipoproteinemia)	1973	1,900	35–59	0.6% over 7.4 yr
Framingham[11] (postmyocardial infarction)	1950	193	35–80	14% over 5 yr 2.3% annually after 30 days
βHAT[12,13] (postmyocardial infarction)	1978	1,556	30–69	5.3–9.6% over 2.1 yr 3.5, 5, and 7% cummulative incidence at 1, 2, and 3 yr

Abbreviations: LRC-CPPT, Lipid Research Clinics Primary Prevention Trial; βHAT, β-Blocker Heart Attack Trial.

mmHg) as the sole identified potential cause of their heart failure, and an additional 29% had hypertension and coronary heart disease (CHD). A recent abstract based on Framingham data suggests that the prevalence of uncontrolled hypertension and rheumatic heart disease decreased from 1950 to 1970, but the incidence of heart failure among those 49 to 62 years of age did not decline.[7] Ischemic and diabetic cardiomyopathy increased somewhat during these three decades. A previous Framingham report had identified insulin-dependent diabetes mellitus (IDDM) as an independent risk factor for heart failure.[8] Similar incidences for men were found in a cohort from Gothenburg, Sweden, diagnosed by different clinical criteria and followed between 1963 and 1980. The annual rates were 1.5, 4.3, and 10.2 per 1,000 for ages 50 to 54, 55 to 60, and 61 to 67, respectively.[9] Ischemic heart disease (59%) and hypertension (43%) were prevalent co-morbidities. Thirteen percent of 67-year-old men had signs and symptoms of heart failure.

The placebo arm of the Lipid Research Clinics Coronary Primary Prevention Trial had 1,900 men with primary type II hyperlipoproteinemia.[10] Patients with a history of heart failure, myocardial infarction (MI), angina, or hypertension were excluded from the investigation. Beginning in 1973, they were followed for 7.4 years, on average. In only 0.6% of this relatively young group did heart failure develop, as defined by unpublished criteria. Once again, this incidence is consistent with the Framingham data of comparable age. Occurrences of cardiovascular disease prior to the onset of heart failure were not discussed; however, approximately 4% of this placebo-treated group died during the follow-up period.

In another Framingham cohort, the incidence of heart failure after a first recognized MI was monitored in 193 men followed from 1950 to 1970.[11] Heart failure developed in 2% of cases within 30 days of MI. Thereafter, in a fairly constant 2 to 3% of cases per year, heart failure developed over a 10-year period.

The β-Blocker Heart Attack Trial also provided incident data concerning heart failure in people who had at least one confirmed myocardial infarction.[12,13] Criteria for definite heart failure were pulmonary rales or vascular congestion on radiography, dyspnea or fatigue, and an S_3 gallop or increased jugular venous pressure. The 1,921 patients in the placebo-treated group were 85% male, with a mean age of 55 years. Enrollment began in 1978 with a minimum follow-up of 12 months and an average follow-up of 25 months. Approximately 9% had a history of heart failure prior to the index MI, and 15% experienced heart failure during the hospital stay. Among the 1,556 subjects in the placebo-treated group without a history of heart failure, chronic heart failure developed in 5.3%. The cumulative incidences at 1, 2, and 3 years were approximately 3.5, 5, and 7%. Another 4.3% had signs and symptoms consistent with heart failure. Treatment with propranolol did not increase these incidence rates, even though there was a lower mortality rate in the treatment group. However, differences in confounders, such as co-intervention, may have developed during the postrandomization period. Combining several similar studies suggests that β-blockers might slightly increase the risk of heart failure postinfarction.[14]

The Multicenter Diltiazem Postinfarction Trial reported a similar 7% crude cumulative risk of new heart failure over an average of 25 months of follow-up among 1,234 subjects in the placebo arm.[15] The criteria for new heart failure were not mentioned. In this sample, the development of new or worsened heart failure was related to the ejection fraction.[16] The incidence was only 4% if the ejection fraction at baseline was greater than or equal to 45%. As the ejection fraction declined from 40 ± 5% to 30 ± 5% to less than 25%, the occurrence of heart failure increased to approximately 6%, 13%, and 18%. Diltiazem increased the occurrence among patients with ejection fractions of less than 35% from 15 to 24%. Since patients with heart failure were not excluded, the groups with poorer left ventricular (LV) systolic function may have had more heart failure prior to enrollment.

The Cardiac Arrhythmia Suppression Trial provided data on the development of symptomatic heart failure up to 1 year after patients were hospitalized for an acute myocardial infarction (AMI) complicated by at least 10 premature ventricular contractions during subsequent 24-hour Holter monitoring.[17] The criteria for heart failure were at least two signs and symptoms that led to new treatment. The average age of the 100 patients in the placebo arm was 60 years, 81 of whom were male.[18] Incidence cases were not separated from those with worsening symptoms of heart failure. Only six had a history of heart failure prior to the index MI, while 19 were treated for heart failure during the period of hospitalization. Their average ejection fraction was 45% with 9 from 21% to 30% and 67 greater than 40%. The probability of new or worsened heart failure during the first year was 21%. This estimate is based on Kaplan-Meier curves with censoring at the times of death, cardiac arrest or a change in protocol-specified antiarrhythmic therapy. Although the numbers were small, an ejection fraction of less than 30% and administration of flecainide therapy tended to increase the risk of heart failure. Shock, pulmonary edema, and treatment for heart failure during the study hospitalization period were not associated with increased risk.

A report from the Mayo Clinic focused on the incidence of idiopathic dilated cardiomyopathy from 1975 to 1984.[19] In contrast to the aforementioned studies, echocardiographic, angiographic, or autopsy information was used to define idiopathic dilated cardiomyopathy, and 12% of the cases were not symptomatic. The overall incidence rates were 7.6 and 2.5 per 100,000 person-years for men and women, respectively, with increasing incidence rates after age 45.

Different patient selection criteria, diagnostic criteria, rates of competing events such as death, length of follow-up, and quantitative methods make synthesis of the available literature concerning the incidence rates and risk factors for heart failure rather hazardous. Nonetheless, the incidence of heart failure does increase with age, particularly after 50 years. The fractional contributions of various primary pathologies remains to be determined. These data confirm the expectation that ischemic heart disease is a major risk factor for symptomatic heart failure. Undoubtedly, the degree of asymptomatic LV dysfunction plays a major role, but the predictive value of various prognostic variables has not been thoroughly evaluated in this group of susceptible patients. Isolated hyperlipidemia does not appear to increase the incidence of heart failure, although a longer follow-up may make a difference. The role of hypertension, which is a primary risk

factor in the development of heart failure, is not clear, especially since more vigorous treatment efforts have become common. The relative contributions of alcohol and diabetes to the incidence of heart failure are also unknown.

As the population ages, preventive efforts should receive more attention. Studies of interventions to prevent or delay the onset of symptomatic heart failure have been initiated. Converting enzyme inhibitors are being evaluated in asymptomatic people with low ejection fractions; efforts to understand and alter the course of myocardial remodeling secondary to damage are under way.[20] Since the incidence of symptomatic heart failure postinfarction is only 2 to 3% annually, more effort toward stratifying the risk is needed to identify patients who will most likely benefit from preventive therapies. Whether thrombolytic therapy for MI decreases, increases, or does not change the incidence of chronic heart failure in the long-term remains to be determined.

PROGNOSIS OF HEART FAILURE

When heart failure becomes clinically evident, the primary prognostic concerns are the patient's functional status and survival time. Many series of cases have been reported describing the probability of survival of selected patients.[21,22]

The Framingham cohort was the only group followed from the onset of symptoms. Whether the 40 to 60% probability of survival after 5 years represents the situation today is not clear.[6] Most other studies have reported an even lower probability of survival among patients who have had various periods of time from symptom onset to the beginning of follow-up.

Numerous variables have been associated with the time to death as listed in Table 21-2. However, the

TABLE 21-2. Factors Associated With the Duration of Survival of Patients With Heart Failure

Atrial fibrillation/flutter	Mean arterial pressure
Arteriolvenous oxygen difference	NYHA classification
Cardiac index	Peak oxygen consumption
Cardiac reserve	Plasma atrial natriuretic
Complex ventricular arrhythmias	peptide concentration
Coronary artery disease	Plasma norepinephrine
Echocardiographic left ventricular	concentration
shortening fraction	Plasma-renin activity
Ejection fraction (left and right)	Right atrial pressure
Heart rate	S₃ gallop
Intraventricular conduction delay	Serum sodium
Left ventricular filling and systolic	Stroke work index
pressures	Systemic vascular
Left ventricular mass/volume ratio	resistance
	Ventricular tachycardia

diversity of definitions of heart failure, patient selection criteria, procedures, and therapy during follow-up, and the analytic methods as well as the usually modest discrimination available from many prognostic variables, have resulted in a database that is inadequate to substantially reduce the uncertainty of prognostications. Although one may be able to rank the mortality risk by using some prognostic variables, such predictions would be probabilistic in nature and unvalidated in practice.[23] Seemingly, the best we can do at this time is to offer most patients the hope of being one of the longer-term survivors, while informing them of the generally increased risk of death caused by events associated with their heart failure.

EFFECTS OF MEDICAL INTERVENTIONS ON PROGNOSIS

Vasodilators

More recently, information has become available concerning the effects of some interventions on survival. The combination of hydralazine and isosorbide dinitrate has been shown to reduce the cumulative mortality rate from 19.5% and 34.3% at 1 and 2 years to 12.1% and 25.6%, respectively, in a randomized controlled study[24] (Fig. 21-1). Prazosin did not prolong survival. These vasodilators were added to digoxin and diuretic therapy in men with chronic symptomatic class II and III heart failure of varying duration. Subjects were excluded from the trial if they had experienced a MI within 3 months or required long-acting nitrates, calcium antagonists, β-blockers, or antihypertensive agents other than diuretics. None of the baseline variables, including ejection fraction and peak oxygen consumption, could be used to identify patients who would not have an increased chance of survival with hydralazine and isosorbide dinitrate treatment.[25]

The addition of a converting enzyme inhibitor to digitalis and diuretic therapy has also been shown to prolong survival in severe class IV heart failure.[26] Most of these patients had a long history of symptomatic heart failure. The cumulative mortality rate was 44% and 52% in the placebo-treated group at 6 and 12 months, respectively. These rates are substantially greater than the study previously cited, as was the av-

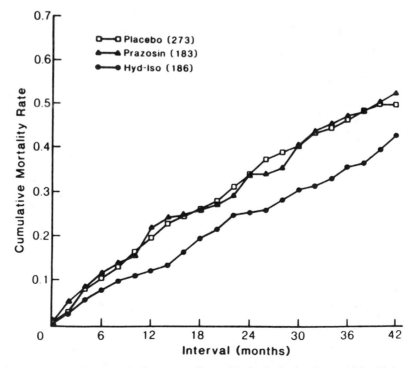

Fig. 21-1. Improvement in cumulative mortality with hydralazine-isosorbide dinitrate therapy. (From Cohn et al.,[24] with permission.)

erage age of approximately 70 years. The group that was randomly assigned to enalapril experienced significantly lower mortality rates of 26% and 36%, respectively. The mortality curves are shown in Figure 21-2. Approximately 45% of each group were also being treated with isosorbide dinitrate; the enalapril effect on survival was similar regardless of concurrent vasodilator therapy.

In view of the documented benefit on survival of different vasodilators in different samples, the evidence that functional status can be improved with converting enzyme inhibitors, and the relatively minor and mostly manageable adverse effects, the potential benefits outweigh the risks of administering vasodilators to all patients with heart failure. Extrapolation of these findings to patients not being treated with digitalis and diuretics would require further study.

As reviewed by others, patients with symptomatic heart failure have a substantial risk of sudden death, with approximately 41% of all deaths categorized as sudden.[27] Unfortunately, useful predictors of who will experience a presumably arrhythmia-related death before terminal progression of the cardiac pumping function are not available, nor has any pharmacologic therapy been proved to reduce the incidence of sudden death in this patient population. Those who survive an episode of sudden death or who experience symptomatic ventricular arrhythmias may have a better prognosis with implantable defibrillators. More research is clearly needed, however, to assess the benefit-to-risk ratio of interventions directed at the common occurrence of arrhythmia-related deaths in patients with heart failure.

Cardiac Transplantation

The development of cardiac transplantation has focused attention on two key prognostic issues. The primary indication for this intervention has been to prolong survival. The effect of cardiac transplantation on survival appears to be extraordinary. The probability of survival 1, 2, and 3 years after heart transplantation has been reported to be as high as 92, 87, and 85% in one large series.[28] Others have cited an 80% probability of survival at 1 year.[29,30] Notwithstanding the variable selection criteria for performing a heart trans-

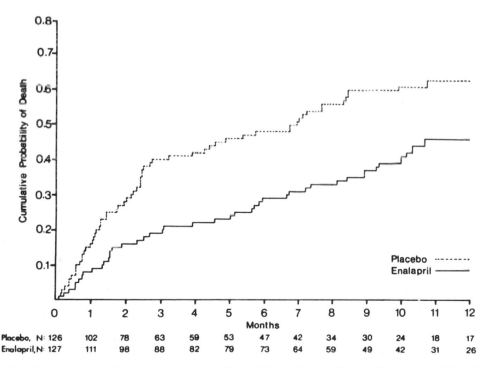

| Placebo, N: | 126 | 102 | 78 | 63 | 59 | 53 | 47 | 42 | 34 | 30 | 24 | 18 | 17 |
| Enalapril,N: | 127 | 111 | 98 | 88 | 82 | 79 | 73 | 64 | 59 | 49 | 42 | 31 | 26 |

Fig. 21-2. Improvement in cumulative mortality with enalapril. (From Consensus Trial Study Group,[26] with permission.)

plant, the procedure appears to carry a far better prognosis than does medical therapy, with which many tertiary referral centers report a 40% or greater 1-year mortality. The registry of the International Society of Heart Transplantation has reported 5- and 10-year survival rates of greater than 70% after transplantation.[31]

The second important prognostic issue is accurately predicting short-term mortality among individuals on transplant lists in order to help prioritize allocation of relatively scarce donor hearts. Aside from patients who cannot be weaned from intensive hemodynamic support, this complex prognostic decision is not supported by rigorous prognostic studies. Many patients referred for urgent cardiac transplantation can be stabilized and discharged on a lower-priority waiting list.[32] Variables that have been useful in predicting survival of patients with dilated cardiomyopathy have been examined in an effort to identify patients with the poorest prognosis among potential heart transplant candidates.[22] Among the 232 patients the 31% who were dependent on intravenous inotropes experienced only a 41% 1-year survival compared with approximately 80% for others in the sample. Other variables, including the ejection fraction, pulmonary capillary wedge pressure, ventricular tachycardia, plasma norepinephrine, and atrial natriuretic factor, were once again significantly associated with survival but did not have sufficient sensitivity and specificity for short-term survival predictions. More recently, a peak oxygen consumption above 14 ml/kg/min has been proposed as a criterion for deferring cardiac transplantation.[33]

SUMMARY

Heart failure is a symptomatic syndrome associated with a poor long-term outcome. The prevalence of heart failure appears to be increasing, perhaps because of the prolongation of life in patients with ischemic heart disease and the aging of our population. The effects of efforts to delay or prevent heart failure by altering risk factors have not been clearly established. Although symptom relief and improved quality of life remain important goals in the management of this syndrome, prolongation of survival must be considered a key endpoint for an effective therapy. To this end, vasodilator therapy and cardiac transplantation have enhanced our ability to improve the prognosis of patients with heart failure.

REFERENCES

1. Hlatky MA, Fleg JL, Hinton PC et al: Physician practice in the management of congestive heart failure. J Am Coll Cardiol 8:966, 1986

2. Marantz PR, Tobin JN, Wassertheil-Smoller S et al: The relationship between left ventricular systolic function and congestive heart failure diagnosed by clinical criteria. Circulation 77:607, 1988

3. Stevenson LW, Perloff JK: The limited reliability of physical signs for estimating hemodynamics in chronic heart failure. JAMA 261:884, 1989

4. Jafri SM, Lakier JB, Rosman HS et al: Symptoms and tests of ventricular performance in the evaluation of chronic heart failure. Am Heart J 112:194, 1986

5. Engler R, Ray R, Higgins CB et al: Clinical assessment and follow-up of functional capacity in patients with chronic congestive cardiomyopathy. Am J Cardiol 49:1832, 1982

6. McKee PA, Castelli WP, McNamara PM, Kannel WB: The natural history of congestive heart failure: the Framingham Study. N Engl J Med 285:1441, 1971

7. Kannel WB, Pinsky J: Trends in cardiac failure—incidence and causes over three decades in the Framingham Study. J Am Coll Cardiol 17:87A, 1991

8. Kannel WB, Hjortland M, Castelli WP: Role of diabetes in congestive heart failure: the Framingham Study. Am J Cardiol 34:29, 1974

9. Eriksson HE, Svardsudd K, Larsson B et al: Risk factors for heart failure in the general population: the study of men born in 1913. Eur Heart J 10:647, 1989

10. Lipid Research Clinics Program: The lipid research clinics coronary primary prevention trial resutls: reduction in incidence of coronary heart disease. JAMA 251:351, 1984

11. Kannel WB, Sorlie P, McNamara PM: Prognosis after initial myocardial infarction: the Framingham Study. Am J Cardiol 44:53, 1979

12. β-Blockers Heart Attack Trial Research Group: A randomized trial of propranolol in patients with acute myocardial infarction: morbidity results. JAMA 250:2814, 1983.

13. Chadda K, Goldstein S, Byington R, Curb JD: Effect of propranolol after acute myocardial infarction in patients with congestive heart failure. Circulation 73:503, 1986

14. Yusuf S, Peto R, Lewis J et al: Beta-blockade during and after myocardial infarction: an overview of the randomized studies. Prog Cardiovasc Dis 27:335, 1985

15. The Multicenter Diltiazem Postinfarction Trial Research Group: The effect of diltiazem on mortality and reinfarction after myocardial infarction. N Engl J med 319:385, 1988

16. Goldstein RE, Boccuzzi SJ, Cruess D, Nattel S, and the Multicenter Diltiazem Postinfarction Research Group: Diltiazem increases late-onset congestive heart failure in postinfarction patients with early reduction in ejection fraction. Circulation 83:52, 1991

17. Greene H L, Richardson DW, Hallstrom AP et al: Congestive heart failure after acute myocardial infarction in patients receiving antiarrhythmic agents for ventricular premature complexes (Cardiac Arrhythmia Pilot Study). Am J Cardiol 63:393, 1989

18. Cardiac Arrhythmia Pilot Study (CAPS) Investigators: Recruitment and baseline description of patients in the cardiac arrhythmia pilot study. Am J Cardiol 61:704, 1988

19. Codd MB, Sugrue DD, Gersh BJ , Melton LJ: Epidemiology of idiopathic dilated and hypertrophic cardiomyopathy: a population-based study in Olmsted County, Minnesota, 1975–1984. Circulation 80:564, 1989

20. Lamas GA, Pfeffer MA: Left ventricular remodeling after acute myocardial infarction: clinical course and beneficial effects of angiotensin-converting enzyme inhibition. Am Heart J 121:1194, 1991

21. Francis GS, Kubo SH: Prognostic factors affecting diagnosis and treatment of congestive heart failure. Curr Probl Cardiol 14:631, 1989

22. Keogh AM, Baron DW, H ickie JB: Prognostic guides in patients with idiopathic or ischemic dilated cardiomyopathy assessed in cardiac transplantation. Am J Cardiol 65:903, 1990

23. Cohn JN, Rector TS: Prognosis of congestive heart failure and predictors of mortality. Am J Cardiol 62:25A, 1988

24. Cohn JH, Archibald DG, Ziesche S et al: Effect of vasodilator therapy on mortality in chronic congestive heart failure: results of a Veterans Administration Cooperative Study. N Engl J Med 314:1547, 1986

25. Cohn JN, Archibald DG, Francis GS et al: Veterans Administration Cooperative Study on vasodilator therapy of heart failure. influence of prerandomization variables on the reduction of mortality by treatment with hydralazine and isosorbide dinitrate. Circulation Suppl 75: IV–49, 1987

26. Consensus Trial Study Group. Effects of enalapril on mortality in severe congestive heart failure: results of the Cooperative North Scandinavian Enalapril Survival Study. N Engl J Med 316:1429, 1987

27. Podrid PJ, Wilson JS: Should asymptomatic ventricular arrhythmia in patients iwth congestive heart failure be treated? An antagonist's viewpoint. Am J Cardiol 66:451, 1990

28. Olivari MT, Kubo SH, Braunlin EA et al: Five-year experience with triple-drug immunosuppressive therapy in cardiac transplantation. Circulation, 80:II-526, 1989

29. Uretsky BF, Murali S, Reddy PS et al: Development of coronary artery disease in cardiac transplant patients receiving immunosuppressive therapy with cyclosporine and prednisone. Circulation 76:827, 1987

30. McGregor CGA, Jamieson SW, Oyer PE et al: Heart transplantation at Stanford University. J Heart Transplant 4: 31, 1984

31. Fragomeni LS, Kaye MP: The registry of the International Society for Heart Transplantation: fifth official report—1988. J Heart Transplant 7:249, 1988

32. Stevenson LW, Dracup KA, Tillisch JH: Efficacy of medical therapy tailored for severe congestive heart failure in patients transferred for urgent cardiac transplantation. Am J Cardiol 63:461, 1989

33. Mancini DM, Eisen H, Kussmaul W et al: Value of peak exercise oxygen consumption for optimal timing of cardiac transplantation in ambulatory patients with heart failure. Circulation 83:778, 1991

22

Risk Assessment and Prognosis of Patients With Hypertrophic Cardiomyopathy

Peter J. Counihan
William J. McKenna

HISTORICAL PERSPECTIVE

The clinical and pathologic features of hypertrophic cardiomyopathy (HCM) were recognized by French workers during the mid-eighteenth century, but it was not until the description in 1958 by the pathologist Donald Teare of nine young subjects who had died suddenly that HCM was characterized as a clinical entity.[1,2] Over the past 30 years, our knowledge has progressed from recognition of the most obvious clinical and morphologic features of asymmetric septal hypertrophy, left ventricular (LV) gradients, and sudden death to our current perspective of the natural history and diversity of morphologic and hemodynamic abnormalities with which hypertrophic cardiomyopathy may manifest.[3,4] This review focuses on our current understanding of the pathophysiologic aspects of the condition and in particular discusses our understanding of the factors underlying prognosis and sudden death.

DEFINITION

The World Health Organization (WHO) defines HCM as an idiopathic heart muscle disease character-

ized by inappropriate and unexplained hypertrophy of the ventricular myocardium.[5] By this definition, the diagnosis excludes specific cardiac and systemic causes of ventricular hypertrophy. These conventional diagnostic criteria may make diagnosis difficult when there are other potential causes of left ventricular hypertrophy (LVH), including obesity, athletic training, and hypertension.

DIAGNOSIS

Currently the diagnosis requires the demonstration of a hypertrophied and nondilated left ventricle or right ventricle, or both.[5] It is recognized, however, that hypertrophy may be absent or mild. This is particularly so in younger patients, in whom hypertrophy may not manifest until completion of the adolescent growth phase.[6,7] In addition, families with a high incidence of sudden death who have histologic features of HCM with widespread areas of myocardial disarray in the absence of LVH or increased myocardial mass have been described.[8] Conventional light and electron microscopic findings in tissue obtained from patients with HCM demonstrate extensive areas of disorganization or disarray of the normal myocyte and myofibrillar architecture.[9,10] The finding of extensive myocyte disarray, the characteristic histologic feature of HCM in the absence of clinical or echocardiographic evidence of hypertrophy, suggests that ventricular hypertrophy is a marker of the underlying disease but may not be essential for the diagnosis; such patients are likely to carry the gene for HCM but do not fulfill conventional diagnostic criteria. This discrepancy between the extent and severity of hypertrophy and myocyte disarray may account for some of the apparently sporadic cases of HCM described. The extent and severity of the disarray are variable in any individual heart, but there is increasing evidence that it is not necessarily confined to areas of macroscopic hypertrophy[11]; in addition myocyte disarray is not uniform throughout the myocardium or in the areas of hypertrophy, precluding reliance on endomyocardial biopsy for the diagnosis.[10,11]

Clinical and pathologic studies suggest that the presence and extent of myofibrillar disarray are both characteristic of the condition and are likely to be an important determinant of the clinical features, particularly sudden death.[9–11] This difficulty of the diagnostic criteria for HCM underscores the need to identify the genetic basic of the disease to permit a definitive diagnosis to be made on molecular, rather than morphologic, criteria.

INCIDENCE

The incidence of unexplained LVH in the general population ranges from as low as 3 in 100,000 to as high as 5 in 1,000; the lower figure represents the annual detection of LVH in the Olmstead County, Minnesota, study in a population with an average age of 19 years.[12] This incidence is considerably lower than that described for the Framingham population, in which the average age was 55 years and the incidence of unexplained LVH was 5 of 1,000.[13] This discrepancy between the two studies may be explained by differences in age, diagnostic criteria, and diagnostic criteria.

GENETICS

The familial nature of HCM was recognized by Teare and was subsequently shown to have an autosomal dominant pattern of inheritance.[2,14–17] Sporadic cases also occur, but it remains unclear whether these cases represent new mutations or diagnostic errors or are due to errors inherent in clinical genetic studies hampered by the limitations of the diagnostic criteria dis-

cussed above, the variable expression of the disease from one generation to the next, and the inability to screen all first degree relatives; particularly parents who may have died.[17–19]

Genetic linkage analysis of a large kindred showed that the gene responsible for familial HCM lies on chromosome 14 [band q1].[20,21] Subsequent studies have identified errors within the DNA code for cardiac β heavy-chain myosin in other families with HCM.[22,23] The finding of abnormalities in the DNA sequences of the heavy-chain myosin gene complex in patients with HCM offers the tantalizing prospect of finding a molecular test that would reliably diagnose HCM and possibly predict patients at high risk of sudden death.

NATURAL HISTORY

The determination of the natural history of HCM is confounded by the fact that the only large studies are based solely on hospital populations and are thus biased in favor of symptomatic patients and/or patients from families with an adverse history of the condition.[3,4,24–26] More recent studies based on well-defined populations with unexplained LVH and using specific diagnostic criteria suggest that HCM is a relatively common disease with a more benign course than was previously suggested by hospital-based studies.[27,28] Nevertheless in most HCM populations examined, it is the high incidence of sudden death that remains the most consistent feature.

Prognosis

In adults, the symptomatic course is variable. In most cases, symptoms are mild or paroxysmal, and deterioration is gradual over many years of follow-up.[4,24–26,28] In a retrospective series of 254 patients, the mean age of onset of symptoms was 29 years, with approximately one-half the patients having some functional limitation with either chest pain or dyspnea, or both.[29] A minority (less than 10%) of this series were severely symptomatic at presentation or became severely limited during follow-up.

This relatively benign symptomatic course, however, is punctuated by a high incidence of sudden death[3,4,29–31]; 58 of the 254 patients died during a median 6-year follow-up, and 32 of these were sudden and unexpected. The causes of death in the remaining 26 were congestive heart failure (CHF) (n = 6), perioperative death following myotomy/myectomy (n = 9), other cardiac causes (n = 4), and noncardiac causes (n = 7). In this series, the annual mortality from sudden death was 2.5%, which is similar to that of other large hospital-based series.[3,4]

The clinical presentation in children resembles that

in adults, with most asymptomatic or only mildly symptomatic.[32,33] In our series of 37 young patients (aged 1 to 14 years; median 9 years), only 18 were symptomatic at diagnosis, and only 2 patients were severely limited.[32,34,35] Despite this seemingly benign course of the disease, 50% died suddenly over a 9-year follow-up, representing an annual mortality from sudden death of approximately 4.8%. A similarly high annual mortality was described in the only other large childhood based series, followed up for 7 years.[33]

Diagnosis made in infancy carries a poor prognosis; Maron et al.[36] reviewed the data from 20 patients for whom the diagnosis was made during the first year of life. Fourteen cases were diagnosed because of heart murmurs and three because of CHF. Patients were followed for a mean of 5.5 years, during which nine died: five from progressive heart failure, two following surgery for relief of heart failure and outflow tract obstruction, and two suddenly. One patient died of noncardiac disease. Of interest, the 10 survivors were the least symptomatic at diagnosis and remained asymptomatic during the follow-up period.

In most published natural history studies of both adults and children, the striking features are that those who die suddenly are often those without prominent symptoms and that hypertrophy may be mild or severe but is associated with more extensive and severe myocyte disarray.[37] Those patients with marked symptoms and severe hypertrophy at diagnosis are more likely to die from progressive heart failure.[4,36]

Symptoms

HCM presents with a wide variety of symptoms and signs.[3,4] In most patients, there is a gradual decline in functional class over many years. In a few of patients (less than 10%), however, severe symptoms develop; in this latter group, the deterioration in functional class is usually associated with progressive wall thinning and concomitant loss of systolic function.[38,39] Prospective evaluation of children and adolescent patients demonstrates that hypertrophy may progress to reach a maximum or become evident de novo, at the end of the rapid adolescent growth phase. Beyond the cessation of somatic growth, cardiac hypertrophy does not seem to progress.[40] The true natural history of LVH is unclear; there are scant serial prospective data on the regression of LVH or evaluation of LV systolic performance, but what evidence there is suggests that the natural history is one of progressive deterioration in functional class with a small minority of patients also demonstrating wall thinning and decline in left ventricular ejection fraction (LVEF).[38–40] Clinically, these changes may manifest as a symptomatic "honeymoon" when the patient with symptoms initially related to LVH and diastolic dysfunction enters a rela-

tively asymptomatic phase, albeit with decreased exercise tolerance, prior to the onset of heart failure symptoms secondary to systolic impairment.

On the basis of these studies of natural history, it is apparent that the clinical symptomatic course of HCM in most affected patients is relatively benign; however, superimposed on this seemingly innocent course is a significant incidence of sudden death. Identification of the high-risk patient is therefore the most important problem in the management of patients with HCM.

SUDDEN DEATH

Mechanisms

Given the high incidence of sudden death in patients with HCM at all ages, the most difficult problem in management is the reliable identification of those at increased risk. In the characterization of patients at increased risk, it is necessary to be aware of the potential mechanisms of sudden death: conduction disturbances such as complete heart block, asystole, and sinus node disease; supraventricular arrhythmias with or without accelerated atrioventricular (AV) node conduction or accessory pathways have all been documented as antecedent events of sudden death.[41–44] Primary ventricular arrhythmias or primary circulatory collapse, whether from systolic shutdown, reduced ventricular filling, acute massive myocardial infarction, or inappropriate peripheral vascular responses, are also potential causes of sudden death.[45–49]

Despite the myriad of potential mechanisms of sudden death in HCM, a precise mechanism is only rarely identified in any individual case. It is likely that a combination of electrical and hemodynamic factors are important and isolated case reports of patients suffering sudden death coincidentally wearing Holter-monitoring devices lend support to this view.[47,50]

Clinical Profile

Sudden death is most common in children and young adults; the vast majority of these cases are asymptomatic or minimally symptomatic during life and in whom the disease has often not been clinically recognized.[4,37] Approximately 40% of cases of sudden death occur during or immediately after vigorous exercise.[37,51] Morphologic study of these victims of sudden death may indicate mild or severe ventricular hypertrophy, but there is often more widespread myocyte and myofibrillar disarray than is seen in patients who die of CHF or other noncardiac causes[37,51]

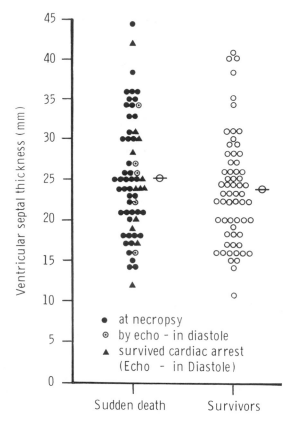

Fig. 22-1. Interventricular septal thickness in 62 patients with hypertrophic cardiomyopathy who died suddenly or had cardiac arrest compared with a control group of 62 age- and gender-matched surviving patients with hypertrophic cardiomyopathy. Mean values are indicated. (From Maron et al.,[37] with permission.)

(Fig. 22-1). It therefore seems likely that the degree and extent of myocardial disarray predispose to the development of electrical instability and also perhaps to hemodynamic collapse.

RISK STRATIFICATION

Identification of High-Risk Adults

Extensive retrospective analysis of clinical, hemodynamic, and echocardiographic measurements fails to provide an accurate clinical algorithm for the identification of high-risk patients.[29] In the retrospective series of 254 children and adults with HCM conducted by McKenna et al.,[29] (see earlier discussion, under Natural History) there were 32 sudden deaths. Discriminant analysis of 24 clinical, electrocardiographic (ECG), and hemodynamic variables demonstrated that a combination of young age at diagnosis, recur-

rent syncope, and a family history of HCM and sudden death were sensitive and specific for the occurrence of sudden death but with a low positive predictive accuracy of only 24%. In a subsequent study, indices of LV function obtained from radionuclide angiograms were analyzed; patients with evidence of impaired diastolic function were at increased risk of sudden death, while those with systolic impairment were more likely to die from progressive heart failure.[52] The predictive value of these findings, however, was similarly low.

Ventricular Arrhythmias

Episodes of nonsustained ventricular tachycardia occur in approximately 25% of adults with HCM but are uncommon in adolescents and rare in children. The importance of finding nonsustained ventricular tachycardia in adults was emphasized by two independent studies of prolonged ambulatory ECG monitoring (24 to 72 hours)[53–55] demonstrating that most episodes were usually slow (median heart rate 140 bpm) and were invariably asymptomatic. They occurred during periods of relative bradycardia with 40% of episodes occurring at night and not associated with ST segment change or QT interval prolongation. These studies demonstrated that the finding of nonsustained ventricular tachycardia on Holter monitoring represented the best single marker of the high-risk adult. Of 170 consecutive unoperated patients from the two largest Holter series, 13 died suddenly during 3-year follow-up. Nine of these 13 patients had nonsustained ventricular tachycardia on Holter monitoring. In both studies, this arrhythmia was significantly more common in those who subsequently succumbed to sudden death. Among those with ventricular tachycardia, the annual mortality was 8.6%, compared with an annual mortality of less than 0.5% among those without this arrhythmia.

The finding of nonsustained ventricular tachycardia represents the best single marker for subsequent sudden death in adult patients, with a sensitivity of 69% and specificity of 80%. The high negative predictive accuracy (97%) of Holter monitoring without this arrhythmia is reassuring, but the positive predictive accuracy of nonsustained ventricular tachycardia is poor (22%), reflecting the fact that 32 of the 41 patients with this arrhythmia survived during 3 years of follow-up evaluation[53] (Table 22-1). In the analysis of the two studies, there did not appear to be any clinical, echocardiographic, or hemodynamic feature to distinguish those patients with ventricular tachycardia who had died from those who had survived. Subsequent study of digitized angiograms in a subset of 14 patients with ventricular tachycardia demonstrated that the peak LV ejection rate was reduced in those with ventricular tachycardia who died suddenly compared with those

TABLE 22-1. Predictive Accuracy of Holter Monitoring for Nonsustained Ventricular Tachycardia as a Marker for Sudden Death[a]

	Sudden Death	
	+	−
VT+	9	32
VT−	9	124

[a] Sensitivity 69%; specificity, 80%; positive predictive value, 22%; negative predictive value, 97%
(Modified from McKenna and Alfonso,[102] with permission.)

who survived.[56] Irrespective of ventricular function, the finding of nonsustained ventricular tachycardia on ambulatory ECG represents a sevenfold increase in risk of sudden death over the succeeding 3 years. It is important to emphasize that the finding of nonsustained ventricular tachycardia does *not* imply a causal relationship between primary ventricular arrhythmia and sudden death, but rather represents a clinical marker of electrical instability and increased risk.

In the assessment of adults, therefore, the high negative predictive accuracy of the Holter monitor is reassuring, whereas the low positive predictive accuracy of nonsustained ventricular tachycardia on Holter monitoring implies that further risk factor stratification is warranted.

Identification of High-Risk Children and Adolescents

The finding of nonsustained ventricular tachycardia on Holter monitoring is a useful marker of the adult at increased risk. However, in many respects, adults with HCM must be considered survivors of the condition, having an overall annual mortality approximately one-half that of younger patients[29,32,34] (Fig. 22-2). In children, spontaneous arrhythmias are rare, and other clinical features are of greater predictive value[29,35]; patients with a family history of multiple sudden deaths, recurrent syncope, or resuscitation from out-of-hospital ventricular fibrillation are recognized to be at particular risk.[57] These clinical features, however, do not identify the majority of young pa-

tients who die suddenly. Children and adolescents without such a malignant family or clinical history still have an annual mortality from sudden death in excess of 4%. Recurrent syncopal episodes in younger patients also imply increased risk; in a retrospective study of 37 children, syncope was 86% specific for subsequent sudden death.[29,34,58] Other clinical, echocardiographic, and hemodynamic measurements, however, were similar for those who died suddenly and for those who survived, and these measurements were not useful in identifying the high-risk young patient. In the assessment of younger patients with HCM who are known to be at greater risk than adults, there is as yet no reliable clinical algorithm that reliably predicts increased risk (Table 22-2).

Of the numerous potential mechanisms of sudden death to consider, it is well recognized that tachycardia, whether physiologic or secondary to an arrhythmia, may be associated with hypotension, ischemia, or symptoms of impaired consciousness. Stafford et al.[47] documented the case of a 15-year-old patient with nonobstructive hypertrophic cardiomyopathy who presented with cardiac arrest and ventricular fibrillation. Electrophysiologic study induced sustained atrial fibrillation with a ventricular response of 170 bpm. Ventricular arrhythmias were not induced by programmed stimulation, and there was no evidence of an accessory pathway. The development of atrial fibrillation in this case was associated with hypotension and evidence of myocardial ischemia and degenerated into ventricular fibrillation. This case suggested that hemodynamic collapse could occur at physiologic heart rates in susceptible patients, leading to progressive myocardial ischemia, and could provide a substrate for lethal ventricular arrhythmia. Similar cases of rapid atrial rhythms precipitating hemodynamic collapse and ventricular fibrillation have been reported in patients undergoing electrophysiologic study.[59,60]

Abnormal hemodynamic responses to exercise in HCM are well recognized; we recently demonstrated exercise hypotension during treadmill testing in one-third of more than 100 consecutive patients with drops in systolic blood pressure of 20 to 110 mmHg (median 40 mmHg) from the peak recorded blood pressure.[48] It

TABLE 22-2. Incidence of Arrhythmia in Relationship to Age in 177 Patients With Hypertrophic Cardiomyopathy

	Age (yr)				
	≤15 (n = 20)	16–30 (n = 50)	31–45 (n = 32)	46–60 (n = 52)	≥60 (n = 23)
Atrial fibrillation	0	0	2 (6%)	4 (8%)	2 (9%)
Supraventricular tachycardia	1 (5%)	8 (16%)	12 (40%)	17 (35%)	8 (38%)
Ventricular tachycrdia	0	8 (16%)	10 (31%)	14 (27%)	6 (26%)

TABLE 22-3. Programmed Electrophysiologic Studies in Hypertrophic Cardiomyopathy

Study	Pts	Age (yr) mean (range)	History	Holter	PVS 2ES	PES 3ES	PAS	FU (mo)	Comments
Ingham et al. (1978)[64]	13	51 (25–74)	Syncope Presyncope	SVA-7[a] NSVT-3	—	—	Dual AV node 7/12 (no induced SVA)	0	—
Anderson et al. (1983)[62]	17	46 (15–74)	Syncope-5 CA-1	—	17 Polym VT/VF-3	14 VT/VF-11	—	0	PVS performed preop under GA
Kowey et al. (1984)[63]	54	54 (25–75)	CA-4 Presyncope-2 Seizure-1	NSVT-3 T de P-1	4 VT-3	1 VF-1	SVA-2	6–30 (mean 17)	PES useful in identification cause of symptoms; no events during FU on antiarrhythmic Rx
Schiavone et al. (1986)[61]	26	51 (18–77)	Syncope-14	NSVT-7 SVA-7	26 VF-1	5 VF-0	26 SVA-17	0	Syncope best predicted by hypotension during SVA
Borggrefe et al. (1986)[65]	31	Syncope-21 VT/VF-5 Presyncope-5	NSVT-9	31 SMVT-2 SPVT/VF-5	—	31 Acc P/AVNT-3 AFib-8	—	0	EPS identified possible cause of syncope in 52%
Kunze et al. (1986)[66]	26	45(–)	Syncope-4 VF-2	—	26 VF-3	23 VF-7	—	32 ± 5	No events during FU; patient with syncope or VF Rx with Am
Watson et al (1987)[67]	17	34 (14–63)	Syncope-4 VT-9 CA-2	—	17 VF-5	12 VF-3	VF-1	0	—
Fananapazir et al. (1989)[60]	155	(7–72)	Syncope-55 CA-22	NSVT-89 SVA-31	16 VT-16	44 Polyn/VT/VF	SMVT-2 AF-1	0	Polymorphic VT on PES marker increased risk

[a] Numbers represent number of patients, unless otherwise stated in column headings.

Abbreviations: A Fib, atrial fibrillation; Acc P, accessory pathway; AV, atrioventricular; AVNT, atrioventricular nodal tachycardia; CA, cardiac arrest; EPS, electrophysiologic study; ES, extra stimuli; FU, follow-up; GA, general anesthesia; NSVT, nonsustained ventricular tachycardia; PAS, programmed atrial stimulation; PES, programmed electric stimulation; Polym VT, polymorphic ventricular tachycardia; PVS, programmed ventricular stimulation; Rx, therapy; SMVT, sustained monomorphic ventricular tachycardia; SPVT, sustained polymorphic ventricular tachycardia; SVA, supraventricular arrhythmia; VF, ventricular fibrillation; VT, ventricular tachycardia.

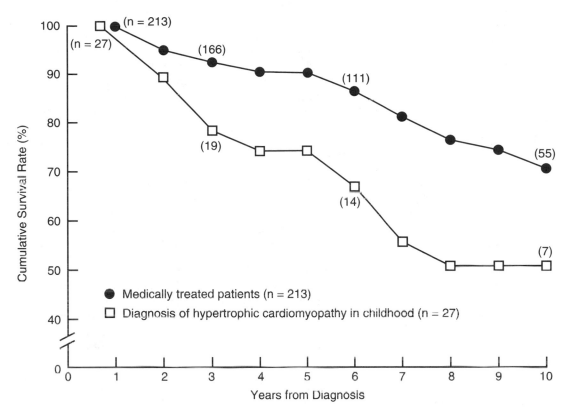

Fig. 22-2. Cumulative survival rate from the year of diagnosis for 213 medically treated adults and 27 children with hypertrophic cardiomyopathy. The probability of death = the total number of deaths per year divided by the adjusted number at risk, minus the number of deaths due to other causes. (Adapted from McKenna et al.,[29] with permission.)

has long been assumed that patients with HCM were unable to maintain stroke volume, and thus cardiac output, during rapid heart rates and that this was the cause of exercise hypotension. We examined this hypothesis by performing invasive hemodynamic monitoring in 10 patients with a normal blood pressure response and in 10 patients with exercise hypotension. Cardiac output increased appropriately and similarly in both groups and attained levels similar to that found in normal controls. In the 10 patients with exercise hypotension, there was an excessive and exaggerated fall in systemic vascular resistance, as compared with those with a normal blood pressure response. Subsequent investigation of the behavior of the peripheral circulation during exercise suggested that the exaggerated drop in systemic vascular resistance relates to inappropriate vasodilation of the regional beds responsible for maintaining peripheral resistance during exercise.[49] Although both observations of abnormal hemodynamics were more frequent in younger pa-

tients and in those with a family history of premature sudden death, the precise prognostic significance of these observations remains to be determined.

The association of nonsustained ventricular tachycardia and the occurrence of sudden death in adults, together with the assumption that all sudden death must in some way relate to a lethal primary ventricular arrhythmia, has led investigators to examine the electrical stability of the myocardium (Table 22-3). Programmed electrical stimulation is of value in the diagnosis and management of patients at risk of syncope and sudden death in association with a variety of cardiac diseases; several investigators have examined the role of electrophysiologic testing in assessing risk in patients with HCM. Many of the initial studies of electrophysiologic testing in HCM included small numbers of patients already known to be at high risk, having experienced frequent syncope or previous cardiac arrest prior to study.[61–65] These studies used a variety of stimulation protocols, and most concluded that patients with HCM had increased susceptibility to ventricular arrhythmia, particularly in the presence of ischemia or hemodynamic collapse. Kuck et al.[59] performed programmed electrical stimulation on 54 consecutive patients, including 3 resuscitated from out-of-hospital ventricular fibrillation, 8 with recurrent syncope, and 43 without documented or suspected ventricular arrhythmia. Programmed stimulation was performed from both atria and from both ventricles using up to two extrastimuli during sinus rhythm and during three paced drive cycles. Sustained monomorphic or polymorphic ventricular tachycardia or ventricular fibrillation was induced in only 8 (15%) patients. Of these 8, only one had previously sustained out-of-hospital cardiac arrest, and in this patient sustained ventricular tachycardia degenerating into ventricular fibrillation was induced by rapid atrial pacing and not by programmed ventricular stimulation.

More recently, investigators at the National Institutes of Health (NIH) have suggested that the predictive value of programmed stimulation may be improved by using a more aggressive stimulation protocol.[60] Fananapazir et al. reported induction of "sustained" ventricular arrhythmia (defined as 30 or more consecutive beats) in 66 of 155 (43%) predominantly high-risk patients. In 48 (73%) of these 66 patients, the induced arrhythmia was polymorphic ventricular tachycardia. The interpretation of these results was that ventricular arrhythmia induced by an aggressive stimulation protocol represented a potential marker of increased risk. This interpretation may be misguided, however. First, it is generally agreed that the specificity of electrophysiologic study and, in particular, the interpretation of induced polymorphic ventricular tachycardia declines with increasingly aggressive stimulation protocols.[66–68] Second, the results of the electrophysiologic study were applied to the patients retrospectively. Third, more than one-half the patients participating in this study had clinical and ECG evidence of increased risk prior to electrophysiologic testing, and the results of the study did not alter the risk profile or suggest an appropriate therapy.

Despite these criticisms Fananapazir's study is of particular interest in that it confirmed a number of preconceptions. First, the use of two extrastimuli produced significant arrhythmia in only 16% of patients, a result similar to that obtained by Kuck et al.[59] Second, the study demonstrated a high incidence of sinus node and conduction system disease in HCM, suggesting that in at least a proportion of patients heart block will develop as a mechanism for syncope and sudden death. Third, of perhaps greatest importance, the study confirmed the value of finding nonsustained ventricular tachycardia on Holter monitoring, particularly in symptomatic patients; 46 of the 66 (70%) pa-

tients in whom "sustained" ventricular tachycardia was induced also demonstrated nonsustained ventricular tachycardia on ambulatory ECG monitoring. Given that spontaneous arrhythmias are rare in young patients with HCM and that nonsustained ventricular tachycardia on ambulatory ECG monitoring is only a reliable marker of the adult patient likely to die, the role of electrophysiologic testing and programmed stimulation in the assessment of high-risk children and the refinement of risk in adults remains to be established in a prospective study. In the face of these observations, many investigators continue to believe that in all patients, be they young or old, the initiating mechanism for sudden death is a primary ventricular arrhythmia, most often polymorphic ventricular tachycardia. In our view, and especially regarding younger patients, the initiating mechanism is primarily a hemodynamic event. These apparently opposing views of the primary hemodynamic and electrical mechanisms of sudden death can be reconciled. We speculate that, in susceptible patients, the initiating event is most likely to be hemodynamic collapse during periods of rapidly changing autonomic balance. This may manifest as rapidly swinging heart rates and blood pressure, whether physiologic in response to exercise or emotion or pathologic in response to a primary supraventricular tachyarrhythmia. These rapid changes in heart rate and blood pressure result in hemodynamic instability and progressive myocardial ischemia (particularly in areas of extensive myocyte disarray) and provide the trigger for fatal arrhythmia (Fig. 22-3). The outcome from these events—survival or death—will ultimately depend on the electrical stability of the underlying myocardium.[69] In support of this hypothesis, Nicod et al.[50] reported the case of a 30-year-old man who died suddenly while wearing a Holter monitor. These investigators concluded that death was due to ventricular fibrillation caused by primary polymorphic ventricular tachycardia. A review of the ECG data, however, suggests an alternative conclusion; that is, that sinus tachycardia led to myocardial ischemia with subsequent marked, nonphysiologic, slowing of the heart rate and a period of junctional escape rhythm, resulting in syncope and reassertion of sinus tachycardia, followed by sudden onset of polymorphic ventricular tachycardia and death. The implication of this report is of a hemodynamic event precipitating myocardial ischemia and a catastrophic ventricular arrhythmia.[70]

Recently, the high-gain, signal-averaged ECG has been evaluated as a noninvasive adjunct to electrophysiologic testing for a variety of cardiac conditions. Initial studies of HCM suggest that the finding of late potentials on signal-averaged ECG correlates with the finding of nonsustained ventricular tachycardia on Holter monitoring.[71] The value of these ECG findings

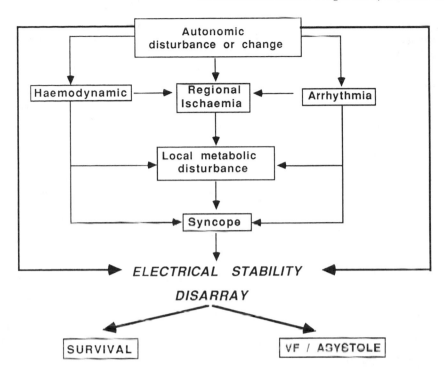

Fig. 22-3. Schematic representation of potential initiating mechanisms of sudden death. It is hypothesized that the outcome of a trigger, be it ischemic, hemodynamic, or arrhythmic, is dependent on the electric stability of the underlying myocardium, which in turn is related to the extent and severity of myocardial disarray. (From Counihan and McKenna,[101] with permission.)

in younger patients who do not demonstrate Holter arrhythmias remains to be determined.

INFLUENCE OF TREATMENT ON PROGNOSIS

Surgery

Surgical therapy for symptomatic relief in HCM (usually septal myotomy) has largely been reserved for patients who demonstrate evidence of outflow tract "obstruction" and in whom medical therapy has failed. Surgery, although having no effect on the underlying morphologic abnormality, undoubtedly has benefit on functional class in selected patients with Doppler or catheter evidence of an LV outflow tract gradient.[72–74] In most patients with severe symptoms and evidence of LV outflow tract gradient, surgery produces considerable symptomatic improvement. To date there is no convincing evidence that surgery improves the overall prognosis, although a decreased occurrence of syncope in some operated patients have been reported.[75] One of the disadvantages of surgery is the appreciable perioperative mortality, which

ranges in the literature from 2.5 to 15%. At the five leading surgical centers, the perioperative mortality was 8.5% and the overall mortality 17% (mean follow-up 6 years).[76] This outcome with surgery is similar to the overall mortality of 16% recorded in medically treated patients of similar functional class. Data from the NIH, the largest published series, fail to demonstrate any evidence that surgery is protective against subsequent sudden death; however, clear evaluation of surgical results from different centers where indication, surgical experience, expertise, and techniques differ is not possible.[73,77]

Pharmacologic Therapy

β-Adrenergic Blocking Drugs

In the belief that the pathophysiology of HCM was attributable to increased sensitivity to catecholamines, β-adrenergic blocking drugs were introduced early in the management of patients with HCM.[78] Since the original introduction of propranolol, β-adrenergic blocking drugs have been shown to improve symptoms by reducing resting heart rate and blunting the heart rate response to physiologic stress, and also by their significant negative inotropic effect. Frank et al.[79] used "complete" β-blocking doses of propranolol (mean 462 mg/day) in a prospective study of 22 symptomatic patients and compared results with 14 retrospective nonrandomized control patients. All the propranolol-treated patients improved by a mean of 58% compared with improvement in only 1 of the 14 controls. During follow-up (mean 5 years), 4 of the control group died suddenly, but all patients in the propranolol-treated group survived. These results suggested that propranolol might have a beneficial effect on mortality. However, this apparent benefit of propranolol may have been influenced by the concomitant administration of specific antiarrhythmic agents to those demonstrating "life-threatening" arrhythmias. As yet there is no clear evidence that β-blockers alter the prognosis of HCM. In a nonrandomized study from our institution 18 of 164 (11%) of patients treated with β-blockers died suddenly during a mean follow-up of 6 years.[25,80] A similar nonrandomized study of 77 patients, by Loogen et al.,[81] showed a similar 13% mortality from sudden death over approximately 5-year follow-up. Despite the disappointing lack of an obvious modifying effect of β-blockade on prognosis, all these studies confirm a beneficial effect on symptoms.

Calcium Antagonists

Reports of the beneficial effects of verapamil on symptoms and clinical features in HCM first appeared during the mid-1970s.[82] These drugs have since come to play an important role in medical therapy for patients with HCM. Recent evidence of disordered calcium flux in myocytes supports the long established clinical evidence that calcium antagonists are effective in improving symptoms in most patients.[83-87] Hopf and Kaltenbach[88] reported symptomatic improvement in 85% of 101 patients followed for a mean of approximately 6 years with a mean dose of verapamil of 506 mg/day. Despite significant hemodynamic improvement in these patients, there was no reduction in the degree of LVH seen in this study. Rosing and colleagues[87] at the NIH have also reported on the beneficial effects of verapamil in both obstructive and nonobstructive HCM and have suggested that up to 50% of patients can defer surgery with verapamil therapy. These investigators, however, have also reported several cases of increased outflow tract gradient, pulmonary edema, cardiogenic shock, and death occurring in patients receiving high-dose oral verapamil, presumably secondary to the vasodilating and negative inotropic properties of the drug.[87,89]

Despite the proven clinical and hemodynamic benefit of verapamil, there is no evidence that it alters the long-term mortality or frequency of sudden death. Experience with diltiazem, although less than that with verapamil, suggests similar long-term results. Diltiazem has perhaps the advantage of having less peripheral vasodilating effect and is often better tolerated at high dose than is verapamil.

Antiarrhythmic Therapy

Conventional therapy with β-blockers, verapamil, and myectomy provides symptomatic relief but does not appear to reduce the incidence of sudden death. Class 1 agents in general may suppress Holter events and improve symptoms to some degree, but they do not reduce the incidence of sudden death.[76] This is not surprising, given that nonsustained ventricular tachycardia on Holter monitoring is a marker of increased risk and not the cause sudden death.

Although disopyramide is primarily an antiarrhythmic agent, Pollick[90] demonstrated a short-term benefit on symptoms with this agent in patients with LV outflow tract gradients. There are no data on the effect of disopyramide on sudden death; recent concerns regarding class 1 antiarrhythmic drugs in general may discourage further evaluation of this drug in patients without life-threatening arrhythmias.[91]

The increasing use of electrophysiologic testing in the assessment of risk of sudden death and the belief held by some researchers that in all patients, both young and old, the initiating event preceding sudden death is a primary ventricular arrhythmia is likely to promote increasing use of the implantable cardioverter defibrillator device; to date, however, there are few published data on use of this device in HCM. The small number of reports of defibrillator discharges in patients who have been fitted with these devices have presumed that discharge was due to syncope related to malignant ventricular arrhythmia. In the absence of Holter data or device telemetry, or both techniques, this may be a misguided assumption. The commonest reason for syncope in patients with HCM relates to supraventricular arrhythmia, particularly paroxysmal atrial fibrillation, and this arrhythmia in turn is a frequent cause of inappropriate implantable cardioverter/defibrillator discharge.[92,93] Given that most cases of sudden death in young patients with HCM are undiagnosed at the time of death, the fact that the number of patients per year who experience a catastrophic event is small, and the poor predictive accuracy of the currently available investigations—the widespread implantation of cardioverter/defibrillator devices is clearly impractical for most patients.

Amiodarone

Amiodarone is a potent antiarrhythmic agent with many electrophysiologic properties.[94] We have used amiodarone in low dose (200 to 400 mg/day) sufficient to produce plasma levels 0.5 to 1.5 mg/L. At these plasma levels, amiodarone suppresses ventricular tachycardia on Holter monitoring, has few side effects, and has been associated with a reduced incidence of sudden death. In our initial series of 21 patients with nonsustained ventricular tachycardia, there were no deaths in the amiodarone-treated group during 3-year follow-up, compared with a 7% annual mortality in a well-matched control group treated with class 1 agents[95] (Fig. 22-4). In a long-term study, 38 consecutive patients with nonsustained ventricular tachycardia treated with amiodarone were compared with 104 control patients without ventricular tachycardia or amiodarone therapy and followed for 5 years.[96] There were five deaths in the amiodarone-treated group: three heart failures, one perioperative death, and one sudden death. In the group without ventricular tachycardia who did not receive amiodarone, there were 16 deaths, 9 of which were sudden and unexpected.

Of perhaps greater importance is the benefit of amiodarone seen in children and young adults at high risk of sudden death. In 15 high-risk patients (21 years or younger) treated with low-dose amiodarone (<1 g/wk) there were no deaths over 3 years, in contrast to a 4% annual mortality in a similarly aged group without obvious risk factors who did not receive amiodarone[58] (Fig. 22-5). This protective effect of amiodarone at plasma levels of approximately 0.5 mg/L has led to speculation that the influence of amiodarone on prognosis is independent of its conventional antiarrhythmic effect. By prolonging action potential duration, the degree of dispersion of repolarization within the myocardium is reduced, thereby attenuating the

substrate for reentry mechanisms. This "normalization" of dispersion would be sufficient to raise the ventricular fibrillation threshold from a low level apparent during electrophysiologic study to a higher level.[93]

Our policy is to use low-dose amiodarone (median dose 1 g/wk) for adults who demonstrate episodes of nonsustained ventricular tachycardia on ambulatory ECG monitoring and for high-risk young patients with recurrent syncope, out-of-hospital ventricular fibrillation, and/or a malignant family history. The dosage of amiodarone is adjusted following the loading period to produce a trough plasma concentration of ≤1.0 mg/L; at this plasma concentration, side effects are infrequent and minor and rarely require discontinuation of therapy. In the use of low-dose amiodarone, it must be emphasized that the goal of therapy is survival and *not* abolition of arrhythmia on Holter monitoring.

Experience with amiodarone in North America has been less encouraging. The reasons for this are many but may in part relate to empirical administration of much larger doses than are used in Europe and to an apparent difficulty encountered in monitoring plasma concentrations as a predictor of side effects. Fananapazir and collaborators recently reported seven sudden deaths occurring within 6 months of commencing therapy with amiodarone, four of which occurred at less than 3 months. In these patients, the mean dosage of amiodarone administered was 2.5 times more than would be administered within the same period in a European setting. Similarly, in the only four patients in whom plasma concentrations of amiodarone were measured, the mean plasma concentration was within the range usually associated with significant side effects. Given the strong temporal association between the commencement of the drug and death and the amount of drug administered, it is probable that the deaths were related to a pro-arrhythmic effect of amiodarone.[97]

Amiodarone has been associated with frequent adverse effects in many organs.[98] However, many of the data on the serious side effects of amiodarone come from studies in which excessively large doses of amiodarone were used without monitoring plasma levels; this resulted in a high incidence of toxicity, necessitating discontinuation of therapy. Heger et al.[98] reviewed eight clinical studies of amiodarone and noted that withdrawal of the drug was required in 13% of cases. In our experience, withdrawal because of adverse effects is less than 5%. Most investigators now agree that serious adverse effects can be avoided if plasma concentrations are maintained at less than 2 mg/L. At concentrations within these therapeutic guidelines, adverse effects are minor and rarely sufficient to warrant discontinuation of therapy.

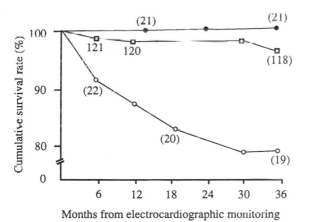

Fig. 22-4. Cumulative survival rate in hypertrophic cardiomyopathy for 24 patients with ventricular tachycardia treated with conventional agents (*open circle*), 21 with ventricular tachycardia treated with amiodarone (*solid circle*), and 122 without ventricular tachycardia (*square*). (Adapted from McKenna et al.,[95] with permission.)

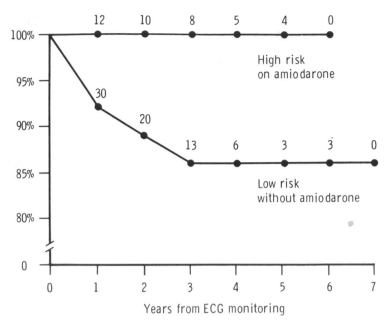

Fig. 22-5. Cumulative survival rate in hypertrophic cardiomyopathy from initial 48-hour ambulatory electro-cardiographic recordings in 15 young "high-risk" patients who received amiodarone and in 37 "low-risk" control patients who received symptomatic treatment. (From McKenna et al.,[35] with permission.)

PROGNOSIS

The high incidence of sudden death in a relatively youthful population makes HCM an important disease in socioeconomic terms. Our ability to determine those adult patients who are at risk is satisfactory, but no specific algorithm to predict those children who are likely to die has yet been established. A confounding factor in our understanding of the mechanism(s) of sudden death in HCM, hence in recommending therapeutic strategies, is the surprising finding that most patients who have been resuscitated from out-of-hospital cardiac arrest do not experience further episodes.[44] Cecchi and colleagues[99] from the NIH reported on the long-term outcome of 33 patients successfully resuscitated from out of hospital cardiac arrest. The mean age of the group was 32 years, followed up for a mean of 7 years. During the follow-up period, 8 patients died of a cardiac-related causes, and in only 4 of these cases was death sudden and unexpected. These results yielded an actuarial survival of 97 ± 3% at 1 year and 74 ± 9% at 5 years, with an event-free survival (without further cardiac arrest or death) of 83 ± 7% at 1 year and 65 ± 9% at 5 years (Fig. 22-6). These results are surprising and are unlike the figures for survivors of cardiac arrest associated with other heart diseases.[100] In HCM, many cases of sudden death appear to be isolated and unexpected events in the natural history of the disease, possibly

the result of several factors simultaneously compounded to produce the substrate for a terminal ventricular arrhythmia. The results from the study conducted by Cecchi's group at the NIH are of importance in planning therapy for patients deemed to be at high risk, particularly in relationship to the implantation of cardioverter/defibrillators. Most patients who sustained cardiac arrest in this study would *not* have required being fitted with such devices.

CONCLUSIONS

Our knowledge of HCM has progressed significantly since the early descriptions of the disease during the 1960s. However, despite improved diagnostic techniques and progress in our understanding of the molecular basis of the disease, our ability to characterize and correctly predict which patients, particularly the young, are likely to die remains unsatisfactory. The finding of nonsustained ventricular tachycardia on ambulatory ECG monitoring, especially in those with evidence of impaired ventricular function, is a useful marker of the at-risk adult patient. Such patients can be effectively managed with low-dose amiodarone and the annual mortality of 9% reduced to less than 1%.

In children and young adults, the annual mortality is approximately twice that of adult patients, but our ability to identify those younger patients who are

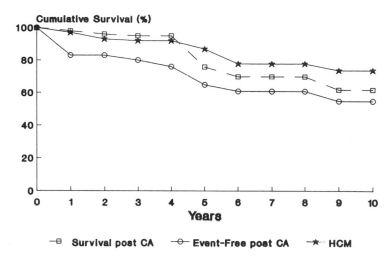

Fig. 22-6. Cumulative survival and event-free survival rates in 33 patients with HCM resuscitated from cardiac arrest and 254 medically treated patients with HCM. (Data from Cecchi et al.,[99] and from McKenna et al.[29])

likely to die remains unsatisfactory. Conventional clinical features of young age at diagnosis, an adverse family history, recurrent syncope, and previous cardiac arrest have low predictive accuracy for subsequent sudden death. Noninvasive assessment with computer-assisted ECG and hemodynamic responses to stress offer some promise for the future but are still under investigation. Prospective evaluation of invasive electrophysiologic testing is awaited. Despite the lack of a useful clinical algorithm with which to identify the youthful patient at risk, the use of low-dose amiodarone suggest improved survival.

In patients who present with severe symptoms at diagnosis or in whom symptoms develop at a young age or postmyectomy, progressive CHF is generally likely to develop. Although there are few data, it seems likely that the prognosis of these patients is similar to that for patients with heart failure from other causes. Cardiac transplantation may be the therapy of choice in such cases.

SUMMARY

Adults with HCM have an overall annual mortality of 2.5 to 3%; the finding of nonsustained ventricular tachycardia on Holter monitoring predicts the majority of those adults who are likely to die. In children and young adults, the annual mortality is approximately 6%; patients with an adverse family history or recurrent syncope or who have been resuscitated from out-of-hospital cardiac arrest are at obvious risk, but the specificity of these clinical features is poor; the annual mortality of young patients putatively at "low

risk" on these criteria remains high, at approximately 4%. Recently, hemodynamic and electrophysiologic responses in patients with HCM have shown promise as possible markers for risk, particularly in younger patients, but prospective evaluation of these results is warranted.

REFERENCES

1. Hallopeau L: Retrecissement ventriculo-aortique. Gaz Med Paris 24:683, 1869
2. Teare RD: Asymmetrical hypertrophy of the heart in young adults. Br Heart J 20:1–8, 1958
3. Frank S, Braunwald E: Idiopathic hypertrophic subaortic stenosis. Clinical analysis of 126 patients with emphasis on the natural history. Circulation 37:759, 1968
4. McKenna WJ, Goodwin JF: The natural history of hypertrophic cardiomyopathy. p. 5. In Harvey P (ed): Current Problems in Cardiology. Vol. VI. Year Book Medical Publishers, Chicago, 1981
5. WHO/ISFC: Report of the WHO/ISFC task force on the definition and classification of cardiomyopathies. Br Heart J 44:672, 1980
6. Maron BJ, Spirito P, Wesley Y, Arce J: Development and progression of left ventricular hypertrophy in children with hypertrophic cardiomyopathy. N Engl J Med 315:610, 1986
7. Spirito P, Maron BJ: Relation between extent of of left ventricular and age in patients with hypertrophic cardiomyopathy. J Am Coll Cardiol 13:820, 1989
8. McKenna WJ, Stewart JT, Nihoyannopoulos P et al: Hypertrophic cardiomyopathy without hypertrophy: two families with myocardial disarray in the absence of increased myocardial mass. Br Heart J 63:287, 1990
9. Maron BJ, Roberts WC: Quantitative analysis of cardiac

muscle cell disorganisation in the ventricular septum of patients with hypertrophic cardiomyopathy. Circulation 59:689, 1979

10. Maron BJ, Anan TJ, Roberts WC: Quantitative analysis of the distribution of cardiac muscle cell disorganisation in the left ventricular wall of patients with hypertrophic cardiomyopathy. Circulation 63:882, 1981

11. Davies MJ: The current status of myocardial disarray in hypertrophic cardiomyopathy. Br Heart J 51:361, 1984

12. Codd MB, Sugrue DD, Gersh BJ, Melton LJ: Epidemiologic features of idiopathic dilated cardiomyopathy and hypertrophic cardiomyopathy: a population based study in Olmstead County, Mn, 1975–1984. Circulation 80:564, 1989

13. Savage DD, Castelli WP, Abbott RD et al: Hypertrophic cardiomyopathy and its markers in the general population: the great masquerader revisited: The Framingham Study. J Cardiovasc Ultrason 2:41, 1983

14. Brent LB, Aburano A, Fisher DL et al: Familial muscular subaortic stenosis. An unrecognised form of "idiopathic heart disease," with clinical and autopsy observations. Circulation 21:167, 1960

15. Hollman A, Goodwin JF, Teare D, Renwick JW: A family with obstructive cardiomyopathy (asymmetrical hypertrophy). Br Heart J 22:449, 1960

16. Pare JAP, Fraser RG, Pirozynski WJ et al: Hereditary cardiovascular dysplasia. A form of familial cardiomyopathy. Am J Med 31:37, 1961

17. Maron BJ, Nichols PF, Pickle LW et al: Patterns of inheritance in hypertrophic cardiomyopathy: assessment by M-mode and two-dimensional echocardiography. Am J Cardiol 53:1087, 1984

18. ten Cate FJ, Hugenholtz PG, van Dorp WJ, Roelandt J: Prevalence of diagnostic abnormalities in patients with genetically transmitted asymettric septal hypertrophy. Am J Cardiol 43:731, 1979

19. Greaves SC, Roche AHG, Neutze JM et al: Inheritance of hypertrophic cardiomyopathy: a cross sectional and M-mode echocardiographic study of 50 families. Br Heart J 58:259, 1987

20. Jarco JA, McKenna WJ, Pare JAP et al: Mapping a gene for familial hypertrophic cardiomyopathy to chromosome 14q1. N Engl J Med 321:1372, 1989

21. Solomon SD, Geisterfer-Lowrance AAT, Vosberg H-P et al: A locus for familial hypertrophic cardiomyopathy is closely linked to the cardiac myosin heavy chain genes, CRI-L436, and CRI-L329 on chromosome 14 at q11-q12. Am J Hum Genet 47:389, 1990

22. Geisterfer-Lowrance AAT, Kass S, Tanigawa G et al: A molecular basis for familial hypertrophic cardiomyopathy: a beta cardiac myosin heavy chain gene missense mutation. Cell 62:999, 1990

23. Tanigawa G, Jarcho JA, Kass S et al: A molecular basis for familial hypertrophic cardiomyopathy: an alpha/beta cardiac myosin heavy chain hybrid gene. Cell 62: 991, 1990

24. Swan DA, Bell B, Oakley CM et al: Analysis of symptomatic course and prognosis and treatment of hypertrophic cardiomyopathy. Br Heart J 33:671, 1971

25. Shah PM, Adelman AG, Wigle ED et al: The natural (and unnatural) history of hypertrophic obstructive cardiomyopathy. Circ Res, suppl II. 34/35:179, 1974

26. Adelman AG, Wigle ED, Ranganathan N et al: The clinical course in muscular subaortic stenosis. A retrospective and prospective study of 60 haemodynamically proved cases. Ann Intern Med 77:515, 1972

27. Spirito P, Chiarella F, Carratino L et al: Clinical course and prognosis of hypertrophic cardiomyopathy in an outpatient population. N Engl J Med 320:749, 1989

28. Shapiro LM, Zezulka H: Hypertrophic cardiomyopathy: a common disease with a good prognosis: Five year experience of a district general hospital. Br Heart J 50: 530, 1983

29. McKenna WJ, Deanfield J, Faruqui A et al: Prognosis in hypertrophic cardiomyopathy. Role of age, and clinical, electrocardiographic and hemodynamic features. Am J Cardiol 47:532, 1981

30. Wahedra D, Gunnar RM, Scanlon PJ: Prognosis in hypertrophic cardiomyopathy with asymmetric septal hypertrophy. Postgrad Med J 61:1107, 1985

31. Hardarson T, de la Calzada CS, Curiel R et al: Prognosis and mortality of hypertrophic obstructive cardiomyopathy. Lancet 2:1462, 1973

32. Deanfield JE, McKenna WJ: Recognition and management in children. p. 143. In Ten Cate F (ed): Hypertrophic Cardiomyopathy. Marcel Dekker, New York, 1985

33. Maron BJ, Henry WL, Clark CE et al: Asymmetric septal hypertrophy in childhood. Circulation 53:9, 1976

34. McKenna WJ, Deanfield JE: Hypertrophic cardiomyopathy: an important cause of sudden death. Arch Dis Child 59:971, 1984

35. McKenna WJ, Franklin RCG, Nihoyannopoulos P et al: Arrhythmia and prognosis in infants, children and adolescents with hypertrophic cardiomyopathy. J Am Coll Cardiol 11:147, 1988

36. Maron BJ, Tajik AJ, Ruttenberg HD et al: Hypertrophic cardiomyopathy in infants: clinical features and natural history. Circulation 65:7, 1982

37. Maron BJ, Roberts WC, Epstein SE: Sudden death in hypertrophic cardiomyopathy: a profile of 78 patients. Circulation 65:1388, 1982

38. ten Cate FJ, Roelandt J: Progression to left ventricular dilatation in patients with hypertrophic cardiomyopathy. Am Heart J 97:762, 1979

39. Spirito P, Maron BJ, Bonow RO, Epstein SE: Occurrence and significance of progressive left ventricular wall thinning and relative cavity dilatation in patients with hypertrophic cardiomyopathy. Am J Cardiol 60: 123, 1987

40. Spirito P, Maron BJ: Absence of progression of left ventricular hypertrophy in hypertrophic cardiomyopathy. J Am Coll Cardiol 9:1013, 1987

41. Joseph S, Balcon R, McDonald L: Syncope in hypertrophic obstructive cardiomyopathy due to asystole. Br Heart J 34:974, 1972

42. Ciro E, Maron BJ: Unusual long term survival following cardiac arrest in hypertrophic cardiomyopathy. Am Heart J 105:145, 1983

43. Chmielewzki CA, Riley RS, Mahendran A, Most AS: Complete heart block as a cause of syncope in asymmetric septal hypertrophy. Am Heart J 93:91, 1977

44. Krikler DM, Davies MJ, Rowland E et al: Sudden death in hypertrophic cardiomyopathy: associated accessory atrioventricular pathways. Br Heart J 43:245, 1980

45. McKenna WJ, Harris L, Deanfield J: Syncope in hypertrophic cardiomyopathy. Br Heart J 47:177, 1982

46. Maron BJ, Epstein SE, Roberts WC: Hypertrophic cardiomyopathy and transmural myocardial infarction without significant atherosclerosis of the extramural coronary arteries. Am J Cardiol 43:1036, 1979

47. Stafford WJ, Trohman RG, Bilsker M et al: Cardiac arrest in an adolescent with atrial fibrillation and hypertrophic cardiomyopathy. J Am Coll Cardiol 7:701, 1986

48. Frenneaux MP, Counihan PJ, Chikamori T, McKenna WJ: Abnormal blood pressure response during exercise in hypertrophic cardiomyopathy. Circulation 82:1995, 1990

49. Counihan PJ, Frenneaux MP, Webb DJ, McKenna WJ: Abnormal vascular responses to supine exercise in hypertrophic cardiomyopathy. Circulation 84:686, 1991

50. Nicod P, Polikar R, Peterson KL: Hypertrophic cardiomyopathy and sudden death. N Engl J Med 318:1255, 1988

51. Maron BJ, Roberts WC, McAllister HA et al: Sudden death in young athletes. Circulation 62:218, 1980

52. Chikamori T, Counihan PJ, Doi Y, et al: Mechanisms of exercise limitation in hypertrophic cardiomyopathy. J Am Coll Cardiol 19:507, 1992

53. McKenna WJ, England D, Doi YL et al: Arrhythmia in hypertrophic cardiomyopathy. 1. Influence on prognosis. Br Heart J 46.168, 1981

54. Savage DD, Seides SF, Maron BJ et al: Prevalence of arrhythmia during 24 hour electrocardiographic monitoring and exercise testing in patients with obstructive and non obstructive hypertrophic cardiomyopathy. Circulation 59;866, 1979

55. Maron BJ, Savage DD, Wolfson JK, Epstein SE: Prognostic significance of 24 hour ambulatory electrocardiographic monitoring in patients with hypertrophic cardiomyopathy. A prospective study. Am J Cardiol 48:252, 1981

56. Newman H, Sugrue DD, Oakley CM et al: Relation of left ventricular function and prognosis in hypertrophic cardiomyopathy: an angiographic study. J Am Coll Cardiol 5:1064, 1985

57. Maron BJ, Lipson LC, Roberts WC et al: "Malignant" hypertrophic cardiomyopathy: identification of a subgroup of families with unusually frequent premature death. Am J Cardiol 41:1133, 1978

58. McKenna WJ: Sudden death in hypertrophic cardiomyopathy: identification of the "high risk" patient. p. 353. In Brugada P, Wellens HJJ (eds): Cardiac Arrhythmias: Where to Go from Here? Futura, Mount Kisco, NY, 1987

59. Kuck K-H, Kunze K-P, Geiger M et al: Programmed electrical stimulation in patients with hypertrophic cardiomyopathy: results in patients with and without cardiac arrest or syncope. p. 367. In Brugada P, Wellens HJJ (eds): Cardiac Arrhythmias: Where to Go from Here? Futura, Mount Kisco, NY, 1987

60. Fananapazir L, Tracy CM, Leon MB et al: Electrophysiologic abnormalities in patients with hypertrophic cardiomyopathy. Circulation 80:1259, 1989

61. Schiavone WA, Maloney JD, Lever HM et al: Electrophysiologic studies of patients with hypertrophic cardiomyopathy presenting with syncope of undetermined etiology. PACE 9:476, 1986

62. Anderson KP, Stinson EB, Derby GC et al: Vulnerability of patients with hypertrophic obstructive cardiomyopathy to ventricular arrhythmia induction in the operating room. Am J Cardiol 51:811, 1983

63. Kowey PR, Eisenberg R, Engel TR: Sustained arrhythmias in hypertrophic obstructive cardiomyopathy. N Engl J Med 310:1566, 1984

64. Ingham RE, Mason JW, Rossen RM et al: Electrophysiologic findings in patients with idiopathic hypertrophic subaortic stenosis. Am J Cardiol 41:811, 1978

65. Borggrefe M, Podczeck A, Breithardt G: Electrophysiologic studies in hypertrophic cardiomyopathy, abstracted. Circulation, suppl II. 74:II-1922, 1986

66. Kunze K-P, Kuck K-H, Geiger M, Bleifeld W: Programmed electrical stimulation in hypertrophic cardiomyopathy—specificity and sensitivity of different stimulation protocols, abstracted. J Am Coll Cardiol 7:195A, 1986

67. Watson RM, Liberati JM, Schwartz J, et al: Inducible polymorphic ventricular tachycardia and ventricular fibrillation in a subgroup of patients with hypertrophic cardiomyopathy at high risk for sudden deaths. J Am Coll Cardiol 10:761, 1987

68. Wellens HJJ, Brugada P, Stevenson WG: Programmed electrical stimulation of the heart in patients with life threatening ventricular arrhythmias. What is the significance of induced arrhythmias and what is the correct stimulation protocol? Circulation 72:1, 1985

69. McKenna WJ, Camm AJ: Sudden death in hypertrophic cardiomyopathy: assessment of patients at high risk. Circulation 80:1489, 1989

70. Losordo DW, Kosowsky BD: Hypertrophic cardiomyopathy and sudden death. (Letter.) N Engl J Med 319·1091, 1988

71. Cripps TR, Counihan PJ, Frenneaux MP et al: Signal-averaged electrocardiography in hypertrophic cardiomyopathy. J Am Coll Cardiol 7:701, 1986

72. Tajik AJ, Giuliani ER, Weidman WH et al: Idiopathic hypertrophic subaortic stenosis. Long-term surgical follow up. Am J Cardiol 34:815, 1974

73. Morrow AG, Reitz BA, Epstein SE et al: Operative treatment in hypertrophic subaortic stenosis: techniques and the results of pre and post-operative assessments in 83 patients. Circulation 52:88, 1975

74. Beahrs MM, Tajik AJ, Seward JB et al: Hypertrophic obstructive cardiomyopathy: ten- to 21 year follow-up after partial septal myectomy. Am J Cardiol 51:1160, 1983

75. Schulte HD, Bircks W, Lösse B: Surgical results in patients with hypertrophic obstructive cardiomyopathy. p. 122. In Baroldi G, Camerini F, Goodwin JF (eds): Advances in Cardiomyopathies. Springer-Verlag, Heidelberg, 1990

76. McKenna WJ: The natural history of hypertrophic cardiomyopathy. p. 135. In Brest AN, Shaver JA (eds): Cardiovascular Clinics. FA Davis, Philadelphia, 1988

77. Maron BJ, Epstein SE, Morrow AG: Symptomatic status and prognosis of patients after operation for hypertrophic obstructive cardiomyopathy: efficacy of ventricular septal myotomy and myectomy. Eur Heart J, suppl F. 4:175, 1983

78. Perloff JK: Pathogenesis of hypertrophic cardiomyopathy: hypotheses and speculations. Am Heart J 101:219, 1981

79. Frank MJ, Abdulla AM, Canedo MI, Saylors RE: Long-term medical management of hypertrophic obstructive cardiomyopathy. Am J Cardiol 42:993, 1978

80. McKenna WJ, Chetty S, Oakley CM, Goodwin JF: Arrhythmia in hypertrophic cardiomyopathy: exercise and 48 hour ambulatory electrocardiographic assessment with and without beta adrenergic blocking therapy. Am J Cardiol 45:1, 1980

81. Loogen F, Kuhn H, Krelhaus W: Natural history of hypertrophic obstructive cardiomyopathy and effect of therapy. p. 286. In Kaltenbach M, Loogen F, Olsen EGJ (eds): Cardiomyopathy and Myocardial Biopsy. Springer-Verlag, Berlin, 1978

82. Hanrath P, Mathey DG, Kremer P et al: Effect of verapamil on left ventricular isovolumic relaxation time and regional left ventricular filling in hypertrophic cardiomyopathy. Am J Cardiol 45:1258, 1980

83. Pearce PC, Hawkwy C, Symons C, Olsen EGJ: Role of calcium in the induction of cardiac hypertrophy and myofibrillar disarray. Experimental studies of a possible cause of hypertrophic cardiomyopathy. Br Heart J 54:420, 1985

84. Wagner JA, Sax FL, Weisman HF et al: Calcium antagonist receptors in the atrial tissue of patients with hypertrophic cardiomyopathy. N Engl J Med 320:755, 1989

85. Bonow RO, Rosing DR, Bacharach SL et al: Effects of verapamil on left ventricular systolic function and diastolic filling in patients with hypertrophic cardiomyopathy. Circulation 64:787, 1981

86. Kaltenbach M, Hopf R, Kober G et al: Treatment of hypertrophic obstructive cardiomyopathy with verapamil. Br Heart J 42:35, 1979

87. Rosing DR, Kent KM, Maron BJ, Epstein SE: Verapamil therapy: a new approach to the pharmacologic treatment of hypertrophic cardiomyopathy. II. Effects on exercise capacity and symptomatic status. Circulation 60:1208, 1979

88. Hopf R, Kaltenbach M: Medical treatment of hypertrophic cardiomyopathy. p. 103. In Baroldi G, Camerini F, Goodwin JF (eds): Advances in Cardiomyopathies. Springer-Verlag, Heidelberg, 1990

89. McKenna WJ, Harris L, Perez G et al: Arrhythmia in hypertrophic cardiomyopathy. II. Comparison of amiodarone and verapamil in treatment. Br Heart J 46:173, 1981

90. Pollick C: Muscular subaortic stenosis. Hemodynamic and clinical improvement after disopyramide. N Engl J Med 307:997, 1982

91. Cardiac Arrhythmia Suppression Trial (CAST) Investigators: Preliminary report: effect of encainide and flecainide on mortality in a randomised trial of arrhythmia suppression after myocardial infarction. N Engl J Med 321:406, 1989

92. Fananapazir L, Epstein SE: Hemodynamic and electrophysiologic evaluation of patients with hypertrophic cardiomyopathy surviving cardiac arrest. Am J Cardiol 67:280, 1991

93. Fogoros RN, Elson JJ, Bonnet CA: Actuarial incidence and pattern of occurrence of shocks following implantation of the automatic implantable cardioverter defibrillator. PACE 12:1465, 1989

94. Counihan PJ, McKenna WJ: Risk-benefit assessment of amiodarone in the treatment of cardiac arrhythmias. Drug Safety 5:286, 1990

95. McKenna WJ, Oakley CM, Krikler DM, Goodwin JF: Improved survival with amiodarone in patients with hypertrophic cardiomyopathy and ventricular tachycardia. Br Heart J 53:412, 1985

96. McKenna WJ, Adams KM, Poloniecki JD et al: Long term survival with amiodarone in patients with hypertrophic cardiomyopathy and ventricular tachycardia, abstracted. Circulation 80:II-7, 1989

97. Fananapazir L, Leon MB, Bonow RO et al: Sudden death during empiric amiodarone therapy in symptomatic hypertrophic cardiomyopathy. Am J Cardiol 67:169, 1991

98. Heger JJ, Prystowsky EN, Miles WM, Zipes DP: Clinical use and pharmacology of amiodarone. Med Clin North Am 68:1336, 1984

99. Cecchi F, Maron BJ, Epstein SE: Long term outcome of patients with hypertrophic cardiomyopathy successfully resuscitated after cardiac arrest. J Am Coll Cardiol 13:1283, 1989

100. Wilber DJ, Garan H, Finkelstein D et al: Out-of-hospital cardiac arrest; use of electrophysiologic testing in the prediction of long term outcome. N Engl J Med 318:19, 1988

101. Counihan PJ, McKenna WJ: Proceedings of interventional workshop on cardiac arrhythmias, Venice, 1991, pp. 381–393

102. McKenna WJ, Alfonso F: Arrhythmias in the cardiomyopathies and mitral valve prolapse. p. 59. In Zipes DP, Rowlands DJ (eds): Progress in Cardiology. Lea & Febiger, Philadelphia, 1988

23

Risk Assessment and Prognosis in Patients With Pericardial Diseases, Including Cardiac Tamponade

Noble O. Fowler

The prognosis in pericardial disease depends on several considerations. Pericarditis is not a single disease, but has multiple causes. The prognosis is closely related to the cause, to the associated illnesses, if any, and to the underlying status of the patient (e.g., age and whether or not the patient is immunocompromised). In many instances, for example, the pericarditis of acute myocardial infarction (AMI), pericarditis is an incidental finding, and the prognosis is that of underlying coronary artery disease (CAD). By contrast, tuberculous pericarditis is often the principal or only clinical manifestation of the disease, and the prognosis is determined by the course of the pericarditis. Pericarditis attributable to metastatic tumor carries a poor prognosis but, even then, the variety of neoplasm is important (see below).

In considering the risks of pericarditis, one must consider the immediate and short-term risks, as well as the long-term risks. The immediate and short-term risks include those of unrelieved pain, cardiac tamponade, associated myocarditis, and arrhythmia. There is also the added risk of the underlying disease (e.g., sep-

ticemia). Long-term risks include those of relapsing pericarditis, the development of effusive-constrictive pericarditis, and the development of constrictive pericarditis. Also, either chronic effusion without tamponade or adhesive fibrous pericarditis without constriction may appear. These last two conditions usually pose no particular risk to the patient but may lead to radiologically evident pericardial calcification or cardiac enlargement.

PERICARDITIS: PROGNOSIS AND RISK MANAGEMENT

Pericarditis is detected in 1 in 100 to 1 in 1,000 of all general hospital admissions. However, many cases are not clinically evident. According to Roberts and Ferrans,[1] there is evidence of pericardial inflammation in approximately 5% of autopsies. In this discussion, the risk and prognosis are estimated from studies of clinically diagnosed pericarditis.

The risks and prognosis in pericarditis depend so

TABLE 23-1. Etiology of Pericardial Effusion in 215 Patients

Cause	n
Cancer	45
Acute idiopathic	40
Renal failure	21
Dressler's syndrome	18
Chronic idiopathic	16
Postradiation	12
Rheumatoid arthritis	6
Systemic lupus erythematosus	4
Purulent	4
Rheumatic fever	4
Perforated heart or aorta	4
Other	41
Heart failure (19)	
Anticoagulants (2)	
Viral (2)	
Echinococcus (2)	
Unknown (16)	

(From Markiewicz et al.,[26] with permission.)

much on the cause that each etiologic variety of pericarditis must be considered individually. Table 23-1 lists the common causes of pericardial effusion seen in a large hospital in Israel. Table 23-2 lists the causes of pericarditis with cardiac tamponade seen between 1963 and 1986 at our University of Cincinnati Hospitals. On a hospital medical service, the commonest cause is malignant tumor, followed by nonspecific pericarditis. Other very common causes are chronic renal disease, infectious pericarditis, connective tissue disease, and traumatic pericarditis, including that caused by diagnostic and therapeutic procedures.

The risks and prognosis in pericardial disease also depend on patient characteristics. In immunocompro-

TABLE 23-2. Etiology of Cardiac Tamponade in 86 Cases: U.C. Medical Center 1963–1986

Cause	n
Malignant tumor	28
Idiopathic pericarditis	10
Uremia	7
Bacterial infections	7
Anticoagulant therapies	6
Dissecting aneurysm	5
Diagnostic procedures	4
Tuberculosis	3
Postpericardiotomy	3
Trauma	3
Connective tissue disease	3
Radiation	2
Myxedema	2
Cardiac rupture postinfarction	2
Primary chylopericardium	1

(From Fowler,[27] with permission.)

mised patients, purulent pericarditis, infectious pericarditis, and neoplastic pericarditis are more likely. These varieties of pericarditis are more likely to require surgical treatment, and thus have a less favorable outlook. Patients with acquired immune deficiency syndrome (AIDS) have a 30 to 40% prevalence of pericardial effusion, which is often clinically insignificant. By contrast, 5 to 10% of AIDS patients have clinical evidence of pericardial effusion, which may be related to bacterial infection, *Mycobacterium* tuberculosis, *Mycobacterium avium* intracellulare, lymphoma, and Kaposi's sarcoma.[2] Although infectious pericarditis may respond to specific treatment, the ultimate prognosis is for death in 3 to 5 years in most patients with AIDS, irrespective of the presence or absence of clinically evident pericardial effusion.

NATURAL HISTORY AND PROGNOSIS

Idiopathic Pericarditis

Idiopathic or nonspecific pericarditis is diagnosed in 10 to 15% of patients hospitalized for acute pericarditis. Except for pain, fever, and malaise, most cases have a benign course, with resolution in 1 to 3 weeks. However, there are complications, including cardiac tamponade and, when there is associated myocarditis, cardiac arrhythmias and congestive heart failure (CHF) may occur. When there is a viral etiology, chronic CHF caused by cardiomyopathy can be a sequel. Constrictive pericarditis is an uncommon late complication. From 15% to 32% of cases have one or more relapses, usually associated with pain, fever, and malaise, but seldom with other complications, such as tamponade of the heart (Table 23-3). None of our 41 patients with relapsing pericarditis died during a follow-up period of 6 months to 19 years.[3]

Neoplastic pericarditis is the commonest cause of acute pericarditis in hospitalized medical patients,

TABLE 23-3. Idiopathic Pericarditis

Recurrence Rate (No. of Cases)	Source
2 of 8	Nathan and Dathe (1946)[28]
3 of 17	Logue and Wendkos (1948)[29]
3 of 27	Levy and Patterson (1950)[30]
5 of 11	Evans (1950)[31]
1 of 22	Parker and Cooper (1951)[32]
7 of 50	Carmichael et al. (1951)[33]
5 of 24	Krook (1954)[34]
17 of 20	Robinson and Brigden (1968)[35]
20 of 62	Clementy et al. (1979)[36]
20% of 221	Guindo et al. (1990)[25]

comprising 20% or so of instances. There is a high risk of cardiac tamponade, effusive-constrictive, or constrictive pericarditis. Myocardial involvement may lead to CHF or to cardiac arrhythmia. The outlook for long survival is poor, especially when cardiac tamponade is present. In two studies, the mean survival in patients with neoplastic cardiac tamponade was 4 months, with 25% surviving 1 year.[4,5] However, in patients with breast cancer, the survival rate was better, averaging 9 months after surgical treatment of tamponade. In one-half to two-thirds of cancer patients, pericardial effusion is not caused directly by neoplastic invasion of the pericardium.[6,7] Such effusion may be due to radiation, opportunistic infection, chemotherapeutic agents, or incidental causes. In such instances, the prognosis may be more favorable.

Pericarditis With Myocardial Infarction

Early Stage

A pericardial friction rub is found in 7 to 10% of patients with AMI, usually between the second and seventh days of infarction. Pericardial effusion may be found by echocardiogram in 28% of patients with AMI.[8] Early pericarditis does not usually lead to complications and does not contraindicate anticoagulant therapy. However, acute pericarditis tends to occur with larger infarctions and thus to be associated with a higher infarction-related mortality rate.

Late-Stage-Postmyocardial Infarction Pericarditis or Dressler Syndrome

This variety of pericarditis most commonly occurs after the tenth day of AMI, but it may begin earlier, or as late as 2 months postinfarction. Pleuropericardial pain, fever, and leukocytosis generally occur. Anticoagulant therapy may be hazardous in this condition. Dressler's syndrome may cause cardiac tamponade and may be followed by relapsing or recurrent pericarditis. Dressler[9] described recurrences in 35% of 44 cases. Constrictive pericarditis is an extremely rare sequel. The condition usually responds to indomethacin, ibuprofen, or adrenocorticosteroid therapy, although the use of these agents entails some theoretical risk of delayed healing of the MI.[10] Aspirin may be safer. The prevalence of this condition has declined substantially in recent years for unknown reasons.

Uremic Pericarditis

Before the availability of dialysis procedures, uremic pericarditis was usually a terminal event in patients with chronic renal disease, occurring in 35 to 50% of patients with end-stage renal disease and pre-

saging death within 1 to 3 weeks.[7] Today, uremic pericarditis is usually not fatal and is principally seen in patients receiving chronic hemodialysis. The occurrence of uremic pericarditis in patients with end-stage renal disease after the onset of dialysis is said to be within the range of 8 to 12%.[7] Silverberg and associates[11] found uremic pericarditis in 43 of 218 uremic patients undergoing either hemodialysis or peritoneal dialysis, a prevalence of 20%. Dialysis-associated pericarditis can be life-threatening, causing death in 8 to 10% of patients with this complication.[7]

Prognosis

Comty et al.[12] treated 25 patients with uremic pericarditis. These patients were treated with more intensive hemodialysis, employed every 36 to 48 hours. In addition, eight patients received oral prednisone. Four were treated outside the hospital and recovered rapidly. Twenty-one patients were disabled for 1 to 22 weeks. Nine patients had an uneventful recovery. In four cases, cardiac tamponade developed. Three required pericardiectomy. Two died of intractable heart failure. Constrictive pericarditis developed in one patient, and subacute constrictive pericarditis developed in two patients.

Tuberculous Pericarditis

In one current study from Spain, tuberculosis was responsible for 4% of cases of acute pericarditis and for 7% of cases of cardiac tamponade.[13]

Prognosis

In the era before antituberculous chemotherapy (before 1945), tuberculous pericarditis was fatal in as many as 80 to 85% of patients. With modern therapy, the mortality rate is well below 50%, but modern therapy may not prevent later constrictive pericarditis. Eighteen of our 19 patients[14] were treated for tuberculosis. Four received streptomycin alone; 14 received two or more antituberculous drugs for 3 months to 2 years. Four patients also received adrenal steroids to treat unrelieved cardiac compression. One patient died of pulmonary embolism before treatment could be started. Seventeen of 18 treated patients responded satisfactorily, but 7 required later pericardiectomy because of failure to relieve constrictive or effusive-constrictive pericarditis. One patient died in the hospital 23 days after the start treatment.

Postcommissurotomy Syndrome

Postcommissurotomy syndrome, characterized by chest pain, fever, leukocytosis, and a pericardial rub or pericardial effusion, occurs in 10 to 30% of patients who have undergone cardiac surgical procedures. The syndrome usually develops during a period of 10 days to 2 months after the surgical procedure. Most cases respond to indomethacin, ibuprofen, or a brief course of adrenal steroid therapy. The complications are cardiac tamponade, relapsing pericarditis, atrial arrhythmias, and, later, constrictive pericarditis. In a study from Yale University, cardiac tamponade developed in 10 of 1,290 patients who survived a cardiac operation (0.8%).[15] In a small percentage of patients, atrial fibrillation or flutter develops at the time of the attack. Constrictive pericarditis developed following cardiac operation in 0.2% of 5,207 operations, but this percentage is believed to be higher than the usual experience.[16] Engle and Ito[17] described relapses in 4 of 30 patients with postpericardiotomy syndrome.

Infectious Pericarditis

The pericardium may be infected via the bloodstream (septicemia), by spread from infective endocarditis (valvular ring abscess or myocardial abscess), by septic coronary embolism, by spread from contiguous pneumonitis, by invasion through foreign bodies or surgical procedures, or from rupture of an hepatic abscess. *Staphylococcus aureus* and streptococci are the commonest causes in adults. In children, *Staphylococcus aureus* is most common, followed by *Haemophilus influenzae* and *Meningococcus*. Pneumococci are a less common cause than in the era before penicillin. The prognosis depends on the causative organism, the immunologic status of the patient, the source of the infection, and whether purulent pericarditis is present. At one extreme, *Histoplasma* pericarditis usually behaves like nonspecific pericarditis and does not require treatment with ketoconazole or amphotericin B, unless there is disseminated histoplasmosis. Although cardiac tamponade may occur, it is uncommon. Late constrictive pericarditis may occur but is uncommon. Only one of 16 patients whom we reported on required amphotericin B therapy,[18] and in no case did constrictive pericarditis develop. Follow-up studies of 10 patients 6 months to 12 years later showed no instance of constrictive pericarditis or late recurrence of the infection. On the other hand, bacterial infection of the pericardium requires appropriate antibiotic therapy and either needle aspiration or more often surgical drainage of the pericardial space.[19] Purulent pericarditis requires antibiotic therapy and open surgical drainage. Some instances require pericardiectomy for adequate control of the infection. Untreated cases of purulent pericarditis are nearly always fatal. In treated cases, Klacsmann et al.[20] found the mortality rate to be approximately 40%.

Rheumatic Fever

Currently, although still seen in the United States, rheumatic fever is uncommon in children and is rarely seen in adults.[21] As a rule, rheumatic pericarditis is associated with acute rheumatic fever, myocarditis, and valvulitis. Bed rest is indicated. Treatment with oral adrenal corticosteroids is usually indicated when there is evidence of myocarditis, especially with CHF. Penicillin is given for 10 days to eradicate group A β-hemolytic streptococci. Long-term follow-up for evidence of chronic rheumatic valvular disease is required, and long-term prophylactic oral penicillin is required daily. Cardiac tamponade is rare in rheumatic pericarditis, and pericardiocentesis is hardly ever indicated.

Connective Tissue Disease

Pericarditis is a common complication of systemic rheumatoid disease, disseminated lupus erythematosus, and scleroderma. It is less commonly seen with Wegener's granulomatosis and with polyarteritis nodosa. Approximately 30% of patients with systemic lupus erythematosus (SLE) have pericarditis at some time, and in 6% of cases pericarditis may be the initial manifestation of the disease.

Necropsy studies show evidence of pericarditis in roughly 30% of patients with rheumatoid disease, but the clinical incidence is much lower. Echocardiography in asymptomatic patients, however, shows a high prevalence of pericardial effusion. Large pericardial effusions may develop but seldom require pericardiocentesis. In a small percentage of patients, constrictive pericarditis develops, requiring pericardiectomy.

Iatrogenic Pericarditis

Pericarditis may follow a number of diagnostic and therapeutic procedures. Right or left heart catheterization, endomyocardial biopsy, needle puncture of the left ventricle (Brock procedure), and transseptal catheterization of the left atrium may cause intrapericardial bleeding and acute tamponade. At times, relapsing pericarditis follows.

Therapeutic agents and procedures that may cause pericarditis include the following:

1. Drugs that may cause lupus-like syndrome: procainamide, Dilantin, hydralazine, isonicotinic acid hydrazide
2. Antineoplastic drugs: doxorubicin; psicofuranine, cyclophosphamide
3. Miscellaneous drugs: penicillin, phenylbutazone, methysergide
4. Anticoagulants: coumadin, heparin, streptokinase, urokinase, tissue plasminogen activators

5. Radiation
6. Pericardial bleeding following diagnostic catheterization, pacemaker catheter insertion, or needle puncture of the heart; bleeding following insertion of central venous lines for parenteral alimentation

Therapeutic X-irradiation directed toward the mediastinum, in doses of 4,000 rads or more, may be followed by acute pericarditis, pericardial effusion, effusive-constrictive pericarditis, or constrictive pericarditis. In the Stanford series, radiation was a leading cause of constrictive pericarditis.[22] Drugs may cause pericarditis. Intrapericardial bleeding may complicate coumadin overdosage. Thrombolytic therapy for acute cardiac infarction does not appear to increase the prevalence of pericardial effusion. Therapeutic agents that produce the lupus-like syndrome may cause pericardial and pleural effusion. Among these are procainamide, diphenylhydantoin, and hydralazine. Methysergide may cause pericardial fibrosis as well as valvulitis. Therapeutic sclerosis of esophageal varices by needle puncture may be complicated by pericarditis. Cardiac tamponade may complicate the placement of central venous lines for parenteral hyperalimentation.

PROCEDURE RISK THAT MAY AFFECT OUTCOME

In the evaluation of pericardial disease, a number of risk-free noninvasive procedures may be employed, such as physical examination, electrocardiography, chest radiography, and echocardiography. Needle pericardiocentesis is often employed, especially when there is cardiac tamponade, when purulent pericarditis is suspected, or when there is persistence of effusion with constitutional symptoms, and the cause is uncertain. Permanyer-Miralda et al.[13] carried out pericardiocentesis after 7 days of undiagnosed acute pericarditis with persistent pericardial effusion accompanied by constitutional symptoms. Local pericardial surgical drainage was considered after 3 weeks if no diagnosis had been reached. Needle pericardiocentesis may be associated with a 1 to 3% mortality rate; the procedure is more hazardous when there is little or no effusion anterior to the right ventricle on echocardiography, or when there are adhesions, or when both problems exist. The risk of needle pericardiocentesis can be lessened when the procedure is performed only by cardiologists or thoracic surgeons, when it is carried out under echocardiographic monitoring, and when resuscitative equipment is at hand. Callahan et al.[23] reported no deaths in 117 consecutive cases when needle pericardiocentesis was guided by two-dimensional echocardiography. The risk of surgical drainage and biopsy can be reduced by using a subxiphoid approach under local anesthesia, avoiding entry into the pleural space.

TREATMENTS THAT AFFECT OUTCOME

The risks of acute pericarditis are lessened if the patient is hospitalized, especially for an initial attack. Hospitalization permits observation for such complications as cardiac tamponade, myocarditis, or cardiac arrhythmia. Hospitalization permits a complete workup for the cause of pericarditis, which will determine whether a specific treatment directed toward the cause is needed (e.g., infection, neoplasm, connective tissue disease, uremia, or withdrawal of an offending therapeutic agent). Observation of the course, in-hospital, will determine whether pericardial drainage, pericardial biopsy, or pericardial resection is required.

Specific treatments for acute pericarditis are chosen in accordance with the etiology as described under Natural History and Prognosis. Neoplastic pericarditis may be treated with chemotherapy, irradiation, and pericardiocentesis. Pericardial resection may be required when tamponade is present. Infectious pericarditis is treated with pericardial drainage and appropriate antibiotics. Tuberculous pericarditis is treated for 6 to 9 months with triple drug therapy. Iatrogenic pericarditis is treated by withdrawal of the offending agent. Uremic pericarditis is treated with change in the dialysis program to more frequent hemodialysis. At times pericardial drainage, intrapericardial triamcinolone, or pericardial resection is required.

Certain varieties of pericarditis are treated with anti-inflammatory agents or with adrenocorticosteroids. Acute idiopathic pericarditis may respond to aspirin, indomethacin, or ibuprofen. Certain other varieties of pericarditis may respond to these agents but may require prednisone if these remedies fail to provide relief. Relapsing pericarditis, Dressler syndrome, post-traumatic pericarditis, and postpericardiotomy syndrome are in this category. Pericarditis associated with rheumatic fever or connective tissue diseases usually requires prednisone or other adrenocorticosteroid therapy.

Ibuprofen may cause nausea, gastrointestinal ulceration, dizziness, headache, skin rash, tinnitus, pancytopenia, fluid retention, aggravation of CHF, bronchospasm, or acute renal failure. Hepatitis occurs rarely. Indomethacin may cause esophageal, gastric, or duodenal ulcer; fluid retention; gastrointestinal bleeding; headache; dizziness; somnolence; tinnitus; mental confusion; corneal deposits; retinal disturbances; and hepatitis. Drug-related dementia is a common problem in patients over age 65.

Side effects of aspirin include gastritis, gastrointestinal bleeding, and bronchospasm. Aspirin hypersensitivity may cause angioneurotic edema and vasomotor collapse.

Adrenosteroid therapy may be complicated by infections, hypokalemia, alkalosis, fluid retention, decreased glucose tolerance, hypertension, moon facies, hirsutism, buffalo hump, peptic ulcer, poor wound healing, skeletal myopathy, osteoporosis, and aseptic necrosis of the femoral head. Emotional disorders are common. Glaucoma or cataracts may occur.

Pericardial resection is indicated for the following conditions: constrictive pericarditis, effusive-constrictive pericarditis, infectious pericarditis unrelieved by pericardial drainage and antibiotics, neoplastic pericarditis with repeated cardiac tamponade, and uremic pericarditis with repeated tamponade unrelieved by a change in the dialysis program. Occasionally, pericardial resection is indicated for relapsing pericarditis that requires continued high-dose prednisone therapy, that is unrelieved by prednisone, or for which prednisone has produced unacceptable complications. At Emory University, of 102 pericardiectomies performed over a 7.5-year period, relapsing pericarditis was the indication in 15 cases.[24] The mortality rate for pericardial resection in constrictive or effusive-constrictive pericarditis is in the range of 5 to 15%, even in the most experienced medical centers; pericardial resection is less risky in the other settings in which less extensive dissection is necessary. The Mayo Clinic experience from 1936 to 1990 yielded an operative mortality of 14%; the risk was 1% for patients in New York Heart Association (NYHA) class 1 or 2, 10% for those in class 3, and 46% for class 4.[7]

COSTS

The cost of treating a patient with pericarditis will depend on the cause of the disease, on the length of the hospitalization required, on the diagnostic tests that are necessary, and on whether cardiac surgical procedures are required. Several years ago, the estimated cost for treatment of one of our cases of acute idiopathic pericarditis, including a 4-day stay in the coronary care unit, was $4,075. For another patient with constrictive pericarditis who required pericardiectomy, the cost of treatment, including operating room fees, anesthesia fees, recovery room charges, professional fees, and laboratory tests, was $12,696. These costs would undoubtedly be considerably higher today.

REFERENCES

1. Roberts WC, Ferrans VJ: A survey of the causes and consequences of pericardial heart disease. p. 49. In Reddy PS, Leon DF, Shaver JA (eds): Pericardial Disease. Raven Press, New York, 1982
2. Anderson DW, Virmani R: Emerging patterns of heart disease in human immunodeficiency virus infection. Hum Pathol 21:253, 1990
3. Fowler NO, Harbin AD III: Recurrent acute pericarditis. Follow-up study of 31 patients. J Am Coll Cardiol 7:300, 1986
4. Posner MR, Cohen GI, Skarin AT: Pericardial disease in patients with cancer. Am J Med 71:407, 1981
5. Piehler JM, Schaff HV, Orszulak TA et al: Surgical management of effusive pericardial disease. J Thorac Cardiovasc Surg 90:506, 1985
6. Buck M, Ingle JN, Guiliani GR et al: Pericardial effusion in women with breast cancer. Cancer 60:263, 1987
7. Shabetai R (Guest Editor): Diseases of the pericardium. Cardiol Clin 8:579, 1990
8. Galve E, Garcia-del-Castillo H, Evangelista A et al: Pericardial effusion in the course of myocardial infarction: incidence, natural history, and clinical relevance. Circulation 73:294, 1986
9. Dressler W: The post-myocardial-infarction syndrome. A report on forty-four cases. Arch Intern Med 103:28, 1959
10. Brown EJ Jr, Kloner RA, Schoen FJ et al: Scar thinning due to ibuprofen administration after experimental myocardial infarction. Am J Cardiol 51:877, 1983
11. Silverberg S, Oreopoulos DG, Wise DJ et al: Pericarditis in patients undergoing long-term hemodialysis and peritoneal dialysis. Am J Med 63:874, 1977
12. Comty CM, Cohen SL, Shapiro FL: Pericarditis in chronic uremia and its sequels. Ann Intern Med 75:173, 1971
13. Permanyer-Miralda G, Sagrista-Sauleda J, Soler-Soler J: Primary acute pericardial disease: a prospective series of 231 consecutive patients. Am J Cardiol 56:623, 1985
14. Fowler NO, Manitsas GT: Infectious pericarditis. Prog Cardiovasc Dis 16:323, 1973
15. Ofori-Krakye SK, Tyberg TI, Geha AS et al: Late cardiac tamponade after open heart surgery: incidence, role of anticoagulants in its pathogenesis, and its relationship to the postpericardiotomy syndrome. Circulation 63:1323, 1981
16. Kutcher MA, King SB III, Alimurung BN et al: Constrictive pericarditis as a complication of cardiac surgery: recognition of an entity. Am J Cardiol 50:742, 1982
17. Engle MA, Ito T: The postpericardiotomy syndrome. Am J Cardiol 7:73, 1961
18. Picardi JL, Kauffman CA, Schwarz J et al: Pericarditis caused by histoplasma capsulatum. Am J Cardiol 37:82, 1976
19. Okoroma EO, Perry LW, Scott LP III: Acute bacterial pericarditis in children: report of 25 cases. Am Heart J 90:709, 1975
20. Klacsmann PG, Bulkley BH, Hutchins GM: The changed spectrum of purulent pericarditis: an 86 year autopsy experience in 200 patients. Am J Med 63:666, 1977
21. Massell BF, Chute CG, Walker AM et al: Penicillin and the marked decrease in morbidity and mortality from

rheumatic fever in the United States. N Engl J Med 318: 280, 1988

22. Cameron J, Oesterle SN, Baldwin JC et al: The etiologic spectrum of constrictive pericarditis. Am Heart J 113: 354, 1987

23. Callahan JA, Seward JB, Nishimura RA et al: Two-dimensional echocardiographically guided pericardiocentesis: experience in 117 consecutive patients. Am J Cardiol 55:476, 1985

24. Miller JI, Mansour KA, Hatcher CR, Jr: Pericardiectomy: current indications, concepts, and results in a university center. Ann Thorac Surg 34:40, 1982

25. Guindo J, Rodriguez de la Serna A, Ramio J et al: Recurrent pericarditis. Relief with colchicine. Circulation 82: 1117, 1990

26. Markiewicz W, Borovik R, Ecker S: Cardiac tamponade in medical patients: treatment and prognosis in the echocardiographic era. Am Heart J 111:1138, 1986

27. Fowler NO: Pericarditis. New Dev Med 3:41, 1988

28. Nathan DA, Dathe RA: Pericarditis with effusion following infections of the upper respiratory tract. Am Heart J 31:115, 1946

29. Logue RB, Wendkos MH: Acute pericarditis of benign type. Am Heart J 36:587, 1948

30. Levy RL, Patterson MC: Acute serofibrinous pericarditis of undetermined cause. Am J Med 8:34, 1950

31. Evans E: Acute nonspecific benign pericarditis. JAMA 143:954, 1950

32. Parker RC, Jr, Cooper HR: Acute idiopathic pericarditis. JAMA 147:835, 1951

33. Carmichael DB, Sprague HB, Wyman SM et al: Acute nonspecific pericarditis. Circulation 3:321, 1951

34. Krook H: Acute nonspecific pericarditis. Acta Med Scand 148:201, 1954

35. Robinson J, Brigden W: Recurrent pericarditis. Br Med J 2.272, 1968

36. Clémenty J, Jambert H, Dallacchio M: Les péricardites aiguës récidivantes: 20 observations. Arch Mal Coeur 72: 857, 1979

Section V

PROGNOSIS AS RELATED TO CONDUCTION SYSTEM DISEASE ARRHYTHMIAS

24
Prognosis of Patients With Syncope

Wishwa N. Kapoor

Syncope is defined as a sudden transient loss of consciousness associated with loss of postural tone with spontaneous recovery. Syncope should be differentiated from other states of altered consciousness, such as dizziness, presyncope, vertigo, coma, seizures, and narcolepsy, since these entities have markedly different etiologies and prognoses. In addition, patients requiring electrical or pharmacologic cardioversion are considered to have experienced sudden death rather than syncope.

INCIDENCE/PREVALENCE

Syncope is a common medical problem. Studies by questionnaires among U.S. Air Force personnel, college students, and South African men have reported a history of syncope in 12 to 47% of individuals interviewed.[1-3] Approximately one third of these episodes have been post-traumatic and therefore do not meet the definition of syncope. Even excluding these cases, the prevalence of syncope is high in the general population. In a survey of ambulatory patients in Pittsburgh, we found a history of syncope in approximately 25% of those interviewed.

Syncope accounts for approximately 3% of emergency department visits and for approximately 1 to 6% of hospital admissions per year. In the Framingham cohort of 2,336 men and 2,873 women, aged 30 to 62 years at entry into the study, at least one syncopal episode was reported by 71 (3%) of men and 101 (3.5%) of women during the 26-year course of surveillance.[4]

The vast majority of the syncopal episodes (79 to 88%) were classified as isolated syncope, defined as transient loss of consciousness in patients without prior or concurrent neurologic or cardiovascular disease manifestations. The mean age at initial episode for men was 52 years and for women 50 years. More than one episode was reported in 30% of men and in 27% of women with syncope. Table 24-1 shows estimates of isolated syncope by age and sex from the Framingham cohort. There was a significant increase with age in both sexes in prevalence of syncope. Elderly men (at least 75 years of age) had significantly more episodes than did elderly women.

Syncope in the elderly is a particularly worrisome symptom because of the higher prevalence of chronic morbidity in these patients. In a comparative study of syncope in the elderly and young,[5] elderly patients (mean age 71 years) had a threefold higher prevalence of hypertension, a fourfold higher history of myocardial infarction (MI), and a two- to threefold higher history of congestive heart failure (CHF) or diabetes as compared with the young (mean age 39 years). Cerebrovascular disease was present almost exclusively in the elderly group.

In a study of institutionalized elderly with a mean age of 87 years, a 10-year prevalence of syncope of 23% and a 1-year incidence of 7% was found.[6] There was also a 2-year prospective follow-up, which revealed a yearly incidence of 6% and a recurrence rate of 30%. Thus, syncope is also common in multi-impaired, institutionalized elderly and is a likely manifestation of comorbid diseases.

TABLE 24-1. Prevalence of Isolated Syncope

Age (yr)	Prevalence of Isolated Syncope by 1,000 Person-exams	
	Men	Women
35–44	7.4	8.7
45–54	13.9	17.1
55–64	17.1	22.5
65–74	28.3	27.7
≥75	55.9	36.1

(Adapted from Savage et al.,[4] with permission.)

NATURAL HISTORY

The Framingham study of isolated syncope showed that over the 26 years of surveillance in patients without stigmata of neurologic and cardiovascular disease, there was no significant increase in all-cause mortality, cardiovascular mortality, or sudden deaths.[4] These findings, however, are not generalizable, since the patient population consisted of a relatively healthy group who in general did not have underlying co-morbid problems. No other studies are available in comparing the outcomes of syncope patients with patients without syncope.

Recent studies on the outcome of patients with syncope have all evaluated outcomes within subgroups of syncope patients and have not incorporated comparison groups without syncope. The outcome has been evaluated within diagnostic subgroups (i.e., cardiac, noncardiac, or syncope of unknown etiology). In all recent studies, patients with cardiac cause of syncope have had higher mortality as compared with patients with noncardiac etiology or syncope of unknown etiology.[7–10] Figures 24-1 and 24-2 show the mortality and sudden death rates of a subgroup of patients with syncope.[8] In this group, patients with cardiac-related syncope had a markedly higher incidence of sudden death than that of patients with other etiologies of syncope. Even after adjustment for underlying differences in co-morbidity, the differences in mortality and sudden death remained significant.

RELATIONSHIP OF PATIENT CHARACTERISTICS TO MORTALITY

Etiology

A retrospective review of records of 510 patients seen between 1945 and 1957 was the first study of the distribution of causes of syncope.[11] The most common cause

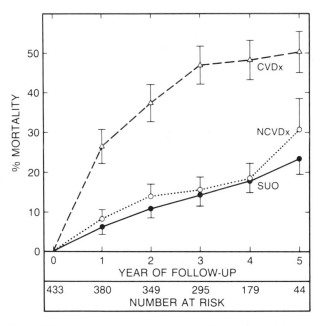

Fig. 24-1. Actuarial mortality rates of patients with cardiac cause of syncope (*triangles*), noncardiac cause of syncope (open circles), and syncope of unknown cause (*solid circles*). The mortality in patients with a cardiac cause of syncope was significantly higher than in patients with noncardiac cause (p <0.00001) or in patients with syncope of unknown cause (p <0.00001). (From Kapoor,[8] with permission.)

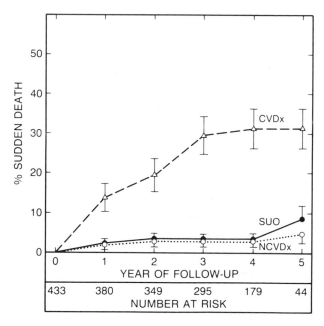

Fig. 24-2. Actuarial incidence of sudden death of patients with cardiac cause of syncope (*triangles*), noncardiac cause of syncope (*open circles*), and syncope of unknown cause (*solid circles*). The incidence of sudden death in patients with cardiac cause of syncope was significantly higher than in patients with noncardiac cause (p <0.00001) or in patients with syncope of unknown cause (p <0.00001). (From Kapoor,[8] with permission.)

was vasovagal syncope, reported in 58% of patients. The vast majority of causes included a variety of noncardiac illnesses, with unknown cause comprising only 5%. This study had several problems, including retrospective review of charts, lack of availability of cardiac monitoring or electrophysiologic testing, and exclusion of 500 patients from analysis because of unsatisfactory records.

During the 1980s, five studies of patients presenting with syncope have been reported,[8–10,12,13] one of which deals exclusively with the elderly.[6] These studies have been retrospective and prospective and include patients from the emergency department,[8,10,13] intensive care unit (ICU),[9] and inpatient services.[8] Large differences in the proportion of patients with cardiac versus noncardiac causes have been noted in these studies. Cardiac causes have been assigned in 8 to 39% of patients in recent studies. These differences are largely due to the co-morbid illnesses of the patients, the source of patient accrual, and the extent of diagnostic workup, since studies reporting the highest rates of cardiac etiologies are those that have evaluated patients more extensively or in the ICU settings.

All studies except one[10] have also shown that, in a large proportion of patients with syncope (38 to 47%), a cause is not established even after a standardized diagnostic evaluation. One study reported unknown diagnoses in 13%, but this report was not comparable to other studies, since approximately 30% of patients were those presenting with a seizure.[10]

The prognosis of patients with syncope has been linked to the etiology of loss of consciousness. The prognosis of patients with vasodepressor syncope, situational syncope, and most of the other noncardiac etiologies is dependent on their underlying co-morbid conditions. Syncope is not known to have any significant impact on their outcome. On the other hand, syncope has important prognostic implications in patients with cardiac disease. For example, in patients with aortic stenosis, the mean survival after syncope is reported to be 2 to 3 years in the absence of valve replacement. Similarly, syncope is considered a marker of worse prognosis in hypertrophic cardiomyopathy. Syncope can be a manifestation of tachyarrhythmia and of bradyarrhythmia. However, it is not known whether the presence of syncope indicates a worse prognosis in patients with arrhythmia. Patients with cardiac etiology have higher mortality and sudden death rates as compared with other patients with syncope[8] (See Fig. 24-1).

Age

In elderly patients, a cardiac cause of syncope is more likely to be diagnosed. In one study, cardiac etiology was diagnosed twice as often in elderly patients as in younger patients (34% vs. 17%).[5] The rate of noncardiac cause was higher in the young (composed primarily of a larger number of patients with vasovagal syncope). In the elderly, syncope more often resulted in trauma, which was often major. The overall mortality and incidence of sudden death in the elderly with cardiac diagnosis were similar to those in the young; however, in the elderly with a noncardiac cause of syncope or syncope of unknown cause, mortality and incidence of sudden death were higher. In multivariate analysis, in patients with noncardiac cause of syncope or syncope of unknown cause, a history of CHF, older age, and male sex were important predictors of mortality.[5]

Outcomes among the institutionalized elderly are somewhat different from outcomes among community elderly. In a 2-year prospective study of institutionalized elderly, it was disclosed that of 46 of 67 patients in whom the cause of syncope was determined, 21% were of cardiac origin and 48% were noncardiac.[6] It was also found that 31% of elderly patients had syncope of unknown etiology. There were no differences in mortality in subgroups of patients with cardiac or noncardiac syncope or syncope of unknown cause. Mortality at 2 years in each of the groups ranged between 40 to 50%. It should be noted, however, that these patients were very elderly, with a mean age of 87 years. These very elderly patients often have multiple other co-morbid illnesses that may have a major impact on survival and tend to mask any effect of cardiac syncope on mortality.

Diagnostic Testing

The issues of the relationship of patient characteristics to mortality in the area of diagnostic testing have primarily centered around the detection of arrhythmias. Studies have involved the detection of arrhythmias by prolonged electrocardiogram (ECG) or by electrophysiologic studies.

Prolonged Electrocardiographic Monitoring

It is well recognized that arrhythmias are frequently found on prolonged ECG monitoring in patients with syncope (11 to 70%). However, most arrhythmias are of short duration and do not produce symptoms during monitoring. The importance of these arrhythmias in determining a cause of prior syncopal episode or in defining a prognosis has been difficult to establish, since similar arrhythmias frequently occur in asymptomatic or normal subjects. However, the finding of certain arrhythmias is associated with worse outcomes. In one study, frequent or repetitive premature ventricular contractions (PVCs) were associated with a threefold or fourfold increased risk of mortality in patients with syncope (adjusted for underlying disease).[14] Similarly, sinus pauses were associated with increased risk of mortality and sudden death.[14]

Electrophysiologic Studies

Electrophysiologic studies are being widely used for evaluation of syncope, especially in patients with underlying organic cardiac disease. No controlled trials with this technology have been conducted. The studies reporting on this issue have been case studies identifying a subset of patients who have abnormal tests (evidence of conduction system disease, inducible tachyarrhythmias, or other abnormalities, such as carotid sinus hypersensitivity). Patients with abnormal tests are treated, and those patients considered to have normal results are followed without specific therapy. The proportion of patients with abnormal results has been variable in these studies. Table 24-2 summarizes the results of some of these recent studies.[15–24]

There is considerable variability in the types of patients and electrophysiologic protocols reported in the literature. First, some studies have only included patients with recurrent syncope, while others have tested patients with one episode and even those not with syncope but with presyncope. Because the patient groups reported on are not comparable, the results of these studies become less generalizable. Second, in some studies, extensive noninvasive evaluation has been done prior to electrophysiologic testing. Others do not report having done ambulatory monitoring or other evaluation prior to electrophysiologic testing. The extent of noninvasive evaluation is likely to affect the reported yield of these studies. Third, most studies have included patients with a wide variety of underlying heart diseases, but some have reported on patients without clinical heart disease[15] and in those with bundle-branch block. The types of heart disease have been heterogeneous, with the largest category being coronary disease. It is expected that the yield may be different in patients with different varieties of heart disease. Patients with cardiomyopathy are likely to have a higher rate of inducible ventricular tachycardia than that of patients with mild degrees of coronary disease and without prior MI. Finally, each laboratory has used its own routine protocol and criteria. The variations have included left ventricular (LV) stimulation, the use of isoproterenol, and a number of extrastimuli for induction of ventricular tachycardia. The criteria for abnormalities as a cause of syncope have also been different in various studies, contributing partly to the difference in the yield of this test from different centers. Similarly, multiple abnormalities are often found, making it difficult to determine which of the findings was the cause of syncope.

In evaluating outcomes, recurrence of syncope and mortality (sudden death, cardiac mortality, or overall mortality) have been used.

Recurrence Rates After Electrophysiologic Studies

The frequency of syncope, before and after therapy, is difficult to analyze statistically, since syncopal events are often sporadic, and it is likely that the most

TABLE 24-2. Results of Electrophysiologic Testing in Patients With Syncope of Unknown Etiology

Investigators	No. of Patients	ABN EP (%)	EP Abnormality[a] SVT (%)	VT (%)	Conduction[b] (%)	Other[c]	Mean Follow-up (mo)	Recurrent Syncope ABN EP (%)	NL EP (%)	Mortality ABN EP (%)	NL EP (%)
DiMarco et al.[16]	25	68	6	53	18	24	18	18	50	6	0
Gulamhusein et al.[17]	34	18	50	0	50	0	15	0	39	0	0
Hess et al.[18]	32	56	61	6	33	0	21	11	29	11	0
Akhtar et al.[19]	30	53	0	68	32	0	17	13	80	0	0
Olshansky et al.[20]	105	50	18	56	22	10	26	28	20	6	0
Doherty et al.[21]	119	66	29	40	11	19	27	32	24	13	4
Denes and Ezri[22]	50	74	12	8	60	24	23	5	8	14	8
Teichman et al.[23]	150	75	11	22	54	12	31	15	47	5	14
Denes et al.[24]	89	71	15	15	41	—	47	11	13	41	9
Bass et al.[15]	70	53	7	80	13	0	30	32	24	48	9
Total No., mean %	704	58	21	35	34	10	25	16	33	14	4

Abbreviations: ABN, abnormal; NL, normal; VT, ventricular tachycardia; SVT, supraventricular tachycardia; EP, electrophysiologic testing.
[a] Patients have more than one abnormality.
[b] Includes abnormal sinus node, atrioventricular node, or His-Purkinje function.
[c] Includes hypervagotonia, carotid sinus hypersensitivity.
(Adapted from Kapoor et al.,[25] with permission.)

recent episode would have precipitated the evaluation and the consequent electrophysiologic testing, resulting in a clustering of the syncopal events just *prior* to electrophysiologic studies. Thus, the assessment of post-treatment efficacy may be difficult.[25] All studies on electrophysiologic testing have used recurrence as an endpoint of efficacy. Recurrences have been lower in patients with positive studies (0 to 32%) as compared with those with negative findings (8 to 80%) in most reports, suggesting that treatment may have had a beneficial effect on this outcome. Several problems make this conclusion difficult, however. First, some of the larger studies show an equal or higher rate of recurrence between patients with negative and positive studies.[15,20,21] Second, the follow-up interval has been variable in different studies, and loss to follow-up is substantial in some studies, potentially leading to biases in reporting recurrence rate. Third, all the studies have used nonblinded assessment of outcome, which can be subject to ascertainment bias.

Mortality Rates After Electrophysiologic Studies

Most reports of electrophysiologic studies have paid less attention to mortality rates. Except for two studies,[15,24] a mortality rate of 0 to 14% is reported over a mean of approximately 2 years. Since cardiac syncope is reported to confer higher mortality, these results appear to be inconsistent, showing a mortality rate similar to that of patients with syncope of unknown origin. One would expect that patients undergoing electrophysiologic testing should have a higher mortality because they have significant heart disease and arrhythmia. The results could be interpreted as showing that treatment of arrhythmia (diagnosed by electrophysiologic testing) has led to improved outcome, but a more likely explanation is that the ascertainment of mortality is incomplete. Incomplete ascertainment seems to be the problem, as studies that have paid specific attention to mortality have reported markedly higher rates in patients with positive electrophysiologic tests. For example, one study showed markedly higher mortality (61% vs. 15% at 3 years) and sudden death rates (48% vs. 9% at 3 years) in patients with positive, as compared with negative electrophysiologic results.[15]

OTHER OUTCOME MEASURES

Recurrences

Among 433 patients who presented with syncope, the recurrence rate was 35.3% over a mean period of follow-up of 40 months.[26] Approximately 61% of all recurrences occurred within 1 year of entry into this

study. Patients with cardiac causes of syncope had a similar rate of recurrence, as compared with those with non-cardiac causes of syncope. Patients with syncope of unknown origin had a higher rate of recurrence, but these patients were not significantly different from the other two groups (Fig. 24-3). Few new etiologies emerged based on evaluation of recurrence. In approximately 10% of patients, new etiologies were found that included seizure disorder, supraventricular tachycardia, and sinus node disease. Recurrence led to major morbidity in 5% of those patients (including fractures of head, leg, face, and arm) and to minor injury in 7% of patients.

Recurrences often have serious implications for physicians, since they could indicate undiagnosed or untreated underlying diseases. As a result, there may be concern that patients with recurrence may be at risk of increased mortality. In one study, recurrences were neither a predictor of overall mortality nor a predictor of sudden death by multivariate analysis.[26]

Other Cardiovascular Outcomes

In patients with isolated syncope as defined in the Framingham cohort, there was no difference in the rate of stroke or MI over the 26-year follow-up between patients with isolated syncope and those without syncope. Similar data are not available in patients with other etiologies of syncope. In our study, rates of multiple different cardiovascular events were higher in patients with cardiac cause of syncope[8] (Table 24-3).

COST ISSUES

Syncope is very costly to evaluate. In 1982, a retrospective review of diagnostic evaluation of admitted patients with syncope (with negative history, physical examination, and ECG) showed that a wide variety of diagnostic tests were done in these patients.[27] The

TABLE 24-3. Other Vascular Endpoints[a]

	5-Year Rates		
	Cardiac (%)	Noncardiac (%)	SUO (%)
Cardiac arrest	4.1[b]	0.8	0
Congestive heart failure	17[c]	5.3	2.5
Transient ischemic attacks	26[c]	5.4	5.2
Stroke	5.6	6.9	8.4
Myocardial infarction	6.0	8.3	5.6

[a] Rates calculated by Kaplan-Meier life-table methods.
[b] Significant (p <0.05) as compared with synocpe of unknown origin.
[c] Significant (p <0.05) as compared with syncope of unknown origin or noncardiac.
(From Kapoor,[8] with permission.)

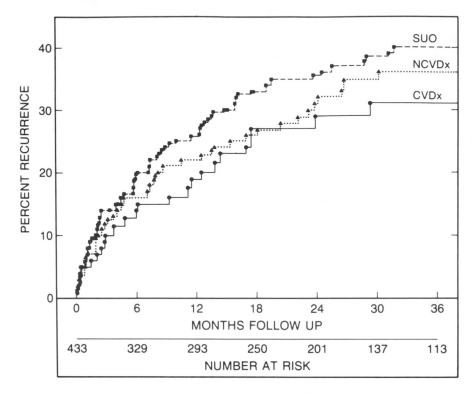

Fig. 24-3. Cumulative incidence of recurrence in patients with syncope of cardiovascular origin (CVDx, circles), syncope due to a noncardiovascular cause (NCVDx, *triangles*), and syncope of unknown cause (SUO, *squares*) (Kaplan-Meier estimates). Patients with an initial diagnosis of a cardiovascular cause of syncope had a recurrence rate of 31%, patients with a noncardiovascular cause had a recurrence rate of 36%, and patients with syncope of unknown origin had a recurrence rate of 43% at 3 years. These differences were not significant, with the minimum for any two-way comparison being p ≥0.11. (From Day et al.,[10] with permission.)

most common tests were prolonged ECG monitoring and electroencephalography (EEG). Patients stayed in the hospital for an average of 9.1 days. In only 13 patients was the cause of syncope assigned on the basis of inpatient evaluation (10 patients with arrhythmias and 3 in whom severe aortic stenosis was documented by cardiac catheterization). At the time, it was estimated that inpatient evaluation resulted in a cost of $23,000 per new diagnosis. There is no evidence that the practice pattern for evaluation of syncope has changed substantially since the 1980s. Clearly, there is a need for more cost-effective approaches to this problem.

REFERENCES

1. Dermksian G, Lamb LE: Syncope in a population of healthy young adults. JAMA 168:1200, 1958
2. Williams RL, Allen PD: Loss of consciousness. Aerospace Med 33:545, 1962
3. Murdock BD: Loss of consciousness in healthy South African men. S Afr Med J 57:771, 1980
4. Savage DD, Corwin L, McGee DL et al: Epidemiologic features of isolated syncope: the Framingham Study. Stroke 16:626, 1985
5. Kapoor W, Snustad D, Peterson J, Karpf M: Syncope in the elderly. Am J Med 80:419, 1980
6. Lipsitz LA, Wei JY, Rowe JW: Syncope in an elderly, institutionalized population: prevalence, incidence, and associated risk. Q J Med 55:45, 1985
7. Kapoor W, Karpf M, Wieand S et al: A prospective evaluation and follow-up of patients with syncope. N Engl J Med 309:197, 1983
8. Kapoor W: Evaluation and outcome of patients with syncope. Medicine (Baltimore) 69:160, 1990
9. Silverstein MD, Singer DE, Mulley A et al: Patients with syncope admitted to medical intensive care units. JAMA 248:1185, 1982
10. Day SC, Cook EF, Funkenstein H, Goldman L: Evaluation and outcome of emergency room patients with transient loss of consciousness. Am J Med 73:15, 1982
11. Wayne HH: Syncope: physiological considerations and an analysis of the clinical characteristic in 510 patients. Am J Med 30:418, 1961

12. Eagle KA, Black HR: The impact of diagnostic tests in evaluating patients with syncope. Yale J Biol Med 56:1, 1983

13. Martin GJ, Adams SL, Martin HG et al: Prospective evaluation of syncope. Ann Emerg Med 13:499, 1984

14. Kapoor W, Cha R, Peterson J et al: Prolonged electrocardiographic monitoring in patients with syncope: the importance of frequent or repetitive ventricular ectopy. Am J Med 82:20, 1987

15. Bass EB, Elson JJ, Fogoros RN et al: Long-term prognosis of patients undergoing electrophysiologic studies for syncope of unknown origin. Am J Cardiol 62:1186, 1988

16. DiMarco JP, Garan H, Harthorne JW, Ruskin JN: Intracardiac electrophysiology techniques in recurrent syncope of unknown cause. Ann Intern Med 95:542, 1981

17. Gulamhusein S, Naccarelli GV, Ko PT et al: Value and limitations of clinical electrophysiologic study in assessment of patients with unexplained syncope. Am J Med 73:700, 1982

18. Hess DS, Morady F, Schierman MM: Electrophysiologic testing in the evaluation of patients with syncope of undetermined origin. Am J Cardiol 50:1309, 1982

19. Akhtar M, Shenasa M, Denker S et al: Role of cardiac electrophysiologic studies in patients with unexplained recurrent syncope. PACE 6:192, 1983

20. Olshansky B, Mazuz M, Martins JB: Significance of inducible tachycardia in patients with syncope of unknown origin: a long-term follow-up. J Am Coll Cardiol 5:216, 1985

21. Doherty JU, Pembrook-Rogers D, Grogan EW et al: Electrophysiologic evaluation and follow-up characteristics of patients with recurrent unexplained syncope and presyncope. Am J Cardiol 55:703, 1985

22. Denes P, Ezri MD: The role of electrophysiologic studies in the management of patients with unexplained syncope. PACE 8:424, 1985

23. Teichman SL, Felder SD, Matos JA et al: The value of electrophysiologic studies in syncope of undetermined origin: report of 150 cases. Am Heart J 110:469, 1985

24. Denes P, Vretz E, Ezri MD, Borbola J: Clinical predictors of electrophysiology findings in patients with syncope of unknown origin. Arch Intern Med 148:1922, 1988

25. Kapoor WN, Hammill SC, Gersh BJ. Diagnosis and natural history of syncope and the role of invasive electrophysiologic testing. Am J Cardiol 63:730, 1989

26. Kapoor W, Peterson J, Wieand HS, Karpf M: Diagnostic and prognostic implications of recurrences in patients with syncope. Am J Med 83:700, 1987

27. Kapoor W, Karpf M, Maher Y et al: Syncope of unknown origin: The need for a more cost-effective approach to its diagnostic evaluation. JAMA 247:2687, 1982

25
Complete Heart Block and Conduction Abnormalities

John H. McAnulty

A review of the recent literature would suggest that our understanding of bradyarrhythmias is nearly complete. There are very few recent studies on the subject. While the prognosis with some of these rhythms has been well defined and, on occasion, measures to assess risk have proved helpful, there is still much room for study. This chapter discusses some of what is known about the prognosis of complete heart block and how it affects management. A discussion of chronic conduction system abnormalities, which in some cases put patients at risk of heart block, follows.

COMPLETE HEART BLOCK

Complete heart block is the complete failure of normal sinus node and atrial activity to reach the ventricle. When present, it is most often a chronic persistent rhythm, although on occasion it can be intermittent. The prognosis is related to at least three features: etiology, site of the block within the conduction system, and rate response of the ventricular rhythm. Each of these is influenced by whether the heart block is congenital or acquired.

Congenital Complete Heart Block

Congenital complete heart block is not a singular entity. Autopsies have revealed different sites of disruption of conduction within the lower atrium, in the atrioventricular (AV) node (or even due to absence of the AV node), in the His bundle, or at the bifurcation of the bundle branches.[1,2] The ventricle is activated from the lower AV node or His bundle and the QRS complex is normally less than 0.10 seconds in duration, with a resting rate of 40 to 60 bpm, increasing to twice that level as a physiologic response to normal chronotropic stimuli. While familial heart block is well recognized[3] (sometimes first occurring late in life), the cause of most congenital heart block is unknown. The heart block is frequently associated with other congenital cardiac abnormalities, which often primarily dictate symptoms and survival. Occasionally, maternal disease is associated with the development of complete heart block in the newborn infant. For example, women with systemic lupus erythematosus (SLE) may have children with complete heart block, possibly from placental transfer of immune complexes.[4,5]

Conventional wisdom has suggested that congenital heart block is benign and asymptomatic. This may not be true. Symptoms and sudden death related to the bradycardia have been well documented.[6–8] A resting heart rate of less than 50 bpm in the young has been used as one early clue to the likelihood that they will develop symptoms and of an increased risk of early death as a result of the rhythm.[9,10] Attempts to define prognosis further in patients with congenital heart block, with the use of electrophysiologic studies, exercise tests, or drug assessment, have added little to an understanding of the ultimate prognosis or the consideration of the need for pacing.

The increasing evidence that hemodynamic function is significantly improved by physiologic pacing suggests that the simple presence of the rhythm itself is a reason to insert a physiologic dual-chamber pacemaker. Symptoms are likely to be eliminated, and this may prevent some of the sporadic deaths that occur with congenital heart block. If an infant is identified as having complete heart block, its size makes pacing less desirable. Only if the heart rate is significantly below 50 bpm should a pacemaker be inserted.

Acquired Chronic Complete Heart Block

Complete heart block can be caused by all forms of acquired heart disease. Coronary artery disease (CAD) is far and away the most common cause in the United States.[1] Defining and correcting the cause may be sufficient evaluation and treatment. While reversible ischemia may explain the rhythm, if the heart block is not part of a myocardial infarction (MI) process, treatment of the ischemia alone will not reliably prevent the bradycardia. Direct treatment of the rhythm itself is required. Hyperkalemia may be the most common recognizable reversible cause of heart block, contributing to almost one-half of the heart block that occurred in a large bundle branch block population.[11] If a drug (Table 25-1) can be stopped, and is a likely cause, further assessment may be unnecessary. While it has been suggested that drugs could be used as a "provocation test" to define those with a variety of cardiac diseases who might be at risk of subsequent

TABLE 25-1. Correctable Causes of Complete Heart Block

Drugs
  Antiarrhythmia agents
  Digitalis
  Calcium-blocking agents
  β-Blocking agents
  Clonidine
  Tricyclic amines
  Phenothiazine

Metabolic abnormalities
  Hyperkalemia
  Hypercalcemia
  Hypermagnesemia
  Severe acid-base disturbances

Endocrine abnormalities
  Hypothyroidism
  Hypoadrenalism

Intracardiac catheters

Ischemia

chronic complete heart block, this claim has never been substantiated. Additional potentially reversible causes include inflammatory diseases (the role of using antiinflammatory agent in terms of long-term prevention of complete heart block is not clearly defined), endocrine abnormalities, and other metabolic abnormalities.

If no clearly reversible cause is found, the ultimate prognosis in terms of both mortality as well as freedom from symptoms is poor.[12] This is due not only to the associated heart disease, but to the rhythm itself. There is some suggestion that the prognosis from the rhythm can be optimally defined by performing an intracardiac electrophysiologic study to determine the site of the block. However, the subsidiary pacemaker (or the site of the escape rhythm) in patients with acquired heart block, whether in the AV node, the His bundle, or the Purkinje system, is unpredictable. Unless there are strong mitigating factors against it, management should include insertion of a permanent pacemaker, as this will minimize symptoms and probably improve survival.[13]

Complete Heart Block With Myocardial Infarction

Complete heart block occurs in approximately 12% of patients with inferior MI and in approximately 5% of patients with anterior MI.[14–18] There are similarities and differences between these two groups. They are similar in that complete heart block with either type of infarction is associated with more myocardial damage, increased incidence of ventricular fibrillation, and increased in-hospital mortality as compared with MI patients without heart block.[13,15,17] Another similarity between inferior and anterior MI overall is that the same clinical and electrocardiographic (ECG) variables will predict those patients in whom heart block will develop (see below).[18] They are different in that the site of block with an inferior MI is most often at the level of the AV node, while with anterior MI, it is more often distal to the His bundle. The bundle branches diverge as they leave the His bundle. Thus, a larger infarction is required to damage enough of the distal conduction system to cause heart block, the probable reason that the in-hospital mortality with an anterior MI with heart block (50 to 70%)[13,16,17] is so much greater than that seen with an inferior MI with heart block (20 to 30 percent).[14,15]

There are multiple causes of heart block with inferior MI, which in turn probably affect the long-term prognosis. Occlusion of flow to the posterior descending artery is the usual cause of an inferior MI and, since the major AV node artery arises from this vessel, ischemic damage of the AV node is one cause. This, however, is less common than might be expected, because the AV node is also supplied by branches of the left coronary artery system. It has been suggested that heart block with an inferior MI is a clue that a patient may have associated left anterior descending (LAD) vessel stenosis,[19] but this has not been substantiated.[17] Increased vagal tone is a likely explanation of the heart block seen during the early postinfarction period (first 6 hours). This block responds to atropine and is shorter in duration than the block that occurs first after 6 hours.[20] Local hyperkalemia and increased adenosine concentrations resulting from cell damage may also explain some heart block.

If first-degree, or Mobitz type 1 (second-degree) AV block occurs with an inferior MI, no treatment is necessary, but each increases the chance that complete heart block will occur. If it does, and the junctional escape rhythm is sufficient to provide adequate hemodynamic function, temporary pacing therapy is unnecessary because this rhythm rarely leads to asystole. It is often difficult to assess perfusion and, if there is concern that the bradycardia is having an adverse effect, a temporary wire can be inserted. This wire should be left in place until 24 to 48 hours after return of AV conduction. Complete heart block usually resolves within 1 week of the MI. While it may eventually resolve in others beyond this point, it is less likely, and keeping a patient in the hospital to wait for this to occur becomes increasingly cost ineffective. This plus the chance that the heart block will persist point to the need to proceed to a permanent pacemaker.

Thrombolysis therapy does not alter the outcome of complete heart block with an inferior MI.[17] The presence of AV block is associated with a higher reocclusion rate after vessel patency (29% versus 16% in those who do not have AV block), with a higher incidence of ventricular fibrillation (36% versus 14% in those who do not have heart block), and with an increased in-hospital mortality (20% versus 4% in those without heart block). The prognosis in those discharged alive that had in-hospital AV block is similar to those who did not have AV block.

In the case of complete heart block complicating an acute anterior MI, the ultimate prognosis is related to the amount of myocardium damaged. This has led to the consideration that there may be no point in using a temporary pacemaker. However, as with an inferior MI, the bradyarrhythmia itself can promote syncope, shock, ventricular fibrillation, and death.[18] Thus, complete heart block causing hemodynamic embarrassment warrants treatment with a temporary pacemaker because some patients will survive the infarction and, in some cases, pacing may promote survival. Again, thrombolysis therapy does not alter the significance or management of heart block.[16,18] Heart block present at 1 week after the infarction requires treatment with permanent pacing.

Retrospective analysis of outcome of patients with transient complete heart block occurring with an anterior infarction and associated bundle branch block has revealed a subsequent high sudden death rate.[21–23] Permanent pacemaker implantation before hospital discharge has been recommended.[21,22] This issue is not fully resolved. Prolonged in-hospital monitoring of this patient group in a study from the Netherlands revealed a 10% incidence of ventricular fibrillation by 6 weeks, unrelated to complete heart block.[24] Had the patients been at home, it might have been assumed that the sudden death events were due to bradyarrhythmia. The single prospective assessment of the role of pacemakers is small, but it did not demonstrate an advantage in patients receiving the device.[25] Measurement of the His to ventricular conduction time (HV interval) may possibly help in the decision about whether to insert a permanent pacemaker. A greatly prolonged HV (i.e., >100 ms), or block below the His bundle with atrial pacing may predict those at risk of subsequent chronic heart block. This assumption has not been proved correct.

CHRONIC CONDUCTION SYSTEM ABNORMALITIES

Selected conduction system abnormalities have repeatedly raised concern that patients are at risk of complete heart block with an associated high mortality. These include first-degree AV block, second-degree AV block, and block in the bundle branches.

First-Degree AV Block

Of least concern is first-degree AV block. Defined as a PR interval greater than 0.20 seconds (although this is somewhat rate dependent), its presence warrants consideration of the cause (often drugs or associated disease). When associated with a narrow QRS complex, the site of block is almost always within the AV node; with a wide QRS complex, it is either in the AV node or in the distal conduction systems. In either event, by itself, the prognosis is only related to the associated disease. No specific treatment is required.

Second-Degree AV Block

The unifying concept of this rhythm is that, each ventricular complex is the result of a P wave, but some P waves do not conduct to the ventricle. Definitions of types of second-degree blocks can be difficult.

Mobitz Type 1 AV Block (Wenckebach Rhythm)

Defined by the gradually prolonging PR interval with a subsequent dropped ventricular beat, this rhythm almost always occurs at the level of the AV node, and the QRS complex is usually narrow. It can be found in healthy young people, presumably the result of high vagal tone, and its prognosis in other populations is only related to the associated heart disease.[26,27] Because it does not put patients at risk, further assessment of the rhythm is not necessary. Treatment is required only if the ventricular response is slow enough to be the clear explanation for symptoms.

Mobitz Type 2 and "High-Degree" AV Block

While difficult to differentiate these two rhythms, Mobitz type 2 and high-degree AV block are associated with syncope caused by complete heart block. Both have a constant PR interval of conducted beats with absence of conduction of some P waves. Mobitz type 2 depicts isolated P waves that do not conduct to the ventricles, while "high-degree" AV block describes more than one P wave in a row without conduction. Both most often occur in patients who have evidence of distal conduction system disease, that is, bundle branch block. The site of the block itself is generally in the His bundle or below. The prognosis for the rate of progression to complete heart block is sufficient to warrant pacemaker insertion even without further evaluation (except for the need to look for a reversible cause).[13]

2:1 AV Block

It is difficult to know whether 2:1 AV block is Mobitz type 1 or Mobitz type 2 second-degree AV block.[28] Associated bundle branch block increases the likelihood that the 2:1 block is within or distal to the His bundle. If the QRS is narrow, the site of block is less predictable. In the patient with 2:1 AV block, evaluation of long rhythm strips may reveal evidence for intermittent, more definite, Mobitz 1 block (e.g., 4:3 or 3:2 AV block), providing reasonable evidence that the block is at the level of the AV node. Assessment of risk may be enhanced by performing an intracardiac electrophysiologic study. If the AV block can be documented as occurring within or below the His potential, the prognosis is sufficiently poor to insert a pacemaker. Should the 2:1 block be above the His bundle, symptoms can dictate the need for further treatment.

Chronic Bundle Branch Block

The concept of the distal conduction system being trifascicular is perhaps too simple, but it has been useful in defining patients at risk of bradyarrhythmia. Unifascicular block (either right bundle branch block, left anterior fascicular block, or left posterior fascicular),

although associated with heart disease, is not a clue for an increased progression to complete heart block.

There is increased concern for patients who have ECG evidence of bifascicular block: left bundle branch block, right bundle branch block with left anterior fascicular block, or right bundle branch block with left posterior fascicular block. Found in up to 2% of a population over 60 years of age,[11,29,30] these ECG patterns indicate block in two of the three major distal conduction pathways. Whether caused by primary scarring or fibrosis of the conduction system or by associated disease, most often in the coronary arteries, damage to the remaining fascicle would lead to complete heart block.

This is not simply theoretical. While complete heart block occurs in only isolated cases of bifascicular block patients identified by community screening,[29] it has been documented to occur at a rate of 1 to 2%/year in similar patients identified in routine hospital screening.[11,30,31] Efforts have been made to identify which bifascicular patients will develop heart block. The type of bundle branch block (left bundle versus right bundle with fascicular block), the presence of associated first degree AV block, and the type of clinical heart disease were not helpful. A previous history of transient neurologic symptoms, including syncope, did not define those in whom complete heart block subsequently developed or who died suddenly.[11,30,32] Resting HV intervals in this population not being evaluated for recent transient neurologic symptoms also did not help define which patients would go on to experience these serious events. If atrial pacing caused atrioventricular block distal to the His bundle, subsequent clinical heart block occurred in almost 50%, but this finding occurs in less than 4% of the bundle branch block patients.[30,33]

Concern about complete heart block should be greater in bifascicular block patients presenting for medical care because of near syncope or syncope. Complete heart block has been shown to be the likely cause of the symptoms in up to 5% of this group.[31] Still, this incidence of heart block is not high enough to warrant putting a pacemaker in all patients, purely on the basis of symptoms. Electrophysiologic testing can help define those at particularly high risk. Patients with a resting HV interval of 70 to 100 ms have up to a 5 to 8% yearly chance of progressing to complete heart block,[11] and this increases to 25% when the HV interval is greater than 100 ms.[31] Thus, in patients presenting with bundle branch block and unexplained global neurologic symptoms, electrophysiologic studies can define those who might benefit from pacemaker insertion. In addition, these patients are at risk of tachyarrhythmia; the results of programmed ventricular stimulation can define those in need of treatment for tachyarrhythmia. Drug provocation studies to bring out atrioventricular block have also been tried. Ajmaline and other drugs have shown some potential prognostic value; the studies have been too limited to know how to apply their use in general.

Identification of bundle branch block patients in whom complete heart block will develop would seem important, but it could be argued that recognized complete heart block is not a concern—once it develops, a permanent pacemaker can be inserted. Of greater concern is recognition of bundle branch block patients who will die as a result of heart block—a death that theoretically could be prevented if patients were treated with prophylactic pacemakers. The mortality rate in patients with bifascicular block is 7%/year.[11,30,31] Death caused by the conduction abnormality would seem more likely to be arrhythmic and thus, sudden. This type of death occurs at a rate of approximately 3%/year.[30] When sudden deaths documented to be due to causes other than a bradyarrhythmia are excluded, deaths demonstrated, or judged possibly, to be due to complete heart block occur at a rate or 1.2%/year.[30] While the same evaluations of distal conduction reviewed for predicting complete heart block can be performed, treatment based on the results has not been shown to alter mortality significantly.

In summary, patients identified to have chronic bundle branch who have unexplained transient neurologic symptoms require further evaluation or assessment of arrhythmia. Those with symptoms possibly attributable to intermittent heart block should undergo ambulatory rhythm monitoring consisting of 48 to 72 hours of Holter monitoring if presenting with recent symptoms, or with 1 to 2 months of event monitor evaluation if symptoms are infrequent (Fig. 25-1). Electrophysiologic assessment may provide evidence of bradycardias or tachycardias if monitoring fails to provide the explanation for the symptoms.

Prognosis in Patients with Bundle Branch Block in Selected Clinical Situations

Cardiac Catheterization

A right ventricular catheter, touching the intraventricular septum, can cause right bundle branch block. In a patient with left bundle branch block, this can result in complete heart block, which may not clear immediately with repositioning of the catheter. The same complete heart block can occur in a patient with right bundle branch block undergoing left heart catheterization. Since this occurs in fewer than 10% of patients with either of the bundle branch blocks and since catheter withdrawal quickly corrects the problem in most cases, temporary pacemaker insertion on a prophylactic basis is not required. Because complete heart block can persist despite catheter removal, intra-

venous (IV) access and the availability of a temporary pacing unit should be ensured in bundle branch block patients undergoing these procedures.

General Surgery

The stress of surgery and anesthesia could potentially cause heart block in patients with bifascicular block. Although the risk of this is small (less than 2%[34-36]), IV access and availability of temporary pacing are appropriate when these patients undergo surgery.

Cardiac Surgery

Bundle branch block occurs in up to 38% of patients during coronary artery bypass surgery.[37-39] It is transient in more than two-thirds of those affected. While progression to complete heart block is rare (isolated cases), the new bundle branch block is associated with up to a fourfold increased risk of perioperative MI and an even greater risk of perioperative sudden death—not related to heart block. Because the progression to complete heart block is rare, diagnostic evaluation other than perioperative rhythm monitoring is not useful, even in those with persistent bundle branch block.

New right or left bundle branch block develops in 2 to 3% of patients undergoing mitral valve surgery: progression to complete atrioventricular block occurs in fewer than 0.5% of patients.[40,41] Postoperative complete heart block occurs in 1 to 10% of aortic valve replacements.[41,42] Clinical, hemodynamic, or ECG variables, including bundle branch block, do not define those in whom this rhythm will develop. If the complete heart block persists, management is clear: a permanent pacemaker is needed. It is more difficult to know what to do with patients who have transient complete heart block. While its value is not clearly defined, measuring an HV interval may be helpful with a greatly prolonged interval (i.e., >80 to 100 ms) or block below the His bundle with atrial pacing being used as a reason to consider a pacemaker.

New right bundle branch block, often with associated left anterior fascicular block is the rule after surgery for tetralogy of Fallot. The subsequent sudden death rate has raised the concern about late heart block, but on review the deaths are more often due to ventricular tachyarrhythmias. Measurement of the HV interval has been of limited value in predicting subsequent heart block, but block below the His bundle with atrial pacing may be more predictive.[43]

Antiarrhythmic Drugs

All the standard antiarrhythmic drugs can prolong distal conduction. The incidence of progression to complete heart block with use of these drugs is small.

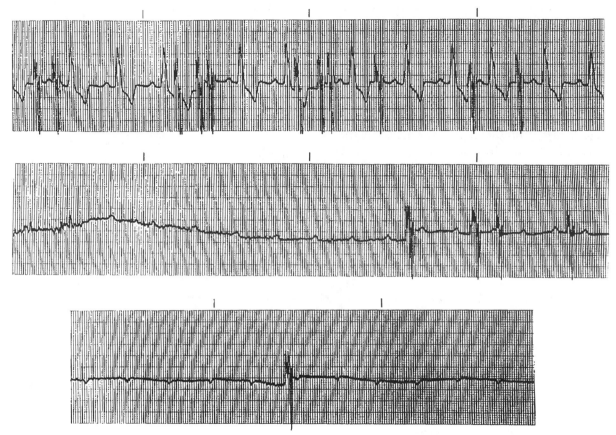

Fig. 25-1. This tracing from an ambulatory event monitor is presented to make three points. First, in this man with syncope, known left bundle branch block, and subsequently documented complete heart as the cause (based on this tracing), an intracardiac electrophysiological study 1 month earlier was negative. Second, these event monitors can define the cause of syncope (a family member pushed the recording button when the patient lost consciousness). Finally, it shows that while useful, the tracing may have artifacts and be difficult to read. The tracings are from a continuous recording made after the event button was pushed. The tracings were cut and mounted by a monitoring reading company before being sent to us, so the beginning of the ventricular standstill was not saved. The top tracing reveals sinus rhythm with normal conduction and artifact. Only P waves are recorded on the bottom two strips (with a change in P wave morphology; the leads were not mismounted). (From McAnulty,[46] with permission.)

While there is disagreement about whether hospitalization is required for initiating antiarrhythmic therapy in general, the presence of bifascicular block is a reason to consider hospital admission. A measurement of distal conduction times before and after drug administration can be used in the most fragile to determine whether the relative safety of the drug is worth its value.

Exercise

Bundle branch block (like complete heart block) brought out with exercise testing is not a clue for a subsequent bradycardia death.[44,45] While pacemaker treatment is indicated for heart block, it is not indi-

cated for bundle branch block. The bundle branch block may be, but is not necessarily, the result of ischemia.

Bundle Branch Block and Acute Myocardial Infarction

Conduction system abnormalities increase the chance that complete heart block will occur in the acute phase of an MI. Since the development of the block can be abrupt with prolonged asystole, efforts to identify those who would benefit from a prophylactic temporary pacemaker have been performed.[18,23] Until more is known, perhaps the most useful results and rules come from the Multicenter Investigators of the

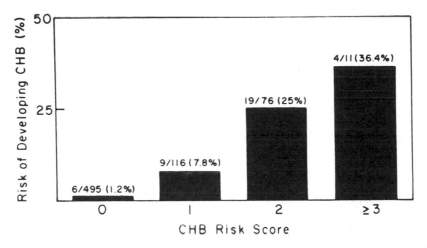

Fig. 25-2. Risk of the development of complete heart block in a patient with an acute myocardial infarction, with each risk score (see text) depicted graphically. (From Lamas et al.,[18] with permission.)

Limitation of Infarct Size (MILIS Study).[18] They are in agreement with, and are "validated" by, comparison with other large studies.[23] In MILIS, each of the following was given a "risk score" of one: first-degree AV block, Mobitz type 1 second-degree AV block, Mobitz type 2 second-degree AV block, left anterior fascicular block, left posterior fascicular block, right bundle branch block, and left bundle branch block. When applied to infarctions of any location, the risk of progressing to complete heart block is as presented in Figure 25-2. In those with a complete heart block risk score of 2 or more, based on the initial ECG, a prophylactic temporary pacemaker is recommended. In those with a risk score of 1, with about an 8% chance of heart block, a pacemaker could be inserted but availability of an external pacing unit is an acceptable management alternative (remembering that the external device does not always work and it invariably makes patient and ECG assessment difficult). If a patient with bundle branch block develops transient complete heart block and survives the infarction, the need for permanent pacemakers should be considered, but its value is unclear.

REFERENCES

1. Davies MJ, Anderson RH, Becker AE: The Conduction System of the Heart. Butterworth, London, 1983
2. Lev M: The conduction system in congenital heart disease. Am J Cardiol 21:619, 1968
3. Perloff JK: Congenital complete heart block. pp. 43–56. In The Clinical Recognition of Congenital Heart Disease. WB Saunders, Philadelphia, 1978
4. Scott JS, Maddison DJ, Taylor PV et al: Connective tissue disease, antibodies to ribonucleoprotein, and congenital heart block. N Engl J Med 309:209, 1983
5. Litsey SE, Noonan JA, O'Connor WN et al: Maternal connective tissue disease and congenital heart block. N Engl J Med 312:98, 1985
6. Reid JM, Coleman EN, Doig W: Complete congenital heart block: report of 35 cases. Br Heart J 48:236, 1982
7. Karpawich PP, Gilette PC, Garson A et al: Congenital complete atrioventricular block: clinical and electrophysiologic predictors of need for pacemaker insertion. Am J Cardiol 48:1098, 1981
8. Pinsky WW, Gilette PC, Garson A et al: Diagnosis, management, and long-term results of patients with congenital complete atrioventricular block. Pediatrics 69:728, 1982
9. Besley DC, McWilliams GJ, Moodie DS et al: Long-term follow-up of young adults following permanent pacemaker placement for complete heart block. Am Heart J 103:332, 1982
10. Dewey RC, Capeless MA, Levy AM: Use of ambulatory electrocardiographic monitoring to identify high-risk patients with congenital complete heart block. N Engl J Med 316:835, 1987
11. Dhingra RC, Palileo E, Strasberg D et al: Significance of the HV interval in 517 patients with chronic bifascicular block. Circulation 64:1265, 1981
12. Rosen DM, Dhingra RC, Loeb HS et al: Chronic heart block in adults: clinical and electrophysiological observations. Arch Intern Med 131:663, 1973
13. Dreifus LS, Fisch C, Griffin JC et al: Guidelines for implantation of cardiac pacemakers and antiarrhythmia devices: a report of the American College of Cardiology/American Heart Association Task Force on Assessment of Diagnostic and Therapeutic Cardiovascular Procedures (Committee on Pacemaker Implantation). Circulation 84:455, 1991
14. McDonald K, O'Sullivan JJ, Conroy RM et al: Heart block as a predictor of in hospital death in both acute inferior and acute anterior myocardial infarction. Q J Med 74:277, 1990
15. Berger PB, Ryan TJ: Inferior myocardial infarction: High risk subgroups. Circulation 81:401, 1990

16. Wilber D, Walton J, O'Neill W et al: Effects of reperfusion on complete heart block complicating anterior myocardial infarction. J Am Coll Cardiol 6:1315, 1984

17. Clemmensen P, Bates ER, Califf RM et al and the TAMI Study Group: Complete atrioventricular block complicating inferior wall myocardial infarction treated with reperfusion therapy. Am J Cardiol 67:225, 1991

18. Lamas GA, Muller JE, Turi ZG, et al and the MILIS Study Group: A simplified method to predict occurrence of complete heart block during acute myocardial infarction. Am J Cardiol 57:1213, 1986

19. Bassan R, Maia IG, Bozza AA et al: Atrioventricular block in acute inferior wall myocardial infarction: Harbinger of associated obstruction of the left anterior descending coronary artery. J Am Coll Cardiol 8:773, 1986

20. Feigl D, Ashkenazy J, Kishion Y: Early and late atrioventricular block in acute inferior myocardial infarction. J Am Coll Cardiol 4:35, 1984

21. Atkins JM, Leshin SJ, Blomquist G et al: Ventricular conduction blocks and sudden death in acute myocardial infarction: potential indications for pacing. N Engl J Med 6:281, 1973

22. Waugh RA, Wagner GS, Haneg TL et al: Immediate and remote prognostic significance of fascicular block during acute myocardial infarction. Circulation 47:765, 1973

23. Hindman MC, Wagner GS, Jaho M et al: The clinical significance of bundle-branch block complicating acute myocardial infarction. II. Indications for temporary and permanent pacemaker insertion. Circulation 58:689, 1978

24. Lie KI, Liem KL, Schiulenberg RM et al: Early identification of patients developing late in-hospital ventricular fibrillation after discharge from the coronary care unit: a 5½ year retrospective and prospective study of 1897 patients. Am J Cardiol 41:674, 1978

25. Watson RDS, Glover DR, Page AJF et al: The Birmingham Trial of Permanent Pacing in Patients with Intraventricular Conduction Disorders After Acute Myocardial Infarction. Am Heart J 108:496, 1984

26. Strasberg B, Amat-Y-Leon F, Dhingra RC et al: Natural history of chronic second-degree atrioventricular nodal block. Circulation 63:1043, 1981

27. Young D, Eisenberg R, Fisch B et al: Wenckebach atrioventricular block (Mobitz type 1) in children and adolescents. Am J Cardiol 40:393, 1977

28. Barold SS: Narrow QRS Mobitz type 2 second-degree atrioventricular block in acute myocardial infarction: true or false? Am J Cardiol, 67:1291, 1991

29. Schneider JF, Thomas HE, Jr, Dreger DE et al: Newly acquired right bundle-branch block: the Framingham study. Ann Intern Med 90:303, 1979

30. McAnulty JH, Rahimtoola SH, Murphy E et al: Natural history of "high-risk" bundle-branch block: final report of a prospective study. N Engl J Med 307:137, 1982

31. Scheinman MM, Peters RW, Sauvé MJ et al: The value of the HQ interval in patients with bundle branch block and the role of prophylactic pacing. Am J Cardiol 50:1316, 1982

32. Dhingra RC, Denes P, Wu D et al: Syncope in patients with chronic bifascicular block: Significance, causative mechanisms and clinical implications. Ann Intern Med 81:302, 1974

33. Dhingra RC, Wyndham C, Bauernfeind R et al: Significance of block distal to the His bundle induced by atrial pacing in patients with chronic bifascicular block. Circulation 60:1455, 1979

34. Goldman L, Caldera DL, Southwich FS et al: Cardiac risk factors and complications in non-cardiac surgery. Medicine (Baltimore) 57:357, 1978

35. Santini M, Carrara P, Benhar M et al: Possible risks of general anesthesia in patients with intraventricular conduction disturbances. PACE 3:130, 1980

36. Mikell FL, Weir EK, Chesler E: Perioperative risk of complete heart block in patients with bifascicular block and prolonged PR interval. Thorax 36:14, 1981

37. O'Connell JB, Wallis D, Johnson SA et al: Transient bundle branch block following use of hypothermic cardioplegia in coronary artery bypass surgery: high incidence without perioperative myocardial infarction. Am Heart J 103:35, 1982

38. Wexelman W, Lichstein E, Cunningham JN et al: Etiology and clinical significance of new fascicular conduction defects following coronary bypass surgery. Am Heart J 111:923, 1986

39. Caspi J, Amar R, Elami A et al: Frequency and significance of complete atrioventricular block after coronary artery bypass grafting. Am J Cardiol 63:526, 1989

40. Brodell GK, Cosgrove D, Schiovone W et al: Cardiac rhythm and conduction disturbances in patients undergoing mitral valve surgery. Cleve Clin J Med 58:397, 1991

41. Keefe DL, Griffin JC, Harrison DC et al: Atrioventricular conduction abnormalities in patients undergoing isolated aortic or mitral valve replacement. PACE 8:393, 1985

42. Shandling AH, Braithwaite J, Crump R et al: Atrioventricular conduction block early after aortic valve replacement: are there predictive perioperative factors? J Invas Cardiol 3:115, 1990

43. Friedli B, Bolens M, Taktak M: Conduction disturbances after correction of tetralogy of fallot: are electrophysiologic studies of prognostic value? 11:162, 1988

44. Woelfel AK, Simpson RJ, Gettes LS, Foster JR: Exercise-induced distal atrioventricular block. J Am Coll Cardiol 2:578, 1983

45. Wayne VA, Bishop RL, Cook L, Spodick DH: Exercise induced bundle branch block. Am J Cardiol 52:283, 1983

46. McAnulty JH: Syncope. p. 390. In Narccarelli GV (ed): Cardiac Arrhythmias: A Practical Approach. Future, Mount Kisco, New York, 1991

26

Atrial Fibrillation: Prognostic Significance and Therapeutic Implications

Jack J. Farahi
Bramah N. Singh

As life expectancy in recent decades has increased significantly in the wake of advances in the palliation and control of ischemic heart disease, hypertension, congenital heart disease, heart failure of varied etiology, and numerous lesser disorders, atrial fibrillation has emerged as the commonest cardiac arrhythmia requiring treatment. The disorders that most commonly form the substrate for the arrhythmia (e.g., those causing ventricular and atrial dysfunction) are, for the most part, irreversible. Therefore, while it is usually possible to convert sustained atrial fibrillation to sinus rhythm by chemical or electrical means, maintaining stability of sinus rhythm to any length of time is often exceedingly difficult and success over long term is variable. As a result, the prognosis of atrial fibrillation is inextricably linked to the underlying disease predisposing the patient to recurrences of the arrhythmia. Atrial fibrillation has often been regarded as a relatively benign disorder; however, many patients with chronic atrial fibrillation need long-term treatment with potent antiarrhythmic and anticoagulant drugs, which themselves may produce major adverse reactions including death. For example, the presence of chronic atrial fibrillation places a patient at a significantly increased risk of arterial thromboembolism. There is growing evidence that sustained uncontrolled ventricular response per se may impair ventricular function and augment existing dysfunction. In many patients, the arrhythmia interferes with the well-being of the patient and may lead to impaired exercised capacity.

The purpose of this chapter is threefold. The first is to discuss briefly the salient features of the current concepts of the genesis of atrial fibrillation. This may provide the basis for understanding the circulatory and electrophysiologic perturbations that follow when the atria fibrillate. The second, and the main, objective is to discuss the prognostic significance of atrial fibrillation with a particular reference to the development of ventricular dysfunction, systemic emboli, and, in particular, the impact of the arrhythmia on cardiovascular mortality. Finally, the issue of whether the natural history of the disorder might be influenced by different modalities of drug therapy is discussed. The major focus is on the relative merits of delaying conduction versus prolonging refractoriness in effecting the chemical conversion of the arrhythmia to sinus rhythm and maintaining its stability over long periods by prophylactic pharmacologic therapy. The maintenance of sinus rhythm is clearly an important therapeutic goal, as it might reduce the morbidity and mortality that results from the development of atrial fibrillation in the context of various cardiovascular disorders.

MECHANISMS OF ATRIAL FIBRILLATION: ELECTROPHYSIOLOGIC AND ELECTROPHARMACOLOGIC CONSIDERATIONS

In recent years, considerable advances have been made in our understanding of the mechanisms that underlie the genesis of atrial fibrillation.[1] Many of the observations have stemmed from experimental studies using a variety of in vitro and in vivo animal models of atrial fibrillation and flutter.[1] There is reasonably compelling evidence that atrial fibrillation arises essentially from a myriad of randomly generated atrial reentrant wavelets as originally suggested by Moe[2] based on his observations using a computer model of atrial fibrillation. The central feature of this model is shortening of the effective refractory period and the need for the presence of a certain critical mass of tissue. These observations are consistent with the knowledge that sustained atrial fibrillation can readily be produced during vagal stimulation, which markedly abbreviates the atrial action potential duration,[3] and hence the voltage-dependent refractory period. Moreover, the arrhythmia rarely occurs in small animals, in which atrial size is unusually small.

Support for the multiple wavelet hypothesis has been derived from in vitro as well as in vivo experimental models.[1] These studies have indicated that there are three types of reentry: (1) those that use circuits based on macro-anatomic pathways, (2) those that are functionally determined in the syncytium of myocardial cells without gross anatomic pathways and (3) reentrant circuits occurring in uniform and nonuniform anisotropic tissues.[4] The latter two forms of reentry are the most likely basis for the genesis of atrial fibrillation at least in the experimental model.[1] It is clear that, in all such models of reentry, the excitation wave is the critical determinant for initiating and perpetuating of reentrant impulse propagation. Thus, when the wavelength (i.e., the product of refractory period and conduction velocity) is prolonged, an extensive area of unidirectional block of the impulse may be necessary for the impulse to reenter itself. Conversely, when the refractory period is short, or when there is slowed conduction, areas of depressed conduction will be conducive to initiating reentrant circuits.

The size of the excitation wavelength is crucial in sustaining a reentrant arrhythmia; this is of particular significance in the pharmacologic termination and prevention of atrial flutter and fibrillation. For example, in the case of the leading circle hypothesis, interventions that augment the size of the wavelength will increase the minimal size of intra-atrial circuits. In the presence of an excitable gap in the reentrant loop, prolongation of the wavelength (e.g., with interventions that lengthen the action potential duration) will progressively reduce, and finally close, the excitable gap. This will result in instability of the reentrant circuit, with the likelihood of complete block and termination of the arrhythmia. These considerations are especially germane to the issue of initiation, perpetuation, and termination of atrial fibrillation, in which the basis is multiple reentering wavelets. A prolongation of the wavelength will result in an increase in the average size of the reentrant circuit.

Because the tissue mass involved in the arrhythmia at a given time is likely to remain constant, there is a high probability that the net number of wandering impulses will diminish and that fusion and extinction of excitatory wavelets will increase if wavelength is prolonged. These considerations, supported by numerous experimental observations, permit certain conclusions and provide an explanation for a number of common clinical observations. First, it is clear that any interventions that prolong the wavelength during atrial fibrillation may result in termination of the arrhythmia. Second, interventions that shorten the wavelength are likely to stabilize the reentrant circuit by increasing the excitable gap or may lead to a degeneration into multiple smaller circuits, resulting in fibrillation. Since the wavelength may increase markedly if the action potential duration is lengthened, even in the absence of a change in conduction velocity (i.e., a "pure" class 3 effect), drugs (class 1A, class 3) that exert such an effect are likely to terminate atrial fibrillation and maintain the stability of sinus rhythm. It is of interest that in the atria, class 1C agents, which are also known to be effective in terminating atrial fibrillation, increase the action potential duration and refractoriness markedly at fast cycle lengths.[5] They are likely to be potent in converting atrial flutter and fibrillation to sinus rhythm and also in maintaining stability of sinus rhythm. Electrophysiologically, this is a unique situation in the atria and is not evident in the ventricular tissue, where the bulk of the proarrhythmic actions of this class of agents is associated with life-threatening proarrhythmic reactions.

It is common clinical knowledge that atrial fibrillation occurs frequently in patients with hyperthyroidism, in which atrial repolarization and effective period are markedly shortened.[6] Conversely, in hypothyroidism, in which the duration of the atrial action potential is markedly increased, atrial fibrillation rarely occurs. Within this context, it is noteworthy that patients who are susceptible to atrial fibrillation tend to have a shorter action potential duration when these are recorded by the monophasic potential recordings.[7] Similarly, after direct current (DC) cardioversion to sinus rhythm, patients who have a shorter action potential duration are more likely to relapse sooner to atrial fibrillation than are those who have longer action potential durations.[7] These electrophysiologic observations have a bearing on the choice of interventions that might be most appropriate in the acute conversion of atrial fibrillation to sinus rhythm, and especially for maintaining the stability of sinus rhythm during prophylactic pharmacologic therapy.

CAUSES AND PREVALENCE OF ATRIAL FIBRILLATION

Atrial fibrillation is a common arrhythmia with an overall prevalence of 2% in the general population.[8] Its importance therefore pervades much of internal medicine, emphasized clearly by the knowledge of its association with 6 to 24% of ischemic strokes and with about 50% of cardioembolic strokes.[9]

During the 30-year follow-up of the Framingham Study, atrial fibrillation was diagnosed in 193 of 2,336 men and in 183 of 2,873 women, for an overall incidence of 7.2%.[10] Atrial fibrillation increases sharply with age in both sexes.[10] From 1959 to 1960, Ostrander et al.[11] found atrial fibrillation in 2.3% of men and in 2.5% of women aged 60 to 69 years, while the prevalence increased to 3.0% in men and to 5.0% in women in the population aged 70 to 79 years. The incidence of atrial fibrillation increases sharply in patients with heart disease. About 4.0% of all cardiac patients and 40% of patients with overt heart failure also suffer from atrial fibrillation.[12]

Although atrial fibrillation can occur as a primary electrical disorder of the atria in the absence of myocardial dysfunction, the occurrence of the arrhythmia increases with age and the nature and the severity of associated cardiac disease. The relative prevalence of associated disorders in patients with atrial fibrillation is shown in Table 26-1, in which the relative prevalence of the arrhythmia in disease is also presented.[13]

The two most common causes are ischemic heart disease, followed by hypertensive heart disease.[14–16] It is common in patients in whom ischemic heart disease and hypertensive heart disease coexist. Until recently, rheumatic heart disease (RHD) was the most common cause of atrial fibrillation.[17] Other causes of atrial fibrillation include hyperthyroidism, chronic obstructive airway disease, hypertrophic cardiomyopathy,

TABLE 26-1. Diseases Associated With Atrial Fibrillation

Disease	Prevalence in Patients With Atrial Fibrillation (%)	Prevalence of Atrial Fibrillation in Each Disease (%)
Valvular heart disease		
Rheumatic valvular heart disease	20–30	20
Nonvalvular heart disease		
Coronary artery disease	50–60	1
Hypertension	40–60	5–10
Pericarditis	<1	1
Cardiomyopathy		
Dilated	<1	20
Hypertrophic	<1	10
Alcohol (the holiday heart syndrome)	<1	40
After coronary bypass surgery	<5	30–40
Conductive system disease (sick sinus syndrome, the Wolff-Parkinson-White syndrome)	<5	<5
Pulmonary embolism	<1	3
Lone atrial fibrillation	10	—
Hyperthyroidism	2.5	20–30

(Adapted from Albers et al.,[13] with permission.)

and overt heart failure with end-stage heart disease of varied etiology.[14,16] Transient atrial fibrillation is also common in pericarditis, pulmonary embolus, myocardial infarction (MI), following cardiothoracic surgery, and intrathoracic infections such as pneumonia. In addition, atrial fibrillation is seen in sick sinus syndrome, myopericarditis, constrictive pericarditis, specific cardiac muscle disease, atrial septal defect, and acute and chronic alcohol abuse.[16,18,19] In a significant proportion of cases of atrial fibrillation, no specific etiology is identified. These cases have been broadly categorized as "lone" atrial fibrillators.[20–22] There are also published reports of familial preponderance of atrial fibrillation,[23] presumably occurring on the basis of either inherited electrophysiologic or myocardial disorder predisposing to the development of atrial fibrillation.

An important form of atrial fibrillation is paroxysmal. As pointed out by Coumel et al.,[24] a number of such cases occur in association with vagomimetic states and in others in association with sympathetic stimulation. The percentage of outpatients with paroxysmal atrial fibrillation is not known. However, 35% of all atrial fibrillation in the inpatient population is paroxysmal.[25] In many patients, paroxysmal atrial fibrillation ultimately develops into chronic atrial fibrillation. The transition rate from paroxysmal to chronic atrial fibrillation varies significantly, depending on the underlying etiology. In approximately 27% of patients with ischemic heart disease, 40% of patients with hypertensive heart disease, and 66% of patients with rheumatic heart disease who have paroxysmal atrial fibrillation, chronic atrial fibrillation eventually develops.[25] The precise incidence is also dependent on the duration of the paroxysmal atrial fibrillation; if the duration of atrial fibrillation is less than 2 days, chronicity develops in only 31%, as opposed to those with durations longer than 2 days, in whom chronic atrial fibrillation develops in 46%. It is clearly important to distinguish between paroxysmal from chronic atrial fibrillation, since the overall complication rates and prognosis differ significantly between the two forms of arrhythmia.

The presence of atrial fibrillation has been shown to be associated with increased morbidity and mortality.[10] The precise manner by which atrial fibrillation increases mortality is unclear. However, for the most part, regardless of etiology, atrial fibrillation is a marker for underlying heart disease. The mortality rate in patients with atrial fibrillation depends on the age of the patient, underlying etiology, and the degree of ventricular dysfunction coexisting with the arrhythmia.[25] It should be emphasized, however, that recent data suggest that the uncontrolled ventricular rate in the case of the arrhythmia itself may induce or aggravate existing left ventricular (LV) dysfunction.

PROGNOSTIC SIGNIFICANCE OF ATRIAL FIBRILLATION: IMPACT ON MORTALITY

Although an extensive database is available on the prognostic significance of atrial fibrillation, few large prospective, stringently controlled, studies have been conducted. Three issues are of particular importance: increased mortality, thromboembolism, and impaired exercise capacity with or without the development or deterioration of ventricular dysfunction. This chapter focuses primarily on the impact on mortality and on the development of systemic embolism, the latter being the most serious morbid event complicating the course of atrial fibrillation. The effect on mortality is discussed here and will be highlighted further within the context of individual underlying causes of arrhythmia. The issue of thromboembolism is dealt with relative to the question of the impact of anticoagulation on the overall incidence.

Petersen and Godtfredsen[26] pooled the available data from several discrete studies and found mortality rates ranging from 0.2% to 16%, depending on the population studied (Table 26-2). The Framingham Study,[10] which included only patients with chronic atrial fibrillation, revealed a very poor prognosis for patients with atrial fibrillation. In such patients, mortality was twofold higher compared with matched controls. By the end of the study period (30 years), 60% of the men and 45% of women with atrial fibrillation were dead. The average time span between the diagnosis of atrial fibrillation and death was 6 years.

In the follow-up of 1,212 patients with atrial fibrillation, Godtfredsen[25] also found a significant difference in the mortality between patients with atrial fibrillation and the matched general population (Fig. 26-1). In addition, patients above 70 years of age had a significantly higher mortality than did those below age 70. There was no difference in mortality between men and women (Fig. 26-2).

Kulbertus et al.[27] followed 193 ambulatory patients with atrial fibrillation, most of whom were above 70 years of age, for an average of 4.3 years. When com-

TABLE 26-2. One-Year Mortality in Atrial Fibrillation

Investigators	Study Design	Follow-up (yr)	No. of Pts.	Type of AF	Age at Onset (yr)	Yearly Mortality (%)
Godtfredsen[25]	Retrospective Clinical	13	1,212	All types	>70	16
					<70	10
	Hospital based		231	All types	<70	11
Kulbertus et al.[27]	Prospective Epidemiologic	6	193	Chronic	>70	8
Kannel et al.[10]	Prospective Epidemiologic	16.5	98	Chronic	<70	5
Gajewski and Singer[28]	Retrospective Insurance	7	3,099	Chronic	<70	3.7
				Chronic	<70	2.6
				Paroxysmal	<70	0.6
				Paroxysmal	<70	0.2
Flegel et al.[29]	Prospective civil service personnel	15	80		<70	7

(Modified from Petersen and Godtfredsen,[26] with permission.)

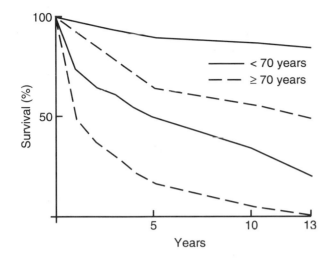

Fig. 26-1. Survival in patients with atrial fibrillation (1958–1967): 261 patients <70 years of age and 273 patients ≥70 years of age. Curves indicated by the solid lines are from the general population of similar ages. (Redrawn from Godtfredsen,[25] with permission.)

pared with age-matched controls, 35% of patients with atrial fibrillation and 18% of the controls died during the follow-up period.

These data are also supported by other studies involving younger patient populations. For example, in a retrospective analysis of life insurance company records, Gajewski and Singer[28] identified 3,099 subjects with atrial fibrillation. In this study, 85% of patients were below 60 years of age. The annual mortality of patients with atrial fibrillation with other associated conditions was 3.7%, as opposed to the expected 0.5%.

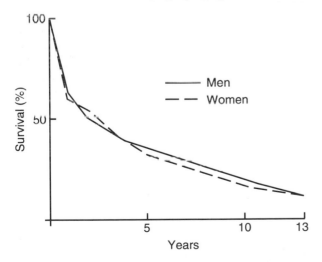

Fig. 26-2. Survival in atrial fibrillation (1958–1967): 266 men and 268 women. There were no differences. (Redrawn from Godtfredsen,[25] with permission.)

In the prospective study of civil service personnel in England, Flegel et al.[29] found 80 men with nonrheumatic atrial fibrillation out of a screened population of 19,018. At the end of 15 years, only 33% of the subjects survived, compared with 82% in the control group.[29]

Despite the fact that these five studies (see Table 26-2) are based on different methodologies, all show a significant increase in mortality associated with atrial fibrillation. The differences in the mortality seen among them might be related to the lack of homogeneity in the population mix for individual studies. Hospital-based populations tend to be older with more serious associated conditions, such as severe CHF, which increase the baseline mortality rate. Thus, an accurate assessment of the prognosis of any patient with atrial fibrillation requires taking cognizance of the multiplicity of complex interdependent factors that affect morbidity and mortality.

The Cox multivariate model showed that patient age, severity of congestive heart failure (CHF) at the onset of atrial fibrillation, cardiomegaly, hypertension, and the etiology of the underlying heart disease (excluding thyrotoxicosis) were statistically significant factors influencing mortality.[30]

HYPERTENSION AND HYPERTENSIVE HEART DISEASE

In the Framingham Study,[14] hypertensive heart disease was the commonest predisposing disorder for the development of atrial fibrillation, occurring in 37% of men and in 50% of the women in whom atrial fibrillation developed. Hypertensive heart disease was diagnosed if a patient had hypertension and had either left ventricular hypertrophy (LVH) as gauged by electrocardiography, cardiomegaly on chest radiography, or clinical heart failure. Interestingly, hypertension without evidence of ventricular hypertrophy as defined by the above criteria was only a weak predictor for the development of atrial fibrillation, highlighting the importance of myocardial damage as a prerequisite. Hypertension was also the most common cause of atrial fibrillation in the study of life case studies cases,[28] being responsible for 16.3% of all chronic and 12.2% of all paroxysmal atrial fibrillation. Other studies have also confirmed that hypertension is one of the commonest causes of atrial fibrillation.[25]

The development of atrial fibrillation in a patient with hypertension is associated with a substantive increase in mortality. In his study of 1,212 cases, Godtfredsen[25] found a 5-year survival rate of only 57% for patients with hypertensive heart disease. In the study of life insurance cases,[28] patients with atrial fibrillation and hypertension had a mortality ratio of observed to expected deaths (matched by exposure, age, and sex) of 721% and an annual excess death rate (defined as observed minus expected deaths per 1,000 exposed to risk per year) of 38. Hence, the development of atrial fibrillation in hypertensive patients is far from "benign"; it may portend a serious prognostic change during the course of the disease. It is not clear, however, whether the prevention of LVH by aggressive therapy with effective regimens might delay or prevent the development of the arrhythmia, its attendant complications or impact on associated mortality.

CORONARY ARTERY DISEASE AND ATRIAL FIBRILLATION

Standard reference sources indicate that atrial fibrillation occurs commonly in patients with coronary artery disease (CAD).[19] The Framingham Study[14] showed that CAD is a "significant precursor of atrial fibrillation." CAD occurred in 25% of men and in 14% of women with atrial fibrillation. CAD was associated with both chronic and paroxysmal atrial fibrillation. It doubled the risk of both chronic and paroxysmal atrial fibrillation in men and increased the risk of paroxysmal atrial fibrillation fourfold in women. CAD was also found to be a common cause of atrial fibrillation in several other studies.[16,25,28] Comparative mortality results in the Framingham Study showed that after excluding other predisposing factors, such as hypertensive heart disease, CHF, and rheumatic heart disease, atrial fibrillation caused by CAD was associated with 4.6 times greater mortality than with CAD alone.[14] In Godtfredsen's study, patients with atrial fibrillation caused by CAD had the worst 5-year prognosis of any group.[25] In the life insurance study,[28] atrial fibrillation associated with CAD had a mortality ratio of 700%, with an annual excess death rate of 30. Thus, there is a undeniable association between early death and atrial fibrillation in CAD (Fig. 26-3). However, the precise basis for such an increase risk is unclear. Data from the Coronary Artery Surgery Study (CASS)[31] showed that the frequency of atrial fibrillation rose linearly with the number of major coronary arteries with greater than 70% stenoses.

The frequency of occurrence of atrial fibrillation in the setting of acute myocardial infarction (AMI) is well recognized. However, transient atrial fibrillation during AMI needs to be distinguished from that occurring in the setting of ventricular dysfunction remote from the acute incident. Supraventricular arrhythmias have been reported in as many as 44% of patients with AMI.[32-35] Atrial fibrillation most commonly occurs within the first 72 hours of infarction. It is more common in older patients and in those with elevated right

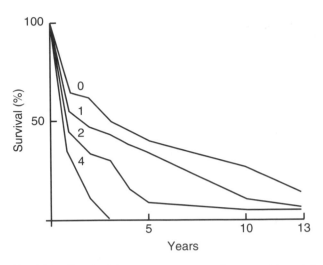

Fig. 26-3. Survival in coronary artery disease with atrial fibrillation (1958–1967): effect of degree of heart failure (CHF) − 0 = no CHF(n = 152); 1 = slight CHF (n = 237); 2 = moderate CHF (n = 117); 4 = severe CHF (n = 21). The vertical bars shown represent 95% confidence limits by Greenwood's estimate. (Redrawn from Godtfredsen,[25] with permission.)

and/or left atrial pressures.[36] The etiology of atrial fibrillation in AMI is probably multifactorial, including atrial ischemia or infarction, CHF, alteration in the autonomic nervous system, and drugs.[37]

Atrial fibrillation in the setting of acute myocardial infarction is associated with 35 to 40% inhospital mortality.[32-36] Interestingly, in patients with AMI and ventricular tachycardia, the mortality was 54% if the ventricular arrhythmia was concurrent with atrial fibrillation, as compared with 27% for patients with ventricular tachycardia without atrial fibrillation. Such an association might reflect the overall severity of myocardial damage sustained during coronary occlusion. This increase in mortality was still present at the end of 1 year postinfarction.[35] Again, as in the case of hypertensive heart disease, it is not known whether early, successful control of the arrhythmia in the setting of CAD or AMI reduces the associated morbidity and mortality resulting from atrial fibrillation.

RHEUMATIC HEART DISEASE AND ATRIAL FIBRILLATION

Despite its decline as the most common cause of atrial fibrillation,[17] RHD is still one of most potent risk factors for atrial fibrillation.[17] Within this context, mitral valve disease is the most common cause of atrial fibrillation, while aortic valve disease has a low propensity for causing atrial fibrillation.[38] Patients

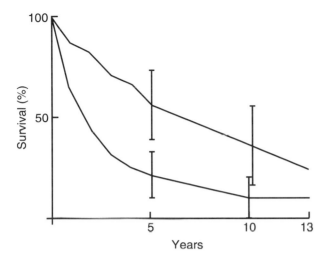

Fig. 26-4. Survival curve in rheumatic heart disease with atrial fibrillation (1958–1967). Upper curve: No or slight congestive heart failure (CHF) at onset of atrial fibrillation, 28 patients. Lower curve: Moderate CHF at onset of atrial fibrillation, 52 patients. (From Godtfredsen,[25] with permission.)

with RHD and atrial fibrillation also have poorer prognosis than do their counterparts without atrial fibrillation. In studies from the database of life insurance records, patients with mitral stenosis and atrial fibrillation had the highest mortality, with a mortality ratio of 1,737% and annual excess death rate of 81[38] (Fig. 26-4). This translates into a 5-year survival rate of 64.1%, as compared with a 5-year standard expected rate of 97.6%. In Godtfredsen's study[25] of 1,212 cases, patients with atrial fibrillation attributable to mitral disease had a "reasonably good" 5-year prognosis of more than 50%. However, patients with aortic valve disease and atrial fibrillation had a "poor" prognosis, that is, a 5-year survival of less than 50%. The worst prognosis was noted in patients when severe congestive heart failure was present before or at the onset of atrial fibrillation.[25] It is widely recognized that the onset of atrial fibrillation in the setting of valvular disease is associated with a sudden, marked deterioration of functional status, which may exert a secondary effect on the overall prognosis.

ATRIAL FIBRILLATION IN CONGESTIVE HEART FAILURE

Atrial fibrillation is a very common finding in patients with CHF. However, its clinical significance in this subgroup of patients is less clear and is still somewhat controversial. In the Framingham study,[10] CHF and RHD were the two strongest predictors for the

development of atrial fibrillation. It is also well established that the degree of CHF before, and at the onset of, atrial fibrillation is the best predictor of prognosis in patients with atrial fibrillation of other etiologies.[25] Hence, in patients with atrial fibrillation caused by CAD or RHD, the more severe the CHF before or at onset of the arrhythmia, the higher the mortality (Fig. 26-5). However, whether atrial fibrillation per se is the independent determinant of worse prognosis in patients with CHF is less certain. Clearly, a long-term controlled study of patients with a defined degree of heart failure with sinus rhythm and another with atrial fibrillation will help resolve this issue.

The data on the prognosis of atrial fibrillation in patients with CHF have been contradictory. Most investigators, however, have found a decreased survival rate.[39, 44] Others have found no effect on the prognosis.[45–48] Oddly, several investigators have reported beneficial outcome in CHF with atrial fibrillation.[49,50] Most recently, a study of 390 consecutive patients with advanced heart failure showed a 1-year survival rate of 52% with atrial fibrillation, as compared with 71% with normal sinus rhythm.[39] This difference was significant in patients with a pulmonary capillary wedge pressure (PCWP) of less than 16 mmHg. In the group with higher wedge pressures, atrial fibrillation did not have a poor prognostic significance. On balance, the data indicate that atrial fibrillation is a marker for poor outcome in patients with advanced heart failure. It should be emphasized, however, that the occurrence of atrial fibrillation and its frequency is inextricably

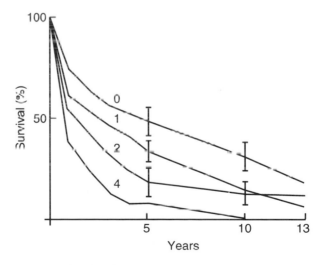

Fig. 26-5. Survival in atrial fibrillation (1958–1967): effect of congestive heart failure (CHF). Degree of CHF before. 0, no CHF (n = 152); 1, slight CHF (n = 237); 2, moderate CHF (n = 117); 4, severe CHF (n = 21). Vertical bars denote 95% confidence limits. (Redrawn from Godtfredsen,[25] with permission.)

linked, as is the case with life-threatening ventricular arrhythmias, to the severity of heart failure and the degree of disorganization of the ventricular function. The control of either form of the arrhythmias is often unsuccessful. Whether such arrhythmias are independent markers of enhanced risk of mortality remains conjectural. Only the availability of agents that are safe and effective in restoring and maintaining rhythm in the case atrial fibrillation and flutter and a complete suppression of ventricular arrhythmias will permit testing of the hypothesis that such arrhythmias are independent markers of prognosis in patients with heart failure.

THYROTOXICOSIS

Thyrotoxicosis is an important cause of atrial fibrillation, occurring in 5 to 30% of all cases.[16,50–53] The electrophysiologic basis for the arrhythmia is well established, since thyroid hormone is known to shorten the refractory period in the atria. While atrial fibrillation is the most common arrhythmia found in patients with thyrotoxicosis, other rhythm abnormalities are also found in this patient population. These include sinus tachycardia, paroxysmal supraventricular tachycardia, atrial flutter, bradycardia-tachycardia syndrome, and even ventricular tachycardia.[53] In patients in whom atrial fibrillation develops as a result of thyrotoxic heart disease, the prognosis is excellent after the return to biochemical euthyroidism after effective treatment. In the Godtfredsen study of 1,212 patients with thyrotoxicosis, the 5-year and 10-year survival was 78% and 59%, respectively.[25] This survival rate was very close to the control population.

SICK SINUS SYNDROME AND ATRIAL FIBRILLATION

The relationship between bradycardia and paroxysmal supraventricular arrhythmias was originally described by Short in 1951.[54] The term sick sinus syndrome (SSS) was subsequently coined by Lown,[55] after his observations of rhythm abnormalities following DC cardioversion of chronic atrial fibrillation. SSS is defined as intermittent episodes of atrial bradycardia, supraventricular tachycardia, and sinus rhythm, all occurring in the same patient. The prevalence of SSS increases with advancing age, with a mean age of 70 in affected patients. Paroxysmal atrial fibrillation is a common occurrence is this syndrome, especially during the earlier phases of the disorder. The true incidence of atrial fibrillation is however still unclear. In a recent review of 1,171 cases of SSS, atrial fibrillation was seen in 15.8% of patients.[56] Owing to the high inci-

dence of paroxysmal atrial fibrillation, these patients are at increased risk of thromboembolic events. However, the survival rates of patients with the bradycardia-tachycardia syndrome are 86%, 73%, and 62%, at 1 year, 3 years, and 5 years, respectively.[56,57]

ALCOHOL INGESTION AND ATRIAL FIBRILLATION

Alcohol and binge drinking are recognized causes of new-onset atrial fibrillation.[19] Ettinger et al.[58] reported 32 episodes of arrhythmias, including 12 with atrial fibrillation, in a group of patients with history of heavy drinking and without any history of cardiomyopathy. These investigators noted that a disproportionate number of these patients were admitted after weekends and holidays; they coined the term "holiday heart syndrome" for the syndrome. The precise incidence of alcohol-related atrial fibrillation is unknown. However, because of the high prevalence of alcoholism in the United States and many European countries, alcohol is probably a very significant cause of atrial fibrillation. Indeed, in a study reported by Lowenstein et al.,[59] 35% of patients who presented to their public hospital with new-onset atrial fibrillation were intoxicated. The mechanism by which alcohol causes atrial fibrillation is unclear. It is probably a combination of a direct effect of alcohol on the atrial muscle, an indirect effect through an increased amount of catecholamine release, and an early cardiomyopathy in those with a long history of heavy drinking and electrolyte imbalance. Rich et al.[60] compared 64 cases of new-onset atrial fibrillation with 64 age- and sex-matched controls. Approximately 62% of cases with atrial fibrillation and 33% of controls had history of heavy drinking. There was no difference in the two groups with respect to the clinical evidence of CHF, electrocardiographic (ECG) abnormalities, heart size, or response to therapy. Hence, in this study alcohol-induced atrial fibrillation could not be attributed solely to alcoholic cardiomyopathy. In patients with alcohol-induced atrial fibrillation, the prognosis is favorable once they abstain from alcohol. This is also true for patients with atrial fibrillation and alcoholic cardiomyopathy.[45]

HYPERTROPHIC CARDIOMYOPATHY

Atrial fibrillation is a common finding in patients with hypertrophic obstructive cardiomyopathy (HOCM). In a study at the National Heart and Lung Institute, 16 of 167 (10%) patients with HOCM suffered from atrial fibrillation.[61] The arrhythmia developed late in the course of the disease (average duration of 16 years after diagnosis, probably attributable to progression of the disease). The development of atrial fibrillation was an ominous event, with severe deterioration in the patients' clinical condition. The average duration of follow-up was 5 years from the onset of atrial fibrillation. During the observation period, 3 of the 16 patients died as a result of their heart disease, and cerebral emboli developed in 4 patients. Hence, in patients with HOCM, atrial fibrillation is associated with an unusually severe worsening of symptoms and prognosis.

WOLFF-PARKINSON-WHITE SYNDROME

Atrial fibrillation is a common arrhythmia in patients with Wolff-Parkinson-White (WPW) syndrome with an incidence of up to 32% of patients.[62,63] In the absence of overt heart disease and atrial enlargement, the possible etiologies for the development atrial fibrillation are reciprocating tachycardia, intrinsic atrial properties predisposing to the arrhythmia, or the bypass tract itself. Atrial fibrillation can be life-threatening in these patients if anterograde conduction occurs over the accessory pathway. Indeed, patients with WPW syndrome who are at increased risk for the development of ventricular fibrillation and sudden cardiac death have a history of atrial fibrillation and tend to conduct rapidly over an accessory pathway during the atrial fibrillation.[64]

LONE ATRIAL FIBRILLATION

Lone atrial fibrillation is defined as atrial fibrillation without any predisposing conditions, with structural heart disease or thyrotoxic heart disease. Since its original description by Evans and Swann,[21] others have described it as idiopathic, functional, and even benign.[65,66] Among patients with atrial fibrillation in the Framingham Study, lone atrial fibrillation occurred in 16.6% of men and in 6% of women, with mean ages of 70 and 68 years, respectively.[20] In the life insurance case study, the percentage of patients with lone atrial fibrillation was significantly higher 41%.[28] Kopecky et al.[22] found lone atrial fibrillation in only 97 of 3,623 patients with atrial fibrillation (2.7%) who were 60 years old or younger at diagnosis. There is a significant disagreement in these studies as to the prognosis of patients with lone atrial fibrillation. In the Framingham study, the investigators found a fourfold higher stroke rate in the lone atrial fibrillation group, as compared with matched controls.[20] In the life insurance study,[28] patients with chronic lone atrial fibrillation had a 5-year survival rate of 85%, as opposed to 97.6% for the standard insurance tables. In the Mayo Clinic study, however, patients with lone atrial fibrillation had an excellent prognosis, with 10- and 15-year survival rates of 98% and 94%, respectively. In the mean follow-up time of 14.8 years, embolic stroke developed in only 4 of 97.[22] This was also seen in another study of flight personnel with atrial fibrillation who also had a good prognosis.[67] The mean age of the affected individuals was 37 years. The reason for the difference in these observations are unclear. One of the reasons is the difference between the populations studied. In the Framingham study, patients with lone atrial fibrillation were older, and 32% had history of hypertension. Hence, younger patients with lone atrial fibrillation might be expected to have a better prognosis.

PAROXYSMAL VERSUS CHRONIC ATRIAL FIBRILLATION

It is important to distinguish between chronic and paroxysmal atrial fibrillation. In Godtfredsen's study,[25] 35% of all cases of atrial fibrillation were paroxysmal. In his study, patients with paroxysmal atrial fibrillation with transition to chronic atrial fibrillation had a significantly higher 5-year survival rate than that of patients with chronic atrial fibrillation (Fig. 26-6). These patients were slightly younger than those with chronic atrial fibrillation, 63 years versus 68 years. Interestingly, in this study, patients with transient atrial fibrillation (i.e., one single episode and

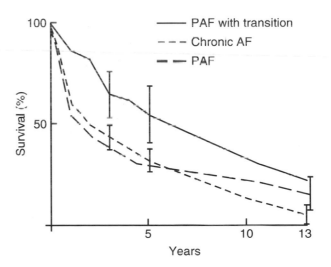

Fig. 26-6. Survival in atrial fibrillation relative to the mode of presentation (1958–1967). Paroxysmal atrial fibrillation (PAF) with transition, 57 patients; chronic AF, 313 patients; PAF, 164 patients. Vertical bars represent 95% confidence limits. (Redrawn from Godtfredsen,[25] with permission.)

probable sinus rhythm for the remainder of the follow-up), had a 5-year survival rate of only 26%.

In the life insurance company study, 90% of all cases were paroxysmal, with most (59%) having no known associated condition (lone atrial fibrillation). In this study, patients with paroxysmal atrial fibrillation without any associated condition had a normal mortality rate.[28] Those with paroxysmal atrial fibrillation attributable to other associated conditions had a significant excess mortality, with a ratio of 199% and an excess death rate of 3.3 per 1,000 per year. However, this excess in mortality was only 27% of the mortality ratio of the comparable group with chronic atrial fibrillation.

In the Framingham study, subjects with paroxysmal atrial fibrillation attributable to CAD also had a significantly lower mortality than that of patients with chronic atrial fibrillation caused by CAD.[4] Again, these data are at variance with those published by the Mayo Clinic, in which among patients with lone atrial fibrillation, there was no significant difference in mortality among the different subgroups with isolated, recurrent, and chronic atrial fibrillation.[22]

These data indicate that, at least in patients with paroxysmal atrial fibrillation resulting from other conditions, mortality is higher than their comparable cohort without atrial fibrillation. But their prognosis is significantly better than those with chronic atrial fibrillation. In addition, patients with paroxysmal atrial fibrillation have lower rate of thromboembolic complications.[68]

ATRIAL FIBRILLATION: OCCURRENCE OF THROMBOEMBOLISM

Thromboembolic disease is one of the major complications associated with atrial fibrillation. Atrial fibrillation is associated with loss of effective atrial contractions and subsequent atrial enlargement.[69] In turn, this results in stagnation of blood and clot formation, which can embolize and cause cerebral and, less often, systemic infarction.[70] Thromboembolism is a major clinical problem that can have disastrous consequences. Emboli to the brain can cause severe and, at times, disabling neurologic deficits, and even death. Of those patients who survive the original insult, more than one-half die of further emboli to the brain with or without clinical evidence of peripheral embolism.[71] It is well established that atrial fibrillation caused by RHD is associated with increased risk of stroke.[71–85] In multiple studies, as many as 20 to 40% of patients with RHD and atrial fibrillation have a history of cerebral infarction.[70–85] Until recently, RHD was the most

common cause of cardiogenic thrombi.[73] However, with the decreasing prevalence of RHD, atrial fibrillation of other etiologies is now the major clinical disorder responsible for 45% of all cases of cardiac thrombi.[74] It is estimated that nonvalvular atrial fibrillation affects more than 1 million Americans and is associated with more than 75,000 cases of stroke annually, with one-half of all cases caused by cardiogenic thromboembolism.[75] Since a limited effect is expected from therapy for embolic strokes after the catastrophe, prevention either by anticoagulation or the stability of sinus rhythm by drug therapy appears to be the only major approach to make an inroad into the morbidity and mortality figures associated with atrial fibrillation.

Evidence that the presence of atrial fibrillation further increases the risk of embolism associated with RHD is compelling. Coulshed et al.[76] were among the first to link atrial fibrillation to an increased risk of embolism in RHD. They reported that, in 737 patients with mitral stenosis, the incidence of embolism was 8% for patients with normal sinus rhythm and 31.5% for those with atrial fibrillation. In subjects with mitral incompetence, the figures were 0.7% and 22%, respectively. Of the 157 patients with emboli, only 20% were in sinus rhythm. Coulshed and co-workers concluded that atrial fibrillation was the main cause of thromboembolism.[76] Other studies have confirmed the high incidence of atrial fibrillation in patients with RHD and a history of thromboembolism. As many as 64 to 100% of all patients with RHD who had a history of embolism were in atrial fibrillation.[71,76–83] In the Framingham Study, the risk of stroke in patients with atrial fibrillation, compared with controls, was 5.6 times higher in those with non-RHD and 17.6 times higher in those with RHD.[77]

Autopsy and angiographic data have provided further evidence. Hinton et al.[70] reported that, in 333 autopsy cases with atrial fibrillation, 41% of all symptomatic emboli with surgical or pathologic confirmation occurred in patients with mitral valve disease. Aberg[84] studied 642 autopsy cases and found left atrial thrombi in 30% of patients with a history of atrial fibrillation and in only 2% of controls. Using cardiac angiography, Parker et al.[85] found left atrial thrombi in 8 of 113 patients with mitral stenosis. This was confirmed in all 6 patients who subsequently underwent surgery. Two others had atrial thrombi, which was diagnosed only at surgery. All 10 patients had atrial fibrillation. Given this high incidence of thromboembolism in patients with atrial fibrillation and RHD, chronic long-term oral anticoagulant therapy as a preventive measure appears to be mandatory.

There is also substantive evidence that atrial fibrillation caused by nonvalvular heart disease is associated with a greater incidence of thromboembolism.

Hinton et al.[70] found that the rate of symptomatic emboli in atrial fibrillation with ischemic heart disease was almost as high as with RHD, that is, 35% versus 41%. The incidence in the control group was 7%. Aberg[73] reported that in 506 autopsy cases of atrial fibrillation caused by nonvalvular heart disease, embolic phenomena were present in 41.7%, as opposed to 18.7% in the control group.

Clinical and epidemiologic data also support the notion that atrial fibrillation per se predisposes patients to stroke. For example, in a study of 30 patients with atrial fibrillation caused by thyrotoxicosis, 12 (40%) and none of the control suffered from arterial embolism.[86] Hurst et al.[87] reported that, in their patients with atrial fibrillation, embolism was more common in those with ischemic heart disease than in those with mitral valve disease. Fairfax et al.[88] found evidence of embolism in 16 of 100 patients with chronic sinoatrial disorder, compared with 1.3% of controls with chronic atrioventricular block and normal atrial rhythm. Fifteen of the 16 patients with embolism had the bradytachycardia syndrome, and 10 of 16 were found to have paroxysmal atrial flutter of atrial fibrillation.

During 22 years of follow-up in the Framingham study, the risk of stroke in patients with atrial fibrillation caused by nonvalvular heart disease was 5.6 times higher than controls.[77] During the 30-year follow-up, this was confirmed; it was further reported that a clustering of the strokes occurred with the onset of atrial fibrillation.[89] In another large epidemiologic study, the Regional Heart Study,[29,90,91] only one stroke occurred in patients with atrial fibrillation, resulting in a relative risk of 2.3, which was not statistically significant. The Whitehall Study of 19,018 London civil servants confirmed the Framingham results; it showed an age-adjusted risk of stroke for men with nonrheumatic atrial fibrillation, in 6.9% of those without atrial fibrillation.[29,92]

As in the case of mortality, the data on the risk of stroke in lone atrial fibrillation are conflicting. During the 30-year follow-up of the Framingham study, the risk of stroke was 28% in patients with lone atrial fibrillation and 7% in controls.[11] By contrast, in the Mayo Clinic Study of subjects with lone atrial fibrillation, the risk of stroke was only 1.7% at 15 years of follow-up.[22] Patients in the Mayo Clinic study were significantly younger (44 years) than those in the Framingham Study (mean age of 64 years); they were excluded if they had other medical conditions, leaving only 3% of patients categorized as having lone atrial fibrillation. This indicates that only young patients with atrial fibrillation and without other medical illness are at low risk of thromboembolism.

The risk of stroke in patients with paroxysmal atrial fibrillation is less than in those with chronic atrial fibrillation. In a retrospective study of 426 patients with paroxysmal atrial fibrillation and 786 with chronic atrial fibrillation, the risk of stroke during the first month was 6.8% and 8.2%, respectively. The risk was 2% and 4%, respectively, for the next 2 to 5 years.[68]

The risk of recurrence of stroke after the initial event is very high in patients with atrial fibrillation. Of the 500 cases of patients with mitral valve disease, 25% suffered from systemic embolus.[82] In this study, 30% of patients had more than one embolus. Of these recurrences, 35% occurred within the first month and 58% within 12 months of the first episode. In the Framingham Study, the risk of recurrent stroke after the initial event was 47% for those with atrial fibrillation, as compared with 20% for those without atrial fibrillation.[89] This risk is the same for both chronic as well as paroxysmal atrial fibrillation.[93]

IMPACT OF ANTICOAGULATION ON THROMBOEMBOLISM

There is general consensus in the literature that patients with RHD complicated by atrial fibrillation should be treated with long-term oral warfarin therapy. The consensus is based on clinical experience,[93–99] rather than on randomized placebo-controlled trials. The experience is so compelling that a randomized trial would appear unethical. Nevertheless, several studies demonstrate the efficacy of anticoagulation in RHD (Table 26-3). However, these studies have major limitations, namely the patients were not randomized and not matched against controls; in many cases, the studies failed to address specifically the issue of atrial fibrillation in these patients. Nonetheless, these studies do show that prophylactic anticoagulation produced a striking decrease in the number of strokes, providing a compelling basis for the use

TABLE 26-3. Effect of Anticoagulant on Frequency of Thromboembolism in Patients With Rheumatic Heart Disease[a]

Investigators	Without AC		With AC	
	n	TE	n	TE
McDevitt et al.[93]	51	113	51	3.6
Cosgriff[94]	28	37.4	28	2.1
Foley and Wright[95]	29	15.3	29	1.3
Askey[96]	14	6.0	14	1.0
Owren[97]	17	2.3	15	0.9
Szekely[81]	46	0.8	23	0.3
Griffith et al.[98]	48	38%	90	7%
Carter[99]	33	67%	18	17%

Abbreviations: TE, thromboembolism; AC, anticoagulant.
[a] Frequency is expressed as the number of thromboembolic events per 100 patient-months, except for the last two entries, in which it is the percentage of patients with thromboembolism.
(From Abernathy and Willis,[73] with permission.)

TABLE 26-4. Clinical Trials of Warfarin in Patients With Nonvalvular Atrial Fibrillation

	BAATAF	AFASAK	SPAF
n (warfarin)	335	210	212
n (aspirin)	336	346,[a] 206[b]	
n (control)	336	357,[a] 211[b]	212
Age	74.2	67	68
Follow-up time (y)	2	1.3	2.2
Goal pretrial	1.5–2.0	1.3–1.8	1.2–1.5
Stroke rate/y (%)			
Warfarin group	2.0	2.3	0.41
Aspirin group	5.5	3.6	3.99
Control group	5.5	6.3,[a] 7.4[b]	2.98
Reduction of stroke in warfarin group	64%	67%	86%
Serious bleeding/y (%)			
Warfarin group	3.0	1.5	0.9
Aspirin group	0.3	1.4	
Control group	0.0	1.6	0.5
Fatal bleeding/y (%)			
Warfarin group	0.0	0.5	0.5
Aspirin group	0.0	0.4	
Control group	0.0	0.4,[a] 0.0[b]	0.5
Total death rate/y (%)			
Warfarin group	No difference	2.2	2.25
Aspirin group	No difference	5.3	
Control group	No difference	6.5,[a] 3.1[b]	5.97

Abbreviations: AFASAK, Copenhagen Atrial Fibrillation ASAK Study; SPAF, Stroke Prevention Atrial Fibrillation Investigators; BAATAF, Boston Area Anticoagulation Trial for Atrial Fibrillation Investigators.
[a] Aspirin-treated group.
[b] Warfarin-treated group.

of anticoagulants in all patients with RHD and atrial fibrillation.

By contrast, the use of anticoagulants in the more common problem of atrial fibrillation in patients with nonvalvular heart disease has been controversial. However, the increased risk of thromboembolism has been widely recognized for a number of years. Recently, three major randomized controlled trials have recently demonstrated the substantial benefit of long-term warfarin therapy in reducing the risk of stroke in patients with nonvalvular atrial fibrillation.[100–102] An additional study, Canadian Atrial Fibrillation Anticoagulation (CAFA) was prematurely terminated when the data from the others reached statistical significance.[103] The salient efficacy data of these trials are summarized in Tables 26-4 and 26-5 and the effect of anticoagulant therapy in curtailing the incidence of strokes is shown in Figure 26-7.

In the AFASAK study, the investigators randomized 1,007 patients to warfarin, aspirin (75 mg), or placebo.[100] At the end of the 2-year follow-up period, patients on warfarin had significantly fewer strokes than did those on aspirin or placebo. There was no difference between patients receiving 75 mg of aspirin and placebo. Although patients in the warfarin group had more serious bleeding, there was no fatality. Hence, the risk/benefit ratio favored the use of warfarin anticoagulant therapy.[100]

The Stroke Prevention in Atrial Fibrillation (SPAF) study examined two groups of patients on the basis of their eligibility for warfarin therapy. The first group comprised those patients in whom warfarin was not contraindicated. These 627 patients were randomized

TABLE 26-5. Efficacy of Warfarin for the Prevention of Stroke[a]

Variable	AFASAK	SPAF[b]	BAATAF	CAFA
Control group[c]				
Person-years of follow-up	413	244	435	250
Strokes, n	19	17	13	9
Stroke events/100 person-years	4.6	7.0	3.0	3.6
Warfarin				
Person-years of follow-up	412	260	487	240
Strokes, n	8	6	2	5
Stroke events/100 person-years	1.9	2.3	0.4	2.1
Risk reduction (95% CI)	58 (7–81)	67 (21–86)	86 (51–96)	42 (−68–80)
p-value[d]	0.03	0.01	0.002	<0.2

Abbreviations: AFASAK, Copenhagen Atrial Fibrillation, Aspirin, Anticoagulation Study; SPAF, Stroke Prevention in Atrial Fibrillation Study; BAATAF, Boston Area Anticoagulation Trial for Atrial Fibrillation; CAFA, Canadian Atrial Fibrillation Anticoagulation (study).
[a] Intention-to-treat analysis. Strokes represent all strokes, regardless of suspected cause. Transient ischemic attacks, systemic emboli, and intracranial hemorrhages are not included.
[b] Data are from group 1 only (see text).
[c] Controls received placebo in all studies except BAATAF; in BAATAF, 46% of control patients took aspirin and 54% received "no treatment."
[d] By chi-square analysis.

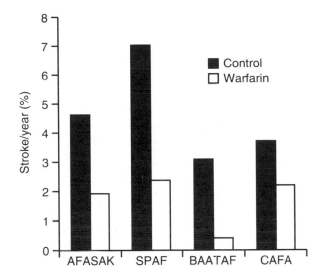

Fig. 26-7. Stroke prevention in atrial fibrillation (AF) patients receiving warfarin and in concurrent controls. Anticoagulant studies: AFASAK, Copenhagen Atrial Fibrillation, Aspirin, Anticoagulation Study; SPAF, Stroke Prevention in Atrial Fibrillation (study); BAATAF, Boston area Anticoagulant Trial for Atrial Fibrillation Study; CAFA, Canadian Atrial Fibrillation Anticoagulant (study). (Adapted from Albers et al.,[13] with permission.)

equally to open-label warfarin (prothrombin time, 1.3 to 1.8 × control, INR, 2.8 to 4.5) or double-blind to aspirin (enteric coated, 325 mg) or placebo. The second group included those patients who were ineligible for warfarin therapy and who were randomly assigned, in a double-blind fashion, to aspirin (enteric-coated, 325 mg) or placebo. At the end of 1.3 years of follow-up, patients in group 1 who were on warfarin had a significant reduction in stroke as compared with those on placebo, 2.3% and 7.4%, respectively. Comparison data between the warfarin and aspirin-treated patients in the first group are not yet available. In group 2, patients who were on aspirin group did better (3.6%) than did those on placebo (7.4%).

There was no significant difference in serious bleeding among the four groups. Interestingly, the rate of serious bleeding in SPAF was less than that reported in the AFASAK study. This is probably due to younger patient population and lower goal for prothrombin time. Again, in the SPAF study, warfarin was significantly better than placebo in preventing strokes. The principal outcome was also reduced by aspirin as compared with placebo. The risk/benefit ratio favored the use of aspirin, but the benefit was much less marked than that for warfarin. However, the effects of warfarin and aspirin were evaluated in two different patient populations, and the data from a direct comparison are not yet available.

The Boston Area Anticoagulation Trial for Atrial Fibrillation (BAATAF) randomized 420 patients equally to open-label warfarin and placebo.[102] At the end of the 2.2-year follow-up period, warfarin again was associated with a significant reduction in the incidence of stroke as compared with placebo. Major bleeding plus transfusion was increased by an absolute amount of about 0.4% per year (see Table 26-3) in the warfarin-treated group. In this study, patients were not assigned to aspirin. However, 46% of all patient-years in the placebo-treated group were contributed by those who were taking aspirin. Eight of the 13 strokes (total) in the control group occurred among the patients who were taking aspirin, for an incidence of 3.99% per year. As with other studies, warfarin was significantly better in reducing the incidence of stroke, a consistent observation of much clinical importance.

On the basis of these three studies, warfarin is the drug of choice for reducing the stroke rate. The use of aspirin is still somewhat controversial. Both the AFASAK and BAATAF studies showed that warfarin was superior to aspirin. However, in the AFASAK study 75 mg of aspirin was used, and in the BAATAF study there was no separate aspirin treatment arm. Clearly, there is a certain patient population that would benefit from aspirin. Indeed, a subgroup analysis from the preliminary report of the SPAF study[75] showed that the benefit of aspirin is confined to patients under the age of 75 years. Until further studies define its possible role, aspirin should only be used in patients in whom warfarin therapy cannot be used safely.

The population most likely to benefit from long-term warfarin therapy appears to be patients with paroxysmal or chronic atrial fibrillation in whom anticoagulation therapy is not contraindicated. Patients below 50 years of age with lone atrial fibrillation are at a low risk of stroke[22] and probably require anticoagulant therapy rarely.

Anticoagulation therapy is the only question regarding therapeutic modalities in atrial fibrillation that has received enough attention to result in randomized, placebo-controlled trials. It is noteworthy that remarkably little research has been conducted on the issue of optimal drug regimens for controlling ventricular rate, conversion, or the maintenance of sinus rhythm after conversion. Therefore, the treatment of atrial fibrillation remains difficult despite new therapeutic options.

IMPACT OF CONTROLLING VENTRICULAR RESPONSE VERSUS MAINTAINING STABILITY OF SINUS RHYTHM

The primary aim of medical treatment is dependent on the clinical presentation and the underlying cause of the atrial flutter-fibrillation. In all types of atrial fibrillation, the initial goal of therapy is to restore normal sinus rhythm. Drug treatment is therefore directed toward conversion and maintenance of normal sinus rhythm, especially in the presence of a correctable underlying cause.

Controlling Ventricular Response

In many patients, atrial fibrillation is chronic and stable. In this situation, conversion may be neither indicated nor successful. In these patients, the main goal of therapy is simply to control ventricular rate and decrease the risk of thromboembolism with chronic oral anticoagulant therapy.

Three classes of drugs are currently available for controlling ventricular response; all reduce the ventricular rate by increasing the extent of the AV nodal conduction block through different mechanisms.

Digoxin

Digoxin, which has been in clinical use for the past 200 years, is widely considered the drug of choice for control of ventricular rate. Cardiac glycosides, such as digoxin, exert their effect by prolonging AV nodal refractoriness through an indirect vagomimetic and presumably weak antiadrenergic action.[104,105] Hence, in the resting digitalized patient, the vagal effect on the AV node is enhanced, and ventricular rate is slowed. It is clearly established that digoxin does not convert atrial fibrillation to normal sinus rhythm.[106] The objective of digoxin therapy is thus to slow ventricular rate to 90 bpm or lower at rest. At this rate, there is an acceptable control with the least compromise of cardiac output.[107]

There is little doubt that in patients with CHF and atrial fibrillation, digoxin is the preferred drug, but there are no controlled data that address whether the drug influences total or cardiovascular mortality (favorably or adversely). In these patients, digoxin improves hemodynamics both by slowing the ventricular rate and by possibly a direct effect on the myocardium. However, there are many clinical situations in which digoxin is ineffective, and possibly harmful.

During exercise, intrinsic vagal tone is withdrawn and sympathetic activity increased. Hence, the beneficial effect of the drug, which is mediated through enhanced vagal tone, is not maintained.[108,109] This results in excessive tachycardia during exercise and even during average daily activity, which may cause symptoms of palpitations, shortness of breath, and fatigue. Digoxin may not be an ideal agent in a young, active patient with normal ventricular function. Other clinical situations in which digoxin should not be used include atrial fibrillation with WPW syndrome.[110] By blocking the AV node and increasing the anterograde

conduction over the bypass tract, digoxin may accelerate the ventricular response and induce ventricular fibrillation that is already high. In addition, in patients with infarction and atrial fibrillation, digoxin can decrease the ventricular fibrillation threshold.[111] Moreover, in patients with HOCM, in whom the drug induces cardiac contractility, the beneficial effect of digoxin is outweighed by its ability to decrease the ventricular rate.[112] Vagally induced atrial fibrillation is another situation in which the use of digoxin is of little value, as it may sustain the arrhythmia by shortening the atrial effective refractory period.[113] In patients in renal failure, digoxin should be used with caution, as it the drug is cleared by the kidneys and is not dialyzable.

Digoxin is usually well tolerated, but adverse effects such as nausea or other gastrointestinal (GI) disturbances are common. There are also reports that digoxin may have direct effects on the central nervous system (CNS) and may alter memory or mood.[114] In addition, digoxin has a narrow therapeutic-to-toxic ratio; toxicity may be associated with potentially serious arrhythmias although ventricular pro-arrhythmic reactions as a result of digoxin toxicity have not been well documented. Hence, because of its inability to control the ventricular rate effectively during exercise, as well as contraindications to its use in several important clinical situations and its potential for untoward effects, many believe that digoxin should not be the drug of choice in atrial fibrillation.[115] However, in certain clinical situations digoxin has an important role in the treatment of atrial fibrillation, in particular, in the setting of ventricular dysfunction, and especially in patients with clinically significant CHF and ventricular dilation.

Calcium-Channel Blockers and β-Adrenergic Blocking Agents

Given some of the limitations in the use of digoxin, the other two classes of drugs have now been advocated as the drugs of choice, individually or in combination with digoxin, to control the ventricular rate in atrial fibrillation: rate-lowering calcium-channel blockers such as diltiazem and verapamil, and β-adrenergic blocking agents. The former exert their salutary effect by inhibiting calcium influx at the AV node, thereby increasing the AV nodal refractory period and decreasing conduction, producing slowing of the ventricular rate.[116] These drugs exert additional nonspecific antiadrenergic actions. Their efficacy in controlling ventricular rate has been well documented.[108,116–118] In contrast to digoxin, calcium-channel blockers exert their effect directly on the myocardium, and their efficacy is influenced less by changes in the autonomic nervous system. Hence, these agents achieve better control of ventricular rate during exercise than is produced by digoxin.[108,119] Several studies have also shown the superiority of combination therapy with verapamil-digoxin or diltiazem-digoxin over digoxin alone, with respect to control of ventricular rate, both at rest and during exercise, as well as marked improvement in exercise capacity.[108,117,119] Thus, some investigators advocate combination therapy as the treatment of choice.[120]

Calcium-channel blockers are also well tolerated with minor GI side effects in 3 to 9% of patients.[121] However, because of their negative inotropic effect on the myocardium, these drugs should be used with caution in patients with CHF of New York Heart Association (NYHA) class 1 and 2 and should be avoided in those with NYHA class 3 and 4.[112] Other clinical situations in which their use is contraindicated include hypotension, SSS, and WPW syndrome.[112]

β-Blockers are the third class of drugs used to control ventricular rate in atrial fibrillation. Unlike calcium-channel blockers, they act by blocking sympathetic impulse traffic in the AV node. Hence, they are very effective in controlling heart rate both at rest and with exercise.[122–124] The use of β-blockers as adjuvant therapy to digoxin has also been studied and shown to be effective.[125] However, the use of β-blockers can be associated with decreased exercise capacity and increased perception of the severity of the exercise.[124] In addition, these compounds have negative inotropic effects, contraindicating their use in patients with CHF. Moreover, β-blocker therapy can cause both peripheral and CNS side effects, which again may prevent their use in some patients.[126] Another important side effect of β-blockers in patients with atrial fibrillation is that those agents that lack partial agonist activity (e.g., propranolol, atenolol) can cause nocturnal bradycardia.[123,124]

A recent metanalysis of 24 randomized control trials of efficacy of digoxin, verapamil, and β-blockers in preventing supraventricular arrhythmias after coronary artery bypass surgery showed that neither digoxin nor verapamil reduced the incidence of atrial fibrillation.[127] β-Blockers, however, were significantly effective in preventing the development of supraventricular tachycardia postoperatively, with an odds ratio of 0.28.

There is no ideal drug therapy for the control of ventricular rate in atrial fibrillation. The choice of specific drug or combination regimen should be tailored to the clinical presentation of the patient, underlying cause of atrial fibrillation, and the relevance of the pharmacodynamic actions of the drug to the clinical setting.

In most patients, controlling the ventricular rate and oral anticoagulation to decrease the risk of thromboembolism constitutes adequate treatment of their atrial fibrillation. In some patients, however, there are clear indications for restoring and maintaining normal sinus rhythm, if this can be accomplished safely and at an acceptable risk/benefit ratio. The major reasons for converting atrial fibrillation are as follows:

1. New-onset atrial fibrillation
2. Relief of symptoms of palpitations, dyspnea, or angina
3. Hypotension
4. Decreased risk of embolic stroke
5. Improved overall cardiac function
6. Improved exercise tolerance

The appropriateness of these goals will vary relative to the clinical circumstances.

CARDIOVERSION AND MAINTAINING STABILITY OF SINUS RHYTHM

With the advent of DC cardioversion by Lown et al.[128] conversion of atrial fibrillation has become immediate, easily accessible, safe, and successful. Studies over the past three decades have shown the initial success rate of DC cardioversion to be 80 to 90%.[129–131] DC cardioversion is safe and usually well tolerated. The most life-threatening side effect of DC cardioversion is the development of ventricular fibrillation.[129–133] This usually occurs with improper technique and in patients with digoxin or quinidine toxicity. Another important complication of cardioversion is risk of embolization. The incidence of embolism after either electrical or pharmacologic cardioversion ranges from 1.1 to 5.3%.[87,134–136] The incidence of embolization in anticoagulated patients can be decreased from 5.3% to 0.8%[137] It is currently accepted medical therapy to anticoagulate patients with atrial fibrillation of more than 3 days with warfarin for at least 2 weeks prior to conversion.

Unfortunately, the recurrence rate of atrial fibrillation after cardioversion is very high.[87] Strong predictors of early relapse include left atrial size greater than 45 mm, duration of atrial fibrillation of more than 3 months, and failure of the A wave on Doppler echocardiography to increase by more than 10% over 24 hours after cardioversion.[137] To prevent relapse, one must either correct the underlying cause or initiate antiarrhythmic therapy. It is generally accepted, however, that all patients with new-onset atrial fibrillation should be cardioverted at least once initially, since approximately 25% of all cases remain in normal sinus rhythm at the end of the first year.

Although DC cardioversion is safe and effective, it is not always looked on favorably by some patients. In addition, it requires hospitalization, the use of light anesthesia, and close monitoring. Hence, pharmacologic cardioversion may be preferred in certain situations. In addition, the use of antiarrhythmic therapy increases the likelihood of maintaining normal sinus rhythm.

Currently, several different classes of antiarrhythmic drugs are available for chemical cardioversion of atrial fibrillation and maintenance of normal sinus rhythm, but they are far from ideal. Most have a low efficacy rate and a high incidence of cardiac and extracardiac side effects, and some are associated with increased mortality when used chronically. Hence, one has to weigh carefully the benefits of maintaining normal sinus rhythm against the risks associated with the use of antiarrhythmic drug therapy. Converting atrial fibrillation results in a decreased rate of thromboembolic phenomena and, at times, improvement in patient symptoms. However, no studies are available to show that conversion of atrial fibrillation and maintenance of normal sinus rhythm can favorably influence the observed increase in mortality associated with atrial fibrillation. Indeed, studies show increased mortality with the use of certain classes of antiarrhythmic drugs.

Despite widespread belief, there is no evidence that digoxin, calcium-channel blockers, or β-blockers convert atrial fibrillation to sinus rhythm. This is not unexpected, as none of these classes of drugs exerts antifibrillatory activity in the atrial muscle.

Class 1A drugs, such as quinidine, procainamide, and disopryamide, have been used extensively for chemical cardioversion of atrial fibrillation[138-164] (Tables 26-6 and 26-7). However, several significant side effects limit their use in many patients. In addition, this class of drugs can accelerate AV nodal conduction, leading to increased ventricular rate.

TABLE 26-6. Efficacy Rate of Different Antiarrhythmic Agents in Converting Atrial Fibrillation in Patients With Paroxysmal and Recent-Onset Atrial Fibrillation

Drugs	Success (%)	References
Digitalis	20–85	138, 139
Quinidine + digitalis	70–88	138, 140
Procainamide	40–43	138, 141
Ajmaline	79	138
Verapamil	10–16	142, 143, 144
Diltiazem	6.5–17	145
β-Blockers	16	122, 147
Amiodarone	48–81	147, 162, 163
Disopyramide	30–75	147
Flecainide	61–92	145, 149, 150
Propafenone	45	147, 151
Verapamil + quinidine	50–92	143, 145, 152, 153

(Modified from Bolognesi,[112] with permission.)

TABLE 26-7. Efficacy Rate of Antiarrhythmic Agents in Converting Atrial Fibrillation in Patients With Chronic Atrial Fibrillation

Drugs	Success (%)	References
Quinidine	62	154
Digitalis + quinidine	50–90	155
Amiodarone	48–81	144, 148, 162, 163, 164
Amiodarone + digitalis	50	148
Amiodarone + quinidine	94	148
Disopyramide	43–76	147, 156
β-Blocker + quinidine	61	157
Verapamil + quinidine	60–84	143, 145, 156, 158,
Procainamide	57	159, 160, 161

(Modified from Bolognesi,[112] with permission.)

Flecainide, a class 1C drug, is very effective in converting atrial fibrillation with minimal side effects. However, this drug should be used very cautiously in light of the Cardiac Arrhythmias Suppression Trial (CAST).[165] Indeed, there are several reports of the proarrhythmic effects of this agent in patients with and without overt heart disease.

Amiodarone, a class 3 agent, is probably the most potent antiarrhythmic available in the treatment of supraventricular and ventricular arrhythmias. This is a very safe drug with minimal risk of proarrhythmia. Unfortunately, when used chronically, it can cause significant pulmonary, dermatologic, and thyroid toxicity, preventing its widespread use.

Irrespective of the method used to convert atrial fibrillation, most patients revert to atrial fibrillation unless prophylactic antiarrhythmic therapy is used. Even with the use of drug prophylaxis, maintaining stable sinus rhythm is not uniformly or predictably successful in most patients treated long term; drug regimens are often associated with serious complications. Studies have shown that maintenance of sinus rhythm is dependent on several factors, including age, underlying etiology, duration of atrial fibrillation, size and function of the heart, and left atrial dimension.[166-171] It is well documented that older patients with an enlarged left atrium, a dilated and poorly functioning left ventricle, and atrial fibrillation duration of more than 1 year have a very low probability of staying in normal sinus rhythm, despite medical therapy.

Only three classes of drugs are available to maintain normal sinus rhythm: class 1A, class 1C, and class 3. Quinidine, class 1A, is the most commonly used drug for prophylaxis of atrial fibrillation. There are many studies conducted to determine the efficacy of quinidine. They have reported an efficacy rate of 8 to 74% at the end of 1-year, as compared with 0 to 60% for the untreated group.[166,169,172-176] With longer follow-up, these efficacy rates drop to 11 to 33% and 25%, respectively.[174,177] Hence, quinidine does not prevent relapse in most patients. It merely delays the recurrence of atrial fibrillation. Unfortunately, most of these studies were inadequately designed; most had small numbers of patients, some were not randomized, and only a few were double-blind.

In a metanalysis of randomized placebo-controlled trials, Coplen et al.[178] showed a 1-year efficacy rate of 50% for quinidine and of 25% for placebo. Hence, quinidine is more effective than placebo in delaying recurrence. However, quinidine-treated patients had significantly increased mortality, 2.9% versus 0.8%. Thus, increased efficacy was associated with a significant cost of increased fatality. This increased mortality in quinidine-treated patients has also been also reported by other investigators.[166,179,180] Indeed, Radford and Evans[179] considered quinidine therapy too dangerous to justify its continued use in attempting to maintain normal sinus rhythm. Hence, they prematurely stopped their study. In a study[180] of 367 advanced heart failure patients, those treated with class 1 drugs had a 1-year risk of 24% as compared with 15% for amiodarone and 14% for no antiarrhythmic therapy. Another metanalysis of studies comparing quinidine with other class 1 drugs, including flecainide, for the treatment of nonsustained ventricular arrhythmia showed that quinidine is more likely to cause death than other drugs already known to be proarrhythmic.[181]

In addition to proarrhythmia, quinidine is associated with other side effects, including GI complications (e.g., diarrhea), dermatologic problems, and pyrexia. They are common findings in patients taking quinidine, requiring its discontinuation in a significant percentage of patients.[178,182] Hence, quinidine is far from an ideal "drug of choice" for the treatment of atrial fibrillation.

Very limited data are available on the efficacy and safety of procainamide. In one study, procainamide alone or in combination with propranolol was successful in delaying relapse of atrial fibrillation at 1 month after cardioversion. Unfortunately, at the end of 1 year, 77% of those on procainamide and 100% of those on no drug therapy had reverted to atrial fibrillation.[169] In another small study, the 6-month efficacy rate for procainamide was only 13%.[169] Disopyramide is another class 1A drug used to maintain normal sinus rhythm. Hartel et al.[183] reported a 3-month efficacy rate of 72% for patients on disopyramide, as compared with 30% for the control group. In addition, patients tolerated the antiarrhythmic agent well. In another study,[184] however, there was no difference between quinidine, disopyramide, and placebo in maintaining normal sinus rhythm at the end of 6 months of follow-up, but side effects were less in the disopyramide group as opposed to the quinidine group, 8% versus 15%. The difference between the two studies could be attributable to the large number of patients with valvular heart disease in the latter study. In the Hartel study, only 23% of patients had RHD, whereas in the latter study, 76% of all patients had valvular heart disease. There is no data available on the long-term efficacy of disopyramide.

Flecainide is a class 1C antiarrhythmic agent, originally synthesized for the treatment of ventricular arrhythmias. However, it has also found proved very effective in the treatment of supraventricular arrhythmias.[185] Studies have shown long-term efficacy rates of flecainide alone or in combination with other antiarrhythmic drugs in the treatment of chronic and paroxysmal atrial fibrillation to be 31 to 82%,[186-189] in line with the electrophysiologic effects of the drug. In contrast to its action in the ventricular myocardium, Wang et al.[5] showed that in a variety of mammalian atria including humans, flecainide increased the action potential duration and the effective refractory period as the stimulation frequency was increased. In this regard, the effect of flecainide in atrial flutter and fibrillation is unique, as it appears to function as a pure class 3 agent at short cycle lengths. Such an effect will not be conducive to prompt termination of the arrhythmia but also will contribute the stability of sinus rhythm once conversion has occurred. In addition, flecainide is usually well tolerated. However, the major limitation of the compound, despite being well tolerated, is its propensity to induce atrial and ventricular proarrhythmic reactions, many of which may lead to fatality, especially in patients significant structural heart disease.[165] Various studies have reported proarrhythmic effects of flecainide within the range of 0 to 20% in patients with atrial fibrillation.[186-193] These proarrhythmic effects occur at both the atrial and ventricular levels. Patients at high risk of aggravation of ventricular arrhythmia usually have a history of CAD, structural heart disease, history of ventricular arrhythmia, and impaired LV function.[194] Unfortunately, it is generally very difficult to determine the high-risk group of patients with atrial fibrillation in whom proarrhythmic effects may develop. Studies have documented proarrhythmia in patients with atrial fibrillation of various underlying etiologies and in those with lone atrial fibrillation. These adverse effects have been very serious in many instances and have resulted in sudden death in some. Hence, flecainide, as well as quinidine, should be used with caution in patients with atrial fibrillation, regardless of the underlying heart disease. With regard to flecainide (and probably quinidine) therapy, there are no high-risk and low-risk patients. It is likely that other class 1C agents, such as propafenone, will exhibit similar antiarrhythmic and proarrhythmic profiles.

Because of major shortcomings of class 1 drugs, attention has recently shifted to class 3 agents.[196,197] Of the class 3 agents, sotalol is somewhat different. It has both β-blocking, as well as class 3, effects.[185] In an open parallel study comparing sotalol versus quinidine, Juul-Moller et al.[182] showed a 6-month efficacy rate of 52% and 48% for sotalol and quinidine, respectively. Hence, there was no significant difference in efficacy between these two agents. However, sotalol was tolerated much better. Of note, there was one death in each group. Another study reported the same efficacy rate for sotalol and propafenone, with a good side effect profile.[195] Hence, sotalol is probably not more efficacious, but better tolerated, than quinidine.

Amiodarone, another unique class 3 antiarrhythmic agent, was originally marketed as an antianginal drug.[186] In recent years, the efficacy of the drug in life-threatening ventricular arrhythmias has been established, albeit in systematic but uncontrolled clinical trials. The drug has been found to be effective in more than 60% of patients when conventional class 1 agents have failed.[198–208] Less attention has focused on the potential of the drug to maintain stability of sinus rhythm in patients with atrial fibrillation converted to sinus rhythm by DC cardioversion or in those experiencing paroxysmal atrial fibrillation/flutter. However, studies have indicated that amiodarone is effective in maintaining normal sinus rhythm in 60 to 92% of patients.[199–207] This finding is in line with a number of clinical observations suggesting the importance of prolonging the refractory period in atria as a basis for providing stability of sinus rhythm. Studies conducted in Scandinavia[7] indicated that, in patients converted to sinus rhythm by DC cardioversion, the relapse rate to sinus rhythm was higher in patients who had a shorter action potential duration than in those with longer action potentials, as determined by the monophasic potential recordings. In the case of amiodarone, during chronic administration of the drug, the maintenance of the stability of sinus rhythm was correlated with the prolongation of the action potential duration.[209] These overall observations are consistent with the data on the importance of the prolonged refractory period in the case of class 1A agents, flecainide (at fast rates), and class 3 agents including sotalol and amiodarone as a crucial determinant for the conversion of atrial fibrillation and flutter and the maintenance of sinus rhythm. These clinical observations are in line with comparable experimental observations.[210,211]

While the available experimental and clinical data clearly suggest the superiority of amiodarone therapy in maintaining stability of sinus rhythm and its effectiveness in the control of life-threatening ventricular arrhythmias, the difficulty of direct studies to compare the efficacy of the drug to other agents should be appreciated. A direct comparison between amiodarone and quinidine showed amiodarone to be significantly better in maintaining normal sinus rhythm with much better side effect profile.[206] Of importance, the efficacy of amiodarone is not influenced by patient's age, duration of atrial fibrillation, type of underlying heart disease, or degree of LV dysfunction. Indeed, left atrial size does not seem to be a very important factor in determining the efficacy rate of amiodarone.[203]

The side effect profile of amiodarone has been the limiting factor in using this drug. Studies have reported minor side effects in 30 to 75% of patients and serious side effects requiring termination of therapy in 4 to 15% of patients.[199–207] However, the lower maintenance dose of 200 to 400 mg/d required to control atrial tachyarrhythmias is generally well tolerated and is associated with fewer side effects. Of importance, proarrhythmia and exacerbation of CHF, a common and serious side effect of other antiarrhythmic agents, is rarely seen in patients on amiodarone.[180,208] Indeed, amiodarone may be one of the safer antiarrhythmic agents available.

In treating atrial fibrillation, amiodarone has many advantages over other antiarrhythmic compounds:

1. High efficacy rate in maintaining normal sinus rhythm, but possibly also in converting atrial fibrillation and slowing the ventricular response: unique aggregate of properties in a single agent for use in atrial fibrillation
2. Long therapeutic half-life: makes it possible for amiodarone to be taken once a day
3. High LD_{50}: much higher than that of other antiarrhythmic agents, such as quinidine and procainamide
4. Proarrhythmic effects: very low
5. Side effect profile: low when used at low dosages
6. Variety of clinical conditions in which this drug can be used: factors such as type of underlying heart disease, patient's age, LV function, and left atrial size important only when other antiarrhythmic agents used, but amiodarone safe, and at times ideal, drug in these situations

Nevertheless, it must be emphasized that, to date, no blinded comparisons between amiodarone and quinidine or other conventional agents have been performed to examine the relative potencies of these agents in maintaining the stability of sinus rhythm after cardioversion in patients with atrial fibrillation, nor have there been studies of this kind in patients subject to paroxysmal atrial fibrillation relative to the side effect profiles of the test agents. Such studies will be crucial in defining the role of pharmacologic therapy of atrial fibrillation and flutter with respect to maintaining sinus rhythm.

CONCLUSIONS

Atrial fibrillation is perhaps the most common arrhythmia requiring treatment for relief of symptoms, improvement in morbidity, and reduction in mortality, all of which are significant complications of the disorder. In patients with atrial fibrillation, no single therapeutic approach is universally applicable, and attempts at influencing the natural history of the disease consists of dealing with the underlying disorder, slowing the ventricular response, chemically or electrically converting the arrhythmia, and maintaining the stability of sinus rhythm as might be appropriate in an individual patient. It is unclear whether conversion of atrial fibrillation and maintaining normal sinus rhythm will indeed reduce the increased mortality associated with atrial fibrillation. It is clear, however, that by maintaining normal sinus rhythm, the risk of thromboembolism in most patients can be eliminated. Placebo-controlled studies have confirmed that chronic anticoagulation can reduce this risk significantly.

The ultimate goal in controlling this arrhythmia is the restoration and maintenance of sinus rhythm. The precise efficacy and safety of the conventional regimens to achieve such a goal are not clearly defined but, on the basis of experimental and clinical data, a perspective is developing that both for conversion as well as for maintaining sinus rhythm, drugs that prolong the effective refractory period in the atria are superior to those that act essentially by delaying conduction. In this respect, the perspective is similar, if not identical, to that being developed for life-threatening ventricular arrhythmias. The greatest experience has been with quinidine, which appears to be as effective as sotalol in maintaining sinus rhythm, but much concern has been engendered that the proarrhythmic effect of class 1 agents (even those that have the additional property of prolonging refractoriness) might exceed the potential benefit. It is probably the only agent currently available for which therapy carries a favorable risk/benefit ratio despite the well-recognized list of side effects that make it a less than ideal antifibrillatory drug. Further studies are needed to find a new generation of class 3 antiarrhythmic drugs with an efficacy rate comparable to that of amiodarone but without its side effect profile.

Nevertheless, the precise role of amiodarone in the treatment of atrial fibrillation needs to be defined by controlled clinical trials against either placebo or an active control such as quinidine, or both. It should be emphasized that the drug encompasses a number of properties that might be crucial for testing the hypothesis that the conversion and maintenance of sinus rhythm in patients with recurrent or chronic atrial fibrillation will favorably influence the mortality and morbidity associated with the arrhythmia.

REFERENCES

1. Allessie MA, Rensma PL, Brugada RJ et al: Pathophysiology of atrial fibrillation. p 548. In Zipes DP, Jalife J (eds): Cardiac Electrophysiology: From Cell to Bedside. WB Saunders, Philadelphia, 1990
2. Moe GK: On the multiple wavelet hypothesis of atrial fibrillation. Arch Int Pharm Ther 140:183, 1962
3. Burn JR, Vaughan Williams EM, Walker EM: Effects of acetylcholine in the heart-lung preparation including production of auricular fibrillation. J Physiol (Lond) 28:277, 1955
4. Spach MS, Miller WT, Dolber PC: The functional role of structural complexities in the propagation of depolarizations in the atrium of the dog. Cardiac conduction disturbances due to discontinuities of effective axial resistivity. Circ Res 50:175, 1982
5. Wang Z, Pelletier LC, Talajic M, Nattel S: Effects of flecainide and quinidine on human atrial action potentials. Circulation 82:274, 1990
6. Freedberg AS, Papp JG, Vaughan Williams EM: The effect of altered thyroid state on atrial intracellular potentials. J Physiol (Lond) 207:357, 1970
7. Olsson SB, Cotoi S, Varnauskas E: Monophasic action potentials and sinus rhythm stability after conversion of atrial fibrillation. Acta Med Scand 190:381, 1971
8. Dunn M, Alexander J, de Silva R, Hildner F: Anti-thrombotic therapy in atrial fibrillation. Chest 95:1185, 1989
9. Cerebral Embolism Task Force: Cardiogenic brain embolism. The second report of the Cerebral Embolism Task Force. Arch Neurol 46:727, 1989
10. Kannel WB, Abbott RD, Savage DD, McNamara PM: Epidemiologic features of chronic atrial fibrillation: the Framingham Study. N Engl J Med 306:1018, 1982
11. Ostrander LD, Brandt RL, Kjelsberg MO, Epstein FH: Electrocardiographic findings among the adult population of a total natural community, Tecumseh, Michigan. Circulation 31:888, 1985
12. Ostor E, Schnohr P, Jensen G et al: Electrocardiographic findings and their association with mortality in the Copenhagen City Heart Study. Eur Heart J 2:317, 1981
13. Albers GW, Atwood JE, Hirsh J et al: Stroke prevention in nonvalvular atrial fibrillation. Ann Intern Med 115:727, 1991
14. Kannel WB, Abbott RD, Savage DD, McNamara PM: Coronary heart disease and atrial fibrillation: the Framingham Study. Am Heart J 106:389, 1983
15. Sloan RW: Atrial fibrillation. Am Family Physician 25:165, 1982
16. Davidson E, Weinberger I, Rotenberg Z et al: Atrial fibrillation, cause and time of onset. Arch Intern Med 149:457, 1989
17. Olsson SB: Atrial fibrillation—some current problems. Acta Med Scand 207:1, 1980
18. Bennett D: Atrial fibrillation. Eur Heart J suppl A. 89, 1984

19. Braunwald E: Heart Disease: A Textbook of Cardiovascular Medicine. WB Saunders, Philadelphia, 1988

20. Brand FN, Abbott RD, Kannel WB, Wolf PA: Characteristics and prognosis of lone atrial fibrillation. 30-year follow-up in the Framingham Study. JAMA 254:3449, 1985

21. Evans W, Swann P: Lone auricular fibrillation. Br Heart J 16:189, 1954

22. Kopecky SL, Gersh BJ, McGoon MD et al: The natural history of lone atrial fibrillation. A population-based study over three decades. N Engl J Med 317:669, 1987

23. Gould WL: Auricular fibrillation: Report on a study of a mitral tendency, 1920–1956. Arch Intern Med 100:916, 1957

24. Coumel P, Attuel P, Lavalle JP: Syndrome d'arrhythmie auriculaire d'origine vagale. Arch Mal Coeur 71: 645, 1978

25. Godtfredsen J: Atrial fibrillation: course and prognosis—a follow-up study of 1,212 cases. p. 158. In Kulbertus HE, Olsson SB, Schlepper M (eds): Atrial Fibrillation. AB Hassle, Molndal, Sweden, 1982

26. Petersen P, Godtfredsen J: Atrial fibrillation—a review of course and prognosis. Acta Med Scand 215:5, 1984

27. Kulbertus HE, de Leval-Rutten F, Bartsch P, Petit JM: Atrial fibrillation in elderly, ambulatory patients. p. 148. In Kulbertus HE, Olsson SB, Schlepper M (eds): Atrial Fibrillation. AB Hassel, Molndal, Sweden, 1982

28. Gajewski J, Singer RB: Mortality in an insured population with atrial fibrillation. JAMA 245:1540, 1981

29. Flegel KM, Shipley MJ, Rose G: Risk of stroke in nonrheumatic atrial fibrillation [published erratum appears in Lancet 11:878, 1987]. Lancet 1:526, 1987

30. Petersen P, Godtfredsen J: Risk factors for stroke in chronic atrial fibrillation. Circulation, suppl II. 74:152, 1986

31. Cameron A, Schwartz MK, Kronmal RA, Kosinski AS: Prevalence and significance of atrial fibrillation in coronary artery disease (CASS Registry). Am J Cardiol 61: 714, 1988

32. Klass M, Haywood LJ: Atrial fibrillation associated with acute myocardial infarction: a study of 34 cases. Am Heart J 79:752, 1970

33. Helmers C, Lundman T, Mogensen L et al: Atrial fibrillation in acute myocardial infarction. Acta Med Scand 193:39, 1973

34. Liberthson RR, Salisbury KW, Hutter AM, Jr, DeSanctis RW: Atrial tachyarrhythmias in acute myocardial infarction. Am J Med 60:956, 1976

35. Hunt D, Sutton L, Sloman G, Srinivasan M: The prognosis of atrial fibrillation with acute myocardial infarction. p. 211. In Kulbertus HE, Olsson SB, Schlepper MS (eds): Atrial Fibrillation. AB Hassle, Molndal, Sweden, 1982

36. Sugiura T, Iwasaka T, Ogawa A et al: Atrial fibrillation in acute myocardial infarction. Am J Cardiol 56:27, 1985

37. Alpert JS, Petersen P, Godtfredsen J: Atrial fibrillation: natural history, complication, and management. Annu Rev Med 39:41, 1988

38. Selzer A: Atrial fibrillation revisited. (Editorial.) N Engl J Med 306:1044, 1982

39. Middlekauf HR, Stevenson WG, Stevenson LW: Prognostic significance of atrial fibrillation in advanced heart failure. A study of 390 patients. Circulation 84:40, 1991

40. Romeo F, Pelliccia F, Cianfrocca C et al: Predictors of sudden death in idiopathic dilated cardiomyopathy. Am J Cardiol 63:138, 1989

41. Hoffmann T, Meinertz T, Kasper W et al: Mode of death in idiopathic dilated cardiomyopathy: a multivariate analysis of prognostic determinants. Am Heart J 116: 1455, 1988

42. Fuster V, Gersh BJ, Giuliani ER et al: The natural history of idiopathic dilated cardiomyopathy. Am J Cardiol 47:525, 1981

43. Unverferth DV, Magorien RD, Moeschberger ML et al: Factors influencing the one-year mortality of dilated cardiomyopathy. Am J Cardiol 54:146, 1984

44. Lengyel M, Kokeny M: Follow-up study in congestive (dilated) cardiomyopathy. Acta Cardiol 36:35, 1981

45. Koide T, Kato A, Takabatake Y et al: Variable prognosis in congestive cardiomyopathy. Role of left ventricular function, alcoholism, and pulmonary thrombosis. Jap Heart J 21:451, 1980

46. Carson P, Fletcher R, Johnson G, Cohn J, and the VEHFT I Study Group: Atrial fibrillation/flutter does not decrease survival in congestive heart failure, abstracted. J Am Coll Cardiol 17:90A, 1991

47. Diaz RA, Obasohan A, Oakley CM: Prediction of outcome in dilated cardiomyopathy. Br Heart J 58:393, 1987

48. Kelly TL, Cremo R, Nielsen C, Shabetai R: Prediction of outcome in late-stage cardiomyopathy. Am Heart J 119:1111, 1990

49. Convert G, Delaye J, Beaune J et al: Prognosis of primary non-obstructive cardiomyopathies. [In French.] Arch Mal Coeur Vaisseaux 73:227, 1980

50. Olshausen KV, Stienen U, Schwarz F et al: Long-term prognostic significance of ventricular arrhythmias in idiopathic dilated cardiomyopathy. Am J Cardiol 61: 146, 1988

51. Baker PS, Bohning AL, Wilson FN: Auricular fibrillation in Grave's disease. Am Heart J 8:121, 1982

52. Hoffman I: The electrocardiogram in thyrotoxicosis. Am J Cardiol 6:893, 1980

53. Bromcart M, Hennen G: Atrial fibrillation and thyroid disease. p. 220. In Kulbertus HE, Olsson B, Schlepper M (eds): Atrial Fibrillation. AB Hassel, Molndal, Sweden, 1982

54. Short DS: The syndrome of alternating bradycardia and tachycardia. Br Heart J 16:209, 1951

55. Lown B: Electrical reversion of cardiac arrhythmias. Br Heart J 29:469, 1967

56. Sutton R, Kenny RA: The natural history of sick sinus syndrome. PACE 9:1110, 1986

57. Hauser RG, Jones J, Edward LM, Messor JV: Prognosis of patients paced for AV block or sino-atrial disease in the absence of ventricular tachycardia. PACE 6A:123, 1983

58. Ettinger PO, Wu CF, De La Cruz C, Jr et al: Arrhythmias and the "Holiday Heart": alcohol-associated cardiac rhythm disorders. Am Heart J 95:555, 1978

59. Lowenstein SR, Gabow PA, Cramer J et al: The role of

alcohol in new-onset atrial fibrillation. Arch Intern Med 143:1882, 1983

60. Rich EC, Siebold C, Campion B: Alcohol-related acute atrial fibrillation. A case-control study and review of 40 patients. Arch Intern Med 145:830, 1985

61. Glancy DL, O'Brien KP, Gold HK, Epstein SE: Atrial fibrillation in patients with idiopathic hypertrophic subaortic stenosis. Br Heart J 32:652, 1907

62. Campbell RW, Smith RA, Gallagher JJ et al: Atrial fibrillation in the preexcitation syndrome. Am J Cardiol 40:514, 1977

63. Wellens HJ, Durrer D: Wolff-Parkinson-White syndrome and atrial fibrillation. Relation between refractory period of accessory pathway and ventricular rate during atrial fibrillation. Am J Cardiol 34:777, 1974

64. Klein GJ, Bashore TM, Sellers TD et al: Ventricular fibrillation in the Wolff-Parkinson-White syndrome. N Engl J Med 301:1080, 1979

65. Neufeld HN, Wagenvoort CA, Burchell HB, Edwardo JR: Idiopathic atrial fibrillation. Am J Cardiol 8:193, 1961

66. Levine SA: Benign atrial fibrillation of 40 years duration with sudden death from emotion. Ann Intern Med 58:681, 1983

67. Lamb LE, Pollard CW: Atrial fibrillation in flying personnel. Circulation 29:694, 1964

68. Petersen P, Godtfredsen J: Embolic complications in paroxysmal atrial fibrillation. Stroke 17:622, 1986

69. Sanfilippo AJ, Abascal VM, Sheehan M et al: Atrial enlargement as a consequence of atrial fibrillation. A prospective echocardiographic study. Circulation 82:792, 1990

70. Hinton RC, Kistler JP, Fallon JT et al: Influence of etiology of atrial fibrillation on incidence of systemic embolism. Am J of Cardiol 40:509, 1977

71. Daly R, Mattingly TW, Holt CL et al: Systemic arterial embolism in rheumatic heart disease. Am Heart J 42:566, 1951

72. Ellis LB, Harken DE: Arterial embolization in relation to mitral valvuloplasty. Am Heart J 62:611, 1961

73. Abernathy WS, Willis PW: Thromboembolic complications of rheumatic heart disease. Cardiovasc Clin 5:131, 1973

74. Stratton JR: Common causes of cardiac emboli—left ventricular thrombi and atrial fibrillation. West J Med 151:172, 1989

75. Stroke Prevention in Atrial Fibrillation Study Group Investigators: Special Report: Preliminary Report of Stroke Prevention in Atrial Fibrillation Study. N Engl J Med 332:863, 1990

76. Coulshed N, Epstein EJ, McKendrick CS et al: Systemic embolism in mitral valve disease. Br Heart J 32:26, 1970

77. Wolf PA, Dawber TR, Thomas HE, Jr, Kannel WB: Epidemiologic assessment of chronic atrial fibrillation and risk of stroke: the Framingham Study. Neurology 28:973, 1978

78. Casella L, Abelmann WH, Ellis LB: Patients with mitral stenosis and systemic emboli: hemodynamic and clinical observations. Arch Intern Med 114:773, 1964

79. Harris AW, Levine SA: Cerebral embolism in mitral stenosis. Ann Intern Med 15:637, 1941

80. Rowe JC, Bland EF, Sprague HB, White PD: The course of mitral stenosis without surgery: ten-twenty year perspectives. Ann Intern Med 52:741, 1960

81. Szekely P: Systemic embolism and anticoagulant prophylasix in rheumatic heart disease. Br Med J 1:1209, 1964

82. Fleming HA, Bailey SM: Mitral valve disease, systemic embolism and anticoagulants. Postgrad Med J 47:599, 1971

83. Wood P: An appreciation of mitral stenosis. Part I. Clinical features. Br Med J 1:1051, 1953

84. Aberg H: Atrial fibrillation. I. A study of atrial thrombosis and systemic embolism in a necropsy material. Acta Med Scand 185:373, 1969

85. Parker BN, Friedenberg MJ, Templeton AW, Burford TH: Preoperative angiocardiographic diagnosis of left atrial thrombi in mitral stenosis. N Engl J Med 273:136, 1965

86. Bar-Sela S, Ehrenfeld M, Eliakim M: Arterial embolism in thyrotoxicosis with atrial fibrillation. Arch Intern Med 141:1191, 1981

87. Hurst JW, Paulk EA, Jr, Proctor HD, Schlant RC: Management of patients with atrial fibrillation. Am J Med 37:728, 1964

88. Fairfax AJ, Lambert CD, Leatham A: Systemic embolism in chronic sinoatrial disorder. N Engl J Med 295:190, 1976

89. Wolf PA, Kannel WB, McGee DL et al: Duration of atrial fibrillation and imminence of strokes: the Framingham Study. Stroke 14:664, 1983

90. Pocock SJ, Shaper AG, Cook DG et al: British Regional Heart Study: geographic variations in cardiovascular mortality, and the role of water quality. Br Med J 280:1243, 1980

91. Shaper AG, Pocock SJ, Walker M et al: British Regional Heart Study: cardiovascular risk factors in middle-aged men in 24 towns. Br Med J 283:179, 1981

92. Sage JI, Van Uitert RL: Risk of recurrent stroke in patients with atrial fibrillation and non-valvular heart disease. Stroke 14:537, 1983

93. McDevitt E, Carter SA, Gatze BW et al: Use of anticoagulants in treatment of cerebral vascular disease. JAMA 166:592, 1958

94. Cosgriff SW: Chronic anticoagulant therapy in recurrent embolism of cardiac origin. Ann Intern Med 38:278, 1953

95. Foley WT, Wright IS: The use of anticoagulants. An evaluation. Med Clin North Am 40:1339, 1956

96. Askey JM: Systemic Arterial Embolism. Modern Medical Monograph No. 14. Grune & Stratton, Orlando, Fl, 1957

97. Owren PA: The results of anticoagulant therapy in Norway. Arch Intern Med 111:240, 1963

98. Griffith GC, Stragnell R, Levinson DC et al: A study of the beneficial effects of anticoagulant therapy in congestive heart failure. Ann Intern Med 37:867, 1952

99. Carter AV: Prognosis of cerebral embolism. Lancet 2:514, 1965

100. The Copenhagen AFASAK Study: Placebo-controlled, randomized trial of warfarin and aspirin for prevention of thromboembolic complications in chronic atrial fibrillation. Lancet 1:175, 1989

101. Stroke Prevention Atrial Fibrillation Investigators: Stroke Prevention in atrial fibrillation study. Final results. Circulation 84:527, 1991
102. The Boston Area Anticoagulation Trial for Atrial Fibrillation Investigators: The effects of low-dose warfarin on the risk of stroke in patients with non-rheumatic atrial fibrillation. N Engl J Med 323:1503, 1990
103. Connolly SJ, Laupacis A, Gent A et al: Canadian atrial fibrillation anticoagulation (CAFA) study. J Am Coll Cardiol 18:349, 1991
104. Mendez C, Aceves J, Mendez R: Inhibition of adrenergic cardiac acceleration by cardiac glycosides. J Pharmacol Exp Ther 31:191, 1961
105. James TN, Nadeau PA: The chronotropic effect of digitalis studied by direct perfusion of sinus node. J Pharmacol Exp Ther 139:42, 1963
106. Falk RH, Knowlton AA, Bernard SA et al: Digoxin for converting recent-onset atrial fibrillation to sinus rhythm. A randomized, double-blinded trial. Ann Intern Med 106:503, 1987
107. Rawles JM: What is meant by a "controlled" ventricular rate in atrial fibrillation? Br Heart J 63:157, 1990
108. Lewis RV, Irvine N, McDevitt DG: Relationships between heart rate, exercise tolerance and cardiac output in atrial fibrillation: the effects of treatment with digoxin, verapamil and diltiazem. Eur Heart J 9:777, 1988
109. Beasley R, Smith DA, McHaffie DJ: Exercise heart rates at different serum digoxin concentrations in patients with atrial fibrillation. Br Med J 290:9, 1985
110. Storstein L: Role of digitalis in ventricular rate control in atrial fibrillation. p. 285. In Kulbertus HE, Olsson SB, Schlepper M (eds): Atrial Fibrillation. AB Hassle, Molndal, Sweden, 1982
111. George A, Spear JR, Moore EN: The effects of digitalis glycosides on the ventricular fibrillation threshold in innervated and denervated canine hearts. Circulation 50:353, 1974
112. Bolognesi R: The pharmacologic treatment of atrial fibrillation. Cardiac Drugs Ther 5:617, 1991
113. Coumel P, Leelerg JF, Attvel P: Paroxysmal atrial fibrillation. p. 158. In Kulbertus HE, Olsson SB, Schlepper M (eds): Atrial Fibrillation. AB Hassle, Molndal, Sweden, 1982
114. Tucker AR, Ng KT: Digoxin-related impairment of learning and memory in cardiac patients. J Psychopharmacol 81:86, 1983
115. Falk RH, Leavitt JI: Digoxin for atrial fibrillation: a drug whose time has gone? Ann Intern Med 114:573, 1991
116. Klein HO, Kaplinsky E: Digitalis and verapamil in atrial fibrillation and flutter. Is verapamil now the preferred agent? Drugs 313:185, 1986
117. Lang R, Klein HO, Weiss E et al: Superiority of oral verapamil therapy to digoxin in treatment of chronic atrial fibrillation. Chest 83:491, 1983
118. Ochs HR, Anda L, Eichelbaum M, Greenblatt DJ: Diltiazem, verapamil and quinidine in patients with chronic atrial fibrillation. J Clin Pharmacol 25:204, 1985
119. Lang R, Klein HO, DiSegni E et al: Verapamil improves exercise capacity in chronic atrial fibrillation: double-blind crossover study. Am Heart J 105:820, 1983
120. Pomfret SM, Beasley CR, Challenor V, Holgate ST: Relative efficacy of oral verapamil and digoxin alone and in combination for the treatment of patients with chronic atrial fibrillation. Clin Sci 74:351, 1988
121. Drug Information: American Hospital Formulary Service, 1991
122. Coumel P, Leclercq JR, Escoubet B: Beta-blockers: use for arrhythmias, suppl A. Eur Heart J 8:41, 1987
123. Harrison DC, Griffin JR, Fiene TJ: Effects of beta adrenergic blockade with propranolol in patients with atrial fibrillation. N Engl J Med 273:410, 1965
124. Atwood JE, Sullivan M, Forbes S et al: Effect of beta-adrenergic blockade on exercise performance in patients with chronic atrial fibrillation. J Am Coll Cardiol 10:314, 1987
125. David D, Segni ED, Klein HO, Kaplinsky E: Inefficacy of digitalis in the control of heart rate in patients with chronic atrial fibrillation: beneficial effect of an added beta adrenergic blocking agent. Am J Cardiol 44:1378, 1979
126. Lewis RV, McDevitt DG: Adverse reactions and interactions with beta-adrenoceptor blocking drugs. Med Toxicol 1:343, 1986
127. Andrews RC, Reinold SC, Berlin KA, Antman EM: Prevention of supraventricular arrhythmias after coronary artery bypass surgery: a meta-analysis of randomized control trials, suppl III. Circulation 84:236, 1991
128. Lown B, Amarasingham R, Neuman J: New method for terminating cardiac arrhythmias. Use of synchronized capacitor discharge. JAMA 182:548, 1962
129. DeSilva RA, Graboys TB, Podrid PJ, Lown B: Cardioversion and defibrillation. Am Heart J 100:881, 1980
130. Byrne-Quinn E, Wing AJ: Maintenance of sinus rhythm after DC reversion of atrial fibrillation. A double-blind controlled trial of long-acting quinidine bisulphate. Br Heart J 32:370, 1970
131. Morris JJ, Jr, Peter RN, McIntosh HD: Electrical conversion of atrial fibrillation: immediate and long-term results and selection of patients. Ann Intern Med 65:216, 1966
132. Rabbino MD, Likoff W, Dreifus LS: Complications and limitations of direct-current countershock. JAMA 190:417, 1964
133. Ross EM: Cardioversion causing ventricular fibrillation. Arch Intern Med 114:811, 1964
134. Aberg H, Cullhed I: Direct current conversion of atrial fibrillation—long-term results. Acta Med Scand 184:433, 1968
135. McCarthy C, Varghese RJ, Barritt DW: Prognosis of atrial arrhythmias treated by electrical counter shock therapy. A three-year follow-up. Br Heart J 31:496, 1969
136. Bjerkelund CJ, Orning OM: The efficacy of anticoagulant therapy in preventing embolism related to D.C. electrical conversion of atrial fibrillation. Am J Cardiol 23:208, 1969
137. Dethy M, Chassat C, Roy D, Mercier LA: Doppler echocardiographic predictors of recurrence of atrial fibrillation after cardioversion. Am J Cardiol 62:723, 1988
138. Weiner P, Bassan MM, Jarchovsky J et al: Clinical course of acute atrial fibrillation treated with rapid digitalization. Am Heart J 105:223, 1983

139. Botti G, Visloli, Bianchi C: Farmacologia clinica dei farmacia antiarritmisi e terapia medica delle arritmia. p. 226. In Atti del 26 Congresso della Societa Italiana di Cardiologica. Vol. II. Cagliari 1985. Roma Il Pensicro Scientifico, 1965

140. Katz AM (ed): Disorders of Cardiac Rhythm. Focus on Disopyranide. ADIS Press, Auckland, 1983, p. 143

141. Halpern SW, Ellrodt G, Singh RN, Mandel WJ: Efficacy of intravenous procainamide infusion in converting atrial fibrillation to sinus rhythm. Relation to left atrial size. Br Heart J 44:489, 1980

142. Milazzotto F, DiMarco Tullio G, Uguccion M: I calcioantagonisti nel trattamento del flutter e della fibrillazione atriale. p. 74. In Fazzini PF, Abbate C, Colo A (eds): Il punto Su: I calcioantagonisti in cardiologia. O.I.C. Medical Press, Florence, 1986

143. Bolognesi R, Tsialtas D, Vasini P et al: Effetti del verapamil e della combinazione verapamil-chinidina nel trattamento delle fibrillazioni atriali. In 48° Congresso Nazionale SIC, Roma 1987, suppl 12. Cardiologia 32: 111, 1987

144. Singh BN, Mandel WJ: Antiarrhythmic drugs: basic concepts and their actions, pharmacokinetic characteristics and clinical applications. p. 550. In Medical WJ (ed): Cardiac Arrhythmias. JB Lipincott, Philadelphia, 1980

145. Steinbeck G, Doliwa R, Bach P: Cardiac glycosides for paroxysmal atrial fibrillation? p. 471. In Erdmann E, Greeff K, Skon JC (eds): Cardiac Glycosides 1785–1985. Springer-Verlag, New York–Verlag Darmstadt, Steinkopff, 1986

146. Betriu A, Chaitman BR, Bourassa MG et al: Beneficial effect of intravenous diltiazem in the acute management of paroxysmal supraventricular tachyarrhythmias. Circulation 67:88, 1983

147. Carlier J: Disopyramide in the treatment of supraventricular arrhythmias. p. 121. In Katz AM (ed): Disorders of Cardiac Rhythm. Focus on Disopyramide. ADIS Press, Auckland, 1986

148. Harris L, Michat L: Clinical efficacy. Arrhythmias. p. 137. In Harris L, Roncucci R (eds): Amiodarone. MEDSI Paris, 1986

149. Bolognesi R, Tsialtas O, Manca C, Visioli O: Effetti della flecainide nel trattamento delle fibrillazioni atriali parossistiche o di recente origine. Cardiologica 34: 173, 1989

150. Anderson JL, Jolivette DM, Fredell PA: Summary of efficacy and safety of flecainide for supraventricular arrhythmias. Am J Cardiol 62:62D, 1988

151. Coumel P, Leclercq JF, Assayag P: European experience with the antiarrhythmic efficacy of propafenone for supraventricular and ventricular arrhythmias. Am J Cardiol 54:60D, 1984

152. Bender F: Modern therapy of cardiac arrhythmias (Ger) Schweiz Med Wochenschr 103:272, 1973

153. Klienebenne A, Mannebach H, Gleichmann U: Chinidin und verapamil kombinations therapie zur behandlung von vorhofrhythmusstorungen. Fortschr Med 99:1569, 1981

154. Cramer G: Early and late results of conversion of atrial fibrillation with quinidine, suppl 1. Acta Med Scand 4: 490, 1986

155. Anderson JL, Gilbert EM, Alpert BL et al, and the Flecainide Supraventricular Tachycardia Study Group: Prevention of symptomatic recurrences of paroxysmal atrial fibrillation in patients initially tolerating antiarrhythmic therapy. Circulation 80:1557, 1989

156. Beck OA, Gunther R, Hochrein H: Konversionbehandlung von chronischem vorhofflimmern und-flattern mit disopyramid und einer verapamil-chinidin-kombination. Dtsch Med Wochenschr 107:1419, 1982

157. Levi GF, Proto C: Combined treatment of atrial fibrillation with quinidine and beta-blockers. Br Heart J 34: 911, 1972

158. Bolognesi R, Licogna R, Monca C et al: Associazione verapamil-chinidina nel trattamento della fibrillazioni atriali. 46° Congresso Nazionale SIC, Roma 1985, suppl II. Cardiologia 30:28, 1985

159. Ochs HR, Anda L, Eichelbaum M, Greenblatt DJ: Diltiazem, verapamil, and quinidine in patients with chronic atrial fibrillation. J Clin Pharmacol 25:204, 1985

160. Belz GG, Olesch K, Schmidt-Voigt J: Die behandlung des chronischer vorhoffimmerns mit einer kombination von chinidin und verapamil. Med Welt 21:1670, 1970

161. Grogan EW, Waxman FL: Management of supraventricular arrhythmias. p. 261. In Dreifus L (ed): Cardiac Arrhythmias: Electrophysiologic Techniques and Management. FA Davis, Philadelphia, 1985

162. Faniel R, Schoenfeld P: Efficacy of i.v. amiodarone in converting rapid atrial fibrillation and flutter to sinus rhythm in intensive care patients. Eur Heart J 4:180, 1989

163. Straberg B, Arditti A, Sclarovsky S et al: Efficacy of intravenous amiodarone in the management of paroxysmal or new atrial fibrillation with fast ventricular response. Int J Cardiol 7:47, 1985

164. Haines DE, DiMarco JP: Use of new and investigational drugs in treating cardiac arrhythmias. p. 87. In Yu PN, Goodwin JF (eds): Progress in Cardiology. Lea & Febiger, Philadelphia, 1987

165. CAST Investigators—Preliminary Report: Effect of encainide and flecainide on mortality in a randomized trial of arrhythmia suppression after myocardial infarction. N Engl J Med 321:406, 1989

166. Waris E, Kreus KE, Salokannel J: Factors influencing persistence of sinus rhythm after DC shock treatment of atrial fibrillation. Acta Med Scand 189:161, 1971

167. Oram S, Davies JP: Further experience of electrical conversion of atrial fibrillation to sinus rhythm: analysis of 100 patients. Lancet 1:1294, 1964

168. Ewy GA, Ulfers L, Hager WD et al: Response of atrial fibrillation to therapy: role of etiology and left atrial diameter. J Electrocardiol 13:119, 1980

169. Szekely P, Sideris DA, Batson GA: Maintenance of sinus rhythm after atrial defibrillation. Br Heart J 32:741, 1970

170. Brodsky MA, Allen BJ, Capparelli EV et al: Factors determining maintenance of sinus rhythm after chronic atrial fibrillation with left atrial dilatation. Am J Cardiol 63:1065, 1989

171. Cramer G: Early and late results of conversion of atrial fibrillation with quinidine. A clinical and hemodynamic study. Acta Med Scand 490:5, 1968

172. Normand PJ, Legendre M, Kahn JC et al: Comparative efficacy of short-acting and long-acting quinidine for maintenance of sinus rhythm after electrical conversion of atrial fibrillation. Br Heart J 38:381, 1976

173. Hall JI, Wood DR: Factors affecting cardioversion of atrial arrhythmias with special reference to quinidine. Br Heart J 30:84, 1968

174. Stern S: Treatment and prevention of cardiac arrhythmias with propranolol and quinidine. Br Heart J 33: 522, 1971

175. Sodermark T, Jonsson B, Olsson A et al: Effect of quinidine on maintaining sinus rhythm after conversion of atrial fibrillation or flutter. A multicentre study from Stockholm. Br Heart J 37:486, 1975

176. Hillestad L, Bjerkelund C, Dale J et al: Quinidine in maintenance of sinus rhythm after electroconversion of chronic atrial fibrillation. A controlled clinical study. Br Heart J 33:518, 1971

177. Gunning JF, Kristinsson A, Miller G, Saunders K: Long-term follow-up of direct current cardioversion after cardiac surgery with special reference to quinidine. Br Heart J 32:462, 1907

178. Coplen SE, Antman EM, Berlin JA et al: Efficacy and safety of quinidine therapy for maintenance of sinus rhythm after cardioversion. A meta-analysis of randomized control trials. [Published erratum appears in Circulation 83:714, 1991] Circulation 82:1106, 1990

179. Radford MD, Evans DW: Long-term results of DC reversion of atrial fibrillation. Br Heart J 30:91, 1968

180. Middlekauf HR, Stevenson WG, Stevenson LW, Saxon LA: Antiarrhythmic drug therapy in 367 heart failure patients: class I drugs but not amiodarone are associated with increased sudden death risk, abstracted. J Am Coll Cardiol 17:92A, 1991

181. Morganroth J, Goin JE: Quinidine-related mortality in the short-to-medium-term treatment of ventricular arrhythmias. A meta-analysis. Circulation 84:1977, 1991

182. Juul-Moller S, Edvardsson N, Rehnquist-Ahlberg N: Sotalol versus quinidine for the maintenance of sinus rhythm, after direct current conversion of atrial fibrillation. Circulation 82:1932, 1990

183. Hartel G, Louhija A, Kolittinen A: Disopyramide in the prevention of recurrence of atrial fibrillation after electrocardioversion. Clin Pharmacol Ther 15:551, 1974

184. Lloyd EA, Gersh BJ, Forman R: The efficacy of quinidine and disopyramide in the maintenance of sinus rhythm after electroconversion from atrial fibrillation. A double-blind study comparing quinidine, disopyramide and placebo. S Afr Med J 65:367, 1984

185. Furlanello F, Vergara G, Bettini R et al: Flecainide and encainide, suppl A. Eur Heart J 98:33, 1987

186. Chouty F, Coumel P: Oral flecainide for prophylaxis of paroxysmal atrial fibrillation. Am J Cardiol 62:350, 1988

187. Epstein M, Jardine RM, Obel IW: Flecainide acetate in the treatment of resistant supraventricular arrhythmias. S Afr Med J 74:559, 1988

188. Sihm I, Hansen FA, Rasmussen J, Pedersen AK, Thygesen K: Flecainide acetate in atrial flutter and fibrillation. The arrhythmogenic effects. Eur Heart J 11: 145, 1990

189. Anderson JL, Gilbert EM, Alpert BL et al: Prevention of symptomatic recurrences of paroxysmal atrial fibrillation in patients initially tolerating antiarrhythmic therapy. A multicenter, double-blind, crossover study of flecainide and placebo with transtelephonic monitoring. Flecainide Supraventricular Tachycardia Study Group. Circulation 80:1557, 1989

190. Falk RH: Flecainide-induced ventricular tachycardia and fibrillation in patients treatment for atrial fibrillation. Ann Intern Med 111:107, 1989

191. Feld G, Chen PS, Nicod P, Fleck RP, Meyer D: Possible atrial proarrhythmic effects of class 1C antiarrhythmic drugs. Am J Cardiol 66:378, 1990

192. Neuss H: Long term use of flecainide in patients with supraventricular tachycardia. Drugs 29:21, 1985

193. Berns E, Rinkenberger PL, Jeang MK et al: Efficacy and safety of flecainide acetate for atrial tachycardia or fibrillation. Am J Cardiol 59:1337, 1987

194. Morganroth J: Risk factors for the development of proarrhythmic events. Am J Cardiol 59:32E, 1987

195. Antman EM, Beamer AD, Cantillon C et al: Therapy of refractory symptomatic atrial fibrillation and atrial flutter: a staged care approach with new antiarrhythmic drugs. J Am Coll Cardiol 15:698, 1990

196. Singh BN, Nadamanee K: Sotalol: a beta blocker with unique antiarrhythmic properties. Am Heart J 114:121, 1987

197. Charlier R, Deltour G, Baudine A, Chaillet F: Pharmacology of amiodarone, and anti-anginal drug with a new biological profile. Arzneimittelforschung 18:1408, 1968

198. Heger JJ, Prystowsky EN, Zipes DP: Clinical efficacy of amiodarone in treatment of recurrent ventricular tachycardia and ventricular fibrillation. Am Heart J 106:887, 1983

199. Haffajee CI, Love JC, Canada AT et al: Clinical pharmacokinetics and efficacy of amiodarone for refractory tachyarrhythmias. Circulation 67:1347, 1983

200. Rosenbaum MB, Chiale PA, Halpern MS et al: Clinical efficacy of amiodarone as an antiarrhythmic agent. Am J Cardiol 38:934, 1976

201. Fogoros RN, Anderson KP, Winkle RA et al: Amiodarone: clinical efficacy and toxicity in 96 patients with recurrent, drug-refractory arrhythmias. Circulation 68: 88, 1983

202. Harris L, Michat L: Clinical efficacy. Arrhythmias. p. 137. In Harris R, Rongucci R (eds): Amiodarone. MEDSI, 1987

203. Brodsky MA, Allen NJ, Walker CJ et al: Amiodarone for maintenance of sinus rhythm after conversion of atrial fibrillation in the setting of a dilated left atrium. Am J Cardiol 60:572, 1987

204. Gold RL, Haffajee CI, Charos G et al: Amiodarone for refractory atrial fibrillation. Am J Cardiol 57:124, 1986

205. Rowland E, McKenna WJ, Harris L et al: Amiodarone in the prophylaxis of atrial fibrillation. p. 262. In Atrial Fibrillation. Kulbertus HE, Olsson SB, Schlepper M (eds): Kiruna, Sweden, 1981

206. Vitolo E, Tronci M, Larovere MT et al: Amiodarone versus quinidine in the prophylaxis of atrial fibrillation. Acta Cardiol 36:431, 1981

207. Graboys TB, Podrid PJ, Lown B: Efficacy of amiodarone

for refractory supraventricular tachyarrhythmia. Am Heart J 106:870, 1983

208. Mason JW: Drug therapy: amiodarone. N Engl J Med 316:455, 1987

209. Olsson SB, Brorson L, Varnauskas E: Class III antiarrhythmic action in man. Observations from monophasic action potential recordings in man and amiodarone treatment in man. Br Heart J 35:1255, 1973

210. Feld GB, Venkatesh N, Singh BN: Pharmacologic conversion of atrial flutter. Circulation 74:147, 1985

211. Singh BN, Sarma JSM, Zhang Zi-hao, Takanaka C: Controlling cardiac arrhythmias by lengthening repolarization: rationale from experimental findings and clinical considerations. Ann NY Acad Sc 644:187, 1992

27

Risk Assessment and Prognosis of Patients With Supraventricular Tachyarrhythmias

Michael de Buitleir
Fred Morady

The most common form of paroxysmal supraventricular tachycardia (PSVT) is atrioventricular (AV) node reentry, which accounts for about 50% of all cases of PSVT. A further 30% of cases is due to AV reentry, sometimes referred to as orthodromic reciprocating tachycardia. In AV reentry, the tachycardia circuit involves both the AV node and an accessory AV bypass tract. The presence of an accessory AV connection may be inferred from the 12-lead electrocardiogram (ECG) in sinus rhythm in which case the typical Wolff-Parkinson-White (WPW) pattern may be seen. In many cases, however, the accessory pathway conducts only in the retrograde direction, thus, no delta wave is apparent in sinus rhythm. Less common forms of PSVT are those due to intra-atrial reentry, sinus node reentry, automatic atrial foci and reentry involving Mahaim fibers.

INCIDENCE

The exact incidence of AV node reentry tachycardia in the general population is unknown, partly because mildly symptomatic patients may not present for med-

ical attention, and, if they do, they are infrequently referred for further evaluation. It is seen in patients of all ages and typically, although not exclusively, in the absence of structural heart disease. By contrast, the incidence of the WPW syndrome is 0.1 to 3 per 1,000 ECGs[1,2] and 12 to 80% of these patients will have symptoms at one time or another.[3] Among patients who present with PSVT under the age of 21 years, the incidence of the WPW syndrome is higher than among patients who present with PSVT for the first time when they are over 21 years of age.[3] WPW syndrome may occur in association with structural heart disease, for example, Ebstein's anomaly, which is associated with right-sided accessory pathways. Mitral valve prolapse may be accompanied by left-sided accessory pathways; hypertrophic cardiomyopathy is also associated with the WPW syndrome.

In contrast to AV node and AV reentry tachycardia, intra-atrial reentry tachycardia is more often than not accompanied by structural heart disease, typically of the kind that results in atrial enlargement. These patients will often have a history of atrial fibrillation or flutter in addition to their atrial tachycardia.[4]

ETIOLOGY

Reentry is the mechanism underlying the majority of supraventricular tachycardias. Thus, in the case of AV node reentry (Fig. 27-1), the AV node is believed to consist of tissues with disparate properties of conduction and refractoriness. For reentry to occur, these tissues or pathways must communicate proximally and distally, and unidirectional block must occur in one limb. The reentrant tachycardia is often initiated by a premature atrial impulse that blocks in one pathway, conducts antegradely in the other so-called "slow" pathway, and reenters the initially blocked "fast" pathway in the retrograde direction. If the conduction and refractoriness properties of the two pathways are compatible, the returning retrograde wavefront of activation may reenter the antegrade pathway, initiating the reentrant circuit and tachycardia. In the case of orthodromic reciprocating tachycardia, the two limbs of the tachycardia circuit are the AV node (antegrade limb) and the accessory pathway (retrograde limb) (Fig. 27-2).

It is believed that the substrate for reentrant PSVT, at least in the case of WPW syndrome and probably in the case of AV node reentry, occurs as a congenital anomaly. Whether PSVT occurs subsequently depends on other factors, such as autonomic influences and the presence of atrial and ventricular premature beats as potential triggers. Other types of PSVT, such as intra-atrial reentry or automatic atrial tachycardia, are acquired disorders associated with underlying structural heart disease.

NATURAL HISTORY

The natural history of PSVT depends on the rate and mechanism of the tachycardia and the type of any underlying heart disease.

AV Node Reentry Tachycardia

In the case of AV node reentry tachycardia, at one end of the spectrum, patients with slow and infrequent bouts of PSVT are unlikely to present for medical attention and will have a normal life expectancy. Other patients with more frequent and rapid bouts of tachycardia will present early for diagnosis and definitive treatment. In general, however, these patients will also have a normal life expectancy and excellent prognosis.

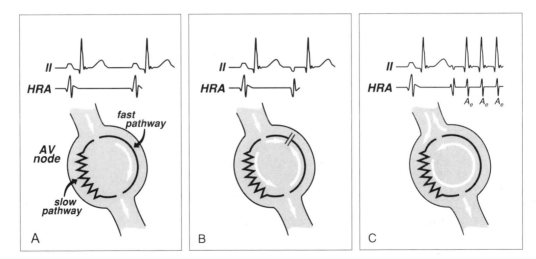

Fig. 27-1. Schematic representation of dual AV nodal pathways and the initiation of AV node reentry tachycardia. (**A**) Conduction through the AV node during sinus rhythm (*white arrow*) over the fast AV nodal pathway. (**B**) Atrial premature beat blocking the fast pathway because of its longer refractory period, but conducting to the ventricle over the slow pathway. The activation wavefront can reenter the fast pathway in the retrograde direction but will block if the fast pathway has not had adequate time to recover excitability. (**C**) Yet an earlier atrial premature beat. In this case, the initial sequence is the same as that seen in Fig. B, but now both the retrograde fast and antegrade slow pathways have had sufficient time to recover excitability so that the reentrant circuit is established and AV node reentry tachycardia begins. Note the occurrence of atrial echo beats as each returning wavefront activates the atrium. Included are electrocardiographic lead II and an intra-cardiac recording from the high right atrium (HRA).

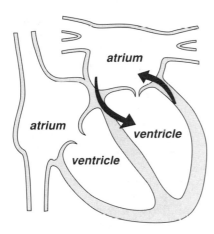

Fig. 27-2. Schematic representation of the reentrant circuit in orthodromic reciprocating tachycardia (AV reentry tachycardia). The antegrade limb is the AV node and the retrograde limb in this case is a left lateral accessory pathway. The accessory pathway can be located at any site around the AV ring.

WPW Syndrome

The natural history of the WPW syndrome depends almost exclusively on the accessory pathway or pathways: the number, the location and the electrophysiologic properties of conduction and refractoriness. In its most severe form, the initial presentation of the WPW syndrome may be ventricular fibrillation and sudden death.[5] Ventricular fibrillation occurs during atrial fibrillation with rapid conduction over the accessory pathway. Klein et al.[6] compared the clinical and electrophysiologic features of two groups of patients with the WPW syndrome; one group presented with ventricular fibrillation, and the other group presented with arrhythmias other than ventricular fibrillation. These investigators[6] found that patients who presented with ventricular fibrillation had a higher prevalence of both reciprocating tachycardia and atrial fibrillation and multiple accessory pathways. In addition, the mean and shortest pre-excited R-R interval during atrial fibrillation was less in patients with ventricular fibrillation.

Wellens and Durrer[7] demonstrated a strong correlation between the antegrade effective refractory period of the accessory pathway and the shortest R-R interval and mean ventricular rate during atrial fibrillation. Patients with a short effective refractory period of the accessory pathway (≤250 ms) displayed almost exclusive and rapid conduction over the accessory pathway. By contrast, patients with an accessory pathway antegrade effective refractory period of more than 250 ms displayed a combination of conduction over the accessory pathway and AV node and a slower ventricular rate during atrial fibrillation.

Most patients with WPW syndrome or a concealed accessory pathway present with AV reentry tachycardia. The rate of this tachycardia is usually faster than AV node reentry, and typical symptoms include palpitations, dyspnea, chest pain, lightheadedness, syncope, and presyncope. If the tachycardia is sustained, the patient may present to the emergency department for treatment. Once the acute episode has been treated, an electrophysiologic study is indicated to establish the tachycardia mechanism, localize the accessory pathway(s), and permit definitive catheter ablation therapy. Until recently, the therapeutic options for these patients consisted of either drugs or surgery, with catheter ablation an option for a minority of patients. During the past 2 years, however, the treatment of these patients has been revolutionized with the increasing use of radiofrequency catheter ablation, allowing cure during the diagnostic electrophysiologic test in most patients.[8,9]

What is the natural history of asymptomatic patients with the WPW ECG pattern? Klein et al.[10] performed electrophysiologic studies on two occasions at least 36 months apart, in 29 such patients. Twenty-seven patients remained asymptomatic, and sustained supraventricular tachycardia developed in two patients (7%) during the follow-up period. Nine patients (31%) lost the capacity for pre-excitation and antegrade conduction over the accessory pathway. The other patients had little change in the conduction rate over the accessory pathway. Patients who lost accessory pathway conduction tended to be older and to have a longer baseline antegrade refractory period than that of patients who retained pre-excitation (414 ± 158 versus 295 ± 27 ms). Klein et al.[10] concluded that a considerable number of asymptomatic patients with the WPW pattern lose the capacity for antegrade conduction over the accessory pathway. Furthermore, these investigators postulated that this loss of capacity probably contributes to the low mortality among asymptomatic patients.

In a follow-up essay,[11] Klein's group stated that mass screening and aggressive investigation of asymptomatic WPW patients are not justified by epidemiologic data. However, for such patients who request risk stratification, Klein et al.[11] suggested some guidelines and approaches to management based on the shortest R-R interval during induced atrial fibrillation.

Intra-atrial Reentry

In contrast to AV node and AV reentry tachycardia, patients with intra-atrial reentry are generally older at presentation. Their prognosis is also much poorer, mainly because of their concomitant structural heart disease. Haines and DiMarco[4] studied 19 patients with intra-atrial reentry tachycardia and found that 90% of the patients had structural heart disease, including valvular, congenital, myopathic, and coronary disease. Despite good control of their arrhythmia, 50% of the patients were dead within approximately 2.5 years of presentation from a variety of causes, including congestive heart failure (CHF), pulmonary embolism, ventricular tachycardia, and noncardiac disease.[4]

EVALUATION OF RISK

Patients with AV node reentry tachycardia are at lower risk of adverse events than are those with WPW syndrome, but certain potential for morbidity and mortality exists. Patients with rapid PSVT may present with syncope, which can result in serious injury. Although most patients present with more benign symptoms, a recent report[12] described a series of 13 patients who presented with aborted sudden death and in whom the etiology was a supraventricular tachyarrhythmia. These 13 patients accounted for 4.5% of a series of 290 patients who presented with aborted sudden death over an 11-year period. Three of the 13 patients (23%) had typical AV node reentry tachycardia that degenerated into ventricular fibrillation. The mean cycle length of the AV node reentry tachycardia was 293 ms (range 270 to 310). Six of the 13 patients (46%) had an accessory AV pathway and either atrial fibrillation (5 patients) or AV reentry tachycardia (1 patient) that progressed to ventricular fibrillation. Four patients (31%) had atrial fibrillation and enhanced AV node conduction that deteriorated to ventricular fibrillation.

Tachycardia-Induced Cardiomyopathy

Incessant PSVT is an unusual presentation that, left untreated for months or years, has the potential to result in a tachycardia-induced cardiomyopathy. This rare event is most often associated with the permanent form of junctional reciprocating tachycardia[13,14] in which the reentry circuit consists of the AV node (antegrade limb) and a slowly conducting or atypical posteroseptal accessory pathway (retrograde limb). Tachycardia-induced cardiomyopathy may resolve once the incessant PSVT is cured.[13,14]

Proarrhythmia

The risk posed to these patients by the proarrhythmic effects of antiarrhythmic drug therapy was of greater concern in the past than it is today. Antiarrhythmic drugs are now used much less frequently in these patients than they were in the past, related in part to the results of the Cardiac Arrhythmia Suppression Trial[15] but also to the increasing availability and acceptance of curative catheter ablation techniques.[16] However, if antiarrhythmic drug therapy is being considered for a patient with PSVT, the small risk of a proarrhythmic response should be borne in mind, although this adverse reaction is relatively rare in patients without structural heart disease.

The adverse effects sometimes seen with the use of intravenous verapamil in patients with PSVT are occasionally catastrophic. Thus, for example, there are case reports[17] of patients presenting with narrow complex AV reentry tachycardia who, when given intravenous verapamil, have converted to atrial fibrillation with rapid conduction over an accessory pathway with associated hypotension and hemodynamic instability. When intravenous verapamil is administered to a patient with atrial fibrillation and rapid conduction over an accessory pathway, the outcome can potentially be fatal.[18] By blocking conduction through the AV node, verapamil in this situation promotes conduction over the accessory pathway, which results in a still more rapid ventricular rate. By virtue of its peripheral vasodilatory properties, verapamil aggravates the already existing hypotension and frequently results in cardiovascular collapse. For these reasons, the use of intravenous verapamil in this situation is strictly contraindicated.[18]

Procedural Risk

An electrophysiologic study (EPS) is an essential step in the evaluation of any patient with recurrent symptomatic PSVT. Horowitz et al.[19] examined the risks and complications of EPS in 1,000 consecutive patients undergoing the procedure. Most of these patients were men (73%); the mean age was 58 years. Coronary artery disease (CAD) was present in 56%, and 20% had no structural heart disease. The indication for EPS was a ventricular tachyarrhythmia or cardiac arrest in 58%. In approximately 10% of patients, the indication for EPS was PSVT or the WPW syndrome. During the course of these 1,000 studies, there was one death (0.1%). Other major complications included arterial injury (0.4%), thrombophlebitis (0.6%), systemic arterial embolism (0.1%), pulmonary embolism (0.3%), and cardiac perforation (0.2%). Significant arrhythmic complications included catheter-induced permanent third-degree AV block in one patient, nonclinical atrial fibrillation requiring therapy in 10 patients, and severe proarrhythmic events in 12 (3%) of 397 patients undergoing electropharmacologic testing for tachyarrhythmias. Horowitz et al.[19] concluded that, although EPS is associated with complications, the risks are small and acceptable.

Although helpful in illustrating the general low-risk

nature of EPS, the indication for EPS in the above study was PSVT only in 10% of the patients. In patients with PSVT, the risks of EPS are even lower than in the above study, given the predominant absence of structural heart disease and LV dysfunction. In fact, Kadish et al.[20] have shown that outpatient EPS can be performed with safety in selected patients, including those with PSVT.

TREATMENT

Drugs

Mention has already been made of the risks associated with the use of intravenous (IV) verapamil in patients with PSVT or in patients with the WPW syndrome and atrial fibrillation. In the former situation the current acute treatment of choice is therefore 6 to 12 mg of adenosine given by rapid IV bolus with continuous cardiac monitoring. In the latter circumstance, IV procainamide is used unless the patient is hemodynamically unstable, in which case synchronized cardioversion is indicated. Chronic antiarrhythmic drug therapy carries a small risk of proarrhythmia in these patients; other disadvantages include inconvenience, recurring expense, and frequent suboptimal control of symptoms. For these reasons, radiofrequency catheter ablation has become the treatment of choice for symptomatic patients with PSVT or the WPW syndrome.

Radiofrequency Ablation

Lee et al.[21] performed radiofrequency modification of the AV node to eliminate rapid pathway conduction in 39 patients with AV-node reentry tachycardia. They reported a success rate of 82% at a mean follow-up of 8 months, but in three patients (8%) complete AV block developed requiring permanent pacemaker placement. In two patients (5%) deep venous thrombosis developed at the site of femoral venipuncture. Jackman et al.[8] performed radiofrequency ablation of accessory pathways in 166 patients, with success in 99%. During a mean follow-up of 8 months, pre-excitation or AV reentry tachycardia recurred in 15 patients (9%), all of whom had a successful second ablation. Complications in three patients (1.8%) included AV block, pericarditis, and cardiac tamponade. No deaths were reported. Calkins et al.[9] reported a success rate in excess of 90%, using radiofrequency ablation in 106 patients with PSVT. Most patients in this study had the WPW syndrome or AV node reentry tachycardia.[9] The only complications were one instance of left circum-

flex (Cx) coronary artery occlusion, resulting in acute myocardial infarction (AMI) and one instance of complete AV block.[9]

With increasing experience, the few complications noted in the above series now appear to be even less frequent. To minimize the risk of heart block in patients with AV-node reentry tachycardia, an alternate approach is to attempt slow pathway modification in which radiofrequency lesions are delivered away from the region of the His bundle and closer to the os of the coronary sinus. Complete heart block seems to be very rare with this latter method, and slow pathway modification is now the initial approach of choice in patients with AV node reentry tachycardia.[21a,21b]

Bolling et al.[22] recently reviewed their experience with surgical treatment of the WPW syndrome and compared it with their more recent experience with radiofrequency catheter ablation. These authors investigators[22] found that surgical and radiofrequency ablation offer an excellent success rate with low morbidity; furthermore, they concluded that, in the future, surgery in the WPW syndrome will probably be indicated only in cases of radiofrequency ablation failure, multiple accessory pathways or when additional cardiac surgical procedures are required.

AV Junction Ablation

In the case of intra-atrial reentry tachycardia, type 1 antiarrhythmic drugs are infrequently effective in controlling symptoms.[4] In patients who are intolerant or unresponsive to antiarrhythmic drugs, catheter ablation of the AV junction, followed by permanent pacemaker placement can provide excellent symptom relief.[23]

Until recently, direct current (DC) shock ablation was the method of choice to achieve therapeutic complete heart block. However, a recent study[24] described the outcome of this procedure in 136 patients and reported a success rate of approximately 85%. However, 8 patients died during hospitalization for ablation, and in 7 (5%) it was deemed that the ablation may have contributed to their deaths. Causes of death included ventricular fibrillation in 5 patients, progressive heart failure in 1 patient, and respiratory failure in 2 patients. Compared with survivors, the patients who died had a higher incidence of markedly impaired LV function, congestive heart failure (CHF), cardiomyopathy, and prior aborted sudden death. On the basis of these findings, Evans et al.[24] concluded that DC shock ablation of the AV junction carries a significant, previously unrecognized risk of death (5%), especially from lethal arrhythmias, when used in patients with severe LV dysfunction. Evans and colleagues[24] advised great care in these seriously ill patients to guard against postablation ventricular arrhythmias.

In view of this experience with DC shock ablation of the AV junction, radiofrequency ablation is now the method of choice to achieve therapeutic complete heart block.[25,26] Radiofrequency ablation can be performed using either a standard right atrial approach to the His bundle or an approach from the left side of the intraventricular septum[27] in more resistant cases. Only future studies will reveal whether radiofrequency ablation of the AV junction carries a similar or lower risk than shock ablation in patients with severe LV dysfunction.

Cost Issues

De Buitleir et al.[28] compared the cost of the catheter versus surgical ablation in the WPW syndrome. At the time this retrospective study was performed in 1988, DC shock was the energy modality in use; de Buitleir and co-workers compared the cost of catheter ablation of a posteroseptal accessory pathway in 11 patients with that of surgical ablation in another 11 patients. The total cost of therapy was significantly lower in the catheter ablation group ($14,000 versus $34,000), but the mean hospital stay at 6 days and 8 days, respectively, was not significantly different. The mean time lost from work as a result of the procedure was significantly shorter for catheter ablation (10 days versus 60 days).

In a follow-up study[29] the same investigators compared the cost of radio-frequency catheter ablation of accessory pathways in 25 patients with that of surgical ablation in another 25 patients. In this study,[29] catheter ablation cost approximately $15,000 compared with $53,000 for surgical ablation. Duration of hospitalization for the procedure was also substantially shorter for catheter ablation (3 days versus 9 days). As in the first study,[28] time lost from work because of the procedure was predictably much shorter with catheter ablation. This latter study[29] demonstrated that catheter and surgical ablation have a similar success rate, but clearly the catheter method finds greater acceptance among patients. Thus, the advantages of catheter ablation of accessory pathways include a high success rate in achieving complete cure, reduction in medical care cost, and a high degree of patient acceptance when compared with surgical therapy.

Rosenqvist et al.[30] examined the long-term follow-up of patients after transcatheter DC ablation of the AV junction. The procedure was successful in more than 80% of the patients with symptomatic improvement in the majority. Furthermore, health care utilization decreased significantly after the procedure as manifested by the number of hospital admissions per year before and after ablation (2.4 ± 2.0 versus 0.3 ± 0.5, p <0.001). Thus, in suitable patients with atrial tachycardia or atrial fibrillation refractory to medical therapy, AV junction ablation is an effective procedure which has the additional advantage of reducing health care costs.

REFERENCES

1. Averill KH, Fosmoe RJ, Lamb LE: Electrocardiographic findings in 67,375 asymptomatic subjects. IV. Wolff-Parkinson-White syndrome. Am J Cardiol 6:108, 1960
2. Chung KY, Walsh TJ, Massie E: Wolff-Parkinson-White syndrome. Am Heart J 69:116, 1965
3. Wellens HJJ, Farré J, Bar FWHM: The Wolff-Parkinson-White syndrome. p. 274. In Mandel WJ (ed): Cardiac Arrhythmias. Their Mechanisms, Diagnosis and Management. 2nd Ed. JB Lippincott, Philadelphia, 1987
4. Haines DE, DiMarco JP: Sustained intraatrial reentrant tachycardia: Clinical, electrocardiographic and electrophysiologic characteristics and long-term follow-up. J Am Coll Cardiol 15:1345, 1990
5. Dreifus LS, Haiat R, Watanabe Y et al: Ventricular fibrillation. A possible mechanism of sudden death in patients with Wolff-Parkinson-White syndrome. Circulation 43:520, 1971
6. Klein GJ, Bashore TM, Sellers TD et al: Ventricular fibrillation in the Wolff-Parkinson-White syndrome. N Engl J Med 301:1080, 1979
7. Wellens HJ, Durrer D: Wolff-Parkinson-White syndrome and atrial fibrillation: relation between refractory period of accessory pathway and ventricular rate during atrial fibrillation. Am J Cardiol 34:777, 1974
8. Jackman WM, Wang X, Friday KJ et al: Catheter ablation of accessory atrioventricular pathways (Wolff-Parkinson-White syndrome) by radiofrequency current. N Engl J Med 324:1605, 1991
9. Calkins H, Sousa J, El-Atassi R et al: Diagnosis and cure of the Wolff-Parkinson-White syndrome or paroxysmal supraventricular tachycardias during a single electrophysiologic test. N Engl J Med 324:1612, 1991
10. Klein GJ, Yee R, Sharma AD: Longitudinal electrophysiologic assessment of asymptomatic patients with the Wolff-Parkinson-White electrocardiographic pattern. N Engl J Med 320:1229, 1989
11. Klein GJ, Prystowsky EN, Yee R et al: Asymptomatic Wolff-Parkinson-White. Should we intervene? Circulation 80:1902, 1989
12. Wang Y, Schermann MM, Chien WW et al: Patients with supraventricular tachycardia presenting with aborted sudden death incidence, mechanism and long-term follow-up. J Am Coll Cardiol 18:1711, 1991
13. Cruz FES, Cheriex EC, Smeets JLRM et al: Reversibility of tachycardia-induced cardiomyopathy after cure of incessant supraventricular tachycardia. J Am Coll Cardiol 16:739, 1990
14. Brown JM, Grosso MA, Reiter MJ et al: Chronic supraventricular tachycardia can cause severe ventricular dysfunction, which can be surgically repaired. J Thorac Cardiovasc Surg 96:796, 1988
15. The Cardiac Arrhythmia Suppression Trial (CAST) Investigators: Preliminary report: effect of encainide and flecainide on mortality in a randomized trial of arrhythmia

suppression after myocardial infarction. N Engl J Med 321:406, 1989

16. Ruskin JN: The Cardiac Arrhythmia Suppression Trial (CAST). (Editorial) N Engl J Med 321:386, 1989

17. Garratt C, Ward D, Camm AJ: Degeneration of junctional tachycardia to pre-excited atrial fibrillation after intravenous verapamil. (Letter) Lancet 2:219, 1989

18. McGovern B, Garan H, Ruskin JN: Precipitation of cardiac arrest by verapamil in patients with Wolff-Parkinson-White syndrome. Ann Intern Med 104:791, 1986

19. Horowitz LN, Kay HR, Kutalek SP et al: Risks and complications of clinical cardiac electrophysiologic studies: a prospective analysis of 1,000 consecutive patients. J Am Coll Cardiol 9:1261, 1987

20. Kadish A, Calkins H, de Buitleir M, Morady F: Feasibility and cost savings of outpatient electrophysiologic testing. J Am Coll Cardiol 16:1415, 1990

21. Lee MA, Morady F, Kadish A et al: Catheter modification of the atrio-ventricular junction with radiofrequency energy for control of atrioventricular nodal reentry tachycardia. Circulation 83:827, 1991

21a. Jazayeri MR, Hempe SL, Sra JS et al: Selective trans catheter ablation of the fast and slow pathways using radiofrequency energy in patients with atrioventricular nodal reentrant tachycardia. Circulation 85:1318, 1992

21b. Kay GN, Epstein AE, Dailey SM, Plumb VJ: Selective radiofrequency ablation of the slow pathway for the treatment of atrioventricular nodal reentrant tachycardia. Evidence for involvement of perinodal myocardium within the reentrant circuit. Circulation 85:1675, 1992

22. Bolling SF, Morady F, Calkins H et al: Current treatment for Wolff-Parkinson-White syndrome: results and surgical implications. Ann Thorac Surg 52:461, 1991

23. Kay GN, Bubien RS, Epstein AE, Plumb VJ: Effect of catheter ablation of the atrioventricular junction on quality of life and exercise tolerance in paroxysmal atrial fibrillation. Am J Cardiol 62:741, 1988

24. Evans GT, Jr, Scheinman MM, Bardy G et al: Predictors of in-hospital mortality after DC catheter ablation of atrioventricular junction. Results of a prospective, international, multicenter study. Circulation 84:1924, 1991

25. Langberg JJ, Chin MC, Rosenqvist M et al: Catheter ablation of atrio-ventricular junction with radiofrequency energy. Circulation 80:1527, 1989

26. Jackman WM, Wang X, Friday KJ et al: Catheter ablation of atrioventricular junction using radiofrequency current in 17 patients. Comparison of standard and large-tip catheter electrodes. Circulation 83:1562, 1991

27. Sousa J, El-Atassi R, Rosenheck S et al: Radiofrequency catheter ablation of the atrioventricular junction from the left ventricle. Circulation 84:567, 1991

28. De Buitleir M, Bove EL, Schmaltz S et al: Cost of catheter versus surgical ablation in the Wolff-Parkinson-White syndrome. Am J Cardiol 66:189, 1990

29. De Buitleir M, Sousa J, Bolling SF et al: Reduction in medical care cost associated with radiofrequency catheter ablation of accessory pathways. Am J Cardiol 68:1656, 1991

30. Rosenqvist M, Lee MA, Moulinier L et al: Long-term follow-up of patients after transcatheter direct current ablation of the atrioventricular junction. J Am Coll Cardiol 16:1467, 1990

28

Prognostic Importance of Ventricular Premature Beats

Philip J. Podrid
Seth D. Bilazarian
Therese Fuchs

It has been well recognized that the most frequent etiology of sudden cardiac death is a sustained ventricular tachyarrhythmia, primarily ventricular tachycardia or ventricular fibrillation.[1] Among patients with heart disease, regardless of the etiology, the most frequent cause of mortality is sudden cardiac death.[2] Over the past decade, there has been growing recognition of the importance of ventricular premature beats (VPBs), largely resulting from their association with sudden cardiac death.

Despite this association, VPBs are ubiquitous in the population and are frequently documented in those with and without heart disease. In view of this, their very presence cannot be the important factor associated with their significance. It has now become clearer that certain types of VPBs may be of particular importance.

The purpose of this chapter is to review the frequency and prognostic significance of VPBs in different subsets of patients. This is particularly important, since the first step in antiarrhythmic treatment is identification of the patient for whom therapy may be indicated, and the first and most frequent intervention is pharmacologic therapy using antiarrhythmic drugs. The growing recognition of the potential hazards of these agents and the absence of data about their beneficial role in preventing sudden death mandate a clearer understanding of the importance of VPBs and a more careful selection of patients who are candidates for such therapy.

RELATIONSHIP BETWEEN SUDDEN DEATH AND VENTRICULAR ARRHYTHMIA

Sudden death claims more than 400,000 lives each year in the United States. The majority (more than 95%) of victims have some type of underlying heart disease that damages and alters the ventricular myocardium, rendering it electrophysiologically unstable.[1,2] As a result of the disease process, the electrophysiologic properties of the myocardium are altered nonuniformly, providing the basis for reentry, the mechanism most often responsible for the occurrence of sustained ventricular tachycardia or ventricular fibrillation.[3,4] The most frequent process resulting in this electrophysiologic abnormality is coronary artery disease (CAD), but any disease affecting the ventricular myocardium can be an etiologic factor. In an animal model, the evaluation of the unstable myocardium and its potential to fibrillate involves basic electrophysiologic measurements, in particular the ventricular fibrillation threshold.[5] This is not usually possible in the intact human heart, and there is no simple way to establish the stability of the myocardium. Clinically, certain types of VPBs have been associated with sudden death and have been established as markers of myocardial electrophysiologic instability and an increased risk for ventricular fibrillation. Alternatively, it has been proposed that VPBs are triggers and, by activating a latent reentrant circuit, can provoke a sustained ventricular tachyarrhythmia.[6,7]

Despite this association, it remains uncertain whether VPBs themselves are primarily implicated. The fact that VPBs are frequent in the population makes their very presence less important. While the vast majority of patients with and without heart disease have frequent VPBs, sudden death due to ventricular fibrillation is uncommon and unpredictable, suggesting that VPBs alone are not the critical factor for its occurrence or for exposing the patient at risk. There are other important factors that can affect the underlying myocardial substrate and its stability, altering the potential for the occurrence of a serious ventricular arrhythmia. Such transient factors include the sympathetic nervous system,[8] circulating catecholamines, pH changes, electrolyte fluxes,[9] and ischemia,[10] as well as many others. Several interrelated factors are responsible for the occurrence of a sustained ventricular arrhythmia and sudden death: (1) the presence of an abnormal substrate, a result of damage by some disease process, which is capable of sustaining reentry; (2) triggering factors, including spontaneously occurring ventricular arrhythmia, which can influence the substrate and activate reentry; and (3) transient modulating factors, which can change the frequency of the triggers or the stability of the substrate and thereby alter the potential for the generation and establishment of a sustained arrhythmia.

Despite the fact that there are a number of components to the problem of sudden death, spontaneously occurring or inducible ventricular arrhythmia have been and remain the most important clinical feature upon which management is based.[11] The patient for whom therapy may be indicated is identified by the presence of arrhythmia; therapy is guided by arrhythmia suppression.

VPB MORPHOLOGY AND RELATIONSHIP TO HEART DISEASE

Although VPBs are ubiquitous in the population, occurring in those with and without heart disease, it has been observed that some morphologic feature of VPBs are associated with the presence of heart disease and an abnormal myocardium. In an early study, Soloff[12] reported that VPBs with an exceptionally wide QRS complex or that are bizarre and that have a distorted configuration are more suggestive of underlying myocardial disease than those with a smooth pattern. In a recent study by Moulton and co-workers,[13] this relationship was examined more closely in 100 patients who underwent echocardiography, cardiac catheterization, or nuclear angiography to document left ventricular (LV) function and hemodynamic status. Patients were classified on the basis of the QRS morphology of the VPB. Group 1 patients (50%) had a smooth, uninterrupted QRS contour or narrow (<40 ms) notching of the complex, while the 50 group 2 patients had VPBs with broad (>40 ms) notching or shelves. The QRS duration was greater in the group 2 patients (181 versus 134 ms, p = 0.0001). The group 2 patients had a greater frequency of congestive heart failure (CHF) (66% versus 12%, p = 0.0004), an underlying dilated cardiomyopathy (38% versus 2%, p = 0.0005), and mitral regurgitation (58% versus 13%, p = 0.001). Group 2 patients also had a greater end-diastolic volume index and lower left ventricular ejection fraction (LVEF) (34% versus 59%). Moulton et al. concluded that a broadly notched VPB with a QRS of long duration (>160 ms) was a marker for a dilated and globally hypokinetic left ventricle attributable to any etiologic factor, while a VPB with a smooth contour QRS, with narrow notching and of short duration, reflects a heart of normal size and near-normal LV function.

Many patients with VPBs have multiform QRS complexes, and their meaning has been uncertain. It is not clear whether the multiple configurations represent different ectopic foci or are manifestations of multiple conduction pathways and reentrant circuits within the diseased myocardium. In support of multiple reentry circuits, Kessler and co-workers[14] reported that multiform VPBs may be a transitional arrhythmia as most patients with such forms also have repetitive VPBs as well as a variability in the coupling intervals of the VPBs. In addition, Kessler et al.[15] observed that there is a differential response of these various QRS morphologies to antiarrhythmic drug. Independent of frequency, VPBs with one QRS morphology may be suppressed by an antiarrhythmic drug while another morphology persists.

Although QRS morphology and VPB multiformity may be markers for the extent of disease and the degree of LV dysfunction, there may not always be a similarity between spontaneous VPB morphology and that of the sustained ventricular tachycardia induced in the electrophysiology laboratory. Anderson and co-workers[16] reported that in only 13% of patients was the VPB morphology identical to the induced ventricular tachycardia. However, the patients in this study had multiform VPBs (average 12 QRS morphologies/patient) and several morphologies of ventricular tachycardia. The meaning of these observations is therefore, unclear.

VPB morphology and multiformity may be markers of more extensive disease and LV dysfunction, but it is not certain whether this is associated with a poorer prognosis independent of the extent of underlying myocardial disease.

INCIDENCE OF ARRHYTHMIA IN DIFFERENT PATIENT POPULATIONS

The incidence of arrhythmia in the population and its frequency in an individual patient depend on the method used for exposure.[17] A simple 12-lead electrocardiogram (ECG) or rhythm strip is generally recorded over 1 to 2 minutes; these are insensitive techniques for documenting ventricular arrhythmia. As expected, the incidence of VPBs when these methods are used is very low. As the period of observation is increased to 6, 12, or 24 hours, using an extended ambulatory (Holter) ECG recording, the exposure of VPBs is enhanced and the incidence in the population increased. Currently, most clinical studies involve at least 24 hours of ambulatory monitoring for documenting and quantifying arrhythmia.

Exercise testing is another useful noninvasive method for exposure of ventricular arrhythmia.[18] Ob-servation of the rhythm during exercise testing is generally over a period of 30 to 60 minutes and, as expected, arrhythmia is less frequently observed when compared with the use of ambulatory monitoring, which involves a longer period of observation.[19] Although of briefer duration, exercise testing may be useful to expose more complex arrhythmia, particularly repetitive forms.[20] In general, exercise testing serves as an adjunctive method for arrhythmia exposure.

The role for exercise testing is based on the normal and physiologic changes that occur as a result of exercise (Fig. 28-1). There is withdrawal of vagal tone, but more importantly, sympathetic neural traffic and circulating catecholamines increase. Sympathetic activation and stimulation have significant effects on the ventricular myocardium, important for arrhythmogenesis.[8] There are hemodynamic changes as a result of the increase in heart rate, blood pressure or afterload, and myocardial inotropy. These factors increase myocardial work and oxygen demands and, when heart disease is present, ischemia may develop that can cause electrophysiologic and mechanical alterations, including LV stretch, contraction abnormalities, and dysfunction, important for the induction of arrhythmia. There are also chemical alterations during exercise testing, including changes in electrolytes, pH, and oxygen demand and supply, which have important effects on the myocardium and its electrophysiologic properties. These changes often result in arrhythmia. Lastly, sympathetic stimulation activates or augments the basic mechanisms responsible for arr-

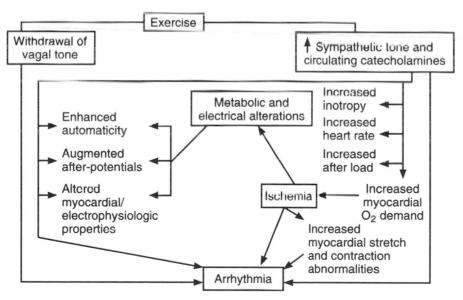

Fig. 28-1. Physiologic changes occurring with exercise. The most important effect of exercise is activation of the sympathetic nervous system and an increase in circulating catecholamines. This results in mechanical, electrical and metabolic changes that can affect arrhythmia.

hythmogenesis, including enhanced automaticity, triggered automaticity, and reentry, as a result of changes in conduction velocity and refractory periods.

As with ambulatory monitoring, the documentation of arrhythmia during exercise testing depends on the duration of exposure. If ECG monitoring of the rhythm is only episodically performed, arrhythmia is infrequently observed. By contrast, arrhythmia is more commonly observed when continuous monitoring is used.[21]

VARIABILITY OF VPB FREQUENCY

Although extended ambulatory monitoring has become an established approach for exposing ventricular arrhythmia, its use has lead to the recognition that there is great daily as well as hourly random changes in the presence, frequency and complexity of VPBs[22–24] (Table 28-1). This spontaneous variability of VPBs has complicated the identification of patients who are at an increased risk and has imposed limitations on the usefulness of noninvasive techniques, which evaluate spontaneous arrhythmia, as a guide to the selection of an effective antiarrhythmic drug. It has been reported that, as with other physiologic changes, such as heart rate and blood pressure, there is diurnal variability in VPB frequency.[25] VPBs are more frequent in the morning than in the evening. Variability is also present over briefer periods of observation, and Winkle[24] has reported wide variability of VPB frequency during sequential half-hour periods. Therefore, the duration of monitoring necessary for evaluation of patients for risk stratification or for assessing drug efficacy is uncertain and relates to the density of arrhythmia present and its daily reproducibility. Winkle and co-workers[26] evaluated 51 patients with an acute myocardial infarction (AMI) and obtained three consecutive ambulatory monitors. These investigators

observed that the prevalence of complex VPBs increased with the duration of monitoring and that low-frequency arrhythmia was poorly reproducible from day to day. This finding suggested that it might be difficult to stratify patients on the basis of a single 24-hour monitor and that potentially serious arrhythmia may be very infrequent, highly variable, and often missed. Similar data were reported by Pratt and co-workers[27] in 26 patients with chronic underlying heart disease. These investigators withdrew antiarrhythmic drugs after 1 year of continuous antiarrhythmic therapy and repeated 24-hour ambulatory monitoring after an appropriate washout period. In 50% of patients VPBs were no longer present or were of a reduced level, meeting criteria for drug efficacy. Couplets were absent or significantly reduced in 65% of patients, while nonsustained ventricular tachycardia (NSVT) was absent or decreased in 83%. These data are supported by a work of Toivouen,[28] who evaluated 20 patients hospitalized for arrhythmia. Two 24-hour ambulatory monitors separated by 4 days were obtained and two additional baseline 24-hour ambulatory monitors were obtained 6 to 12 months later. These investigators reported significantly less variability of VPBs and repetitive forms when patients were evaluated over short periods of time, while it was greater when observations were made over long intervals. The coefficient of variation for VPB frequency over a short period was 22% compared with 71% when the interval was long ($p < 0.001$). The coefficients for repetitive forms were 51% and 92%, respectively ($p < 0.01$). Similar results were reported by Anastasiou-Nana and co-workers,[29] who evaluated 47 patients with chronic arrhythmia using 24-hour ambulatory monitoring obtained in a drug-free state. Multiple recordings were obtained after periods ranging from 1 day to more than 1 year. Variability of VPBs was determined after intervals of 1 day, 1 week, 2 weeks, 3 weeks, 4 weeks, and 1 year or longer. The percentage

TABLE 28-1. Variability of Arrhythmia: Minimal Reduction (%) Necessary to Define Drug Efficacy

Study	n	Interval	Minimal Reduction (%)		
			VPBs	Couplets	NSVT
Morganroth[22]	15	1 day	83	—	—
Michelson[32]	20	1 day	—	75	65
Sami[139]	21	2 wk	65	85[a]	—
Pratt[23]	110	1 day	78	83	77
Pratt[28]	26	17 mo	50	65	83
Pratt[30]	388	8 days	95	88	—
Toivonen[28]	20	4 days–9 mo	65–100	78–100	—
Raeder[25]	75	1 day	64	83	90

a Repetitive forms.
Abbreviations: NSVT, nonsustained ventricular tachycardia; VPBs, ventricular premature beats.

reduction of VPBs required to exceed the 95% confidence limits of spontaneous variability at these intervals was 55%, 85%, 86%, 93%, 96%, and 96%, respectively. For repetitive arrhythmia, the necessary reduction was 75%, 95%, 92%, 95%, 94%, and 98%, respectively. Variability was independent of the nature of the heart disease or LV function and similar to the study of Toivouen, variability was greater as the duration between observations increased, especially when the duration was more than 1 week. In one of the earliest reports dealing with this problem, Morganroth and co-workers[22] evaluated 15 patients with chronic heart disease who had frequent VPBs defined as more than 30/h. Patients were monitored for 3 consecutive days. Using an analysis of variance (ANOVA) these investigators observed a significant degree of daily variability in VPB frequency and concluded that if 48 hours of monitoring were obtained at baseline and 48 hours during a drug intervention, at least 83% reduction of VPBs was necessary to establish the drug as effective. In this group of patients, a percentage reduction that was less than this could be attributed to random variability. However, these investigators also reported that there was a direct relationship between the hourly frequency of VPBs present at baseline and daily reproducibility. When there were >300 VPBs/h, reproducibility was greater and the percentage reduction necessary to define drug efficacy was less.

Random variability may be even greater in patients with a recent myocardial infarction (MI). In a study of 88 patients with an AMI, Pratt and co-workers[30] obtained two baseline ambulatory monitors and reported that a 95% reduction in VPBs was required to exclude random variability. In the Cardiac Arrhythmia Pilot Study (CAPS), 100 patients were randomized to placebo and underwent repeated monitoring.[31] At some point during the 1-year follow-up, 37% of these patients had greater than 70% reduction in VPBs, the definition of drug efficacy used by this study.

Complex or repetitive arrhythmia is also quite variable in its presence and frequency. Michelson and Morganroth[32] studied 20 patients with repetitive arrhythmia. When 24 hours of monitoring at baseline and during drug therapy were obtained, a greater than 65% reduction in runs of NSVT and a greater than 75% reduction in couplets were necessary to define drug efficacy. Similar results were reported by Pratt and co-workers,[23] who obtained four consecutive 24-hour ambulatory monitors in 100 patients with frequent VPBs and NSVT at baseline. They observed a greater variability of VPBs in patients with CAD. In order to exclude random variability, a greater than 78% reduction in VPBs, a greater than 83% decrease in couplets and a greater than 77% reduction in runs of NSVT were required.

While random variability is great in patients with frequent VPBs who do not have a history of a sustained ventricular tachyarrhythmia, it is less in patients who have had a serious sustained arrhythmia. Such patients often have more advanced heart disease and LV dysfunction. When spontaneous arrhythmia, including VPBs, couplets, and runs of NSVT, is present and is of high density, it is very reproducible and daily variability is less. Raeder and co-workers[25] obtained two baseline 24-hour ambulatory monitors in 75 patients presenting with either sustained ventricular tachycardia or ventricular fibrillation. In this study, there was good reproducibility in the frequency of VPBs, couplets and runs of NSVT (r = 0.84, 0.81, 0.80, respectively). In order to demonstrate drug efficacy based on 95% confidence limits, a greater than 65% reduction in VPBs, a greater than 84% decrease in couplets and greater than 90% decrease in NSVT was needed. As with other studies, the greater the density of arrhythmia, the less the variability. Variability was also noted to decrease with increasing age.

Therefore, random variability is a major problem when using noninvasive methods for establishing prognosis and identifying high-risk patients as well as when evaluating the response to antiarrhythmic drugs. The longer the monitoring period, the greater the prevalence of arrhythmia, but daily reproducibility is poor. Reproducibility is greater when VPBs are more frequent, the duration between observation periods is shorter, and the patient has a history of a sustained ventricular arrhythmia.

INCIDENCE AND PROGNOSTIC SIGNIFICANCE OF VPBs IN DIFFERENT PATIENT POPULATIONS

Normal Subjects

Until recently, it was assumed that ventricular arrhythmia resulted from cardiac disease and myocardial damage and that VPBs were clinical markers of heart disease. This perception was, in part, due to the fact that VPBs were rarely observed in normal subjects. Early studies involving thousands of normal subjects reported that the incidence of VPBs was only 2 to 5%[33-35] (Table 28-2). Although these studies involved thousands of subjects, screening involved only simple ECGs or brief rhythm strip recordings. These techniques record the rhythm for only several minutes, and the exposure of VPBs is not likely. There are studies in which normal subjects have undergone ambulatory monitoring for 6 to 24 hours, but the number evaluated is small.[36-40] Nevertheless, VPBs are documented in 40 to 80% of normals when the period of observation is extended to 24 hours. It appears that VPB frequency and complexity are also related to age and increase

TABLE 28-2. Prevalence of Ventricular Arrhythmia in Normal Patients

Study	n	Screening Method	Prevalence of VPBs (%)
Averill[33]	67,375	ECG	0.8
Hiss[34]	122,043	ECG	0.6
Chiang[35]	3,624	ECG	5
Hinkle[37]	301	6-hr monitoring	62
Brodsky[39]	50	24-hr monitoring	50
Sobotka[40]	50	24-hr monitoring	50
Fleg[36]	98	24-hr monitoring	80
Kostis[38]	100	24-hr monitoring	39

Abbreviations: ECG, electrocardiogram; VPB, ventricular premature beats.

exponentially from 16 to 74 years.[41] In the older age group, VPBs are more common, documented in 70 to 100% of such patients, while repetitive arrhythmia, including NSVT, is seen in almost 30%.[42-44] While VPBs are commonly observed, repetitive forms are infrequent in this population. VPBs are also often exposed by exercise testing, being present in up to 35% of normal patients, while repetitive forms are less frequent, documented in only 6%.[20,45] It is clear that VPBs are not markers for heart disease but occur commonly in patients with structurally normal hearts. By contrast, repetitive arrhythmia is uncommon in normal patients, although there are no data for the presence of such forms as markers for heart disease.

Although VPBs are frequent in normal patients, the important concern is whether their presence increases the risk of cardiac mortality or an arrhythmic event, especially sudden cardiac death. Unfortunately, there are only a few long-term studies available (Table 28-3). After an 18-year follow-up of normal subjects, Rodstein and co-workers[46] reported that VPBs had no prognostic significance. While this study followed several hundred patients for a long period of time, only ECG screening was used to document the presence of VPBs. Studies by Chiang and co-workers,[35] Desai and

TABLE 28-3. Prognostic Significance of Ventricular Arrhythmia in Normal Patients

Study	Screening Method	Follow-up (yr)	Prognostic Significance
Rodstein[46]	ECG	18	No
Hinkle[37]	24-hr monitoring	2.5	NO
Chiang[35]	ECG	6	NO
Kennedy[51]	24-hr monitoring	6.5	No
Desai[47]	ECG	3.5	NO
Fisher[48]	ECG	11	NO
Blackburn[50]	ECG	5	NO
Califf[53]	Exercise test	3	No

Abbreviation: ECG, electrocardiogram.

co-workers,[47] Fisher and Tyroler,[48] Crow and co-workers,[49] and Blackburn and co-workers,[50] involving thousands of patients with follow-up for up to several years, confirm the report of Rodstein that VPBs were not associated with an increased mortality in normals. Even in the elderly population, Kantilip and co-workers[44] failed to observe an association between VPB frequency or type and an increased risk of sudden death. However, in each of these studies, only ECG screening was used, so that the presence and frequency of VPBs were poorly documented. More recent studies have used 24-hour ambulatory monitoring, but the number of patients involved is small and follow-up relatively brief. Among 73 patients followed for 6½ years, Kennedy and co-workers[51] reported that there was no relationship between VPBs and mortality, confirming the earlier trials. In a study of 54 patients with VPBs, 37% of whom had complex forms, Eklon and co-workers[52] reported no sudden death after a follow-up averaging 8.3 years.

Similar findings have been reported when VPBs have been exposed during exercise testing. In a study of 673 patients without structural heart disease as established with cardiac catheterization, the presence of VPBs during exercise testing did not increase the risk of overall cardiac or sudden death mortality after a 3-year follow-up.[53] Drory and co-workers[54] exercised 76 young men without heart disease. In this study, 34% had VPBs, while 10% had repetitive arrhythmia. After a 6.7-year follow-up, arrhythmia persisted, but there were no cardiac events or deaths.

In conclusion, VPBs are commonly documented in subjects with a structural normal heart, and they are not a marker of heart disease. Their presence in such patients is not associated with an increased risk for sudden death regardless of their frequency or complexity.

Mitral Valve Prolapse

Mitral valve prolapse is a common abnormality; when the diagnosis is based on echocardiography or physical examination, 5 to 15% of the population are found to have this condition.[55] Supraventricular and ventricular arrhythmias are frequent in such patients and it has been assumed that there is causality (Table 28-4). Several studies have suggested that arrhythmia may be a result of a number of factors. It has been shown that delayed after potentials arise from the mitral valve tissue or papillary muscles.[56] Arrhythmia may be due to enhanced automaticity resulting from "stretch," "tugging," or "traction" of the chordae tendinae and papillary muscles.[57] Increased automaticity may result from contraction abnormalities of the ventricular muscle located at the base of the papillary muscle.[58] A reentrant mechanism attributable to the

TABLE 28-4. Arrhythmia in Patients With Mitral Valve Prolapse

Type of Arrhythmia	Patients with Arrhythmic Form (%)				
	Winkle[62] (n = 24)	Savage[63]		Kligfield[65]	
		Prolapse (n = 61)	No Prolapse (n = 179)	No MR (n = 63)	MR (n = 17)
VPBs	75	49	40	63[a]	100[a]
Couplets	50	?	?	6[a]	65[a]
NSVT	38	20	12	5[a]	5[a]
APBs	63	?	?	81	100
Atrial couplets	21	?	?	58	30
SVT	29	25	27	65	32

Abbreviations: APBs, atrial premature beats; MR, mitral regurgitation; NSVT, nonsustained ventricular tachycardia; SVT, sustained ventricular tachycardia; VPBs, ventricular premature beats.

[a] $p < 0.005$.

presence of a localized cardiomyopathy, suggested as the cause of the prolapse, may lead to arrhythmia.[59] It has been reported that many patients have autonomic dysfunction and elevated catecholamine levels that may be a factor in arrhythmogenesis.[60]

While arrhythmia has been believed to be more common in patients with prolapse, most of the studies involve inpatients or outpatients who have come to medical attention because of symptoms suggesting arrhythmia.[61] Most such patients will have frequent VPBs, and many will have runs of NSVT. For example, Winkle[62] reported that 75% of patients with prolapse have frequent VPBs and 38% have runs of NSVT. Unfortunately, those with symptoms from arrhythmia constitute a minority of patients with prolapse. There are only a few studies in which asymptomatic patients, who constitute the majority, have undergone ambulatory monitoring. One outpatient study from the Framingham Heart Study involved 61 patients with mitral valve prolapse documented by echocardiography and 179 patients without a prolapse who underwent 24-hour ambulatory monitoring.[63] The percentage of patients with frequent VPBs (49% in the prolapse group and 40% in the nonprolapse group) and the number of patients with runs of NSVT (20% and 12%, respectively) were not significantly different. However, the subset of patients with redundant leaflets and associated mitral regurgitation did have an increased incidence of frequent VPBs and repetitive forms.[64,65] This is probably due to the hemodynamic abnormality and not the prolapse itself. In another report from the Framingham Heart Study, Kligfield and co-workers[66] compared the ambulatory monitoring data of 63 patients with prolapse unassociated with mitral regurgitation to that obtained in 17 patients with prolapse and mitral regurgitation. The number of patients with frequent VPBs was higher in the group with regurgitation (100%) compared with those without this lesion

(63%). In addition, couplets and runs of NSVT also occurred more frequently in those with regurgitation (65% and 15% versus 6% and 5%, respectively, p < 0.05).

It may be concluded that VPBs and repetitive forms, primarily runs of NSVT, are commonly documented in patients with mitral valve prolapse, but the incidence appears to be similar to that of the normal population. All forms of VPBs are more frequent when mitral regurgitation is present, but this is a result of the hemodynamic abnormality and not of the prolapse. It does not appear that mitral valve prolapse itself is associated with an increased incidence or frequency of ventricular arrhythmia; therefore, patients with prolapse are not different from normal subjects.

Of major concern is whether the presence of such arrhythmia places these patients at an increased risk of sudden death. Unfortunately, data are lacking. It may be inferred that since sudden cardiac death is rarely seen among young women, a group in which mitral valve prolapse is documented in up to 15%, prolapse is not associated with an increased risk of sudden death. Indeed, autopsy studies in patients with sudden death rarely document mitral valve prolapse as the only structural abnormality. The Framingham Heart Study concluded that the risk of sudden death in patients with mitral valve prolapse is the same, perhaps less, than in the normal population.[63] In one long-term study, Nishimura and co-workers[67] reported on 237 patients with a mitral valve prolapse who were followed for up to 8 years (Fig. 28-2). During the follow-up period, overall mortality was 2.5%, identical to an age-matched normal control population. However, in the subset of those patients who had mitral valve leaflets that were redundant, associated with mitral regurgitation, there was a significantly higher mortality compared with those with prolapse who did not have these features (6.2% versus 0%, p < 0.01). The Fram-

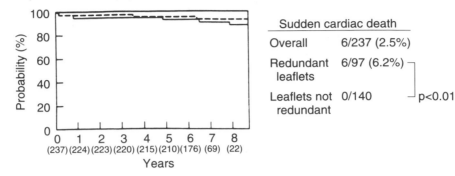

Survival in patients with MVP (solid line)
compared to control population (dashed line)

Fig. 28-2. Survival in patients with mitral valve prolapse (MVP). After an 8-year followup, the survival of patients with MVP valve prolapse is identical to a normal control population. However, those patients with prolapse, redundant leaflets, and mitral regurgitation have an increased sudden death mortality. (From Nishimura et al.,[67] with permission.)

ingham Heart Study also reported that the patients at increased risk of sudden death are the 2 to 4% with hemodynamically severe mitral regurgitation in whom the risk is 50 to 100 times greater than those without mitral regurgitation.[65,68] The increased mortality appears to be the result of the mitral regurgitation. It is, unclear, however, whether there is an association with the increased incidence of NSVT documented in this group.

In conclusion, all forms of ventricular arrhythmia are frequent in patients with mitral valve prolapse, and the prevalence appears to be similar to the normal population. In patients with prolapse, arrhythmia is benign and does not increase total or sudden cardiac mortality. When mitral regurgitation is present, VPBs and runs of NSVT are more common, probably the result of the hemodynamic abnormality, a more severe prolapse or myocardial dysfunction. While those patients with mitral regurgitation have a significantly higher mortality, it is unclear whether the ventricular arrhythmia, particularly NSVT, is predictive or causative.

Cardiomyopathy and Congestive Heart Failure

Patients with a cardiomyopathy, reduced left ventricular ejection fraction (LVEF) and congestive heart failure (CHF), constitute a growing segment of the population with underlying heart disease. There have been several studies in which 24-hour ambulatory monitoring was performed in these patients, although each study involves only a small number (Table 28-5). Nevertheless, the prevalence of frequent VPBs and couplets is high, varying from 70 to 95%.[69–81] Runs of NSVT are also common, documented in 30 to 80% of

such patients. There are many factors that account for this high prevalence of VPBs and repetitive forms.

1. *Underlying structural heart disease.* Patients with a cardiomyopathy have a diffuse underlying disease process that affects the ventricular myocardium. Most often this is CAD, but other etiologies include hypertension, an infectious cause, and an infiltrative process. Not infrequently, it is idiopathic. As a result, there is myocardial damage, necrosis, and scarring which result in an appropriate substrate for the development of ventricular arrhythmia.

2. *Electrolyte abnormalities.* Patients with CHF often have electrolyte abnormalities, especially of potassium, magnesium, and sodium, as a result of renal

TABLE 28-5. Prevalence of Ventricular Arrhythmia in Patients With Congestive Heart Failure

Study	n	% With VPBS or Couplets	% With NSVT
Huang[69]	35	93	60
Wilson[70]	77	71	50
Meinertz[71]	74	87	49
Maskin[81]	35	92	71
Von Olshausen[73]	60	95	80
Holmes[72]	31	87	39
Chakko[75]	43	88	51
Frances[77]	346	81	28
Unverferth[74]	69	NA	41
Costanzo-Nordin[76]	55	76	40
Neri[80]	65	95	80
Gradman[78]	295	46	59
Keogh[74]	137	39	41
Overall	1,322	78	45

Abbreviations: NSVT, nonsustained ventricular tachycardia; VPBs, ventricular premature beats.

dysfunction, increased hormonal activity (renin-angiotension, antidiuretic hormone, atrial naturetic factor, catecholamines), and diuretic use. Although the data are not conclusive, there may be an independent association between electrolyte imbalance, especially hypokalemia and hypomagnesia, VPBs, and an increased risk of sudden death.[9]

3. *Hemodynamic factors.* A number of important hemodynamic factors are associated with ventricular arrhythmia. The left ventricle is dilated and distended, and the resulting myocardial stretch can cause arrhythmia. As a result of the underlying disease process, there are localized or diffuse contraction abnormalities or more severe global LV dysfunction, factors that may result in arrhythmia. When CHF is present, there is additional LV distention caused by the increased diastolic volume and elevated intracardiac pressures, other factors associated with an increase in arrhythmia. In patients with underlying CAD or significant left ventricular hypertrophy (LVH), the development of ischemia may provoke ventricular arrhythmias.

4. *Neurohormonal changes.* Several neurohormonal systems become activated in patients with cardiomyopathy and CHF. The most important are the renin-angiotension and sympathetic nervous systems. The latter is especially important as it has been reported frequently that activation of the sympathetic nervous system and an increase in circulating catecholamines can provoke ventricular arrhythmia, especially repetitive forms.[8] This may be a result of enhanced automaticity, an increase in triggered automaticity, or alterations in membrane conductivity and refractoriness that enhance the potential for reentry. Activation of the renin-angio-

tension system often causes electrolyte alterations, an increase in systemic blood pressure, peripheral vascular afterload and resistance, and a further increase of intraventricular pressure and LV dysfunction that can exacerbate arrhythmias.[82]

5. *Therapeutic interventions.* The very agents used to treat CHF may be responsible for arrhythmogenesis. These include diuretics (which cause hypokalemia and hypomagnesemia), digoxin, β-agonists, phosphodiesterase inhibitors, vasodilators, and perhaps the angiotensin-converting enzyme (ACE) inhibitors.

Although ventricular arrhythmia is common in patients with a cardiomyopathy and CHF, it is unclear whether the VPBs are only a manifestation or marker of the underlying heart disease, related to its extent and the resulting hemodynamic abnormality, or an independent problem associated with an increased risk of total and sudden death mortality. It is well established that there is a high yearly mortality in patients with cardiomyopathy and CHF, averaging approximately 50% and ranging from 11 to 100% in different studies[67,73,75,77,81,83,84] (Table 28-6). While it has been assumed that the major cause of death is progressive CHF and pump failure, more than 40% of these patients die suddenly as a result of a sustained ventricular tachyarrhythmia.[69–73, 83–88] Although it seems well established that there is a significant incidence of sudden death, it is not certain whether spontaneous ectopy is associated with a risk of sudden cardiac death, as studies have reported conflicting data[69–76,78,79,89] (Table 28-7).

The wide variation in the reported total mortality and the incidence of sudden death as well as their rela-

TABLE 28-6. Total Cardiac Mortality and Sudden Death Mortality in Congestive Heart Failure

Study	n	Follow-up (mo)	% Mortality	% Death That Was Sudden
Frances[77]	159	20	46	63
Huang[69]	35	34	11	50
Sakurai[83]	190	NA	46	22
Wilson[70]	77	12	100	25
Mcinertz[71]	74	11	26	63
Maskin[81]	35	NA	71	4
Von Olshausen[73]	60	12	12	43
Holmes[72]	43	14	33	86
Chakko[75]	43	16	37	62
Franciosa[84]	182	12	48	45
Massie[85]	56	13	52	34
Lee[86]	178	36	76	37
Burggraf[87]	28	60	61	53
Cohn[88]	106	1–62	57	47
Gradman[78]	295	16	16	51
Keogh[79]	232	10	33	47
Overall	1,793		52	42

TABLE 28-7. Prognostic Significance of NSVT in Patients with Congestive Heart Failure

Study	n	Follow-up (mo)	NSVT Prognosis of Sudden Death
Huang[69]	35	34	No
Wilson[70]	77	12	No
Meinertz[71]	74	11	Yes
Von Olshausen[73]	60	12	No
Holmes[72]	43	14	Yes
Chakko[75]	43	16	Yes
Unverferth[74]	61	12	Yes
Costanzo-Nordin[76]	55	16	No
Follansbee[89]	19	19	Yes
Gradman[78]	295	16	Yes
Keogh[79]	137	10	Yes

Abbreviations: NSVT, nonsustained ventricular tachycardia.

tionship to spontaneous VPBs is due to the inclusion of patients with various etiologies of heart disease (ischemic and idiopathic) and different degrees in the severity of LV dysfunction as measured by LVEF. Patients have differences in the severity of clinical symptoms ranging from class 2 to class 4 CHF. These factors result in a very heterogeneous population of patients, which may account for the lack of consensus about the prognostic significance of ventricular arrhythmia. Unfortunately, most of these studies involve a small number of patients, and follow-up is usually limited to only 1 to 2 years. In addition, many studies do not independently analyze the role of VPBs and runs of NSVT. Of note is the study of Meinertz and co-workers[71] involving 74 patients, all of whom had an idio-

pathic dilated cardiomyopathy. These workers analyzed the importance of LV ejection fraction, VPBs as well as NSVT. They reported that the presence of NSVT was of prognostic significance for total as well as sudden cardiac death mortality, and this association was independent of LV dysfunction. Patients with NSVT died suddenly, while in the absence of such arrhythmia, death was due to CHF (Fig. 28-3). Holmes and co-workers[72] also reported a statistically significant association between NSVT and an increased risk of sudden cardiac death. These investigators observed that the presence and complexity of arrhythmia were independent of the degree of LV dysfunction and severity of CHF as determined by invasively obtained intracardiac hemodynamic measurements.

In a study by Cleland and co-workers,[90] involving 152 patients with chronic CHF who were followed for 21 months, the clinical variables associated with a poor outcome, in order of importance, were frequent VPBs, nontreatment with amiodarone, low mean arterial pressure, and underlying CAD. Another study from this group involving 84 patients with chronic CHF further evaluated the significance of arrhythmia as well as electrolyte abnormalities.[91] VPBs were the most important predictor of mortality. Hypokalemia and hyponatremia were also associated with a poor prognosis with univariate analysis, but did not provide independent prognostic information. The presence of ventricular arrhythmia was related to the severity of LV dysfunction, exercise tolerance, and neurohormonal activation, but not to electrolyte abnormalities alone.

A recent study reported by Gradman and co-work-

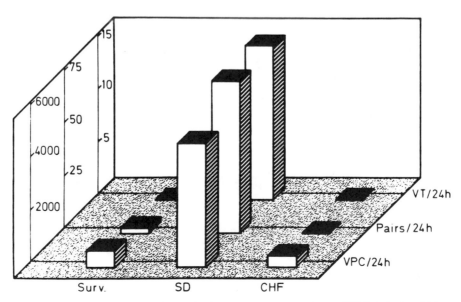

Fig. 28-3. Frequency of different forms of ventricular premature complexes (VPCs) during 24-hour monitoring in those who survived, died from CHF, or died suddenly. (From Meinertz et al.,[71] with permission.)

ers[78] involved 295 patients who were in the placebo group of the VA Cooperative Study in which placebo, captopril, and digoxin were compared. The follow-up was 16 months, and the Gradman et al. reported that the presence and frequency of NSVT were independent predictors of risk, significantly associated with total cardiac mortality (p = 0.008) and sudden death (p = 0.003) (Fig. 28-4). By contrast, the LVEF and New York Heart Association (NYHA) class were not significant predictors of sudden death (p = 0.06 and p = NS, respectively), while they were important predictors of total mortality (p = 0.006 and p = 0.02, respectively). Another recent report from Keogh and co-workers[79] involved 232 patients with a dilated cardiomyopathy referred for consideration of cardiac transplant. Ambulatory monitoring was performed in 137 patients. After a follow-up of 10 months, patients not receiving antiarrhythmic therapy who had runs of NSVT (≥4 consecutive VPBs) had a significantly reduced survival at 1 and 2 years compared with patients without NSVT. No other arrhythmia was related to mortality. There was a significant difference in survival between patients with NSVT compared with those with no VPBs, frequent VPBs, or multiform VPBs (p = 0.03). In addition, survival was significantly decreased as compared with that of patients with couplets (p = 0.02).

It should be pointed out that many of the above studies involved patients with NYHA class 2 and 3 CHF. In these patients, the presence and complexity of arrhythmia were not related to the severity of LV dysfunction and the LVEF. It appears, therefore, that ventricular arrhythmia is not just a marker of poor LV function, but is an independent risk factor for sudden death.

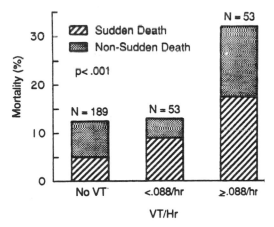

Fig. 28-4. Relationship between presence and frequency of nonsustained ventricular tachycardia (NSVT) at baseline and subsequent mortality rate. (From Gradman et al.,[78] with permission.)

It can be concluded that sudden cardiac death is an important problem in patients with a congestive cardiomyopathy and CHF, and 40% of deaths are arrhythmic. All forms of ventricular arrhythmia are frequent in these patients, and it appears that arrhythmia is independent of the extent of disease, degree of LV dysfunction, or the LVEF. While VPBs are the result of the underlying disease, they are not associated with its severity. In most of the studies evaluating risk factors associated with mortality, it appears that NSVT is an independent predictor of sudden death as well as total cardiac mortality. It is not just a marker of a damaged myocardium and poor LV dysfunction but is important in the genesis of a sustained ventricular tachyarrhythmia and sudden death.

Hypertropic Cardiomyopathy

A specific group of patients with cardiomyopathy are those with a hypertrophic cardiomyopathy. It has been reported that such patients also have an increased risk of sudden death; the annual rate is 2 to 3% in adults, but up to 6% in the young.[92] It has been reported that as many as 90% of such patients have VPBs, while up to 26% have NSVT.[92-96] Ando and co-workers[97] reported that ventricular arrhythmia was more common in patients with segmental dysfunction involving the LV apex (p < 0.001). Maron and co-workers[95] reported that after a 2-year follow-up of 84 patients with a hypertrophic cardiomyopathy treated medically, there were seven deaths (8.3%), of which six were sudden. McKenna and co-workers[94] reported an 8% sudden death rate after a 2.6-year follow-up of 86 patients. As in patients with a congestive, dilated cardiomyopathy, NSVT is the only form of ventricular arrhythmia that has prognostic importance. In the study of Maron and co-workers,[95] the annual mortality in patients with NSVT was 8.6% compared with 1% among those without this arrhythmia. Nienaber and co-workers[98] analyzed 29 patients with hypertrophic cardiomyopathy who underwent noninvasive and invasive testing to establish risk factors for the occurrence of syncope and for sudden death. Three variables were significant predictors of risk, including age under 30 years (p = 0.0007), left ventricular end-diastolic volume index (p = 0.006) and NSVT (p = 0.03).

Hypertension and Left Ventricular Hypertrophy

Patients with hypertension with or without LVH have been reported to have frequent VPBs. The etiology of ventricular arrhythmia in these patients is varied and includes

1. Elevated intraventricular diastolic pressure, which directly produces changes on the endocardium and

probably affects the electrophysiologic properties of the Purkinje fibers[99,100]

2. Presence of LVH, which may directly result in alterations in the electrophysiologic properties of the myocardium or can cause arrhythmia as a result of associated ischemia
3. Distention or stretch of the LV wall as a result of the increased intraventricular pressure
4. Development of hypokalemia, which is often due to diuretic therapy frequently administered to such patients.[101,102]

Although ventricular arrhythmias are observed in hypertensive patients, data about incidence are not well established, since often only brief ECG recordings were used to document the presence, type, and frequency of the arrhythmia. Extended ambulatory monitoring has only infrequently been employed. Therefore, the prevalence of VPBs in this population and their frequency and complexity have not been well established. In a substudy of the Medical Research Council (MRC) Mild Hypertension Trial,[103] the incidence of VPBs, defined as >10 VPBs/100,000 QRS complexes on 24-hour monitoring, was 4.2% in the group receiving placebo. The presence of VPBs has been of growing concern since there is a substantial risk of sudden arrhythmic death in hypertensive patients, especially when LVH is present. Although it has been reported that abrupt changes in ventricular afterload may cause arrhythmias,[100] and acutely unloading the heart by treatment of blood pressure may reduce their frequency,[104] there are as yet no data that chronic blood pressure elevation is associated with ventricular arrhythmia or that its long-term reduction has a beneficial effect.

It is uncertain whether hypertension alone is associated with VPBs. In a study by Dendale and deMeirleir,[105] 50 untreated patients with an exaggerated systolic blood pressure response to exercise were compared with 54 control subjects. VPBs were present in 4% of normals, in 14% of those with rest and exercise-induced hypertension (p <0.01), and in 31% of patients with only exercise hypertension (p <0.01). Similarly, Sideris et al.[100] reported that the acute elevation of systolic blood pressure by metaraminol provoked VPBs in 14 or 15 normotensive patients while the acute reduction of pressure by nitroprusside eliminated VPBs in 8 of 13 hypertensive patients with frequent ectopy. In another study involving animals, Sideris and co-workers[106] reported that the arrhythmogenic effect on the ventricles results from an increase in afterload rather than the increase in the aortic pressure itself or in preload. While an acute change in blood pressure may cause arrhythmia, the role of chronic or sustained hypertension is unknown.

Efforts to reduce blood pressure in hypertensive pa-

tients are aimed at reducing the long-term risk of cardiovascular events and mortality. Although large-scale intervention trials have reported that blood pressure control does reduce the incidence of CHF, malignant hypertension, and stroke, there has not been a reduction in the overall incidence of ischemic heart disease (IHD) and related events, including sudden cardiac death. Indeed, the Multiple Risk Factor Intervention Trial (MRFIT)[107] reported that in the group of hypertensive patients with an abnormal resting ECG who received aggressive therapy, there was a higher mortality from CAD and sudden death as compared with those receiving conventional or no therapy. However, these data are complicated by the fact that such patients often received therapy with diuretics; it was suggested that the adverse outcome and risk of sudden death were due to hypokalemia. In addition, in patients with long-standing hypertension and LVH, there may be abnormalities of lipid or glucose metabolism or the handling of electrolytes such as potassium and magnesium, other factors responsible for the sudden death mortality in this group.[108]

One of the important factors associated with arrhythmia in hypertensive patients is the presence of LVH. Siegel and co-workers[109] monitored 123 men with untreated hypertension. Among the 48 (39%) with LVH, frequent (>30/h) VPBs were observed in 19% and 17% had NSVT. By contrast, VPBs and NSVT were present in only 8% of hypertensive patients who did not have LVH. In addition, arrhythmia was more common in patients over the age of 60 who were more likely to have LVH, compared with the younger group (50% versus 23%). McLenachan and co-workers[110] performed 48 hours of monitoring in 100 patients with hypertension, 50% of whom had LVH. NSVT was present in 50% of patients with LVH and in only 8% of those without LVH (p < 0.05). NSVT was documented in only 2% of a control population. In addition, the runs of NSVT were of longer duration in those with LVH. Patients with NSVT had a greater LV mass and a higher prevalence of ST-T-wave abnormalities on the surface ECG as compared with patients who did not have these forms. The presence of NSVT was unrelated to the measured systolic or diastolic blood pressure, the use of diuretic therapy, or the presence of hypokalemia. These investigators also analyzed coronary angiograms and endomyocardial biopsies in patients with LVH and concluded that the occurrence of complex VPBs could not be attributed to CAD, but to complications of LVH, such as myocardial fibrosis, which were more commonly seen in patients with NSVT. Similar data about LVH and arrhythmia were reported by Levy and co-workers[111] from the Framingham Heart Study, although hypertension was not the only etiology for LVH (Fig. 28-5). Men with LVH on echocardiography (n = 340) had a significantly

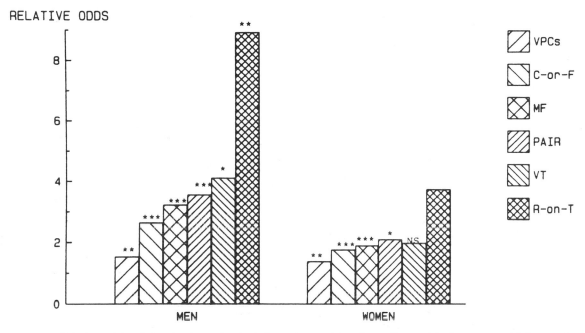

Fig. 28-5. Relative odds of ventricular arrhythmia in patients with echocardiographic documented left ventricular hypertrophy (LVH) (men, 341; women, 502) compared with normal controls (men, 1,829; women, 2,165). VPC, ventricular premature contraction (>1/hr); C or F, complex or frequent VPCs; MF, multiform VPCs; NS, not significant; pair, couplets; VT, NSVT; R on T, early R on T VPCs. *p < 0.05; **p < 0.01; ***p < 0.001. (From Levy et al.,[111] with permission.)

greater prevalence of VPBs (38% versus 30%, p = 0.001), couplets (6.6% versus 2.0%, p < 0.001), and NSVT (1.3% versus 0.3%, p = 0.03) compared with the group without LVH (n = 1829). The same findings were observed in women except that the presence of NSVT was equivalent in those with (n = 502) and without (n = 2,165) LVH. Using echocardiography and 24-hour monitoring, Messerli and co-workers[112] studied 14 normotensive patients, 10 patients with hypertension and no LVH, and 16 patients with hypertension and LVH. There was no difference in the number of hourly VPBs between normotensive and those with hypertension and no LVH (8 versus 10), but there was a significantly greater incidence in hypertensives with LVH (475/h, p < 0.01). Moreover, those with hypertension and LVH had a significantly greater prevalence of multiform VPBs and repetitive forms (p < 0.004).

Although LVH appears to be a factor associated with VPBs in hypertensive patients, the most widely reported abnormality associated with arrhythmia in this group is hypokalemia. In 38 patients with moderate diastolic hypertension, Hollifield and Slaton[102] administered hydrochlorothiazide at an initial dose of 50 mg, titrated up to 200 mg based on blood pressure. Prior to therapy, no VPBs were present at rest or during exercise. However, during diuretic therapy, these patients had a significant increase in VPBs with exercise, and the frequency was directly related to the reduction in the serum potassium level resulting from diuretic therapy. Even when smaller doses of diuretic were administered, hypokalemia occurred and VPB frequency increased. The role of hypokalemia in provoking VPBs is supported by a study of Holland and co-workers,[101] who monitored 21 patients with mild hypertension for 24 hours before and during diuretic therapy. VPBs were present at baseline, but they increased in frequency during diuretic therapy. The frequency returned to the baseline level when potassium supplements were administered. In the large MRFIT report involving 12,866 patients, VPBs on a baseline ECG were present in 1.8% of patients.[107] The presence of VPBs was associated with age, diuretic use, and ECG abnormalities on the resting ECG. However, during follow-up, the prevalence of VPBs increased to 9.1%, primarily related to the level of the diastolic blood pressure, especially in patients receiving diuretic therapy of whom 12.1% had VPBs. In this trial, there was a 28% increase in VPB frequency when serum potassium was reduced by >1 mEq/L during diuretic therapy.

While these studies report an association between VPBs and hypokalemia in hypertensive patients, this is still controversial as other studies do not report such a relationship. In a study by Papademetriou and co-workers,[113] 24 hours of ambulatory monitoring was obtained before and after potassium replacement in 16 patients with diuretic induced hypokalemia. In this study, there was no difference in the type or frequency of arrhythmia when the patients were hypokalemic (K^+ = 2.8 mEq/L) or normokalemic (K^+ = 4.2 mEq/L). Lumme and Jounela[114] reported similar results in a group of 24 hypertensive patients treated for 4 weeks with placebo or one of 3 diuretic programs. This study used a thiazide as well as a potassium-sparing diuretic. There was no difference in VPB frequency or type in any group receiving diuretic therapy as compared with placebo regardless of the potassium level. A third study, by Madias and co-workers[115] involving 20 hypertensive patients, reported the same results.

There are several problems with these many studies. Each included a small number of patients, and the duration of therapy was brief, generally 4 weeks or less. By contrast, studies reporting an association between hypokalemia and arrhythmia have generally been of longer duration (i.e., 24 to 40 weeks). In this regard, the results of the Medical Research Council Hypertension Study[116] are of importance. This trial involved 324 patients who were randomized to diuretic therapy with or without potassium supplementation or with placebo. After a short duration of therapy (9 to 10 weeks), there was no difference in the incidence of VPBs in the treated (37%) or untreated group (29%) as compared with the baseline period (31% versus 37%, respectively). Likewise, there was no difference in incidence at 10 weeks when the placebo and treated groups were compared (29% versus 37%). However, when reevaluated after follow-up was extended to an average of 2 years, patients receiving therapy with diuretics had a significantly greater incidence of VPBs compared with those receiving placebo (61% versus 42%, p = 0.025). The presence of VPBs was related to the serum potassium concentration (p = 0.04). Importantly, complex VPBs were more common in the thiazide-treated group (33% versus 15%).

It appears that hypertensive patients with LVH and resting ECG abnormalities have a higher prevalence of VPBs and complex forms. Such patients also have an increased total cardiac mortality as well as an increased risk of sudden cardiac death. However, it is unknown whether there is a relationship between VPBs or NSVT and the risk of sudden death in such patients. No studies have addressed this issue. It is also uncertain whether therapy, especially nondiuretic drugs, directed at blood pressure reduction will affect the presence, frequency, and complexity of arrhythmia and decrease the incidence of sudden cardiac death.

Coronary Artery Disease

Information about the incidence and prognostic significance of VPBs in patients with chronic CAD, including those with a recent coronary artery bypass grafting (CABG), is limited. Calvert and co-workers[117] performed 24-hour ambulatory monitoring in 124 patients of whom 84 patients had CAD documented by cardiac catheterization. In this study, the overall incidence of VPBs was 83% for the entire group and 86% for patients with CAD. In 75% of those patients, VPBs were present for more than 3 hours during the day. Multiform and repetitive VPBs were documented in 63% of patients with CAD. The frequency and complexity of arrhythmia were related to the extent of CAD, that is, the number of vessels involved. Among the 57 patients with multivessel disease, 42% had repetitive VPBs, while only 15% of those with single vessel disease had these forms (p < 0.02). In addition, the prevalence of advanced grades increased with the level of LV end-diastolic pressure. Runs of NSVT were present in only 4% of those with a normal pressure, but in 25% of patients with a pressure of >19 mmHg (p < 0.02). The presence of repetitive arrhythmia also correlated with the presence and extent of LV asynergy; the incidence was 18%, 27%, and 47% in those with zero, one or two areas of asynergy, respectively (p < 0.005). Madsen and co-workers[118] performed 24-hour ambulatory monitoring in 198 patients with CAD suspected of having an AMI but in whom no MI was confirmed. VPBs occurred in 65% of patients, while complex VPBs were noted in 29%. The presence of VPBs was related to a documented scar from a previous MI, but not to acute ischemia.

There are a few studies in which the relationship between VPBs and the occurrence of active ischemia in patients with CAD has been reported. Hausmann and co-workers[119] studied 97 patients with angiographically proven CAD, stable angina pectoris, and an abnormal exercise test. During 24-hour ambulatory monitoring, there were 573 episodes of ST-segment depression indicating active ischemia. Frequent VPBs occurred during ischemic episodes in only 10 patients (10%) involving 27 (5%) episodes of ischemia. In the remaining 90% of patients, there were no VPBs during the ischemic episodes. There was no significant difference in the extent of CAD or in the hemodynamics between those with and without VPBs. Hausmann and colleagues concluded that VPBs were observed in only a minority patients with stable CAD, unrelated to the severity and extent of the CAD. Mulcahy and co-workers[120] studied 150 patients with stable angina of whom 13 (9%) showed VPBs related to ischemia as determined by ST-segment depression on ambulatory monitoring. In contrast to these studies, a greater incidence of ischemic-related arrhythmia was reported by Carboni and co-workers.[121] In 11 of 31 patients (35%) with stable angina pectoris, 41 of 117 ischemic episodes (35%) were accompanied by VPBs. Banai and co-workers[122] demonstrated an increase in VPBs during ischemic episodes only in those patients who also had VPBs when ischemia was absent. Importantly, no complex arrhythmia was observed in this trial. In a follow-up report from this group, Stern and co-workers[123] conducted a prospective study in 75 consecutive patients with documented CAD who had ischemic episodes (ST-segment depression) observed on 24-hour ambulatory monitoring, positive exercise test, and no known symptomatic or sustained ventricular arrhythmia. A total of 719 ischemic episodes were recorded during 127 monitoring periods. Of the 43 patients without VPBs or <14 VPBs/24 h on ambulatory monitoring, none had an increase in VPBs during ischemic episodes. By contrast, among the 32 patients with ventricular arrhythmia on baseline monitoring (>14 VPBs/24 h), 11 (31%) had an increase in VPBs observed during 47 of 174 (27%) ischemic episodes. There was no correlation between the severity of the ischemic event and the number of VPBs. In a study by Lillis and Hanson,[124] 18 patients with CAD were monitored during a cardiac rehabilitation program. Patients were studied while at rest and during exercise training. Patients considered to be high risk, based on clinical status and cardiac catheterization, had more VPBs during exercise than at rest, as well as during routine daily activities.

In contrast to the findings in patients with underlying CAD and unstable angina, the data are different in patients with variant angina or unstable angina in whom there is a significant increase in VPBs during ischemia.[125-127] In such patients, ventricular arrhythmia increases significantly during active ischemic episodes.

While there are substantial data about the incidence of VPBs in patients with CAD, relatively few studies report the incidence of NSVT in this group of patients. As previously indicated, Calvert and co-workers[117] reported that the presence of repetitive forms, primarily NSVT, was related to the severity of the underlying CAD and were primarily observed in those with multivessel involvement. Quyyami and co-workers[128] used ambulatory monitoring to evaluate 100 consecutive patients with chest discomfort of whom 74 had angiographically documented CAD. Of the 26 patients with normal coronary arteries, none had runs of NSVT on ambulatory monitoring. In the patient group with documented CAD, the frequency of NSVT was associated with the extent of CAD. Thus, only 1 of 22 patients (4.5%) with single vessel disease had NSVT and 1 of 22 patients (4.5%) with two vessel disease and 4 of the

30 patients (13%) with triple vessel disease had runs of NSVT.

Additional information about the incidence of VPBs and CAD are from studies in patients with recent CABG. Ruben and co-workers[129] reported on 92 patients with a normal LVEF who underwent CABG. Complex VPBs were observed in 57%, while almost 22% had NSVT. The presence of such arrhythmia was unrelated to the occurrence of postoperative complications, and there were no sudden deaths in any group during a 16-month follow-up. DeSoyza and co-workers[130] randomized 130 patients with chronic stable angina to medical or surgical therapy. Using 6-hour ECG monitoring, 30% of surgically treated patients had complex VPBs, while 19% of medical patients had such arrhythmia. Complex arrhythmia was not associated with an increase in sudden death in either group, and the mortality was identical in the two groups. Huikari and co-workers[131] evaluated 126 postoperative patients with ambulatory monitoring. These patients underwent cardiac catheterization before and 3 months after surgery. Frequent VPBs (>30/h) or repetitive forms were more common after surgery (39% of patients versus 24% of patients before surgery, p < 0.05). In 18 patients (14%) who had a worsening of arrhythmia after CABG, the LVEF had significantly decreased (56% to 50%, p < 0.05). After a 58-month follow-up, 4 patients died suddenly. While complex arrhythmia was more common in those who died, it did not predict the patient at risk.

A number of studies have reported the prevalence of VPBs during exercise testing in patients with CAD[20,53,132-134] (Table 28-8). Simple VPBs are observed in 23 to 62% of patients, while the incidence of repetitive arrhythmia ranges from 8% to 31%.

VPBs are commonly documented in patients with CAD and occur under a variety of circumstances. However, the association between ventricular arrhythmia and a risk of sudden cardiac death has not been well studied. Data from the Framingham Heart Study[135] reported that VPBs alone in patients with CAD appeared to have only a weak independent influence on incidence of sudden cardiac death and only among men in whom the risk of death was increased twofold (p < 0.002). Ingersler and Bjerragaard[136] studied 73 patients over the age of 85, using ambulatory monitoring. Fifteen patients had IHD, 36 patients had symptoms of a possible cardiac origin, and 22 patients had no known heart disease. Patients with CAD were more likely to have VPBs and ventricular couplets compared with a healthy group. After a 2-year follow-up, four of eight patients (50%) with CAD who had frequent VPBs died suddenly compared with only one death (14%) among those patients who had no VPBs. This study

TABLE 28-8. Prevalence of Ventricular Arrhythmia During Exercise

| Study | % With Arrhythmia | | | |
| | Simple VPBs | | Repetitive VPBs | |
	Normal	Heart Disease	Normal	Heart Disease
Beard and Owen[237]	8.0	—	0.3	—
Master[238]	18.3	—	0.3	—
Whinnery[134]	5.0	50.0	0	15.0
McHenry[133]	34.0	50.0	6.0	22.0
Poblete[132]	7.0	62.0	0	31.0
Ryan[19]	—	55.0	—	20.0
Califf[53]	14	23	2.4	8.2
Jelenik[20]	19.0	36.0	1.8	3.6

Abbreviation: VPBs, ventricular premature beats.

suggests that a high frequency of VPBs in elderly patients with CAD is associated with a poorer prognosis.

Data relating the presence of exercise-induced VPBs with prognosis are also controversial (Table 28-9). Califf and co-workers[53] reported that among 620 patients with documented CAD, the 3-year mortality was 10% among those without exercise-induced arrhythmia, 17% in those with only simple VPBs, and 25% in patients who had repetitive arrhythmia. Udall and Ellestad[137] also reported that exercise-induced VPBs increased the risk of death in patients with CAD, especially of ST-segment depression with exercise was also provoked. In contrast, to this study, Weiner and co-workers[138] reported that among 446 patients with CAD who were treated medically, exercise-induced arhythmias did not affect mortality during a 5.3-year follow-up. Lack of predictive value of exercise-induced ventricular arrhythmia was also reported by Sami and co-workers,[139] who followed 146 patients with CAD for 47 months. Lastly, Nair and co-workers[140] reported no prognostic significance after a 4-year follow-up of exercise induced VPBs in those with or without CAD.

In conclusion, VPBs are common in patients with CAD. Repetitive forms, including NSVT, are also documented in a substantial percentage of such patients. It

is still uncertain whether VPBs are associated with an increased risk of sudden death in such patients, although NSVT appears to be of importance.

Acute Myocardial Infarction

One of the patient groups of most concern are those with a recent MI. These patients have a significantly increased risk of sudden death, especially during the first year after the event. There is a large body of data about the meaning of VPBs in such patients. A number of studies have reported that when 24-hour ambulatory monitoring is used, 80 to 90% of such patients have frequent VPBs, and 30 to 40% will have runs of NSVT.[141–143] Therefore, similar to other groups of patients with heart disease, patients with a recent MI have frequent VPBs including runs of NSVT. VPBs in these patients arise from the surviving Purkinje fibers located within the endocardium.[144] As a result of chronic hypoxia and cellular disruption, the damaged tissue exhibits spontaneous automaticity that may result in the development of ectopic or automatic foci.[145] This diseased and abnormal tissue may also generate triggered automaticity or delayed afterpotentials.[145] Lastly, tissue within and around the infarcted zone

TABLE 28-9. Prognostic Significance of Exercise-Induced Ventricular Premature Beats

| Study | Population | Follow-up (yr) | Mortality (%) | | |
			Simple VPBs	Complex VPBS	Significant
Califf[53]	Normal	3.0	0	0	No
Califf[53]	CAD	3.0	17	25	Yes
Weiner[138]	Significant CAD	4.3	13	?	No
	Minimal CAD	5.0	9	?	No
Udall[137]	CAD − ST	1	15	29	Yes
	CAD + ST	1	33	42	Yes
Weld[155]	Post-MI	1	12	?	Yes
Krone[156]	Post-MI	1	7	13	Yes
Henry[157]	Post-MI	2	25	?	Yes

Abbreviations: CAD, coronary artery disease; VPBs, ventricular premature beats.

and the surviving Purkinje fibers is very heterogeneous as a result of postinfarction cellular damage, chronic ischemia, scarring, fibrosis, and remodeling. This leads to nonuniformity of electrophysiologic properties.[145] It is an important precondition for establishing reentrant circuits and the generation of ventricular arrhythmia caused by reentry. Other variable factors may interact with these mechanism and result in ventricular arrhythmia, including the sympathetic nervous system,[8] circulating catecholamines,[8] hypoxia, hypokalemia,[9] and low magnesium.

An important concern is whether VPBs have prognostic importance in these patients (Table 28-10). In one of the earliest studies, Ruberman and co-workers[143,146] performed 1 hour of sedentary monitoring within 3 months of the MI in 1739 patients. After an average follow-up of 42 months, these investigators observed that there was a significantly increased incidence of sudden death (25%) in patients with complex arrhythmia, primarily NSVT, compared with those with frequent VPBs or no arrhythmias (8%) (Fig. 28-6). Using 24 hours of ambulatory monitoring, Moss and co-workers[142] reported similar results among 978 patients with a recent MI. After an average follow-up of 36 months, the incidence of sudden death was highest (15%) in those with complex VPBs and lowest (4%) in those without arrhythmia. Although mortality was intermediate in patients with frequent VPBs, it was not significantly different from that in the group without arrhythmia. Several other studies have reported the same results.[141,147] In a study by Rappaport and Remedios[140] in which 24-hour ambulatory monitoring was performed in 139 patients, the 12-month sudden death mortality was 34% in patients with complex arrhythmia compared with 6% in those without such arrhythmia. In a larger study of 388 patients entered into the Multicenter Investigators of the Limitation of Infarct Size (MILIS) trial, Mukharji and co-workers[149] reported a 6% sudden death incidence among patients with complex arrhythmia compared with a 3% incidence in those without such arrhythmia. In a large study of 820 post-MI patients who had 24-hour ambulatory monitoring, Bigger and co-workers[150,151] reported a 36% 1-year mortality among patients with runs of NSVT compared with 12% in the absence of such arrhythmia.

From the European Infarction Study Group, Andresen and co-workers[152] reported on 378 placebo patients followed for 2 years. Frequent VPBs (>10/h) were associated with a 4% mortality; couplets or NSVT increased the 2-year mortality to 12.5% and 14.8%, respectively. When NSVT and frequent VPBs were present, the mortality at 2 years was 21.4%. These investigators also observed an association between mortality and the frequency of arrhythmia. When there were <10 couplets per day, the mortality was 9.9% versus 22.2% when there were >10 couplets per day (p < 0.05). When there were <2 runs of NSVT per day, the mortality was 8.5% compared with 25.0% (p < 0.05) when there were >2 runs per day. It has been reported that the incidence of VPBs is related to the severity of underlying CAD but is independent of LVEF.[153] It has also been reported that the prognostic significance of NSVT was independent of extent of the infarction (i.e., Q-wave MI versus non-Q-wave MI.[154] Of 777 patients, 191 had a non-Q-wave MI, 261 had an anterior Q-wave MI, and 325 had an inferior Q-wave MI. Repetitive VPBs (primarily couplets) were observed in 62% of patients with a non-Q-wave MI who died at 1 year compared with 32% of survivors (p < 0.01). No difference was seen between the two Q-wave MI groups. The survival of patients without NSVT was identical in the Q-wave MI and non-Q-wave MI groups (93% and 90%, respectively). By contrast, survival in patients with Q-wave MI and NSVT was 92% compared with 76% in those with a non-Q-wave MI and NSVT (p < 0.001). The poor outcome in those with NSVT and non-Q-wave MI may be related to the presence of ongoing ischemia.

There are data available that exercise-induced arrhythmia in the post-MI patient is also associated with an increased mortality (Table 28-9). Weld and co-

TABLE 28-10. Ventricular Arrhythmia After Myocardial Infarction

Study	n	Duration of Monitoring (hr)	Follow-up (mo)	Sudden Death (%) No Complex VPBs	Complex VPBs
Bigger[150]	820	24	12	12	36
Kotler[147]	160	6	36	20	60
Moss[142]	978	6	36	4	15
Mukharji[149]	388	24	14	3	16
Rappaport[148]	139	24	12	6	34
Ruberman	1,739	1	42	8	25
Vismara[141]	64	20	26	11	30
Schultz[159]	81	24	7	0	28
Andresen[152]	1,741	24	24	4	15

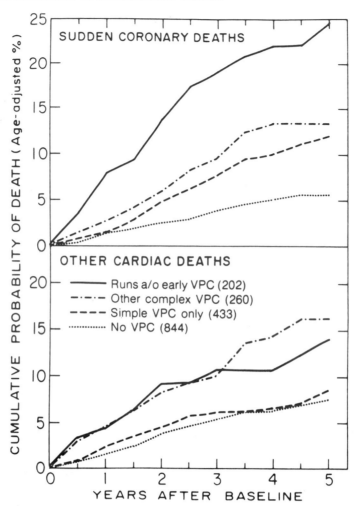

Fig. 28-6. Relationship between type of ventricular premature complex (VPC) documented on 1 hour of monitoring and sudden death or other cardiac death among 1,739 males surviving a myocardial infarction. (From Ruberman et al.,[146] with permission.)

workers[155] observed that exercise-induced arrhythmia increased the risk threefold from 4% in those without exercise-induced VPBs to 12% in those with ectopy. Krone and co-workers[156] performed low-level exercise testing in 667 patients with a recent MI and reported that the occurrence of any VPB during exercise increased the first year mortality from 3% to 7% (p < 0.05). Couplets increased the mortality threefold, from 4% to 13% (p < 0.05). Henry and co-workers[157] reported that the presence of VPBs during exercise testing was the only variable associated with a greater incidence of sudden death (25% versus 8%). Saunamki and Anderson[158] exercised 187 post-MI patients and reported that exercise-induced arrhythmia (>2 VPBs/min or repetitive forms) increased the long-term mortality, especially when associated with a blunted increase in the rate-pressure product during exercise.

The survival at 4.5 years was 49% in those with VPBs and poor heart rate and blood pressure response compared with 85% in those without VPBs and a normal increase in the rate-pressure product.

While these studies all report that the presence of complex arrhythmia, primarily NSVT, increases the risk of sudden death in patients after an AMI, there are other important risk factors that interact with ventricular arrhythmia. Chief among these is LV function (Table 28-11). In an early study by Schultz and co-workers[159] involving 81 patients, the only sudden death mortality was observed in the group of patients with runs of NSVT and a reduced LVEF (less than 40%). In contrast to the 28% mortality in this group, there were no deaths in those without such arrhythmia, regardless of the presence of LV dysfunction. The results from MILIS were identical.[149] The presence of

TABLE 28-11. Relationship Among Ventricular Arrhythmia, LV Function, and Sudden Death in Patients After a Myocardial Infarction

	% Sudden Death			
	No Complex VPBs		Complex VPBs	
Study	LV Intact	LV Dysfunction	LV Intact	LV Dysfunction
Bigger[160]	6	22	12	35
Mukharji[149]	2	7	7	25
Ruberman[143]	3	7	12	22
Schultz[159]	0	0	0	28
Andresen[152]	2	4	4	17

Abbreviations: LV, left ventricle/ventricular; VPBs, ventricular premature beats.

LV dysfunction (ejection fraction less than 40%) was an independent risk factor for sudden death, but the highest mortality (25%) was in those patients with runs of NSVT along with reduced LV function. By contrast, the mortality was 7% when NSVT was absent. Bigger and co-workers[160] reported similar results (Fig. 28-7). LV dysfunction, defined as LVEF less than 30%, increased the sudden death mortality irrespective of the presence of NSVT, but those with a reduced LVEF and runs of NSVT had the highest mortality (35%). Results from the European Infarction Study Group[152] were similar. In the placebo group, the 2-year mortality was 1.9% in those without CHF or NSVT, approximately 4% when either CHF or NSVT was present, but 16.7% when both CHF and NSVT were present. Lastly, using clinical CHF as the definition of LV dysfunction, Ruberman and co-workers[146] reported that the presence of CHF and NSVT was associated with a 22% mortality, compared with 3% when LV function was intact and runs of NSVT were not present. The incidence was intermediate when either factor was present. Although VPB presence and frequency are inde-

pendent of LVEF, their presence and prognostic significance may be related to the severity of the underlying CAD, that is, the number of vessels involved. There also appears to be an interrelationship between the electrical and mechanical abnormalities.

While NSVT is an important independent risk factor that, along with LVEF, identifies a higher-risk group, these values are not as helpful in exposing the individual patient at risk. Other factors have added to the ability to identify the individual patient. Kleiger and co-workers[161] reported on the usefulness of heart rate variability (Fig. 28-8). In this study, heart rate was obtained from ambulatory monitoring and the standard deviation of RR intervals over the 24-hour period determined. Patients with absent heart rate variabil-

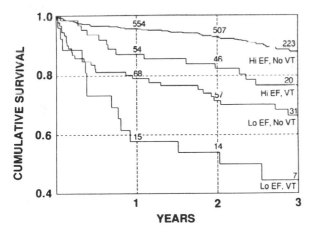

Fig. 28-7. Kaplan-Meier survival curves for patients after a myocardial infarction related to presence or absence of NSVT and ejection fraction (EF <30% or >30%). (From Bigger et al.,[150] with permission.)

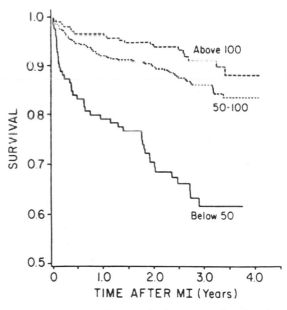

Fig. 28-8. Kaplan-Meier survival curves related to heart rate variability (defined by standard deviation of RR intervals over 24 hours), p < 0.0001 when group with <50-ms variability compared with those with >50-ms variation. (From Kleiger et al.,[161] with permission.)

ity (standard deviation of RR intervals <50 ms) had a significant increase in sudden death mortality compared with the group with intact heart rate variability (>100 ms). Although the absence of heart rate variability was an independent risk factor, it was of particular importance when considered along with LV function and the presence of NSVT during 24-hour ambulatory monitoring.

Another important marker of myocardial instability that has been of help in identifying the high-risk patient is the signal-averaged ECG and the presence of late potentials.[162,163] Late potentials are low-amplitude oscillations located at the end of the QRS complex that represent continuous, delayed, or fragmented electrical activity within a region of damaged myocardium. They occur at a time when myocardial depolarization is completed (i.e., the end of the QRS complex), and the myocardium should be electrically silent, just before repolarization. The presence of late potentials is associated with an increased risk of a serious ventricular tachyarrhythmia and has a predictive accuracy equivalent to that of NSVT.[164] However, its prognostic importance is enhanced if considered along with NSVT and LV dysfunction.

In conclusion, many studies have identified a number of important factors associated with an increased risk of sudden death in the post-MI patient. While they are useful for stratifying these patients into low and high risk, it must be remembered that these data are derived from trials carried out before the use of thrombolytic agents such as streptokinase and tissue plasminogen activator (TPA) or angioplasty. These agents have altered the prognosis and outcome of patients after MI[165] and no doubt will change the significance of these traditional risk factors, including VPBs. Theroux and co-workers[166] evaluated 344 patients presenting with an AMI, of whom 168 (control group) were unsuccessfully treated with streptokinase, while 73 were successfully reperfused and 103 had angioplasty. Revascularization with streptokinase or angioplasty significantly reduced the hourly frequency of VPBs (21 and 17, respectively) compared with control (40, p <0.05). The LVEF was, however, equivalent in the three groups. Other studies have also reported a decreased incidence of late potentials on a signal average ECG in patients receiving thrombolytic agents compared with a control group.[167] Bourke and co-workers[168] reported electrophysiologic data on 87 of 159 patients randomized to therapy with streptokinase (n = 20), aspirin (n = 25), both agents (n = 21), or both placebo (n = 21). Sustained ventricular tachycardia was inducible in eight patients (17%) receiving streptokinase placebo but in no patient receiving streptokinase (p = 0.0005). The use of aspirin did not affect inducibility. During follow-up, there were three arrhythmic events in the streptokinase placebo group but none in those receiving streptokinase (p = NS).

Congenital Heart Disease

Another group of patients reported to be at high risk of sudden cardiac death are those with congenital heart disease, including those who have had surgical repair. Although there is a significantly increased risk of sudden cardiac death in this group of patients, only a few studies have reported the incidence of ventricular arrhythmia in patients with congenital heart disease and its association with sudden death. An additional problem is that there are many diverse congenital abnormalities that result in either right or left ventricular myocardial dysfunction and can be responsible for arrhythmia. A last concern is that conduction abnormalities are also frequent in this group of patients, especially after surgery, and bradyarrhythmias be an important etiologic factor for sudden death.

The majority of reports about the incidence and prognostic significance of VPBs in congenital heart disease involve patients with tetralogy of Fallot, a relatively common congenital abnormality. These studies have primarily reported the incidence of VPBs after surgical repair. Garson and co-workers[169] reported on 207 patients who underwent repair of tetralogy of Fallot. Twenty-one (10.3%) had VPBs on a routine postoperative ECG and eight (38%) of these patients died suddenly 3 months to 10 years after the operation. These investigators reported that all eight patients who succumbed to sudden death had the combination of VPBs and a postoperative right ventricular systolic pressure >70 mmHg. In another study, by Garson and co-workers,[170] 27 patients with tetralogy of Fallot were followed prospectively. In this trial, noninvasive hemodynamic and invasive electrophysiologic data were recorded. These investigators reported that the induction of NSVT or sustained ventricular tachycardia during electrophysiologic testing was associated with a history of syncope, and these patients had a greater prevalence of complex ventricular arrhythmia on 24-hour ambulatory monitoring (63%) compared with those with no inducible arrhythmia in whom complex arrhythmia was absent (p <0.001). While not all patients at risk of syncope and arrhythmia had arrhythmia on ambulatory monitoring, the presence of frequent VPBs was related to the induction of a sustained ventricular tachyarrhythmia. In this study, the role of electrophysiologic testing was uncertain. While Garson et al. recommended that such studies are essential for any patient with syncope, the role in patients with asymptomatic arrhythmia remains undefined.

Chandar and co-workers[171] reported a multicenter retrospective study of 359 patients who underwent surgery for tetralogy of Fallot. On ambulatory monitoring, 48% of patients had spontaneous VPBs, while 17% had sustained monomorphic ventricular tachycardia induced during electrophysiologic study. Spontaneous VPBs and induced ventricular tachycardia were significantly related to a later age at surgery, a longer follow-up interval, symptoms of syncope or presyncope, and right ventricular systolic hypertension. Similarly, VPBs documented on monitoring were more complex when the patient was older at the time of repair and the duration of follow-up increased. Induction of ventricular tachycardia during electrophysiologic study correlated with spontaneous VPBs, particularly the presence of NSVT on ambulatory monitoring. Indeed, ventricular tachycardia was not induced in patients who were asymptomatic, had no arrhythmia on ambulatory monitoring, and had a normal right ventricular systolic pressure. Late sudden death occurred in five patients, most of whom had spontaneous arrhythmia on ambulatory monitoring and a right ventricular diastolic pressure of >8 mmHg. However, none of these patients had ventricular tachycardia induced during electrophysiologic testing. This again suggests that complex arrhythmia, particularly NSVT, is associated with an increased risk of sudden death, but the results of electrophysiologic testing are not helpful.

There appears to be an association between conduction abnormalities, VPBs, and risk of sudden death. Quattlebaum and co-workers[172] followed 243 patients who underwent total correction of a tetralogy of Fallot. The follow-up period in this group of patients averaged 12 years. During this time, there were seven cardiac deaths, four of which occurred in patients with a new right bundle-branch block (RBBB) after surgery. Three of these four patients also had VPBs for more than 1 month postoperatively. VPBs were documented in 10 of 158 patients with a new RBBB and sudden cardiac death occurred in 3 (30%). Three of 10 patients with a RBBB, a left anterior hemiblock, and prolonged PR interval (trifascicular disease) died suddenly. The risk of sudden death seemed to be associated with the presence of VPBs in association with conduction disease. Quattlebaum et al. concluded that the risk of sudden death in patients with a trifascicular disease or RBBB and VPBs after repair of a tetralogy of Fallot is high and that further evaluation is warranted.

These studies do not prove a relationship between VPBs and sudden death, however, and, unfortunately, there are no data about the incidence or type of VPBs in postoperative patients with tetralogy of Fallot. Moreover, the mechanism for sudden death is unclear. While it appears that the cause is a ventricular tachyarrhythmia, a bradyarrhythmia is also possible. Horowitz and co-workers[173] did report the result of EP testing in four patients with surgically corrected tetralogy of Fallot who had spontaneous episodes of sustained ventricular tachycardia. In each patient, endocardial mapping demonstrated that the site of origin of the ventricular tachycardia was the right ventricular outflow tract. Intraoperative mapping confirmed that the reentrant circuit was at this site.

Relationship Between VPBs and Prognosis

It appears from these many studies involving patients with various types of heart disease that the arrhythmia of prognostic significance is NSVT. In the absence of structural heart disease, ventricular arrhythmia, regardless of type or frequency, is of no prognostic importance. The risk of sudden death in these patients is low and is unrelated to ventricular arrhythmia.

An important question relates to why NSVT is an important marker for increased risk of sudden death. There are several potential explanations. It is possible that NSVT is an epiphenomeon, an indicator of the presence and severity of myocardial disease, and that the presence of underlying disease and its severity are the only important factors associated with the increased risk of sudden death. NSVT itself is of no importance. However, most studies have not shown any difference in the extent of disease between patients with and without NSVT. There does not appear to be an association among the presence, frequency, or complexity of VPBs and the extent of heart disease or the degree of LV dysfunction. While the incidence and frequency of NSVT may be greatest in those with more advanced heart disease, NSVT is also common in those with less serious heart disease, and in such patients it is an independent risk factor. In a number of studies there is no association for LVEF, pulmonary artery pressure, or the extent of CAD and ventricular arrhythmia.

It is possible that NSVT serves as a trigger for a sustained ventricular tachyarrhythmia. It has been established that there is a sequential reduction in the threshold of ventricular fibrillation as the number of repetitive VPBs increases.[174] In addition, it has been reported that the chances of activating the reentrant circuit and inducing a reentrant arrhythmia are increased when several premature beats are added in succession.[175] This is important, since the most frequent mechanism for a ventricular tachyarrhythmia is reentry.

Lastly, it is possible that NSVT, a result of reentry that is self-limited, will become a sustained ventricular tachyarrhythmia when the appropriate preconditions are present. These include changes in catecholamine levels, sympathetic tone, electrolyte levels, ischemia, and pH, which provide the appropriate milieu for a reentrant arrhythmia to become sustained (i.e., NSVT converted to a sustained arrhythmia).

DRUG THERAPY FOR THE PREVENTION OF SUDDEN DEATH

Although data now suggest that ventricular arrhythmia, specifically runs of NSVT, is an important indicator of the patient at risk for sudden cardiac death, there are as yet no data to show that therapy based on the suppression of such arrhythmia will prevent this fatal outcome. Unfortunately, only a few studies have addressed this issue, and the majority of these investigations were poorly designed. These studies generally involved patients with structural heart disease, primarily those with a recent MI.

Post-MI β-Blocker Trials

There are now a number of trials that have addressed the role of drug therapy in the post-MI patient for preventing sudden cardiac death. Some of the earliest trials involved the use of β-blocking agents. In an early study carried out by Snow and Manc,[176] propranolol or placebo were administered to 101 patients who were followed for 1 month. Propranolol significantly reduced the incidence of death compared with placebo. However, several studies reported thereafter failed to document any benefit from propranolol.[177–179] More recent studies involving large numbers of patients followed for longer periods of time have reported that many β-blockers are beneficial for reducing cardiac and sudden death mortality in patients after MI[180–187] (Table 28-12). β-Blockers have been acutely administered by the intravenous route[186] or

prescribed as oral therapy. When given acutely, they have reduced the frequency of ventricular arrhythmia and have decreased the incidence of early ventricular tachycardia and ventricular fibrillation.[186] A similar beneficial effect has been reported when long-term oral therapy has been used. The Beta Blocker Heart Attack Trial (BHAT)[180] involved 3,857 post-MI patients randomized to therapy with propranolol or placebo. After a 2-year follow-up, there was a significant reduction in mortality from 9.8% on placebo to 7.2% on propranolol (p <0.01) (Fig. 28-9). A multicenter Norwegian trial[181] involving 560 patients followed for 1 year also reported a significant reduction in mortality (8.2% versus 4.0%, p = 0.038). Other β-blocking agents have been reported to be effective in the post-MI patient. A multicenter Norwegian trial of oral timolol involved 1,884 patients followed for an average of 33 months.[187] The mortality was 13.9% in the placebo group compared with 7.7% in those receiving timolol (p <0.001). Studies involving the use of atenolol,[188] alprenolol,[182–184] practolol,[185] and metoprolol[186] have also reported a similar reduction in mortality resulting from β-blocker therapy. While most β-blockers have been reported to be of benefit for preventing sudden death in the post-MI patient, exceptions are those agents that have intrinsic sympathomimetic activity (ISA), including oxprenolol[189] and pindolol,[190] or agents that have other antiarrhythmic effects, such as sotalol.[191]

Although β-blockers are an effective therapy for preventing sudden death in the post-MI patient, it must be pointed out that there are limitations to these studies.

TABLE 28-12. Randomized Trials of β-Blockers in Patients After a Myocardial Infarction

Study	Drug	n	Duration of Follow-up	Mortality or Sudden Death (%)		p
				Control	Drug	
Snow[176]	Propranolol	101	28 days	12.0	6.0	<0.03
Multicenter[185]	Propranolol	195	28 days	9.3	7.1	NS
Balcon[178]	Propranolol	114	28 days	10.5	12.3	NS
Norris[179]	Propranolol	454	3 wk	7.5	8.8	NS
BHAT[180]	Propranolol	3,857	2 yr	9.8	7.2	<0.01
Norwegian[187]	Propranolol	560	1 yr	8.2	4.0	<0.038
Wilhelmsson[182]	Alprenolol	230	2 yr	9.6	2.6	<0.05
Ahlmark[183]	Alprenolol	162	1 yr	11.1	1.2	<0.05
Andersen[184]	Alprenolol	282	1 yr	20.6	9.2	<0.01
Multicenter[185]	Practolol	3,038	1 yr	3.6	2.0	<0.01
Hjalmarson[186]	Metoprolol	1,395	90 days	8.9	5.7	<0.03
Norwegian[187]	Timolol	1,884	33 mo	13.9	7.7	<0.001
Julian[191]	Sotalol	1,456	1 yr	8.9	7.3	NS
Taylor[189]	Oxprenolol	1,103	6 yr	9.3	8.2	NS
Australian/ Swedish[190]	Pindolol	529	2 yr	18	17	NS

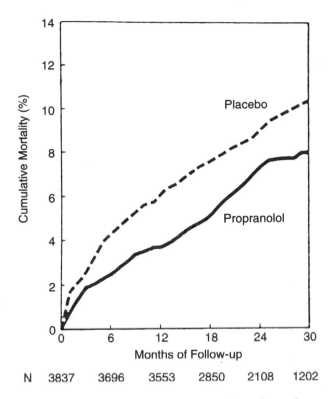

Fig. 28-9. Kaplan-Meier survival curves in patients after a myocardial infarction treated with propranolol or control. (From BHAT,[180] with permission.)

1. Most patients (up to 77% in some trials) were excluded from the study. Reasons for exclusion include a contraindication to β-blocker use, including CHF, hypotension, conduction abnormalities, bradycardia, and lung disease; other conditions requiring β-blocker therapy, including hypertension, angina, and arrhythmia; the use of β-blockers prior to the MI; possible need for surgery; or the need for antiarrhythmic drug therapy because of symptomatic or serious arrhythmia. Therefore, in most of these studies, patients were highly selected and only those at low risk were entered.
2. Most of the studies provide no data about the presence, type, and frequency of arrhythmia before or during therapy.
3. Fixed doses of β-blockers were used. Often, β-blocker therapy was not titrated to their physiologic effect (i.e., heart rate slowing).
4. No data about other therapies, either medical or nonmedical, were used.
5. There is no assessment of patient compliance.

Despite these many limitations, it is clear that the prophylactic use of oral β-blocker in the post-MI patient is associated with an improvement in survival.

The reason for this beneficial effect is uncertain, however, but it does not appear that the mechanism is suppression of arrhythmia. Unfortunately, most studies do not report baseline arrhythmia, nor do they evaluate the effect of β-blockers on arrhythmia. The BHAT trial did perform ambulatory monitoring before and during β-blocker therapy in a subset of patients.[192] Although the survival was better in patients who had less frequent and less serious forms of arrhythmia, this was not associated with the use of β-blockade. β-blockers did, however, prevent the expected increase in arrhythmia frequency during the 6-month follow-up. Proposed mechanisms for the beneficial effect of β-blockers include elevation of the ventricular fibrillation threshold; prevention of ischemia or new MI; interference with the effect of circulating catecholamines on the myocardium that is healing, irritable, and unstable; or perhaps the prevention of catecholamine-induced hypokalemia. While the exact etiology for the beneficial effect of β-blockers is uncertain, it is clear that β-blockers are an important intervention for preventing sudden death in the postinfarction patient.

Antiarrhythmic Drug Therapy in Post-MI Patients

There have been a number of trials in which standard antiarrhythmic drugs have been administered to patients after MI in an attempt to reduce sudden cardiac death (Table 28-13). Probably the most frequently used antiarrhythmic drug during an AMI is intravenous lidocaine.[193–195] Interestingly, only the study of Lie and co workers[196] reported that lidocaine reduced the incidence of ventricular fibrillation or in-hospital mortality. Most of these studies involved small numbers of patients and, as expected, therapy was limited to only a few days. Several long-term studies have used the lidocaine congeners, tocainide,[197,198] mexiletine,[199,200] and aprindine.[201,202] Unfortunately, none reported that these drugs had any beneficial effect on survival. The largest study, IMPACT,[203] actually reported an increased mortality in the patient group receiving mexiletine compared with those on placebo (7.6% versus 4.8%), although this did not reach statistical significance. There have been studies in which quinidine,[204–206] disopyramide,[207,208] procainamide,[209,210] and phenytoin[211,212] have been administered to post-MI patients. In general, these studies reported no beneficial effect for preventing sudden death in the post-MI patient. However, there are a number of methodologic problems with these trials:

1. Generally, small numbers of patients were entered and, since the endpoint (i.e., total cardiac mortality or sudden death mortality) is a relatively low frequency event, many more patients are required if any effect is to be observed.

**TABLE 28-13. Randomized Trials of Antiarrhythmic Drugs in Patients
Postmyocardial Infarction**

Study	Drug	n	Duration	Mortality or Sudden Death (%) Control	Mortality or Sudden Death (%) Drug	p
Morgensen[195]	Lidocaine	79	days	11.0	12.0	NS
Bennett[193]	Lidocaine	610	days	7.0	16.0	NS
Lie[196]	Lidocaine	212	days	10.8	0	<0.05
Ryden[198]	Tocainide	112	6 mo	8.9	8.9	NS
Campbells[199]	Mexiletine	97	4 yr	4.8	2.3	NS
Chamberlain[197]	Mexiletine	344	1 yr	11.6	13.2	NS
IMPACT[203]	Mexiletine	630	1 yr	1.8	7.6	NS
Hugenholtz[201]	Aprindine	193	1 yr	9.3	7.3	NS
Gottlieb[202]	Aprindine	143	1 yr	22.2	17.8	NS
Jones[206]	Quinidine	103	3 days	12.4	8.9	NS
Holmberg[204]	Quinidine	104	15 days	7.2	10.7	NS
Jennings[207]	Disopyramide	95	1 yr	10.2	4.0	NS
Zainal[208]	Disopyramide	60	3 wk	26.7	3.3	<0.05
Kock-Wiser[209]	Procainamide	70	3 wk	6.1	0	<0.05
Kosowsky[210]	Procainamide	78	1 yr	10.3	3.7	<0.05
Collaborative[212]	Phenytoin	560	1 yr	11.0	9.4	NS
Peter[211]	Phenytoin	150	2 yr	18.0	24.0	NS
Burkart[215]	Amiodarone	312	1 yr	16.7	5.1	0.048
CAST[218]	Encainide/flecainide	1,455	10 mo	3.0	7.7	<0.001

2. Baseline arrhythmia was often not evaluated or only poorly documented. Usually, only ECG strips were used for arrhythmia detection and quantification.

3. All patients were entered, irrespective of the type and frequency of arrhythmia present.

4. Reproducibility of arrhythmia was not established. Most of the studies did not use ambulatory monitoring; therefore, there are no available data about this issue.

5. The duration of therapy in most studies was limited to only several weeks or months.

6. A fixed dose of drug was used; often, this dose was subtherapeutic.

7. There was no attempt to titrate dose based on anti-arrhythmia suppression.

8. For the most part, there was no systematic evaluation of drug effect. Ambulatory monitoring was not used for evaluating the effect of drug on arrhythmia frequency.

9. As a rule, drug therapy was continued even if arrhythmia persisted.

10. Side effects from antiarrhythmic drugs were frequent, and withdrawal of patients from studies was common.

11. No information about the addition of other therapies was supplied by these studies.

12. The effect of other intercurrent diseases was not evaluated.

13. Importantly, there was no consideration given for the potential of these drugs to aggravate arrhyth-

mia. This occurs in approximately 9% of patients,[213,214] and this adverse effect certainly could have negated any beneficial effect from the drugs.

Burkart and co-workers[215] recently reported on 312 survivors of an AMI who had complex VPBs (multiform or NSVT) on ambulatory monitoring obtained just before hospital discharge. Patients were randomized to individualized antiarrhythmic drug therapy (group 1, n = 100), low-dose amiodarone (200 mg/day)-(group 2, n = 98), or no antiarrhythmic therapy (group 3, n = 114). After a 1-year follow-up, there were 10 arrhythmic events in group 1, 5 in group 2, and 19 in group 3. Compared with control, amiodarone significantly reduced the risk of an arrhythmic event (p = 0.024) and improved survival (p = 0.048). There was no statistically significant difference between amiodarone and individualized care. These data are suggestive, but not conclusive, since only a small number of patients were involved.

In a meta-analysis performed by Furburg,[216] none of the antiarrhythmic drugs analyzed by subclass was of benefit in preventing sudden death (Table 28-14). Indeed, mortality tended to be higher in those receiving active therapy compared with the placebo group.

Given the lack of meaningful data about the role of antiarrhythmic drugs in post-MI drugs, the National Institutes of Health (NIH) established a pilot protocol, the Cardiac Arrhythmia Pilot Study (CAPS), which was designed to determine the feasibility of performing a large-scale trial to evaluate the role of long-term

TABLE 28-14. Meta-analysis of Post MI Drug Trials

Drug Class	Total n	Mortality (%)			Change in Mortality (%)
		Drug	Control	Odds Ratio	
I (overall)	19,896	5.4	4.8	1.11	+ 12.5
IA	3,693	7.3	7.3	1.01	0
IB	13,801	4.4	4.0	1.08	+ 10
IC	2,395	7.6	5.8	1.42	+ 31
II	53,224	5.4	6.6	0.81	− 12
III	539	12.1	14.6	0.78	− 21
IV	19,532	9.9	9.6	1.03	+ 3.4

(Adapted from Teo et al.,[236] with permission.)

suppression of arrhythmia with antiarrhythmic drugs for preventing sudden arrhythmic death in post-MI patients.[217] In CAPS, 500 patients with >10 VPBs/h documented on ambulatory monitoring were randomized to therapy with encainide, flecainide, moricizine, imipramine, or placebo. The drug used and the dose administered were based on arrhythmia suppression, with efficacy defined as greater than 70% reduction in VPB frequency. This pilot study was not designed as a mortality trial but was simply a feasibility study. Encainide, flecainide, and moricizine were associated with adequate arrhythmia suppression and were well tolerated by patients with a low rate of withdrawal.[31] For this reason, they were selected for use in the definitive mortality trial, the Cardiac Arrhythmia Suppression Trial (CAST).[218] The goal of CAST was the randomization of more than 4,000 patients with a recent MI who had >6 VPBs/h documented on ambulatory monitoring. For those patients with MI within 3 months of entry into the study, the LVEF had to be less than 55%, while it had to be less than 40% if the MI occurred 3 months to 2 years before entry.

The CAST protocol consisted of three periods. The first was a screening phase during which 24-hour ambulatory monitoring was obtained to document arrhythmia frequency and identify candidates for entry. Patients who had an adequate density of arrhythmia entered an open-labeled, non-placebo-controlled dose-titration phase during which one of the three study drugs was administered. The dose was titrated upward until a greater than 80% reduction in VPBs and a greater than 90% decrease in runs of NSVT were achieved. If the agent proved ineffective, an alternative drug was administered. Patients responding to antiarrhythmic therapy entered the double-blind phase and were randomized to treatment with the drug and dose established as effective during the open label phase or to placebo.

In April 1989, after an average follow-up of 10 months, the preliminary results of CAST were reported.[218] At that time, 730 patients were randomized to receive encainide and flecainide, while 725 patients were in the matching placebo group. Patients receiv-

ing encainide or flecainide had a significantly higher total cardiac (7.7%) and sudden death mortality (4.5%) compared with the placebo group (3.0% and 1.2%, respectively, p = 0.0003 and p = 0.0006, respectively) (Fig. 28-10). The relative risk of death from arrhythmia in the drug-treated group was 3.6%, and the relative risk of mortality from all causes was 2.5%. The increased mortality resulting from encainide and flecainide occurred in all subgroups analyzed and was independent of baseline LVEF or VPB frequency.

Implications of CAST

A number of inescapable conclusions can be drawn from CAST. Clearly, encainide and flecainide therapy in patients with a recent MI increases total cardiac mortality, especially sudden death caused by arrhythmia. It would appear that the mechanism for this increased mortality was arrhythmia aggravation although a bradyarrhythmia caused by a conduction abnormality is also possible. However, it is not certain whether these results can be applied to all other class IC agents or, indeed, to all other antiarrhythmic drugs. Unfortunately, there are no similar arrhythmia suppression trials involving the other available agents. It has been well established that the beneficial or adverse effects of one antiarrhythmic drugs do not predict similar effects from any other agent, even if of the same subclass. Therefore, application of the results with these two agents to other drugs has no scientific validity. In addition, it is uncertain whether the results of CAST can be applied to other patient groups. It must be remembered that CAST involved patients with a recent MI, and it has been reported that, in such patients, the myocardial substrate is changing during the follow-up period. The myocardium is undergoing a process of healing, scarring, and remodeling, all of which alter the underlying electrophysiologic properties. Therefore, these patients are different from other patient groups in whom the substrate is relatively stable. Although similar mortality studies in other patient groups are lacking, encainide and flecainide had

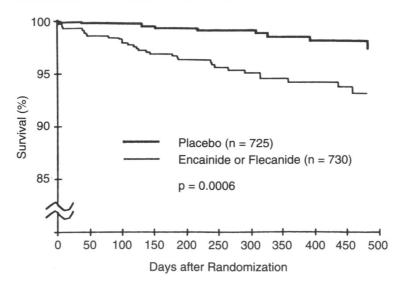

Fig. 28-10. Kaplan-Meier curves based on arrhythmic death or cardiac arrest among 1,455 patients with a recent myocardial infarction randomized to encainide or flecainide or matching placebo. (From CAST,[218] with permission.)

previously been administered to patients with VPBs who had various cardiac diagnosis as part of the development and approval process for these agents. Although the risk of arrhythmia aggravation was known to be high in patients with significant underlying heart disease and with a history of sustained ventricular tachyarrhythmias,[219,220] a similar risk was not observed in other groups of patients with less serious arrhythmias and less advanced heart disease.[221-223] It is important to note that patients with a recent MI were generally excluded these earlier studies and, therefore, data in this group were unavailable.

A second conclusion is that although VPBs were suppressed by encainide and flecainide, the risk of sudden death was increased. It has been suggested that perhaps suppression of VPBs with an antiarrhythmic drug selects out a low-risk group of patients who would do well and do not require antiarrhythmic therapy. It is uncertain whether the results from CAST negate the VPB hypothesis, that is, VPBs are associated with an increased risk of sudden death in the patient with a recent MI. Not only is there uncertainty about the meaning of VPBs in post-MI patients, but CAST has called into question the prognostic meaning of VPBs in those with other forms of heart disease. However, it should be pointed out that in CAST, the average LVEF was 39%, and 52% of patients had an ejection fraction of greater than 40%. In addition, only 20% of patients had runs of NSVT, and in only 10% was there more than one run during the 24-hour monitoring period. This is an important concern, since each of the post-MI trials reported that the increased risk of sudden death was associated with NSVT and an LVEF of less than <40%. In the absence of these two factors,

VPBs themselves, regardless of frequency and multiformity, had no prognosis importance. Therefore, the population entered into CAST was primarily a low-risk group, confirmed by the low mortality in the placebo group. Thus, the role of antiarrhythmic drugs for preventing sudden death in post-MI patients or other groups with a reduced LVEF who have NSVT was not answered by this study.

Another important concern, perhaps accounting for the low mortality in the placebo group, was the use of other interventions such as thrombolysis, angioplasty, bypass surgery, and the administration of β-blockers. It has been reported that these other interventions affect the outcome of the post-MI patient. While only a minority of patients in CAST underwent these interventions, they may have had an important impact on the study and its results. It is likely that these interventions alter prognosis and that new mortality statistics in the post-MI patient are necessary.

A third conclusion is that in the post-MI patient there is an increased risk of arrhythmia aggravation due to encainide and flecainide. In addition, it appears that arrhythmia aggravation is not only an early event, but since it occurred throughout the entire follow-up period, it may also be a late complication. This is in contrast to previous perceptions about arrhythmia aggravation, as observed in other groups of patients, in which it is usually an early complication, occurring during the first few days after the initiation of therapy.[213,224] In fact, all the patients in CAST who were entered into the randomized, double-blind placebo-controlled phase had previously responded to the antiarrhythmic drug. Nevertheless, arrhythmia aggravation occurred during follow-up. Unfortunately, the precise etiology of death in CAST is not certain. While it has been assumed that the mechanism was a ventricular tachyarrhythmia, it is possible that in some patients a bradyarrhythmia occurred, a result of the depressive effects of these drugs on conduction.

Concerns About CAST

Although CAST is a very important study and has provided clinicians with useful data about therapy of VPBs in post-MI patients, a number of important concerns about this trial and its limitations deserve emphasis. Although this study clearly points out that patients with asymptomatic, but frequent, VPBs should not be treated with antiarrhythmic drugs, the role of this therapy in patients with reduced LV function who have NSVT are lacking, and no conclusions can be made based on this study.

The placebo mortality of 3% is the lowest mortality ever reported in a post-MI trail. It is likely that only low-risk patients were entered into CAST as a result of liberal entry criteria and physician bias (i.e., high-risk patients with frequent runs of NSVT and LV dysfunction were not entered). Therefore, the study primarily involved patients with intact LV function who had only frequent VPBs, and these are not the high-risk patients with a substantial mortality for whom drug therapy might be of benefit. This is the most important concern about CAST, as it had been assumed that the mortality in the placebo group would be 11% to 15%. If the placebo mortality had indeed been this high, the study might have had a different outcome.

The use of other interventions such as thrombolysis, angioplasty, surgery, and β-blockers has no doubt affected mortality in the post-MI patients and may have, in part, accounted for the low placebo mortality. Such recent interventions clearly have an important effect on the prognosis of patients after MI; therefore, a new baseline mortality in such patients must be established. In addition, there is growing evidence that the traditional risk factors, important in the post-MI patient for risk stratification (i.e., NSVT, low LVEF, late potentials) have a less important role in the patient who has received thrombolysis.

Other methods of evaluating postinfarction patients, including signal averaging and, importantly, exercise testing, were not used in CAST. Exercise testing has become an important tool in the post-MI patient for risk stratification. More importantly, it is a useful test for providing a complete evaluation of antiarrhythmic drug effect, especially for exposing the potential for arrhythmia aggravation. It has been reported that of those patients who experience arrhythmia aggravation, one-third do so during an exercise test at a time when ambulatory monitoring documents arrhythmia suppression.[219] It is possible that exercise testing would have identified potential problems, es-

pecially during the follow-up period. In addition, in CAST, once an effective drug was identified, ambulatory monitoring during the follow-up period was performed only infrequently. As it is well established that there is considerable random variability of arrhythmia in these patients, it is possible that the drug that was effective during the initial portion of this trial was no longer of benefit during the follow-up period or, indeed, may have been associated with a worsening of arrhythmia. In view of the healing myocardium and changing substrate, such variability is likely to be substantial. It is likely that, as a result of a change in the underlying myocardial electrophysiologic properties, the effect of the drug at one point in time differs from its action at another time.

It must be remembered that CAST involved only post-MI patients and the adverse outcome was reported with only two agents, encainide and flecainide. The third drug, moricizine, was not initially implicated. However, the recent results of CAST II showed that moricizine was also associated with a trend toward an increase in mortality, although this was not statistically significant, and required 3 days to become obvious. At this time, the widespread application of the results of CAST to other patient groups is not appropriate. Nevertheless, CAST has had a major impact on the approach to antiarrhythmic drug therapy for all patients with both ventricular and supraventricular arrhythmia and has influenced the use of all antiarrhythmic drugs.

Antiarrhythmic Therapy in Patients With Chronic CAD

Unfortunately, very few studies have addressed the issue of ventricular arrhythmia suppression and the prevention of sudden cardiac death in patients with chronic CAD. Blevins and co-workers[225] studied 33 patients with CAD who had frequent complex ventricular arrhythmias. Patients who had previously experienced sustained ventricular tachycardia or out-of-hospital sudden cardiac death or who had an AMI were excluded from this trial. Drug selection for the suppression of ventricular arrhythmia was guided by 24-hour ambulatory monitoring. Patients were discharged on the single most effect antiarrhythmic agent; after a 24-month follow-up, 18 patients survived while 15 patients died suddenly. There was no difference between these groups with respect to age, gender, or baseline ventricular arrhythmia. The patients who survived had a higher LVEF (51% versus 34%, p < 0.01) and were more likely to have suppression of complex ventricular arrhythmia (83% versus 40%, p < 0.01). Another study, reported by Hoffmann and co-workers,[226] evaluated 50 patients with CAD who had frequent VPBs and repetitive ventricular arrhythmia. Group 1 patients (n = 39) were those who responded to an antiarrhythmic drug with suppression of ventricular arrhythmia defined as elimination of all repetitive forms and reduction of VPBs to <30/h, while group 2 patients (n = 11) were those in whom antiarrhythmic drugs failed to suppress arrhythmia adequately. After a follow-up of 16 months, patients who did not have complete control of arrhythmia had a higher sudden death mortality (27% versus 3%, p < 0.05). The cumulative probability of survival at 12 months was 0.93 for responders and 0.64 for nonresponders (p < 0.005).

Unfortunately, neither of the above trials was prospective or randomized. Rather, the two groups were defined by response to antiarrhythmic drugs. Therefore, there are no good data about the role of antiarrhythmic drugs for preventing sudden death in patients with chronic CAD.

Antiarrhythmic Drug Therapy in Patients With a Cardiomyopathy and CHF

While it appears that the presence of NSVT in patients with CHF and a cardiomyopathy of any etiology increases the risk of sudden cardiac death, there are as yet limited data about the role of antiarrhythmic drug therapy in such patients. Chakko and Gheorghiade[75] randomized 23 patients with a cardiomyopathy and ventricular arrhythmia to therapy with either procainamide or quinidine, while 20 patients were left untreated. During the follow-up period, there were 16 deaths, 10 of which were sudden. Sudden death, however, was independent of therapy. Unfortunately, the role of antiarrhythmic drugs is uncertain, as therapy in this trial was not guided by arrhythmia suppression. In the report of Unverferth and co-workers,[74] 24 or 69 patients were treated with antiarrhythmic drugs. Although the 1-year mortality was not affected by drug therapy, no conclusions are possible as there was no attempt to suppress arrhythmia with these drugs. Parmley and Chatterjee[227] reviewed the outcome of 26 patients with CHF and complex arrhythmia who were treated with procainamide, quinidine, or amiodarone. Unfortunately, this was not a randomized study, and the effect of the drugs on arrhythmia frequency is not commented on. However, sudden death mortality was decreased in patients receiving antiarrhythmic drug therapy. Neri and co-workers[80] reported on 41 patients with a dilated cardiomyopathy treated with amiodarone. The drug significantly reduced the frequency and complexity of ventricular arrhythmia as well as sudden death (0 versus 4 on placebo). Although patients were not randomized, 91 patients in the study of Keogh and co-workers[79] were taking amiodarone. However, there was no difference in survival when compared with patients on no therapy (p = 0.45). There are, unfortunately, no other studies in which antiarrhythmic therapy has been used. Several ongoing trials are addressing the issue of suppression of arrhythmia in patients with cardiomyopathy, but it will be several years before the data are available.

Preliminary data indicate that β-blockers may have an important effect on survival in patients with cardiomyopathy and CHF. In an early study by Swedberg and co-workers,[228] the survival of 24 patients with CHF treated with metoprolol was improved. Unfortunately, there was no comparative placebo group in this trial; rather, Swedberg et al. compared the results with historic controls. Anderson and co-workers[229] randomly assigned 50 patients with CHF to receive standard therapy alone or therapy along with metoprolol. While there was no difference in outcome between the groups when analyzed by intention to treat, there was a favorable trend in survival in the group receiving metoprolol when analyzed for actual treatment received. In the BHAT report, the greatest impact of propranolol on survival was in those patients with CHF who received the β-blocker.[230,231] The reduction in sudden death was 47% in post-MI patients with CHF receiving propranolol compared with a 13% reduction in the propranolol-treated patients who did not have CHF. Therefore, it would appear that β-blocker therapy in patients with cardiomyopathy and CHF may improve outcome. However, caution is urged, since β-blockers may worsen CHF in this group of patients. Further studies are therefore essential.

INDICATIONS FOR ANTIARRHYTHMIC DRUG THERAPY

There are two general indications for treating patients who have arrhythmia. The first is to relieve symptoms caused by the arrhythmia, and the second is to prevent sudden cardiac death. While antiarrhythmic drugs are effective for the former indication, there are as yet no data indicating that they are of benefit in any group of patients for the prevention of sudden cardiac death. One exception are those patients who have already experienced sudden death because of a sustained ventricular tachycardia or ventricular fibrillation. When antiarrhythmic drug therapy is selected invasively or noninvasively, guided by objective criteria of arrhythmia suppression, a recurrence of arrhythmia can be prevented and life prolonged.[232–235] It is therefore important that the benefit versus risk of therapy be evaluated for each individual patient before antiarrhythmic drugs are administered.

Patients with NSVT who have no heart disease are not at risk of sudden death. When the arrhythmia is asymptomatic, there is no benefit from antiarrhythmic drug therapy. Drug therapy is associated with a risk of arrhythmia aggravation and, although it is low in this group, the risk-benefit ratio is unfavorable. If the NSVT is associated with symptoms, it must be established whether the nature, severity, and frequency of the symptoms and, therefore, the benefits of their relief, are worth the risks, particularly aggravated arrhythmia, involved with antiarrhythmic drug therapy. This requires an individualized decision. Patients with NSVT who have structural heart disease are at an increased risk of sudden death, but there are as yet no data suggesting that therapy, guided invasively or noninvasively, based on the suppression of such forms, will prevent this outcome and prolong life. In the absence of arrhythmia-related symptoms, it is uncertain whether there is any benefit from therapy. In these patients, the use of antiarrhythmic drugs is associated with a moderate risk of arrhythmia aggravation, and other toxicity and cautious use is required. At this time, therapy is not routinely indicated for such patients, although there may be some subgroups who would benefit. Any decision about therapy requires consideration of the individual patient. For patients with symptoms caused by the NSVT, it must determine whether the benefits associated with relief of these symptoms outweighs the risks associated with therapy. As with patients who have no heart disease, the nature, severity, and frequency of the symptoms must be considered.

Patients who have already experienced sudden cardiac death are at significantly increased risk of a recurrence. There is now a substantial body of data indicating that antiarrhythmic drugs can prevent a recurrent episode in this group of patients, when efficacy is based on objective criteria, derived by invasive or noninvasive methods.[232-235] Although the risk of toxicity, particularly aggravated arrhythmia, is high in these patients, it would appear that the benefits outweigh the risks and that antiarrhythmic therapy is indicated for this group.

CONCLUSIONS

The past 20 years have provided the clinician with a great amount of data about the meaning of ventricular arrhythmia in patients with and without heart disease. It has become clear that NSVT, when associated with underlying heart disease, and especially in the setting of LV dysfunction, is associated with an increased risk of sudden cardiac death. Other noninvasive techniques, including the signal-averaged ECG and determination of heart rate variability provided further insight into the identification of the individual at risk. While our ability to identify a high-risk patient group has improved, identification of the individual patient is still a challenge. Moreover, there as are yet no conclusive data that suppression of this arrhythmia will afford protection from a sustained ventricular

tachyarrhythmia and result in prolongation of life. The only placebo-controlled arrhythmia-suppression study to date has been CAST. Unfortunately, the results of CAST do not provide enough data in high-risk patients and therefore, this issue remains uncertain. It is hoped that future studies directed at patients with poor LV function and NSVT will provide necessary data about the role of antiarrhythmic drug therapy for suppression of such arrhythmia.

REFERENCES

1. Lown B: Sudden cardiac death: the major challenge confronting contemporary cardiology. Am J Cardiol 43: 313, 1979
2. Kannel WB, Doyle JT, McNamara PM et al: Precursors of sudden cardiac death. Factors related to the incidence of sudden death. Circulation 51:608, 1975
3. Wit AL, Cranefield PF: Reentrant excitation as a cause of cardiac arrhythmias. Am J Physiol 235:H1, 1978
4. Wit AL, Rosen MR: Pathophysiologic mechanisms of cardiac arrhythmias. Am Heart J 106:798, 1983
5. Harris A, Rojas AG: Initiation of ventricular fibrillation due to coronary occlusion. Exp Med Surg 1:105, 1943
6. El Sherif N, Mehra R, Gough WB, Zuber RH: Ventricular activation patterns of spontaneous and induced ventricular rhythms in canine one day old myocardial infarction. Evidence for focal and reentrant mechanisms. Circ Res 51:152, 1982
7. El-Sherif N, Smith A, Evans K: Canine ventricular arrhythmias in the late myocardial infarction period: epicardial mapping of reentrant circuits. Circ Res 449:225, 1981
8. Podrid PJ, Fuchs T, Candinas R: Role of sympathetic nervous system in the genesis of ventricular arrhythmia. Circulation, suppl I. 82:I-103, 1990
9. Podrid PJ: Potassium and ventricular arrhythmia. Am J Cardiol 65:33E, 1990
10. Patterson E, Holand K, Eller BT, Lucchesi BR: Ventricular fibrillation resulting from ischemia at a site remote from previous myocardial infarction. A conscious canine model of sudden cardiac death. Am J Cardiol 50: 1414, 1982
11. Podrid PJ: Treatment of ventricular arrhythmia. Noninvasive vs invasive approach—applications and limitations. Chest 88:121, 1985
12. Soloff LA: Reference ventricular premature beats diagnostic of myocardial disease. Am J Med Sci 242:315, 1961
13. Moulton KP, Medcalf T, Lazzara R: Premature ventricular complex morphology. A marker for left ventricular structure and function. Circulation 81:1245, 1990
14. Kessler KM, McAuliffe D, Kozlovskis P et al: QRS morphology dependent, concordant frequency distribution of single and repetitive forms of ventricular ectopic activity. Am Heart J 118:58, 1989
15. Kessler KM, McAuliffe D, Kozlovskis P et al: QRS morphology dependent pharmacodynamic in multiform ventricular ectopic activity. Am J Cardiol 61:563, 1988

16. Anderson KP, Lux RA, Dustman T: Comparison of QRS morphologies of spontaneous premature complexes and ventricular tachycardia induced by programmed stimulation. Am Heart J 119:1302, 1990

17. Kennedy HL, Chandra W, Sayther KL: Effectiveness of increasing hours of continuous ambulatory electrocardiography in detecting maximal ventricular ectopy: continuous 48 hour study of patients with coronary artery disease and normal subjects. Am J Cardiol 42:925, 1978

18. Podrid PJ, Vendetti FJ: Evaluation of arrhythmia. Role of exercise testing. Am J Cardiol 62:24H, 1988

19. Ryan M, Lown B, Horn H: Comparison of ventricular ectopic activity during 24 hour monitoring and exercise testing in patients with coronary artery disease. N Engl J Med 292:224, 1975

20. Jelinek MV, Lown B: Exercise stress testing or exposure of cardiac arrhythmia. Prog Cardiovasc Dis 16:497, 1974

21. Antman E, Graboys TB, Lown B: Comparison of continuous to intermittent electrocardiographic monitoring during exercise testing for exposure of cardiac arrhythmias. JAMA 241:2802, 1979

22. Morganroth J, Michelson EL, Horowitz LN et al: Limitations of routine long term electrocardiographic monitoring to assess ventricular ectopic frequency. Circulation 58:408, 1978

23. Pratt CM, Slymen DJ, Wierman AM et al: Analyses of the spontaneous variability of ventricular arrhythmias: consecutive ambulatory ECG recordings of ventricular tachycardia. Am J Cardiol 56:67, 1985

24. Winkle RA: Spontaneous variability of ventricular ectopics frequently mimics antiarrhythmic drug effect. Circulation 57:1116, 1978

25. Raeder EA, Hohnloser S, Graboys TB et al: Spontaneous variability and circadian distribution of ectopic activity in patients with malignant ventricular arrhythmia. J Am Coll Cardiol 12:656, 1988

26. Winkle PA, Peters F, Hall R: Characterization of ventricular tachyarrhythmias in ambulatory ECG recordings in post myocardial infarction patients: arrhythmia detection and duration of recording. Relationship between arrhythmia frequency and complexity and day to day reproducibility. Am Heart J 102:162, 1981

27. Pratt CM, Delclos G, Wierman AM et al: The changing baseline of complex ventricular arrhythmias: a new consideration in assessing long-term antiarrhythmic drug therapy. N Engl J Med 313:1444, 1985

28. Toivonin L: Spontaneous variability in the frequency of ventricular premature complexes over prolonged intervals and implications for antiarrhythmic treatment. Am J Cardiol 60:608, 1987

29. Anastasiou Nana MI, Minlove RL, Nanas JN, Anderson JL: Changes in spontaneous variability of ventricular ectopic activity as a function of time in patients with chronic arrhythmias. Circulation 78:286, 1988

30. Pratt CM, Theroux P, Symen D et al: Spontaneous variability of ventricular arrhythmias in patients at increased risk of sudden death after acute myocardial infarction: consecutive ambulatory electrocardiographic recordings of 88 patients. Am J Cardiol 59:278, 1987

31. The Cardiac Arrhythmia Pilot Study (CAPS) Investigators: Effects of encainide, flecainide, imipramine and moricizine on ventricular arrhythmias during the year after acute myocardial infarction: the CAPS. Am J Cardiol 61:501, 1988

32. Michelson EL, Morganroth J: Spontaneous variability of complex ventricular arrhythmia detected by long-term electrocardiographic recording. Circulation 61:690, 1980

33. Averill KH, Lamb LE: Electrocardiographic findings in 67,375 asymptomatic patients. Incidence of abnormalities. Am J Cardiol 6:76, 1960

34. Hiss RL, Lamb LE: Electrocardiographic findings in 122,043 individuals. Circulation 25:947, 1962

35. Chiang BN, Perlman LV, Fulton M et al: Predisposing factors in sudden cardiac death in Tecumsch Michigan. A prospective study. Circulation 41:31, 1970

36. Fleg J, Kennedy H: Cardiac arrhythmias in a healthy elderly population. Chest 81:302, 1982

37. Hinkle L, Carver ST, Stevens M: The frequency of asymptomatic disturbances of cardiac rhythm and conduction in middle aged men. Am J Cardiol 24:629, 1969

38. Kostis JB, McCrone K, Moreyra AE et al: Premature ventricular complexes in the absence of identifiable heart disease. Circulation 63:1351, 1981

39. Brodsky M, Wu D, Denes P et al: Arrhythmias documented by 24 hour continuous electrocardiographic monitoring in 50 male medical students without apparent heart disease. Am J Cardiol 39:390, 1977

40. Sobotka PA, Mayer JH, Bauernfund RA et al: Arrhythmias documented by 24 hour continuous ambulatory electrocardiographic monitoring in young women without apparent heart disease. Am Heart J 101:753, 1981

41. Sherman H, Sanberg S, Fineberg HV: Exponential increase in age specific prevalence of ventricular dysrrhythmias among males. J Chronic Dis 35:743, 1982

42. Glasser SP, Clark PI, Applebaum HJ: Occurrence of frequent complex arrhythmias detected by ambulatory monitoring. Findings in apparently healthy asymptomatic elderly population. Chest 75:565, 1979

43. Camm AJ, Evans KE, Ward DE, Marben A: The rhythm of the heart in active elderly subjects. Am Heart J 99:598, 1982

44. Kantilip JP, Sage E, Dunchene-Marillaz P: Findings in ambulatory electrocardiographic monitoring in subjects older than 80 years. Am J Cardiol 57:398, 1986

45. Podrid PJ: Role of exercise testing for exposure of arrhythmia. Circulation, suppl IV. 75:60, 1987

46. Rodstein M, Wollock L, Gubner RS: Mortality study of the significance of extrasystoles in an insured population. Circulation 44:617, 1971

47. Desai DC, Hersberg PF, Alexander S: Clinical significance of ventricular premature beats in an outpatient population. Chest 64:564, 1973

48. Fisher FD, Tyroler AA: Relationship between ventricular premature beats on routine electrocardiography and subsequent sudden death from coronary heart disease. Circulation 47:712, 1973

49. Crow R, Prineas R, Blackburn H: The prognostic significance of ventricular ectopic beats among the apparently healthy. Am Heart J 101:244, 1981

50. Blackburn H, Kup A, Taylor HL: The frequency and

prognosis of ventricular ectopic beats in middle aged man. Am J Cardiol 33:127, 1971

51. Kennedy HJ, Whitlock JA, Sprague MT et al: Long term follow-up of asymptomatic healthy subjects with frequent and complex ventricular ectopy. N Engl J Med 312:193, 1985

52. Elkon KB, Swerdlow TA, Myberg DP: Persistant ventricular ectopic beats. A long-term study. S Afr Med J 52:564, 1977

53. Califf AM, McKinnis RA, McNeer F et al: Prognostic value of ventricular arrhythmia associated with treadmill exercise testing in patients studied with cardiac catheterization for suspected ischemic heart disease. J Am Coll Cardiol 2:1060, 1983

54. Drory Y, Pones A, Fisman EZ, Kellermann JJ: Persistance of arrhythmia exercise response in healthy young men. Am J Cardiol 66:1092, 1990

55. Savage DP, Garrison RJ, Devereux RB et al: Mitral valve prolapse in the general population. Epidermiologic features. The Framingham Study. Am Heart J 106:571, 1983

56. Wit AL, Cranefield PF: Triggered activity in cardiac muscle fibers of the simian mitral valve. Circ Res 38:85, 1976

57. Cobb BW, King SB: Ventricular buckling: a factor in the abnormal ventriculogram and peculiar hemodynamics associated with mitral valve prolapse. Am Heart J 93:741, 1977

58. Cipriano PR, Kline JA, Baltaxe HA: An angiographic assessment of left ventricular function in isolated mitral valve prolapse. Invest Radiol 15:293, 1980

59. Gaffney FA, Karlsson ES, Campbell W et al. Autonomic dysfunction in women with mitral valve prolapse syndrome. Circulation 59:894, 1979

60. Boudoulas H, Reynolds JC, Mazzaferri E, Wooley LF: Metabolic studies in mitral valve prolapse syndrome. A neuroendocrine cardiovascular process. Circulation 61:1200, 1980

61. Kramer HM, Kligfield P, Devereux RB et al: Arrhythmias in mitral valve prolapse. Effect of selection bias. Arch Intern Med 144:2360, 1984

62. Winkle RA: Arrhythmia in patients with mitral valve prolapse. Circulation 52:73, 1975

63. Savage PD, Levy D, Garrison RJ et al: Mitral Valve prolapse in the general population III Dysrhythmias: the Framingham Study. Am Heart J 106:582, 1983

64. Nardi E, Alaimo L, Noto G et al: Cardiac arrhythmia in relation to the leaflet morphology in subjects with mitral valve prolapse. Cardiologia 34:797, 1989

65. Kligfield P, Hochreiter C, Kramer H et al: Complex arrhythmia in mitral regurgitation with and without mitral valve prolapse. Contrast to arrhythmias in mitral valve prolapse without mitral regurgitation. Am J Cardiol 55:1545, 1985

66. Kligfield P, Levy D, Devereux RR, Savage DD: Arrhythmias and sudden death in mitral valve prolapse. Am Heart J 113:1298, 1987

67. Nishimura RA, McGoon MD, Shub C et al: Echocardiographically documented mitral valve prolapse. Long term follow-up of 237 patients. N Engl J Med 313:1305, 1985

68. Kligfield P, Hochreiter C, Niles N et al: Relation of sudden death in pure mitral regurgitation with and without mitral valve prolapse to repetitive ventricular arrhythmias and right and left ejection fractions. Am J Cardiol 60:397, 1987

69. Huang SK, Messer JV, Denes P: Significance of ventricular tachycardia in idiopathic dilated cardiomyopathy: observation in 35 patients. Am J Cardiol 51:507, 1983

70. Wilson JR, Schwartz S, St John Sutton M et al: Prognosis in severe heart failure: relation to hemodynamic measurements and ventricular ectopic activity. J Am Coll Cardiol 2:403, 1983

71. Meinertz T, Hoffman J, Kasper W et al: Significance of ventricular arrhythmias in idiopathic dilated cardiomyopathy. Am J Cardiol 53:902, 1984

72. Holmes JR, Kubo SH, Cody RJ, Kligfield P: Milrinone in congestive heart failure: observations in ambulatory arrhythmias, abstracted. Circulation 70:II-11, 1984

73. Von Olshausen K, Schaefer A, Mehmel HC et al: Ventricular arrhythmias in idiopathic dilated cardiomyopathy. Br Heart J 51:195, 1984

74. Unverferth DV, Magorien RD, Moeschberger ML et al: Factors influencing the one-year mortality of dilated cardiomyopathy. Am J Cardiol 54:147, 1984

75. Chakko CS, Gheorghiade M: Ventricular arrhythmia in severe heart failure: incidence, significance and effectiveness of antiarrhythmic therapy. Am Heart J 109:497, 1985

76. Costanzo-Nordin MR, O'Connell JB, Engelmeier RS et al: Dilated cardiomyopathy: functional status, hemodynamics, arrhythmias and prognosis. Cathet Cardiovasc Diagn 11:445, 1985

77. Frances GS: Development of arrhythmias in the patient with congestive heart failure: pathophysiology, prevalence and prognosis Am J Cardiol 57:3B, 1986

78. Gradman A, Deedwania P, Cody R et al: for the Captopril Digoxin Study Group: Predictors of total mortality and sudden death in mild to moderate heart failure. J Am Coll Cardiol 14:564, 1989

79. Keogh AM, Baron DW, Hickie JB: Prognostic guides in patients with idiopathic or ischemic dilated cardiomyopathy assessed for cardiac transplantation. Am J Cardiol 65:903, 1990

80. Neri R, Mestroni L, Salvi A et al: Ventricular arrhythmia in dilated cardiomyopathy: efficacy of amiodarone. Am Heart J 113:707, 1987

81. Maskin CS, Siskind SJ, Lejemtel TH: High incidence of nonsustained ventricular tachycardia in severe congestive heart failure. Am Heart J 107:896, 1984

82. Dzau VJ, Colucci WS, Hollenberg NK, Williams GH: Relation of the renin-angiotension aldosterone system to clinical state in congestive heart failure. Circulation 63:645, 1981

83. Sakurai T, Kawai C: Sudden death in idiopathic cardiomyopathy. Jpn Cardiol J 47:581, 1983

84. Franciosa JA, Wilen M, Ziesche JM, Cohn JN: Survival in men with severe chronic left ventricular failure due to either coronary heart disease or idiopathic dilated cardiomyopathy. Am J Cardiol 51:831, 1983

85. Massie B, Ports T, Chatterjee K et al: Long-term vasodilator therapy for heart failure. Clinical response and its

relationship to hemodynamic measurements. Circulation 63:269, 1981

86. Lee WH, Packer M: Prognosis value of serum sodium concentration in severe heart failure and its modification by converting enzyme inhibition. Circulation, suppl II. 70:II-113, 1984

87. Burggraf GW, Parker JO: Prognosis in coronary artery disease: angiographic, hemodynamic and clinical factors. Circulation 51:146, 1975

88. Cohn JN, Levine TD, Olivari MT et al: Plasma norepinephrine as a guide to prognosis in patients with chronic congestive heart failure. N Engl J Med 311:819, 1984

89. Follansbee WD, Michelson EL, Morganroth J: Unsustained ventricular tachycardia in ambulatory patients. Characteristics associated with sudden cardiac death. Ann Intern Med 92:741, 1980

90. Cleland JG, Dorgie HJ, Ford I: Mortality in heart failure: clinical variables of prognostic value. Br Heart J 58:572, 1987

91. Dargie HJ, Cleland JG, Leckie BJ et al: Relation of arrhythmia and electrolyte abnormalities to survival in patients with severe chronic heart failure. Circulation, suppl IV. 75:IV-98, 1987

92. McKenna WJ, Franklin RL, Nihogannopoulos P et al: Arrhythmia and prognosis in infants, children and adolescents with hypertrophic cardiomyopathy. J Am Coll Cardiol 11:147, 1988

93. Savage DD, Seides S, Maron BJ et al: Prevalence of arrhythmia during 24-hour electrocardiographic monitoring and exercise testing in patients with obstructive and nonobstructive hypertrophic cardiomyopathy. Circulation 59:866, 1979

94. McKenna WJ, Chetty S, Oakley CM, Goodwin JF: Arrhythmia in hypertrophic cardiomyopathy: exercise and 48-hour ambulatory electrocardiographic assessment with and without beta adrenergic blocking therapy. Am J Cardiol 45:1, 1980

95. Maron BJ, Savage DD, Wolfson JK, Epstein SE: Prognosis significance of 24-hour ambulatory electrocardiographic monitoring in patients with hypertrophic cardiomyopathy: a prospective study. Am J Cardiol 48:252, 1981

96. Fleischman C, Gonska BD, Briene S et al: Ventricular arrhythmias and late potentials in patients with hypertrophic cardiomyopathy. Kardiol 79:113, 1990

97. Ando H, Tmaizumi T, Urabe Y et al: Apical segmental dysfunction in hypertrophic cardiomyopathy: subgroup with unique clinical features. J Am Coll Cardiol 16:1579, 1990

98. Nienaber C, Hiller S, Spielmann RP et al: Syncope in hypertrophic cardiomyopathy. Multivariate analysis of prognostic determinants. J Am Coll Cardiol 15:948, 1990

99. Dudel J, Trautwein W: Das aktions-potential und Mechanogramm der Herzmuskels unter dem Einfluss der Dehnung. Cardiologia 25:344, 1954

100. Sideris DA, Kontoyannis DA, Michalis L et al: Acute changes in blood pressure as a cause of cardiac arrhythmias. Eur Heart J 8:45, 1987

101. Holland BO, Nixon JW, von Kuhnert L: Diuretic induced ventricular ectopic activity. Am J Med 70:762, 1981

102. Hollifield JW, Slaton PE: Thiazide diuretics, hypokalemia and cardiac arrhythmias. Acta Med Scand 647:67, 1981

103. Medical Research Council Working Party on Mild to Moderate Hypertension: Ventricular extrasystoles during thiazide treatment: substudy of MRC mild hypertension trial. Br Med J 287:1249, 1983

104. Loaldi A, Pepi M, Agostoni PG et al: Cardiac rhythm in hypertension assessed through 24 hour ambulatory electrocardiographic monitoring. Effects of load manipulation with atenolol, verapamil and nifedipine. Br Heart J 50:118, 1983

105. Dendale P, DeMeirleir K: Prevalence of ventricular premature beats during stress testing in patients with exercise hypertension and the association with a positive family history of established hypertension. Eur Heart J 10:666, 1989

106. Sideris DA, Toumanides ST, Kostos EB et al: Arrhythmogenic effect of high blood pressure: some observations on its mechanisms. Cardiovasc Res 23:983, 1989

107. Multiple Risk Factor Intervention Trial Research Group: Multiple Risk Factor Intervention Trial: risk factor changes and mortality results. JAMA 248:1465, 1982

108. Ames RP: Negative effects of diuretic drugs on metabolic risk factors for coronary heart disease: possible alternative drug therapies. Am J Cardiol 51:632, 1983

109. Siegel D, Cheitlin MD, Black DM et al: Risk of ventricular arrhythmias in hypertensive men with left ventricular hypertrophy. Am J Med 65:742, 1990

110. McLenachan JM, Henderson E, Morris KI, Dargie HJ: Ventricular arrhythmias in patients with hypertensive left ventricular hypertrophy. N Engl J Med 317:787, 1987

111. Levy D, Anderson KM, Savage DD et al: Risk of ventricular arrhythmias in left ventricular hypertrophy. The Framingham Heart Study. Am J Cardiol 60:560, 1987

112. Messerli FH, Ventura HO, Elizardi DJ et al: Hypertension and sudden death. Increased ventricular ectopic activity in left ventricular hypertrophy. Am J Med 77:18, 1984

113. Papademetriou V, Burris JF, Notargiacomo A et al: Thiazide therapy is not a cause of arrhythmia in patients with systemic hypertension. Arch Intern Med 148:1272, 1988

114. Lumme JA, Jounela AJ: Cardiac arrhythmias in hypertensive outpatients on various diuretics. Correlation between incidence and serum potassium and magnesium levels. Ann Clin Res 18:186, 1986

115. Madias JE, Madias NE, Gavras HP: Nonarrhythmogenicity of diuretic induced hypokalemia. Its evidence in patients with uncomplicated hypertension. Arch Intern Med 144:2171, 1984

116. Medical Research Council Working Party: Medical research council trial of treatment of mild hypertension: principal results. Br Med J 291:97, 1985

117. Calvert A, Lown B, Gorlin R: Ventricular premature beats and anatomically defined coronary heart disease. Am J Cardiol 39:627, 1977

118. Madsen JK, Srensen JN, Kromann-Andersen B et al:

Ventricular premature beats on Holter monitoring in patients admitted with chest pain in whom acute myocardial infarction is not confirmed. The prognostic value and relationship to scars or ischemia on thallium-201 scintigraphy. J Clin Cardiol 10:305, 1987

119. Hausmann D, Nikulta P, Trappett J et al: Incidence of ventricular arrhythmias during transient myocardial ischemia in patients with stable coronary artery disease. J Am Coll Cardiol 16:49, 1990

120. Mulcahy D, Keegan J, Crean P et al: Silent myocardial ischemia in chronic stable angina: a study of its frequency and characteristics in 150 patients. Br Heart J 60:417, 1988

121. Carboni GP, Lahiri A, Cashman PMM, Raftery EB: Mechanisms of arrhythmia accompanying ST segment depression on ambulatory monitoring in stable angina pectoris. Am J Cardiol 60:1246, 1987

122. Banai S, Stern S, Keren A, Tzivoni D: Increased ventricular ectopic activity during ischemic episodes in ambulatory patients. J Am Coll Cardiol, abstracted. 13:33A, 1989

123. Stern S, Banai S, Keren A, Tzivoni D: Ventricular ectopic activity during myocardial ischemic episodes in ambulatory patients. Am J Cardiol 65.412, 1990

124. Lillis DL, Hanson P: Ventricular ectopy in cardiac rehabilitation and nonexercising days. J Clin Cardiol 12:569, 1989

125. Araki H, Koiwaye Y, Nakayaki O, Nakamura M: Diurnal distribution of ST segment elevation and related arrhythmias in patients with variant angina: a study by ambulatory electrocardiographic monitoring. Circulation 67:995, 1983

126. Previtale M, Klersy C, Salerno JA et al: Ventricular tachyarrhythmias in Prinzmetal's variant angina: clinical significance and relation to the degree and time course of ST segment elevation. Am J Cardiol 52:19, 1983

127. Nadamanee K, Intarachot V, Josephson M, Singh BN: Characteristics and clinical significance of silent myocardial ischemia in unstable angina. Am J Cardiol 58: 26B, 1986

128. Quyyami AA, Crabe T, Wright C et al: The incidence and morphology of ischemic ventricular tachycardia. Eur Heart J 7:1037, 1986

129. Ruben DA, Nieminski KE, Monteferrante JC et al: Ventricular arrhythmias after coronary artery bypass graft surgery: incidence, risk factors and long-term prognosis. J Am Coll Cardiol 6:307, 1985

130. DeSoyza N, Murphy ML, Bissett JK et al: Ventricular arrhythmias in chronic stable angina pectoris with surgical or medical treatment. Ann Intern Med 89:10, 1978

131. Huikari HU, Yri-May Y, Korhonen UR et al: Prevalence and prognostic significance of complex ventricular arrhythmias after coronary artery bypass graft surgery. Int J Cardiol 27:333, 1990

132. Poblete PF, Kennedy HL, Cavalis DG: Detection of ventricular ectopy in patients with coronary heart disease and normal subjects by exercise testing and ambulatory electrocardiography. Chest 74:402, 1978

133. McHenry PL, Fisch C, Jordan JW: Cardiac arrhythmia observed during maximal exercise testing in clinically normal men. Am J Cardiol 39:331, 1978

134. Whinnery JE: Dysrhythmia comparison in apparently healthy males during and after treadmill and accelerated stress test. Am Heart J 105:732, 1983

135. Kreger BE, Cupples LA, Kannel WB: The electrocardiogram in prediction of sudden death: Framingham Heart Study experience. Am Heart J 113:377, 1987

136. Ingersler J, Bjerragaard P: Prevalence and prognostic significance of cardiac arrhythmias detected by ambulatory electrocardiography in subjects 85 years of age. Eur Heart J 7:570, 1986

137. Udall JA, Ellestad MJ: Prediction implications of ventricular premature contractions associated with treadmill stress testing. Circulation 56:985, 1977

138. Weiner DA, Levine SR, Klein MD, Ryan TJ: Ventricular arrhythmias during exercise testing: mechanism, response to coronary bypass surgery, and prognostic significance. Am J Cardiol 53:1553, 1984

139. Sami M, Chaitman B, Fisher L et al: Significance of exercise-induced ventricular arrhythmia in stable coronary artery disease. A Coronary Artery Surgery Study project. Am J Cardiol 54:1182, 1984

140. Nair CK, Aronow WS, Sketch MH et al: Diagnostic and prognostic significance of exercise induced premature ventricular complexes in men and women: a four year followup. J Am Coll Cardiol 1:1201, 1983

141. Vismara LA, Amsterdam EA, Mason DT: Relation of ventricular arrhythmias in the late hospital phase of acute myocardial infarction to sudden death after hospital discharge. Am J Med 59:6, 1975

142. Moss AJ, Davis HT, DeCamella, Boyer JW: Ventricular ectopic beats and their relation to sudden and non sudden cardiac death after myocardial infarction. Circulation 60:998, 1979

143. Ruberman W, Weinblatt E, Goldberg JD et al: Ventricular premature beats after myocardial infarction. N Engl J Med 297:750, 1977

144. Friedman PL, Stewart JR, Fenoglio JJ, Wit AL: Survival of subendocardial Purkinje fibers after extensive myocardial infarction in dogs: in vitro and invivo correlations. Circ Res 33:579, 1973

145. Wit AL, Rosen MR: Pathophysiologic mechanisms of cardiac arrhythmias. Am Heart J 106:798, 1983

146. Ruberman W, Weinblatt E, Goldberg JD et al: Ventricular premature complexes and sudden death after myocardial infarction. Circulation 64:297, 1981

147. Kotler MN, Tabatznick B, Mower MM, Tominagar S: Diagnostic significance of ventricular ectopic beats with respect to sudden death in the late postinfarction period. Circulation 47:959, 1973

148. Rappaport E, Remedios P: The high risk patient after recovery from myocardial infarction: recognition and management. J Am Coll Cardiol 1:391, 1983

149. Mukharji J, Rude PE, Poole K et al: The MILIS Study Group Risk Factors and sudden death following acute myocardial infarction: two year follow-up. Am J Cardiol 54:31, 1984

150. Bigger JT, Fleiss JL, Rolnitzky LM: The Multicenter post-infarction research group. Prevalence, characteristics and significance of ventricular tachycardia detected by 24 hour continuous electrocardiographic recordings in the late hospital phase of acute myocardial infarction. Am J Cardiol 58:1151, 1986

151. Bigger JT, Weld F, Rolnitzky LM: Prevalence, characteristics and significance of ventricular tachycardia detected with ambulatory ECG recording in the late hospital phase of acute myocardial infarction. Am J Cardiol 48:815, 1982

152. Andresen D, Bethge KP, Borssel JP et al: Importance of quantitative analysis of ventricular arrhythmias for predicting the prognosis in low risk post myocardial infarction patients. European Infarction Study Group. Eur Heart J 11:529, 1990

153. Minisi AJ, Mukharji J, Rehr RB et al: Association between extent of coronary artery disease; ventricular premature beat frequency after myocardial infarction. Am Heart J 115:1198, 1988

154. Collins D, Ross S: Complex ventricular arrhythmias in patients with Q wave versus non Q wave myocardial infarction. Circulation 72:963, 1985

155. Weld FM, Uru KI, Bigger JT, Rolnitzky LM: Risk stratification with low level exercise testing two weeks after myocardial infarction. Circulation 64:306, 1981

156. Krone RJ, Gillespie JA, Weld FM et al: Multicenter Post Infarction Research Group—Low level exercise testing after myocardial infarction—usefulness in enhancing clinical risk stratification. Circulation 71:80, 1985

157. Henry RL, Kennedy GT, Crawford MH: Prognostic value of exercise induced ventricular ectopic activity for mortality after acute myocardial infarction. Am J Cardiol 59:1251, 1987

158. Saunamki KJ, Anderson JP: Post myocardial infarction exercise testing. Clinical significance of a left ventricular function index and ventricular arrhythmias. A prospective study. Acta Med Scand 218:271, 1985

159. Schultz RA, Strauss HW, Pitt B: Sudden death in the year following myocardial infarction. Relation to ventricular premature contractions in the late hospital phase of left ventricular efection fraction. Am J Med 62:192, 1977

160. Bigger JT, Fleiss JL, Kleiger R et al: The Multicenter Post Infarction Study Group. The relationship between ventricular arrhythmias, left ventricular dysfunction and mortality in the two years after myocardial infarction. Circulation 69:250, 1984

161. Kleiger RE, Miller JP, Bigger FT, Moss AJ: The Multicenter Post Infarction Research Group. Decreased heart rate variability and its association with increased mortality after acute myocardial infarction. Am J Cardiol 54:256, 1987

162. Simson MB: Use of signals in the terminal QRS complex to identify patients with ventricular tachycardia after myocardial infarction. Circulation 64:235, 1981

163. Denniss AR, Richards DA, Cody DV et al: Prognostic significance of ventricular tachycardia and fibrillation induced at programmed stimulation and delayed potentials detectable on the signal averaged electrocardiogram of survivors of acute myocardial infarction. Circulation 74:731, 1986

164. Kuehar DL, Thorburn LW, Samuel NL: Prediction of serious arrhythmic events after myocardial infarction: signal averaged electrocardiograms, holter monitoring and radionuclide angiography. J Am Coll Cardiol 9:531, 1987

165. Italian Group for the study of Streptokinase in Myocardial Infarction (GISSI): Effectiveness of intravenous thrombolytic treatment in acute myocardial infarction. Lancet 1:397, 1986

166. Theroux P, Morissette D, Juneau M et al: Influence of fibrinolysis and percutaneous transluminal coronary angioplasty on the frequency of ventricular premature complexes. Am J Cardiol 63:797, 1989

167. Gang ES, Lew SA, Hong M et al: Decreased incidence of ventricular late potentials after successful thrombolytic therapy for acute myocardial infarction. N Engl J Med 314:712, 1989

168. Bourke JP, Young AA, Richards DB, Uther JB: Reduction in incidence of inducible ventricular tachycardia after myocardial infarction by treatment with streptokinase during infarct evolution. J Am Coll Cardiol 16:1703, 1990

169. Garson A, Nihill MR, McNamara DG, Cooley DA: Status of the adult and adolescent after repair of tetralogy of Fallot. Circ 59:1232, 1979

170. Garson A, Porter CJ, Gillette PC, McNamara DG: Induction of ventricular tachycardia during electrophysiologic study after repair of tetralogy of Fallot. J Am Coll Cardiol 1:1493, 1983

171. Chandar JS, Wolff GS, Garson A et al: Ventricular arrhythmias in postoperative tetralogy of Fallot. Am J Cardiol 65:655, 1990

172. Quattlebaum TG, Varghese J, Neill CA, Donahue JS: Sudden death among postoperative patients with tetralogy of Fallot. Circulation 54:289, 1976

173. Horowitz LN, Vetter VL, Harken AH, Josephson ME: Electrophysiologic characteristics of sustained ventricular tachycardia occurring after repair of tetralogy of Fallot. Am J Cardiol 46:446, 1980

174. Axelrod PJ, Verrier RL, Lown B: Vulnerability to ventricular fibrillation during acute coronary arterial occlusion and release. Am J Cardiol 36:776, 1976

175. Moe GK, Cohen W, Vick RL: Experimentally induced paroxysmal AV nodal tachycardia in the dog. Am Heart J 65:87, 1963

176. Snow PJD, Manc MD: Effect of propranolol in myocardial infarction. Lancet 2:551, 1965

177. Multicenter Trial: Propranolol in acute myocardial infarction. Lancet 2:1435, 1966

178. Balcon R, Jewitt DE, Davies JPH, Oran S: A controlled trial of propranolol on acute myocardial infarction. Lancet 2:917, 1966

179. Norris RM, Laughey DE, Scott PJ: Trial of propranolol in acute myocardial infarction. Br Med J 2:398, 1968

180. Beta Blocker Heart Attack Trial Research Group: A randomized trial of propranolol in patients with acute myocardial infarction I. Mortality Results. JAMA 242:1707, 1982

181. Hansteen V, Moinichin E, Lorenstsen E et al: One year's treatment with propranolol after myocardial infarction. Preliminary report of the Norwegian Multicenter Trial. Br Med J 284:155, 1982

182. Wilhelmsson C, Wilhelmsen L, Vedin JA et al: Reduction of sudden death after myocardial infarction by treatment with alprenolol. Lancet 2:1157, 1974

183. Ahlmack G, Saltre H, Korsgren M: Reduction of sudden death after myocardial infarction. Lancet 2:1563, 1974

184. Andersen MP, Frederikson J, Jurgensen HG et al: Effect of alprenolol on mortality among patients with a definite or suspected acute myocardial infarction. Lancet 2: 865, 1974

185. Multicenter International Study: Reduction in mortality after myocardial infarction with long-term beta adrenoceptor blockade. Br Med J 2:419, 1977

186. Hjalmarsen P, Herlitz J, Malek I et al: Effect on mortality of metroprolol in acute myocardial infarction. Lancet 2:823, 1981

187. Norwegian Multicenter Study Group: Timolol induced reduction in mortality and reinfarction in patients surviving acute myocardial infarction. N Engl J Med 304: 801, 1981

188. ISIS-1 Collaborative Group: A randomized trial of intravenous atenolol among 16,027 cases of suspected acute myocarial infarction. Lancet 2:57, 1986

189. Taylor SJ, Silke B, Ebbutt A et al: A long-term prevention study with oxprenolol in coronary heart disease. N Engl J Med 307:1239, 1982

190. Australian and Swedish Pindolol Study Group: The effect of pindolol on the two year mortality after complicated myocardial infarction. Eur Heart J 4:367, 1983

191. Julian DG, Jackson FS, Prescott RJ, Szekeley P: Controlled trial of sotalol of one year after myocardial infarction. Lancet 1:1142, 1982

192. Kostis JB, Wilson AC, Sanders MR, Byington RP: BHAT Study Group. Prognostic significance of ventricular ectopic activity in survivors of acute infarction who receive propranolol. Am J Cardiol 61:975, 1988

193. Bennett MA, Wilner JM, Pentecoste BC: Controlled trial of lidocaine in prophylaxis of ventricular arrhythmias complicating myocardial infarction. Lancet 2:909, 1970

194. Chopra MD, Thadane U, Portal RW, Abu CP: Lignocaine therapy for ventricular ectopic activity after acute myocardial infarction. A double blind trial. Br Med J 3:668, 1971

195. Morgensen L: Ventricular tachyarrhythmias and lignocaine prophylaxis in acute myocardial infarction. Acta Med Scand, suppl. 513:1, 1970

196. Lie KJ, Wellens HJ, VanChampell FS, Durrer D: Lidocaine in the prevention of primary ventricular fibrillation. A double blind randomized study of 212 consecutive patients. N Engl J Med 291:1324, 1974

197. Campbell RWF, Bryson LG, Bailey BJ et al: Oral tocainide in suspected acute myocardial infarction. Circulation, suppl II. 59:II-70, 1979

198. Ryden L, Arnman D, Conradson TB et al: Prophylaxis of ventricular tachyarrhythmias with intravenous and oral tocainide in patients with and recovering from acute myocardial infarction. Am Heart J 100:1006, 1980

199. Campbell RWF, Achuff SC, Pottage A et al: Mexiletine in the prophylaxis of ventricular arrhythmias during acute myocardial infarction. J Cardiovasc Pharmacol 1: 43, 1979

200. Chamberlain DR, Julian DG, Boyle DM et al: Oral mexiletine in high risk patients after myocardial infarction. Lancet 2:1324, 1980

201. Hugenholtz PG, Hagemeijer F, Lubsen J et al: One year follow-up in patients with persistent ventricular dysrythmias aftermyocardial infarction treated with aprindine or placebo. p. 572. In Sandoe E, Julian DG, Bell JW (eds): Management of Ventricular Tachycardia: Role of Mexiletine. Excerpta Medica, Amsterdam, 1978

202. Gottlieb S, Achuff SC, Millets EO et al: Prophylactic antiarrhythmic therapy of high risk survivors of myocardial infarction. Lower mortality at 1 month but not at 1 year. Circulation 75:792, 1987

203. IMPACT Research Group: International mexiletine and placebo antiarrhythmic coronary trial. I. Report on arrhythmia and other findings. J Am Coll Cardiol 4:1148, 1984

204. Holmberg S, Bergman H: Prophylactic quinidine treatment in myocardial infarction. Acta Med Scand 181: 297, 1967

205. Bloomfield SS, Rombilt DW, Chou TL, Fowler NO: Quinidine for prophylaxis of arrhythmia in acute myocardial infarction. N Engl J Med 285:967, 1971

206. Jones DT, Kostuk WJ, Gunton RW: Prophylactic quinidine for the prevention of arrhythmias after acute myocardial infarction. Am J Cardiol 33:655, 1974

207. Jennings G, Jones MBA, Besterman EMM et al: Oral disopyramide in prophylaxis of arrhythmias following myocardial infarction. Lancet 1:51, 1976

208. Zainal N, Griffiths JW, Carmichael DJS et al: Oral disopyramide for the prevention of arrhythmias in patients with acute myocardial infarction admitted to open wards. Lancet 2:887, 1977

209. Kock-Weser J, Klein SW, Foo-Canto LL et al: Antiarrhythmic prophylaxis with procainamide in acute myocardial infarction. N Engl J Med 281:1253, 1969

210. Kosowsky BD, Taylor J, Lown B, Ritchie RF: Long term use of procainamide following acute myocardial infarction. Circulation 47:1204, 1973

211. Peter T, Ross D, Duffield A et al: Effect on survival after myocardial infarction of long term treatment with pheytoin. Br Heart J 42:1356, 1978

212. Collaborative Group: Phenytoin after recovery from myocardial infarction. Controlled trial in 568 patients. Lancet 2:1055, 1971

213. Velebit V, Podrid PJ, Cohen B et al: Aggravation and provocation of ventricular arrhythmias by antiarrhythmic drugs. Circulation 65:886, 1982

214. Podrid PJ, Lambert S, Graboys TB et al: Aggravation of arrhythmia by antiarrhythmic drugs. Incidence and predictors. Am J Cardiol 59:38E, 1987

215. Burkart F, Pfisterer M, Kiowski W et al: Effect of antiarrhythmic therapy on mortality in survivors of myocardial infarction with asymptomatic complex ventricular arrhythmias. Basal Antiarrhythmic Study of Infarct Survival (BASIS). J Am Coll Cardiol 16:1711, 1990

216. Furburg CD: Effect of antiarrhythmic drugs on mortality after myocardial infarction. Am J Cardiol 52:32C, 1983

217. CAPS Investigators: The cardiac arrhythmia pilot study. Am J Cardiol 57:91, 1986

218. Cardiac Arrhythmia Suppression Trial (CAST) Investigators Preliminary Report: Effect of encainide and flecainide on mortality in a randomized trial of arrhythmia suppression after myocardial infarction. N Engl J Med 321:406, 1989

219. Slater W, Lambert SL, Podrid PJ, Lown B: Clinical pre-

dictors of arrhythmia worsening by antiarrhythmic drugs. Am J Cardiol 61:349, 1988

220. Pratt CM, Eaton T, Frances M et al: The inverse relationship between baseline left ventricular ejection fraction and outcome of antiarrhythmic therapy: a dangerous imbalance in the risk-benefit ratio. Am Heart J 118:433, 1989

221. Morganroth J, Horowitz LN: Flecainide—its pro-arrhythmic effect and expected changes on the surface electrocardiogram. Am J Cardiol 53:893, 1984

222. Morganroth J, Horowitz LN: Incidence of proarrhythmic effects from quinidine in the outpatient treatment of benign or potentially lethal ventricular arrhythmias. Am J Cardiol 56:585, 1985

223. Morganroth J: Risk factors for the development of pro-arrhythmia events. Am J Cardiol 59:32E, 1987

224. Minardo JD, Heger JJ, Miles WM et al: Clinical characteristics of patients with ventricular fibrillation during antiarrhythmic drug therapy. N Engl J Med 319:257, 1988

225. Blevins RD, Kerin NZ, Frumin H et al: Arrhythmia control and other factors related to sudden death in coronary disease patients at intermediate risk. Am Heart H 111:638, 1989

226. Hoffmann A, Schutz E, White R et al: Suppression of high grade ventricular ectopic activity by antiarrhythmic drug treatment as a marker for survival in patients with chronic coronary artery disease. Am Heart J 107:1103, 1984

227. Parmley WW, Chatterjee K: Congestive heart failure and arrhythmia. An overview. Am J Cardiol 57:34B, 1986

228. Swedberg K, Hjalmarson A, Waagstein F, Wallentin I: Prolongation of survival in congestive cardiomyopathy by beta receptor blockade. Lancet 1:1374, 1979

229. Anderson T, Lutz JR, Gilbert EM et al: A randomized trial of low dose beta blockade therapy for idiopathic dilated cardiomyopathy. Am J Cardiol 55:471, 1985

230. Chadda K, Goldstein S, Byington R, Curb JD: Effect of propranolol after acute myocardial infarction in patients with congestive heart failure. Circulation 73:503, 1986

231. Furberg CD, Hawkins CM, Lichstein E; for the Beta Blocker Heart Attack Trial Study Group: Effect of propranolol in post-infarction patients with mechanical or electrical complications. Circulation 69:761, 1984

232. Graboys TB, Lown B, Podrid PJ, DeSilva R: Long term survival of patients with malignant ventricular arrhythmias treated with antiarrhythmic drugs. Am J Cardiol 50:437, 1982

233. Vlay SC, Rackman CH, Reid PR: Prognostic assessment of ventricular tachycardia and ventricular fibrillation with ambulatory monitoring. Am J Cardiol 54:87, 1984

234. Horowitz LN, Josephson E, Forshidi A et al: Reccurent sustained ventricular tachycardia: Role of electrophysiologic study in the selection of antiarrhythmic regimins. Circulation 58:986, 1978

235. Swerdlow CD, Winkle A, Mason JW: Determinants of survival in patients with ventricular tachyarrhythmias. N Engl J Med 308:1436, 1983

236. Teo K, Yusuf S, Furberg C: Effect of antiarrhythmic drug therapy on mortality following myocardial infarction (abstract.) Circulation 82(suppl 3):192, 1990

237. Beard EF, Owen CA: Cardiac arrhythmias during exercise stress tests in healthy men. Aerospace Med 44:286, 1983

238. Master AM: Cardiac arrhythmias elicited by two-stage exercise test. Am J Cardiol 32:766, 1973

29

Risk Assessment and Prognosis of Patients After Aborted Sudden Cardiac Death or Suffering From Symptomatic Ventricular Tachyarrhythmias

Hein J. J. Wellens
Luz-Maria Rodriguez
Anton P. M. Gorgels
Joep L. Smeets

For patients resuscitated from sudden death or known to suffer from a symptomatic ventricular tachyarrhythmia (SVT), it is essential to be informed about prognosis in order to select the most appropriate therapy. This chapter addresses the information required to make the most reliable assessment of risk of dying or of having a recurrence of a ventricular tachyarrhythmia in those patients. Recurrence of a sustained ventricular tachycardia should not be equated with sudden death, and parameters predicting risk of dying are different from parameters predicting recurrences of ventricular tachycardia.

RISK STRATIFICATION

Essential in risk stratification is a definition of the different subgroups of patients. A useful first step in classification is to evaluate the patient's heart rhythm, etiology of heart disease, and pump function.

Classification

Rhythm

Resuscitated from sudden death means that no cardiac output was present at the time of resuscitation. The responsible cardiac arrhythmias can be divided into ventricular fibrillation, sustained rapid ventricular tachycardia, and extreme bradycardia or cardiac standstill.

Ventricular tachyarrhythmias include sustained monomorphic ventricular tachycardia, sustained polymorphic ventricular tachycardia, and nonsustained monomorphic or polymorphic ventricular tachycardia lasting long enough to lead to hemodynamic compromise.

Etiology of Heart Disease

Etiology of heart disease plays a major role in risk stratification. But within the same etiology group, prognosis may vary considerably according to the type of arrhythmia and pump function.

Pump Function

Pump function is a major determinant in the prognosis of patients resuscitated from sudden death or suffering from severe ventricular tachyarrhythmias. Pump function can be classified on the basis of the patient's history using the New York Heart Association (NYHA) classification, or by invasive (left ventricular angiogram) and noninvasive measurements (echo-Doppler, nuclear study, heart rate variability, exercise testing).

Prognostic Indicators

The risk of cardiac death in patients resuscitated from sudden cardiac death or suffering from symptomatic ventricular tachyarrhythmia can be prognosticated on the basis of etiology, the clinical history, left ventricular ejection fraction (LVEF), and other factors.

Etiology

Data from our own institution[1-3] indicate that the value of a sustained monomorphic ventricular tachycardia or ventricular fibrillation as a prognostic indicator for cardiac death is totally different in the patient with an old myocardial infarction (MI), as compared with the patient with arrhythmogenic right ventricular dysplasia or without heart disease (so-called idiopathic ventricular tachycardia or ventricular fibrillation). Table 29-1 shows that patients with an old MI have the most ominous prognosis in regard to total and sudden cardiac death, with patients resuscitated from ventricular fibrillation having the worst prognosis.[1] Similar findings regarding prognosis in the different etiology groups have been reported by Leclercq et al.[4] Note from Table 29-1 that the risk of cardiac death is very low in patients suffering from idiopathic ventricular tachycardia. Two of our patients with arrhythmogenic right ventricular dysplasia died, both from pump failure shortly after surgery for arrhythmia.

An interesting group of patients are those having ventricular fibrillation in the absence of overt heart disease. They have been discussed in detail elsewhere.[5] An important lesson from these patients is that sudden death may recur in spite of normal left ventricular (LV) function outside the arrhythmia.

Clinical History

Etiology plays an important role in the prognostic significance of an arrhythmia. Nevertheless, even within a seemingly homogeneous group, such as among patients in whom monomorphic ventricular tachycardia or ventricular fibrillation develops outside the acute phase of MI, marked differences in risk can, and must, be recognized. Recently, we published

TABLE 29-1. Relationship Between Etiology of Ventricular Tachycardia/Ventricular Fibrillation and Arrhythmia Recurrence and Death During Follow-up

	Old MI		ARVD	Idiopathic	
	SMVT	VF	SMVT	SMVT	VF
Total no. of patients	154	52	22	68	9
Total death	32 (21%)	19 (36%)	2 (9%)[b]	1[a]	1
Sudden cardiac death	22 (14%)	9 (17%)	0	0	1
No. of pts with nonlethal VT/VF recurrence	64 (41%)	10 (19%)	15 (70%)	23 (35%)	2 (22%)
Length of follow-up (mo)	40 ± 86	38 ± 72	52 ± 60	96 ± 52	52 ± 46

Abbreviations: ARVD, arrhythmogenic right ventricular dysplasia; MI, myocardial infarction; SMVT, sustained monomorphic ventricular tachycardia; VF, ventricular fibrillation.
[a] Patient died of cancer.
[b] Both patients died during arrhythmia surgery.

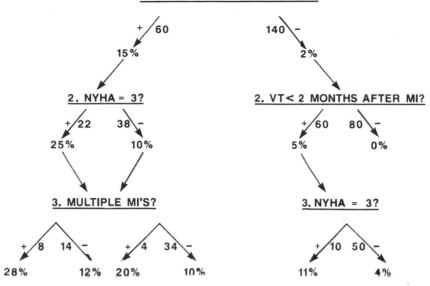

Fig. 29-1. Estimation of risk of sudden death based on the four clinical variables discussed in the text. As shown in this group of 200 consecutive patients with a previous myocardial infarction (MI) developing ventricular tachycardia (VT) or ventricular fibrillation (VF), there was a 6% incidence of dying suddenly within 2 years. NYHA, New York Heart Association classification for dyspnea.

information on the value of the clinical history in assessing the risk of nonsudden and sudden death in such cases. The answers to four questions were found to be of great help[6]: (1) What is the NYHA functional classification outside the arrhythmia? (2) Did the patient lose consciousness during the arrhythmia? (3) Did the first episode of ventricular tachycardia or ventricular fibrillation occur between days 3 to 60 post-MI or later? (4) Has the patient had more than one prior MI?

In 200 consecutive patients with ventricular tachycardia or fibrillation outside the acute phase of MI, we found that these questions were helpful in recognizing patients at low risk of sudden death (i.e., those who did not lose consciousness during the first episode of their spontaneous ventricular tachycardia and in whom the arrhythmia occurred more than 2 months after MI). By contrast, those four questions could also identify patients who had a 25% chance of sudden cardiac death within 2 years (see Fig. 29-1). Using the same information from the clinical history, we found (Fig. 29-2) that pump function is the most important discriminator for risk of nonsudden cardiac death in patients with sustained ventricular tachycardia or ventricular fibrillation after a myocardial infarction. Figure 29-3 demonstrates the value of the total score of the four clinical variables in those 200 post-MI pa-

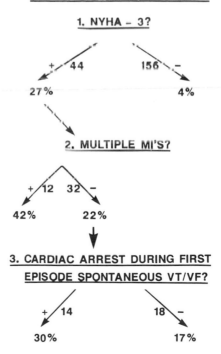

Fig. 29-2. Estimation of risk of nonsudden cardiac death in the same patients as in Figure 29-1. The overall incidence of non-sudden cardiac death at 2 years was 9%. Abbreviations as in Figure 29-1.

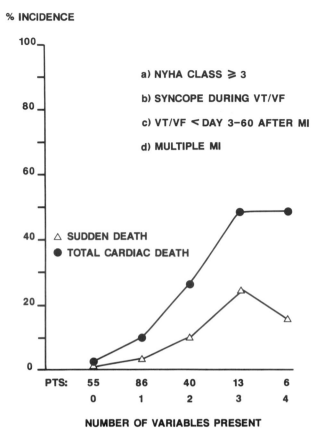

% INCIDENCE

a) NYHA CLASS ≥ 3

b) SYNCOPE DURING VT/VF

c) VT/VF < DAY 3–60 AFTER MI

d) MULTIPLE MI

△ SUDDEN DEATH
● TOTAL CARDIAC DEATH

PTS:	55	86	40	13	6
	0	1	2	3	4

NUMBER OF VARIABLES PRESENT

Fig. 29-3. Incidence of total cardiac death and sudden cardiac death in relation to the total score of four clinical variables in 200 patients (pts) with ventricular tachycardia (169 patients) or ventricular fibrillation (VF) (31 patients) after myocardial infarction (MI). The four clinical variables are listed in the upper right corner of the figure. As shown, depending on the number of variables present, marked differences exist in sudden and total cardiac death after 2 years of follow-up.

tients with ventricular tachycardia or ventricular fibrillation. These four clinical variables permit identification of patients who have a very small chance of dying versus those who have a 50% risk of cardiac death within 2 years.

Left Ventricular Ejection Fraction

Pump function plays an important role in the prognosis of patients with sustained ventricular tachycardia or ventricular fibrillation. The LVEF is therefore an important parameter in risk stratification. In a group of 206 patients who survived sustained ventricular tachycardia (154 patients) or ventricular fibrillation (52 patients), we found that the 3-year incidence of sudden death was 28 of 65 patients with an LVEF

of 40% or greater and was 3 of 141 patients with an LVEF of greater than 40% (p < 0.0001). Interestingly, the incidence of non-sudden cardiac death was 6 of 65 (9%) and 14 of 141 (10%), respectively (p = NS), suggesting that LVEF in this group of post-MI patients with ventricular tachycardia/ventricular fibrillation did not play a role in their risk of non-sudden cardiac death.[7]

Clinical and Electrocardiographic Parameters

Willems et al.[8] reported a prospective study in 1990 on 430 patients with sustained ventricular tachycardia and ventricular fibrillation outside the acute phase of MI. The Cox regression model shows seven clinical and electrocardiographic (ECG) parameters (having a lower limit of the 95% confidence interval of >1) to be predictive of cardiac death during a 2-year follow-up period (Table 29-2). Willems et al.[8] combined the seven parameters to show how patients with ventricular tachycardia or ventricular fibrillation can be classified as to their risk of cardiac death during the 2 years after their first episode (Table 29-3).

Timing of Recurrences of Sudden Death

In patients resuscitated from ventricular fibrillation after a remote MI, we looked at the timing of a recurrence of sudden death.[7] There were two peaks at around 3 and 18 months (Fig. 29-4). Figure 29-5 shows the timing of sudden death in patients with sustained ventricular tachycardia. In those patients there were two peaks, at 3 and 12 months. In patients with ventricular tachycardia or ventricular fibrillation having survived 1 year, sudden death occurred in only 10%

TABLE 29-2. Survival Analysis in the Interuniversity Cardiological Institute of the Netherlands Study on Ventricular Tachycardia/ Ventricular Fibrillation After MI

Variable	Risk Ratio[a]	95% CI	p-value
Age >70 years[b]	2.4	1.6–3.4	0.0001
Killip III/IV[c]	2.2	1.5–3.3	0.0002
Cardiac arrest[b]	1.7	1.2–2.4	0.002
First episode of VT/VF <6 weeks after MI	1.7	1.2–2.3	0.003
Multiple previous MI	1.6	1.1–2.3	0.01
Anterior MI	1.4	1.0–2.1	0.06
Q-wave MI	1.7	0.9–3.0	0.08

Abbreviations: CI, confidence interval; MI, myocardial infarction; VF, ventricular fibrillation; VT, ventricular tachycardia.

[a] The risk was obtained as the exponent of the regression coefficient of the Cox model.
[b] During index arrhythmias.
[c] Within the semi-acute phase of infarction.
(From Willems et al.,[8] with permission.)

TABLE 29-3. Prediction of 2-year Mortality[a]

First VT/VF <6 wk#	Q-wave MI	Multiple MI	Anterior MI	Age >70 yr[b]: +	+	+	+	−	−	−	−
				Killip III/IV[c]: +	+	−	−	+	+	−	−
				Cardiac arrest[a]: +	−	+	−	+	−	+	−
+	+	+	+	99	93	87	69	85	67	57	39
+	+	+	−	96	85	76	57	74	54	45	30
+	+	−	+	94	81	72	52	69	50	41	27
+	+	−	−	86	69	59	41	57	39	31	20
+	−	+	+	94	80	71	51	68	49	40	26
+	−	+	−	85	68	58	40	56	38	30	19
+	−	−	+	82	64	54	36	51	35	28	17
+	−	−	−	70	51	42	27	40	26	20	13
−	+	+	+	93	80	70	51	68	49	40	26
−	+	+	−	85	68	58	40	55	38	30	19
−	+	−	+	82	63	53	36	51	34	27	17
−	+	−	−	70	51	42	27	40	26	20	12
−	−	+	+	80	62	52	35	50	34	27	17
−	−	+	−	69	50	41	26	39	25	20	12
−	−	−	+	65	46	37	24	35	23	18	11
−	−	−	−	52	35	28	18	26	17	13	8

Abbreviations: See Table 29-2.

[a] In percentages; given the presence (+) or absence (−) of seven independent determinants of mortality.

[b] During index arrhythmias.

[c] Within semiacute phase of infarction. According to patient characteristics, a risk profile can be constructed by looking for the related column and row. The numbers represent the mortality (in percentages) within 2 years. See text for further explanation and examples.

(From Willems et al.,[8] with permission.)

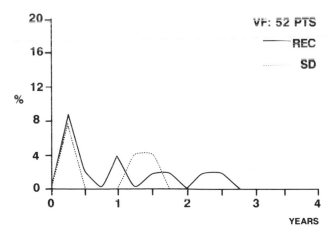

Fig. 29-4. Incidence of sudden death (SD, broken line) and recurrences of nonfatal sustained ventricular tachycardia (REC, solid line) in 52 patients with ventricular fibrillation in the late phase of a myocardial infarction. Note that sudden death had two peaks at 3 and 18 months.

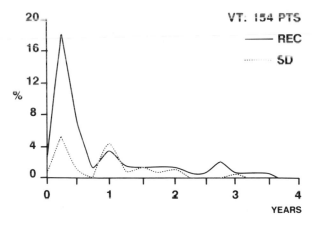

Fig. 29-5. Incidence of sudden death (SD, broken line) and recurrences of nonfatal sustained ventricular tachycardia (REC, solid line) in 154 patients with sustained ventricular tachycardia in the late phase of a myocardial infarction. Sudden death peaked at 3 and 12 months. Recurrences of nonfatal ventricular tachycardia usually occurred in the first year of follow-up.

over the next 3 years. Sudden death occurred more often in the ventricular fibrillation group, but the difference was not statistically significant.

Similar observations of post-MI patients on the improved chance of survival beyond the first year after an episode of sustained ventricular tachycardia or ventricular fibrillation were made by Furukawa et al.[9] Like our patients, most of their patients were on antiarrhythmic drugs. Winkle et al.[10] found a very low defibrillation shock incidence 1 and 2 years after implantation of an automatic defibrillator. These data suggest that risk and therefore therapeutic measures are related to the length of survival after the first episode of ventricular fibrillation or sustained ventricular tachycardia after a remote MI.

Nonfatal Recurrences of Sustained Ventricular Tachycardia

Nonfatal recurrences of sustained ventricular tachycardia are common in patients having ventricular tachycardia of different etiology (Table 29-1).

In contrast to sudden or nonsudden cardiac death, we found that nonfatal recurrences of sustained ventricular tachycardia in patient with a remote myocardial infarction cannot be predicted on the basis of the four clinical variables shown in Figures 29-1 to 29-3. As indicated in Figure 29-6, recurrences of sustained ventricular tachycardia were as common in patients with no or one of the variables as in patients having two to four variables.

Also, LVEF and such parameters as findings on coronary angiography or LV angiography did not prove helpful in predicting nonfatal recurrences of sustained ventricular tachycardia[11] in patients with previous ventricular fibrillation or sustained ventricular tachycardia after a remote MI. We observed recurrences of ventricular tachycardia in 20 of 65 (31%) patients with a LVEF of 40% or less and in 54 of 141 patients (38%) having a LVEF of greater than 40% (p = NS).

Recently, however, our group published[11] a prognostic index based on three clinical variables that was found to be of value in predicting nonfatal recurrences

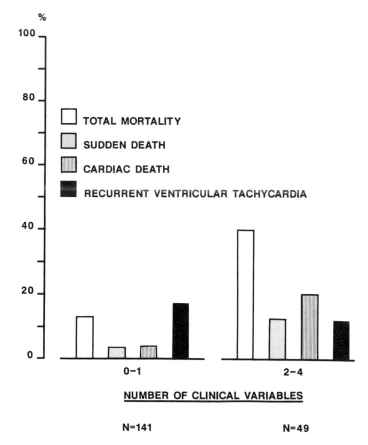

Fig. 29-6. Risk of dying suddenly and nonsuddenly and of recurrent episodes of ventricular tachycardia in relation to the presence of the same four variables shown in Figure 29-3. Recurrences of ventricular tachycardia were at least as common in patients with no or one variable as in patients having two to four variables.

TABLE 29-4. Prognostic Index Using Three Clinical Variables for Risk Estimation for Recurrences of Sustained Ventricular Tachycardia in Patients With Remote MI

Variables	Points
1. Time interval MI to first episode VT/VF	
<2 mo	1
2–6 mo	2
>6 mo	3
2. Drug therapy with or without sotalol	
With	1
Without	2
3. VT or VF as presenting arrhythmia	
VT	1
VF	2

Prognostic index

$3.41 - (0.56 \times \text{time interval}) - (1.44 \times \text{therapy}) + (0.86 \times \text{arrhythmia})$

Negative prognostic index value: 61% risk of VT recurrence
Positive prognostic index value: 4% risk of VT recurrence

Abbreviations: MI, myocardial infarction; VF, ventricular fibrillation; VT, ventricular tachycardia.

of sustained ventricular tachycardia using stepwise logistic discriminant analysis of a study group of 206 patients with ventricular fibrillation or sustained ventricular tachycardia and a remote MI. The prognostic index was constructed by giving points to three variables:

1. Time interval from MI to first episode of ventricular tachycardia or ventricular fibrillation: <2 months, 1 point; 2 to 6 months, 2 points; >6 months, 3 points
2. Drug therapy: with sotalol, 1 point; without sotalol, 2 points
3. Ventricular arrhythmias: ventricular tachycardia/fibrillation at presentation, 1 point; ventricular fibrillation, 2 points

The prognostic index is represented as follows:

$3.41 - (0.56 \times \text{interval}) - (1.94 \times \text{therapy}) + (0.86 \times \text{arrhythmia})$

When prospectively evaluated in a test group of 158 patients with sustained monomorphic ventricular tachycardia or ventricular fibrillation after healing of an acute myocardial infarction (AMI), two risk classes of patients were identified: a high-risk group (61% ventricular tachycardia recurrences in 2 years) corresponding to those with a negative index, and a low-risk group (4% ventricular tachycardia recurrences in 2 years) consisting of those with a positive index.

Thus far, stratification for risk of nonfatal ventricular tachycardia recurrences has only been done in patients with ventricular tachycardia or ventricular fibrillation after healing of an AMI. No information is

yet available concerning patients with idiopathic ventricular tachycardia, arrhythmogenic right ventricular dysplasia, or other causes of ventricular tachycardia.

PRACTICAL IMPLICATIONS

It is of obvious importance to be able to recognize patients with sustained ventricular tachycardia or ventricular fibrillation who are at high or low risk of cardiac death or of having a nonfatal recurrence of ventricular tachycardia. We believe that this is possible in patients with a remote MI. The occurrence of life-threatening ventricular arrhythmias is determined by many factors, chiefly myocardial blood supply, pump function, electrical instability, and neurocontrol (See Fig. 29-7). Some of these factors are present over a long period of time, like the degree of vessel narrowing in chronic coronary artery disease (CAD) or an increased or decreased amount of heart muscle, as in ventricular hypertrophy or after an old MI. Other factors are dynamic, such as changes in platelet function, degree of ischemia, and the neurophysiologic system. First, the physician looking after the patient should not only identify (and possibly correct) static contributing factors but should also control (as far as possible) dynamic changes.

Thereafter, these patients should be stratified as to risk of sudden (arrhythmic) death or of non-sudden death (pump failure). Figures 29-1 to 29-3 indicate factors relevant to recognizing those patients who have suffered a MI followed by ventricular fibrillation or sustained ventricular tachycardia who are at high or low risk of sudden or non-sudden cardiac death. Patients with poor pump function, early onset of a hemodynamically poorly tolerated arrhythmia, and multiple infarctions should be treated by an implantable defibrillator. By contrast, patients with hemodynamically tolerated sustained ventricular tachycardia that develops more than 2 months after a MI must be considered candidates for treatment with antiarrhythmic drugs. Selection of the antiarrhythmic agent should preferably be based on the results from programmed electric stimulation of the heart. Inability to initiate a previously inducible arrhythmia after drug therapy predicts a reduced chance of spontaneous recurrences of ventricular tachycardia.[12–14] Surgical excision or destruction of the area leading to life-threatening ventricular arrhythmias should be limited to patients in whom the site of abnormal impulse function can be localized preoperatively by endocardial mapping.[15] Operative mortality and long-term outcome can be improved by careful selection of patients. Van Hemel et al.[16] reported on the use of a LV segmental wall-motion score for that purpose. They suggested nonsur-

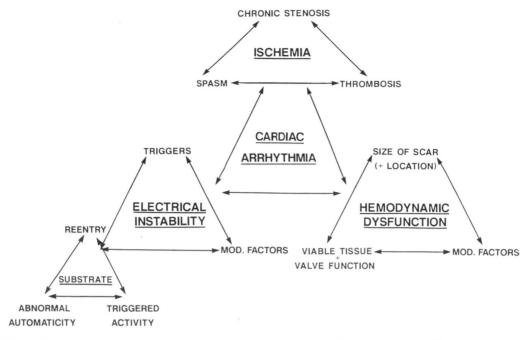

Fig. 29-7. Scheme showing the factors that play a role in cardiac arrhythmias. The basic triangle consists of electrical instability, hemodynamic dysfunction, and ischemia. Each of these three cornerstones has static and dynamic components. Modulating (MOD) factors include the autonomic nervous system, electrolytes, hormones, and drugs. COND, conduction.

gical therapy if fewer than three of nine segments of the left ventricle showed normal motion or slight hypokinesia.

CONCLUSIONS

Stratification for risk of sudden death or recurrences of sustained ventricular tachycardia is possible in some groups of patients who are resuscitated from sudden death or who present with sustained ventricular tachycardia. In those patients, this stratification should be the basis for selecting the most appropriate and cost-effective therapy. Unfortunately, prediction of risk is not possible in other groups of patients. The risk of sudden death rises with decreasing pump function. The finding of poor pump function therefore suggests consideration of the use of an implantable defibrillator. Sudden death may recur, however, in patients with idiopathic ventricular fibrillation and hypertrophic cardiomyoplasty in the presence of normal or near-normal LV function. That observation indicates that a decision to implant a defibrillator should not be based solely on LV function but on the etiology of the arrhythmia as well.

REFERENCES

1. Trappe HJ, Brugada P, Talajic M et al: Prognosis of patients with ventricular tachycardia and ventricular fibrillation: role of underlying etiology. J Am Coll Cardiol 12:166, 1988
2. Lemery R, Brugada P, Della Bella et al: Non-ischemic ventricular tachycardia. Clinical course and long term follow-up in patients without clinically overt heart disease. Circulation 79:990, 1989
3. Wellens HJJ, Brugada P: Treatment of cardiac arrhythmias: when, how and where? J Am Coll Cardiol 14:1417, 1989
4. Leclercq JF, Leenharat A, Ruta I et al: Espérance de vie après une première crise de tachycardie ventriculaire monomorphe soutenue. A propos de 295 patients suivis plus de 5 ans. Arch Mal Coeur 84:1789, 1991
5. Wellens HJJ, Lemery R, Smeets JL et al: Sudden arrhythmic death without overt heart disease. Circulation 85(I): 92, 1992
6. Brugada P, Talajic M, Smeets J et al: Risk stratification of patients with ventricular tachycardia or ventricular fibrillation after myocardial infarction. The value of the clinical history. Eur Heart J 10:747, 1989
7. Rodriguez LM, Smeets J, O'Hara GE et al: Incidence and timing of recurrences of sudden death and ventricular tachycardia during antiarrhythmic drug treatment in patients with sudden death or ventricular tachycardia after myocardial infarction. Am J Cardiol 69:1403, 1992

8. Willems AR, Tijssen JGP, Van Capelle FJC et al: Determinants of prognosis in symptomatic ventricular tachycardia or ventricular fibrillation late after myocardial infarction. J Am Coll Cardiol 16:521, 1990

9. Furakawa T, Rozanski JJ, Nogami A et al: Time-dependent risk of and predictiors for cardiac arrest recurrences in survivors of out-of-hospital cardiac arrest with chronic coronary artery disease. Circulation 80:599, 1989

10. Winkle RA, Mead RH, Ruder MA et al: Long term outcome with automatic implantable cardioverter defibrillator. J Am Coll Cardiol 13:1353, 1989

11. Rodriguez LM, Oyarzun R, Smeets J et al: Identification of patients at high risk for recurrence of sustained ventricular tachycardia after healing of acute myocardial infarction. Am J Cardiol 69:462–464, 1992

12. Fisher JD, Cohen HL, Mehra R et al: Cardiac pacing and pacemakers. II. Serial electrophysiologic-pharmacologic testing for control of recurrent tachyarrhythmias. Am Heart J 93:658, 1977

13. Mason JW, Winkle RA: Electrode-catheter arrhythmia induction in selection and assessment of antiarrhythmic drug therapy for recurrent ventricular tachycardia. Circulation 58:971, 1978

14. Horowitz LN, Josephson ME, Farshidi A et al: Recurrent sustained ventricular tachycardia. 3. Role of the electrophysiologic study in selection of antiarrhythmic regimens. Circulation 58:986, 1978

15. Miller J, Kienzle M, Harken A, Josephson ME: Subendocardial resection for ventricular tachycardia: predictors of surgical success. Circulation 70:624, 1984

16. Van Hemel NM, Kingma JH, DeFauw JAM et al: Left ventricular segmental wall motion score as a criterion for selecting patients for direct surgery in the treatment of postinfarction ventricular tachycardia. Eur Heart J 9: 304, 1989

Section VI

CARDIOVASCULAR PROGNOSIS AS RELATED TO MISCELLANEOUS CONDITIONS

30

Pseudo-Prognosis of Primary Pulmonary Hypertension and Its Impact on Patient Outcome

Robert F. McCauley
Eugene D. Robin

The evolution of management of patients with primary pulmonary hypertension (PPH) provides a useful example of the impact of an erroneous prognostic estimate (pseudo-prognosis) on patient outcome. PPH is a disorder of usually unexplained etiology that affects primarily the precapillary pulmonary vessels, leading to an increase in pulmonary artery pressure and resistance in pulmonary arterioles and ultimately to right heart hypertrophy and cor pulmonale. It is almost certain that the etiology is not homogeneous and, in fact, nosologically the diagnosis is a wastebasket.

Until recently, PPH has been generally regarded as an inexorably progressive disease that is rapidly fatal within a few years. The almost universal acceptance of such a bleak prognosis has resulted in aggressive diagnostic and therapeutic interventions. The implicit theory is that patients with this disorder have little to lose by aggressive approaches. They are doomed by the nature of their disease to an early demise.

This opinion has been summarized by an astute observer (who himself has major reservations about the efficacy and safety of current therapeutic approaches): "In the management of a disease as potentially lethal as PPH, it is difficult to stand by and withhold a promising treatment."[1]

Even the emergence of data obtained from a relatively large group of patients that establishes the fact that a substantial percentage of patients with PPH survive years to decades after the onset of symptoms (or after diagnosis) has done little or nothing to modulate diagnostic or therapeutic aggressiveness.[2] In fact, the improved prognosis has been attributed to the use of current interventions,[3] although many of the long-term survivors were not so treated, and others did not have the so-called benefits of modern treatment during most of the 5, 10, or 15 years of their disease.

EARLY MEDICAL HISTORY

Hippocrates is supposed to have stated: "Desperate diseases demand desperate measures."[4] There is an entire stream in medical history that reflects the application of such an approach. One florid example emanated from Burchhardt, the father of the ill-fated use of psychosurgery in the treatment of schizophrenia. Burckhardt stated: "better a dangerous treatment than no treatment at all."[5]

Systemic lupus erythematosus (SLE) provides a dramatic example. During the late 1930s, it was believed that 80% of patients died within 1 year after the appearance of symptoms. By 1954, it was believed that 50% of patients died within 3 years after the appearance of symptoms. By 1978, it was recognized that less than 20% of patients died within 10 years of the appearance of symptoms. The progressive decline in mortality is now attributed mainly to decreased iatrogenesis and to more selective use of hazardous therapeutic agents.[6]

In cardiovascular disease, the use of thyroidectomy for the treatment of angina and/or congestive heart failure provides another example. The following quotation emphasizes the essence of the concept: "Actually, the operation [thyroidectomy] is a last resort when everything else has been tried and there is nothing more to lose."[7] In fact, there was much to lose. Patients so treated suffered from two diseases: iatrogenic hypothyroidism and coronary artery disease (CAD).

It did not occur to the ancients that estimates of prognosis might be incorrect. Suppose that a generally accepted view of the natural life history of a disease is incorrect. Suppose a significant subpopulation of patients turns out to have a substantially better prognosis than assigned to it by conventional wisdom. These patients may be exposed to avoidable risks based on a fundamental misconception. The fact of early death may turn out to be a self-fulfilling prophesy because of the interaction of the disease and aggressive risky interventions. It will turn out that these general problems apply quite directly to the management of PPH.

The following material was extracted from an excellent historical review of PPH published in 1979.[8] PPH may have been first described in 1891 by Romberg.[9] Arillaga[10] in 1913 believed that the disorder was caused by arteritis of the pulmonary vessels. Dresdale et al.[11] established the disorder as a clinical entity in 1951. They considered "isolated sympathetic overactivity" as the probable etiology. Wood[12] emphasized pulmonary vasoconstriction as a mechanism in the pathogenesis of PPH, using reasoning similar to that used by Prinzmetal in describing vasoconstrictive angina.

The outbreak of an epidemic of pulmonary hypertension in three European countries in 1967 was attributed to (associated with) the ingestion of an appetite suppressant aminorex.[13] Incidentally, this lead to the pathogenesis of the epidemic was not followed up adequately.

The pathologic changes in the pulmonary blood vessels were well documented by Heath and Edwards in 1958[14] and extended by Wagenvoort and Wagenvoort.[15]

Early estimates of prognosis were based on limited numbers of patients with little critical evaluation of the data. For example, Wood[16] reported a mean survival time of 2 to 3 years after diagnosis. This estimate was in accord with most modern estimates. It was not recognized that an accurate determination of prognosis is unusually difficult in PPH. The early symptoms are quite nonspecific. Diagnosis requires right-sided cardiac catheterization, and this is usually not employed until the disease is relatively far advanced. The preliminary diagnosis can only be made by exclusion of other causes of pulmonary hypertension. As a result, the disorder is usually far advanced at the time of diagnosis. The problem of establishing an accurate prognosis is also complicated by the fact that there may be spontaneous regression of PPH (see below). Under these circumstances, the prognosis of the patients becomes that of normals. Spontaneous regression also complicated the interpretation of outcome data related to the use of one therapeutic measure or another. The attribution of efficacy to a given therapy without using adequate data obtained from controls is a general problem in therapeutics. (see below)

Prognostic estimates are also complicated by the effects of treatment. It is generally accepted that for surgical procedures, morbidity and morbidity estimates should include the immediate preoperative (workup) period, the direct operative period, and an arbitrary segment of the postoperative period. In the case of medical treatment, there is no generally accepted approach. It seems reasonable to calculate mortality and morbidity including the pretreatment workup, the rates during treatment, and the posttreatment rate for, again, an arbitrary period. This last calculation can be most difficult, admittedly, especially when long-term harmful effects of diagnostic (e.g., x-ray screening for scoliosis) or therapeutic (e.g., radioiodine therapy for Graves' disease) modalities are involved.

The diagnostic specificity and sensitivity of pathologic changes in the lung have not been clearly established. Although such terms as "unexplained plexogenic pulmonary arteriopathy" have crept into the literature, there is no adequate database to use the presence or absence of such changes for accurate diagnosis.

In any case, ancient medical history provided an impression of a disorder with a very short life expectancy following diagnosis. Moreover, the disorder was assumed to be inexorably and rapidly progressive.

This in turn led to aggressive diagnostic and therapeutic interventions.

It should be emphasized that the belief in a dismal prognosis was not the sole factor in pushing aggressive management for PPH. Physicians and experts caring for these patients were also motivated to provide the best care possible in hopes of extending life expectancy. The assumption of a poor prognosis, however, expanded the boundaries of the permissible. This impact of prognosis on management can be seen now in the management of human immunodeficiency virus (HIV)-positive patients. Therapeutic leads are aggressively pursued.

CONTEMPORARY CRITICAL MEDICAL HISTORY

This segment of analysis begins by arbitrarily using the 1970s as the starting point. During the 1970s and early 1980s, the view of an almost invariably progressive disorder was not seriously challenged. Reports by Fuster et al.,[17] Walcott et al.,[18] Cherian et al.,[19] Wagenvoort and Wagenvoort,[20] and the thoughtful review by Voelkel and Reeves[8] accepted as a given that the prognosis of PPH was bleak. In particular, a large series assembled by Fuster et al.[17] provided evidence for a grim prognosis. This group reported a median survival of 1.9 years after diagnosis. Unfortunately, there was a 5% mortality in the group from diagnostic right-sided catheterization alone.

Almost every study described rare individual patients surviving 5, 10, or 20 years after diagnosis. Such patients were regarded as statistical aberrations or outliers. Individual patients had been described with survivals of 19 to 29 years after diagnosis, but this was considered so unusual as to warrant case reports in the literature.

The first systematic questioning of the duration of survival in patients with PPH was published by Rozkovec et al. in 1986.[21] These data were impressive enough to warrant an editorial in *Lancet* questioning the validity of conventional wisdom about a grim prognosis.[22]

The largest series that confirmed unequivocally that long-term survival in PPH occurred frequently was published in 1987.[2] (The junior author of this chapter [E.D.R.] was a member of the team of investigators and could therefore have an unconscious bias concerning the data.) However, the results are clear cut. The series was large, involving 90 patients. The total of previously published patients including approximately 200 from a National Institutes of Health (NIH) patient registry is less than 1,000 patients. Thus, the series provided data concerning about 10% of all previously reported patients. The diagnosis in each had

been confirmed sufficiently to qualify the patients for consideration of heart-lung transplantation. The degree of abnormality was also deemed sufficient to evaluate each patient seriously for possible heart-lung transplantation.

The series was collected as the result of an incidental set of observations. The survival of some patients with PPH on the active waiting list for transplantation was unexpectedly prolonged. This led to a retrospective analysis of all patients who had been referred for evaluation irrespective of whether they were ultimately selected for active candidacy. The importance of accidental observations is that no member of the investigative team began with a preconception that current dogma was incorrect.

No member of the investigative team had the area of PPH as a major clinical or research interest. The importance of this is that the team of investigators had no conflict of interest involving previous published material affirming or denying the validity of previous published prognostic estimates.

The length of survival following the onset of symptoms was 66 months (>5 years), and the mean survival from diagnosis was 43 months (3.6 years). More significantly by actuarial analysis, 37% of the group lived for 5 years and 15% lived for 10 years following diagnosis. The data fit a continuum so that prolonged survival did not represent a small group of statistical outliers. Most important, if the patients had survived more than 2 to 3 years, there was a high probability that they would survive 5 to 15 years. In fact, the data fit a bimodal distribution. One group of patients of about 20% of the total cohort died within the first 2 years and another group, about 60%, survived as long as 16 years. This finding suggests that, as in the case of systemic hypertension, there is a group of patients that might be diagnosed as having malignant pulmonary hypertension and another group with nonmalignant pulmonary hypertension.[2]

A similar but smaller group of patients was accumulated in England. Of a group of 34 patients, 8 died within 5 years of presentation to a hospital. Twelve patients survived more than 5 years and 4 lived more than 15 years.[21]

In addition to prolonged survival, the evidence for spontaneous reversion of primary pulmonary hypertension independent of treatment is incontrovertible. Spontaneous remissions have been documented by Bourdillon and Oakley[23] by Blount,[8] by Fugii et al.,[24] and in a group of patients with aminorex pulmonary hypertension on withdrawal of anorectics.[25] The precise incidence of spontaneous regression is not known. However, such patients are not included in most prognostic estimates. Their inclusion would lengthen prognostic estimates considerably. More importantly, the death of such patients because of diagnostic or therapeutic misadventures would represent a striking tragedy.

It is therefore clear that PPH is not invariably rapidly fatal, that prior prognostic estimates of what might be termed malignant pulmonary hypertension have dominated the diagnostic and therapeutic efforts of many experts and have led to unwarranted conclusions about the efficacy of various interventions.

There are a number of patients in whom prolonged survival was attributed to the use of various pulmonary vasodilators whose use has been abandoned because of lack of efficacy. A single case report in a prestigious journal describes a patient who showed improvement for 3 years despite progressive disease because of treatment with isoproterenol (now a discredited and abandoned form of treatment).[26] Pietro et al.[27] described a patient with sustained improvement during 6 years of treatment with sublingual isoproterenol. Chann et al.[28] reported reversibility of PPH during 6 years of treatment with another discarded pulmonary vasodilator, oral diazoxide. No one has yet tried snake oil or oil-of-primrose, to our knowledge.

In a disorder with spontaneous remissions, uncontrolled observations of efficacy should always be suspect. The profound limitations of such observations in PPH are demonstrated in a study reported by Danktzer et al.[29] Serial right heart catheterizations were performed in 6 patients with PPH receiving long-term therapy with pulmonary vasodilators. None of the six patients showed a rise in pulmonary artery pressure or pulmonary vascular resistance when vasodilator therapy was withdrawn, nor did these variables fall when therapy was resumed. One would have to believe either that short courses of vasodilators cure PPH indefinitely or that the variability of the disorder makes randomized controlled trials obligatory to assess even the effect of therapy on surrogate criteria (pulmonary vascular resistance and pulmonary artery pressure), let alone patient outcome.

In a thoughtful editorial comment on these studies, Packer[30] summarized a similar sequence in the use of prazosin in the treatment of left ventricular (LV) failure. Uncontrolled nonrigorous studies reported marked hemodynamic improvement accompanied by clear clinical benefit following prazosin. These changes were sustained during long-term therapy.[30] It has now been established by a prospective randomized controlled clinical trial that prazosin produces no patient improvement. Parenthetically, such rigorous trials have not been performed on any pulmonary vasodilator despite the large number of different agents that have, or are being, used.

To document the impact of an erroneous estimate of prognosis on therapy, it is useful to review some of the therapeutic modalities used in the treatment of PPH

TABLE 30-1. Therapeutic Modalities Used in the Treatment of PPH

Therapy	Present Status[a]
1. Steroids	Abandoned
2. Immuran	Abandoned
3. Reserpine	Abandoned
4. Anticoagulants	Largely abandoned
5. Fibrinolysis	Abandoned
6. Sympathectomy	Abandoned
7. Monoamine oxidase inhibitors	Abandoned
8. Antiseritonin	Abandoned
9. Priscoline	Abandoned
10. Nitroglycerine	Largely abandoned
11. Isosorbide dinitrate	Largely abandoned
12. β$_2$-Agonists (isoproterenol, terbutaline)	Abandoned
13. Banthine	Abandoned
14. Oxygen	Abandoned
15. Pulmonary artery banding	Abandoned
16. Hydralazine	Abandoned
17. Captopril	Largely abandoned
18. Diazoxide	Abandoned
19. Epoprostenol	Largely abandoned
20. Calcium-channel blockers, regular dose	Abandoned
21. Calcium-channel blockers, megadose	In use
22. Nitroprusside	Abandoned
23. Phentolamine	Abandoned
24. Phenoxybenzamine	Probably abandoned
25. Prazosin	Abandoned
26. Tolazoline	Abandoned
27. Heart-lung transplant	Actively pursued

[a] For all forms of therapy, the efficacy/safety documented by PRCCT was zero.

(Table 30-1). The first 16 interventions are taken from a table in the review by Voelkel and Reeves.[8] The last 10 have been added by us.

Given a disorder in which the total number of reported cases in the medical literature is less than 1,000, this amounts to one different form of therapy per 30 patients. The exact number of patients harmed by adverse drug effects will never be known.

Another problem is that it is possible that one or more of the listed interventions might be effective, say, in the treatment of malignant PPH. Given the uncontrolled and undisciplined use of these agents, a truly effective and safe form of therapy might have been or could be abandoned.

For example, the potential use of epoprosternol (prostacyclin) to treat PPH and secondary pulmonary hypertension has been suggested.[31] The major problems associated with its use are (1) the requirement for intravenous administration; and (2) the hazards associated with the use of a generalized vasodilator in the face of a high, largely fixed pulmonary vascular resistance and a relatively normal systemic vascular resistance. Vasodilation during exercise can cause systemic pooling of blood and a resultant decrease in cardiac output that can cause hypotension, shock, and death.

Theoretically, it is feasible to administer prostacyclin so that intravenous (IV) infusion is not required, and so that there is first-pass exposure of pulmonary vascular smooth muscle with little or no spillover to systemic arterioles, thus avoiding one of the major risks of pulmonary vasodilator therapy (Robin ED: personal communication). A well-designed PRCCT could explore such a possibility. Such a trial would examine the effects of prostacyclin treatment on patient outcome and not the surrogate criteria of reduced pulmonary vascular resistance or pulmonary artery pressure. In the present setting, it is unlikely such a trial will be organized.

A major error in this smorgasbord of possible therapeutic interventions is that proponents have used only interventions whose safety and efficacy were not validated by a proper prospective randomized controlled trial (despite some promises to do so[32]). No therapeutic interventions have been acceptably validated.

Some comments are in order concerning transplantation either single lung or heart-bilateral lung transplant. When contrasted with an assumed 1- to 2-year mortality of 90%, a favorable risk-benefit balance seemed obvious. Given a substantial 5-year survival rate without surgery, the status of the risk-benefit balance is not as clear. Despite a number of theoretical problems, a well designed PRCCT should be performed.

One major problem has been the nature of the criteria by which to judge therapeutic efficacy. In general, two usually interrelated (but surrogate) criteria have been used. The ability of a given intervention to reduce pulmonary vascular resistance and to reduce pulmonary artery pressure has been substituted for the ability of that agent to prolong patient life or to improve the quality of life. The claim is made that the level of pulmonary vascular resistance is correlated with survival in PPH.[32] In the same communication making this claim, it is stated, "early study evaluating hydralazine did not show improvement in mortality or improved quality of life . . . despite (improvement in hemodynamics)."

To state that the level of pulmonary vascular resistance correlates in untreated patients with survival and hence to imply that reducing pulmonary vascular resistance by drugs improves survival is a variant of a well-known error in logic:

Aristotle is an animal.
A horse is an animal.
Therefore, Aristole is a horse.

Proof of decreased mortality requires a demonstration that the length of survival is increased.

The dependence on surrogate criteria has produced another problem. It appears that the ultimate outcome of patients treated with various pulmonary vasodilators cannot be extracted from the published literature. As a result it is relatively easy to understand why therapy after therapy, pulmonary vasodilator after pulmonary vasodilator has been tried. Involved physicians were attempting to come up with effective treatment for a disease that they considered rapidly and invariably fatal. It is not clear specifically from the published literature why treatment after treatment was abandoned. The number of patients injured during the use of each therapy cannot be estimated from the published literature.

> Monamine begat priscoline.
> Priscoline begat nitroglycerine.
> Nitroglycerine begat isosorbide.
> Isosorbide begat isoproperenol.
> Isoproterenol begat hydralazine.
> Hydralazine begat nitroprusside.
> Nitroprusside begat phentolamine.
> Phentolamine begat phenoxybenzamine.
> Phenoxybenzamine begat normal dose calcium channel blockers.
> Normal dose calcium channel blockers begat mega dose calcium channel blockers.

What in fact happened to patients subjected to these various forms of treatment? It may well require some future medical archeologist to dig through the isoproterenol era and the hydralazine era to determine the fate of those patients managed with specific forms of treatment. Given a disorder believed to be rapidly fatal, it may not have seemed important to determine patient outcome. It may have seemed adequate to determine whether or not pulmonary vascular resistance decreased.

A particular relevant review of the risks associated with some of the drugs that have been employed to treat PPH was contributed by Packer in 1985.[33] These agents included α-adrenergic blockers, parasympathomimetic drugs, β-adrenergic drugs, direct-acting vasodilator drugs, nitroglycerine and nitroprusside, calcium-channel blockers, angiotensin converting enzyme (ACE) inhibitors, prostaglandins, and amrinone. None of these agents was studied by a PRCCT, and none was free of toxicity.

A general phenomenon noted with the use of agents to treat a presumed lethal condition, especially on the basis of surrogate therapeutic goals, involves three practices. One is that many different agents are tried empirically, as has characterized PPH. The second is the use of various combinations of agents. This also has been tried. The third is to use megadoses of a given agent, hoping to find efficacy. Such an approach is now being used with calcium-channel blockers (see below). It is generally not recognized that major increases in dose might not only improve whatever indices are selected for study, but might also increase risks either arithmetically or exponentially.

It is of some interest that a clinical trial that demonstrates unfavorable results, even though the trial falls well short of being an acceptable PRCCT, may not inhibit the use of certain forms of therapy. For example, in a study published by Rich et al. in 1985,[34] 23 patients with PPH were followed. A favorable drug response to nifedipine and hydralazine, defined as a drop in pulmonary vascular resistance of at least 20%, occurred in 18 of the patients. Nine of the patients who exhibited a "favorable" short-term response were treated with long-term pulmonary vasodilator therapy. The nine patients who responded and the five who did not were followed. There was no significant difference in survival between the treated and the untreated groups.

This absence of patient improvement had little if any impact on the use of pulmonary vasodilators in other patients by the investigators who obtained the above data. In fact, the investigators describe long-term favorable effects with diazoxide and nifedipine in isolated patients and speculate: "This raises the question as to whether one must reduce the pulmonary arterial pressure to near-normal levels with therapy before long term clinical benefits will be realized in patients with PPH."

This speculation may have been a factor in the recent use of high-dose calcium-channel blockers in the treatment of PPH. An alternate hypothesis—that pulmonary vasodilators do not prolong life—does not seem to have been seriously considered. Obviously no attention was paid to the possibility that the use of these agents might indeed shorten life expectancy. Such a hypothesis would have been incompatible with the then current view that PPH was rapidly fatal. The point is that without an adequate PRCCT, the ability of any given therapy to lengthen or shorten life expectancy cannot be accurately measured.

In the final analysis, it appears obvious that the plethora of treatments for PPH is partially the result of the presumed poor prognosis of patients with this disease.

DIAGNOSTIC-PHYSIOLOGIC STUDIES

This section discusses some of the diagnostic interventions that have been, or are being, used in patients with PPH. The reader may wish to review the material concerning the criteria to be used in evaluating given medical tests (see Ch. 1). Briefly stated, it must be established by a rigorous clinical trial that (1) the results of the test statistically improve decision making, and (2) improved decision making in turn improves patient outcome. It will become apparent that these criteria have not been achieved by the diagnostic-physiologic approaches used or advocated in patients with PPH.

It may also be useful to review the material on the use of human subjects as experimental subjects (see Ch. 1). It will become obvious that patients with PPH have been and are used in studies involving not only treatment but also testing in which the patients serve primarily as experimental subjects rather than as patients. It is not clear that the two minimal requirements for the employment of human subjects are always met: (1) that truly informed consent is obtained from the subjects, and (2) that there has been institutional clearance to perform the studies. All too often, such studies are performed under the rubric of patient care and not of experimental study. If the patient is suffering from what is believed to be a rapidly fatal disease, it becomes easier to distort patient care and convert the patient into an experimental subject.

These considerations lead to several insights, the first of which is whether diagnosis for the sake of diagnosis is an acceptable practice. There is no simple answer but, in a rational world, a diagnosis would only be pursued when it is highly probable that the establishment of an accurate diagnosis would improve patient outcome. The old Oslerian precept that "medicine is diagnosis, diagnosis, diagnosis"[35] should be replaced by a dictum that medicine must strive for "improved patient outcome, improved patient outcome, improved patient outcome." In a formal sense, the pursuit of specific diagnosis should be guided by acceptable evidence that the risk-benefit balance of the pursuit is favorable for the patient.

Another misconception is that aggressive pursuit of pathophysiology is an acceptable intervention strategy. It is common knowledge that large numbers of effective forms of therapy are introduced and used without knowing the mechanism by which the therapy works. Penicillin was known to be highly effective for pneumococcal pneumonia long before it was recognized that it interfered with bacterial cell wall synthesis. The administration of oxygen was known to be effective long before its role in ATP synthesis was known.

Conversely, an accurate determination of pathophysiology (when that is possible) often leads to no improvement in patient outcome. The fact that adult respiratory distress syndrome (ARDS) is a form of low-pressure pulmonary edema (increased permeability) has been known for about 15 years.[36] This knowledge has not improved the outcome of this disease, whose mortality remains at about 50 to 60% despite improved basic knowledge.[37] A dictum such as that applied to pulmonary hypertension "... most patients should have a catheterization study to characterize the severity and pathophysiology of their disease," should raise the counter question: why? (Rich and Rubin, unpublished observations.) Determination of pathophysiology should be pursued when there is evidence that the pursuit offers a favorable risk-benefit balance for the patient. With this as background, various forms of testing have been and are still advocated for patients with PPH. One driving force has been the view that, given a dismal prognosis, the patient had little to lose.

Lung Biopsy

Open lung biopsy in patients with PPH was in vogue for a number of years. This fad seems to be passing.[31] The ostensible justification for performing a lung biopsy was to eliminate the possibility of a reversible or treatable cause of pulmonary hypertension. This was seldom if ever realized. It has been argued that lung biopsy may permit a distinction between PPH and interstitial or collagen vascular disease. There is no evidence that drawing that distinction would result in a statistical improvement in patient outcome.

There appears to be little doubt that the performance of an open lung biopsy in patients with PPH is more hazardous than in patients with diffuse interstitial lung disease. The operative mortality in patients with interstitial lung disease is generally considered to be about 1.8%.[38] The perioperative mortality in PPH is almost certainly higher.

The nature of the decision-making process with respect to performing open lung biopsy in PPH is illustrated by the following example. An NHLBI-sponsored registry for patients with PPH has been operating for a number of years. Obtaining an open lung biopsy was not an official prerequisite for registering patients, however it was strongly suggested. The strength of the suggestion is reflected in the fact that 10 to 15% of the approximately 200 registered patients underwent this procedure. It seems at least one of the patients may have died as a result of lung biopsy.[39] The suggestion to perform open lung biopsy has been specifically revoked.[40] Both the original decision to recommend lung biopsy and then the decision to disavow lung biopsy were not based on acceptable or substantial evidence. Nor has there been, to the best of our knowledge, an adequate disclosure of the mortality and morbidity of the procedure performed on patients in the federal registry.

The question remains why lung biopsies were ever performed on numerous patients with a presumed diagnosis of PPH. There is no acceptable answer, nor are there acceptable estimates of the mortality and morbidity of open lung biopsy in this group of patients.

Furthermore, repeated emphasis on the need for early diagnosis of PPH is based on the (unsupported) surmise that early diagnosis will—in some unexplained way—benefit patients. It appears that the early diagnosis will, at best, favor data collectors inasmuch as there appears to be little correlation between duration of symptoms before diagnosis and severity of illness at the time of diagnosis.[2,8]

Cardiac Catheterization

The use of cardiac catheterization in patients with suspected PPH runs a wide spectrum of degrees of aggressive patient intervention. On one end of the spectrum is the use of right-sided catheterization to establish or confirm the presence of pulmonary hypertension. On the other end are protocols meant to apply to patients with pulmonary hypertension, whatever the cause (and not only to patients with suspected PPH). Here is an example:

> Should all patients undergo catheterization? Most authorities advise that catheterization of the right side and, if necessary [criteria not stated] the left side of the heart should be performed at some point during clinically significant disease to characterize its severity and pathophysiology. Diagnostic catheterization is crucial [to whom?] with unexplained pulmonary hypertension when you suspect the condition is primary or secondary to congenital heart disease or pulmonary thromboembolism. The need is less crucial when all the non-invasively obtained data including echocardiography are compatible with a straightforward diagnosis of COPD. In older patients, coronary angiography should usually be a part of the catheterization workup.
>
> *(Rich and Rubin, unpublished observations.)*

[And then, in a statement that might daunt the most invasive of invasive cardiologists] A complete study of pulmonary hemodynamics and gas exchange looks at pressures, flows, and shunts. It includes measurement of cardiac output, venous and arterial oxygen saturations, wedge pressure, left and right pulmonary arterial pressures, and left and right intracardiac pressures, and allows the calculation of pulmonary vascular resistance. The data should be sufficient to consider pathophysiology as varied as pulmonary arteriolar atresia, shunts and occult valvular disease.

(Rich and Rubin, unpublished observations.)

In an attempt to determine whether all patients with PPH should undergo cardiac catheterization, one must consider its uses:

1. Confirm a diagnosis of PPH by means of a single isolated right-sided catheterization.
2. Follow the progression of PPH by sequential right-sided catheterization.
3. Estimate the degree of pulmonary vasoconstriction by noting catheterization derived values acutely before and after the use of a putative pulmonary vasodilator. This process is called a drug titration.
4. Evaluate the impact of putative pulmonary vasodi-

lators on pulmonary hemodynamics by repetitive right-sided catheterizations over time.
5. Establish a dose for given pulmonary vasodilators by successive increases in the amount of a given drug required acutely to achieve arbitrary reductions in pulmonary artery pressure or pulmonary vascular resistance.

One immediate question involves the morbidity and mortality associated with right-sided catheterization in PPH. The data in the literature are not reassuring. In one large collated summary series, 31 of 152 (20%) patients catheterized died within 36 hours after catheterization.[8] Some of these patients had more than one catheterization. The series of Fuster et al.[7] reported a 5% mortality associated with a right-sided catheterization in 112 patients with PPH. The increased risk of right-sided cardiac catheterization in children and adolescents were emphasized in 1974[41] and again in 1977.[42] In the latter series, during 30 catheterizations in 22 patients there were five major and six minor complications. One death (4.5%) occurred in the group. A series of right-sided catheterizations were reported by a national registry to collect data on patients with PPH. Ten adverse reactions were noted in the 187 patients catheterized (5.3%) for the purpose of the Registry. No deaths were reported in this series. Six of the adverse reactions included transient hypotension and hemoptysis.[43]

Patients undergoing drug titrations during right-sided catheterization were not as fortunate. Of 163 patients entered into the Registry, only 104 were considered to be acceptable for inclusion into the Registry. In the 104 patients, there were two catheter-associated deaths (1.9%) and 32 adverse effects noted (30.7%). Eight of the patients either died or required treatment for systemic hypotension.[44]

In addition to the high morbidity and mortality, these data pose a puzzling question. Why were the data obtained on 59 of the 163 patients (36%) excluded from the Registry? What was the morbidity and mortality of these patients during single catheterization and during drug titration? Obviously insight into the fate of the total group is required for an accurate estimate of the hazards. It is possible that there were no deaths or complications in the group of the missing 59 patients, but that fact should have been made known, if it is a fact. Because the Registry was supported by federal funds, one would expect particular sensitivity here on the question of complete disclosure.

The failure of adequate disclosure is reminiscent of a similar episode from the great Russian novel, "Dead Souls" by Nicolai Vasilevich Gogal.[45] The hero, Chichikov, organized a scam to acquire title to dead serfs and then sell them. In Czarist Russia, serfs had considerable economic value. After death, the serfs, with their names remaining in the registry, were considered too unimportant to have the fact of their death, much less the mode of death, recorded.

"But allow me first to make a request," he said in a voice in which there was a strange, or almost strange, note, and for some reason he looked round him immediately. Manilov, too, for some reason looked round. "How long is it since you sent off the census list of your peasants?"

"Oh, that must have been some time ago. As a matter of fact, I can't remember."

"And how many of your peasants died since then?"

"I'm afraid I don't know. I expect I'd have to ask my agent about it. You there! Please, call the agent. He should be here today."

The agent appeared. He was a man of about forty who shaved his beard, wore a frock-coat, and apparently led a well-contented life, for he had a plump and well-fed face, and his yellowish complexion and half-shut eyes showed that he was all too familiar with feather beds and bolsters. One could see at once that he had followed his calling as all landowners' agents do: to begin with, he was simply an errand boy in the house who could read and write, then he had married some Agashka, a housekeeper and a favorite of the mistress, had himself become a house steward and, later on, an agent. Having become an agent, he quite naturally did as all agents do: kept company and made friends with the better-off villagers, levied higher taxes on the poorer families, got up at nine o'clock in the morning, waited for the samovar, and drank tea.

"Look here, my dear fellow, how many of our peasants have died since the last census?"

"How many?. Why, lots of them have died since then," said the agent and hiccoughed, covering his mouth slightly with his hand as with a shield.

"Well, I must say, I thought so myself," Manilov interposed. "Yes, yes, lots have died." Then he turned to Chichikov and added, "Yes, indeed, lots, lots have died."

"You don't know the exact figure by any chance?" asked Chichikov.

"Yes, what is the figure?" Manilov put in.

"Well, sir, I'm afraid I can't tell the figure. You see, sir, it's not known how many have died. No one has counted them."

"Yes, that's it," said Manilov turning to Chichikov. "I too thought there had been a high mortality. It's quite impossible to say how many have died."

Finally, it should be emphasized that all catheterization protocols are carried out in the absence of rigorous data that the procedures result in improved patient outcome in PPH or lead to more effective treatment as a result of these studies. It should be emphasized that in many areas of medicine not uncommonly patients who die during diagnostic physiologic or therapeutic studies are simply excluded from the final statistical evaluation of a given intervention (see Ch. 1). These poor souls are even less fortunate than Chichikov's dead serfs.

Ventilation-Perfusion Scans and Pulmonary Angiography

Lung scanning is commonly performed as a routine in patients with suspected PPH. The rationale is that the differential diagnosis of PPH includes pulmonary embolic disease. It is usually not recognized that perfusion scanning is probably more hazardous in patients with restricted pulmonary circulation than in other patients.[46] Perfusion scanning is based on the production of multiple microemboli in the pulmonary circulation that are rapidly biodegradable. Although the risks associated with this procedure are in general exceedingly small, the added risk in pulmonary hypertension should be explicitly recognized.

More important are the limitations of lung scanning. These are not usually emphasized and are often poorly understood. A normal or near-normal perfusion lung scan has high sensitivity (with or without a ventilation scan) and therefore a normal perfusion scan rules out pulmonary clot-obstructive disease with a probability of about 95%. However a positive $\dot{V}/\dot{Q}$ scan whether low probability, intermediate probability or high probability usually lacks sufficient specificity to serve as the basis for important therapeutic decisions.

For example, the summary of the results of one careful prospective study states: "Clinical assessment combined with the ventilation/perfusion scan established the diagnosis or exclusion of pulmonary embolism only for a minority of patients—those with clear and concordant clinical and ventilation/perfusion scan findings."[47]

Given these problems, the demonstration of an abnormal lung scan is often followed by pulmonary angiography. The mortality of pulmonary angiography in a mixed population of patients is probably less than 1%.[48] Among patients suspected of having pulmonary embolism, some with and some without pulmonary hypertension, a positive pulmonary angiogram leads to the use of an effective form of therapy, anticoagulants (which do have their own risks). As a result, the performance of pulmonary angiograms in such a population appears to have a highly favorable risk-benefit ratio.

It is likely that the morbidity and mortality of pulmonary angiography in patients with PPH are substantially higher than in a mixed population[8] thus reducing the possibility of a favorable risk-benefit ratio for angiography in these patients (i.e., increased risk). Likewise, there has been no rigorous demonstration that we have an effective and safe form of therapy for PPH. Thus, the contribution of pulmonary angiography in this disorder, subjected to further risk-benefit analysis (i.e., essentially no benefit), plummets from "questionably favorable" to "grossly unfavorable." None of these considerations seems to have made a significant impact on decision making by some experts in PPH.[3]

Recently a new rationalization has appeared for extensive imaging studies of the pulmonary circulation in PPH. This involves the use of surgical endarterectomy for chronic large pulmonary artery embolism.[3] This rationalization is discussed below.

Miscellaneous studies have been suggested: echocardiography, thallium scanning, measurements of right ventricular ejection fraction, exercise gallium scanning, and bronchial lavage are all potential approaches to patients with PPH of undocumented value in that disease.

For those interested in cost containment or cost-benefit analysis, a number of technological advances are waiting in the wings to be applied to patients with PPH.

Magnetic resonance imaging (MRI) could provide excellent views of the pulmonary circulation. Magnetic resonance spectroscopy (MRS) could provide exciting data on the metabolic events in the hypertensive lung. Positron emission tomography (PET) could provide color pictures that differentiate areas of high, low, or unusual metabolic activity.

Single photon emission computed tomography scanning could be used to supplement the data obtained from the other methods. The point is that, in the absence of a requirement for rigorous evidence, with the use of a given technology improving patient outcome, there is almost no limit to the number and kind of diagnostic tests that can be performed.

As with therapeutic interventions, the paradigm of a rapidly progressive disease with an almost invariably fatal prognosis has fueled the aggressive use of a variety of diagnostic studies, some of which have contributed to a rapid and high mortality.

Impact of the New Prognostics

Evaluation of cultural lag within medicine requires an estimate of how rapidly medical thinking and medical practice change in response to new data. It is difficult to make accurate estimates because there tends to be a heterogeneous response among various experts in a given field. In the specific area of PPH, it should be emphasized that various experts may not have heard about the recent data on prognosis, and some who have been exposed to these data do not accept or believe the new information.

The failure to change is illustrated by a recent article written for primary care physicians. Published in a magazine *Patient Care*, it provides strong evidence that new data have made little impact.[3]

From the standpoint of testing, only the use of open lung biopsy has been downgraded. The degree of aggressive cardiac catheterization has, if anything, been accentuated by coupling drug titration to another—inadequately tested—form of vasodilator therapy.

In a stirring appeal, primary care physicians are encouraged to refer their patients to specialized centers for the benefits of modern management[3]:

> The past decade has seen great strides in the understanding and management of pulmonary hypertension (PH). As the primary care physician, you are the major participant in the management of your patients with this disease, day in and day out on the front line of clinical medicine. By referring patients to specialized centers for evaluation and initiation of therapy and by encouraging their enrollment in clinical trials and research protocols, you can help ensure that they receive the most current therapy.

Aside from various forms of lung transplantation, these current forms of therapy include three modalities: (1) aggressive oxygen treatment, (2) surgical treatment of major pulmonary vessel thromboembolic disease, and (3) megadose treatment of PPH with calcium-channel blockers along with aggressive oxygen therapy.

Aggressive Oxygen Therapy

This approach is recommended not for PPH but for secondary pulmonary hypertension associated with arterial hypoxemia or PPH in patients with PaO_2 values of 59 mmHg or less. No evidence is cited to support the selection of a PO_2 of 59 mmHg or less. The value is simply provided ex cathedra. There is an instructive history dealing with the use of oxygen in both PPH and in the secondary pulmonary hypertension related to chronic obstructive lung disease. That history goes back well beyond the current decade.

Oxygen inhalation rapidly reverses increased pulmonary artery pressure associated with hypoxemia.[49] It therefore seemed rational to try oxygen inhalation as a pulmonary vasodilator in patients with PPH and presumed pulmonary vasoconstriction.

An instructive case report appeared in 1978. Nagasaka et al.[50] observed a beneficial effect (prolonged survival in a single patient with PPH). This was a single, uncontrolled study in a patient being treated with oxygen and other modalities. The report must have been considered worthy of publication because of the long-term survival of a patient on this form of therapy in a disease that was "known" to be rapidly and progressively fatal. This so-called knowledge impressed not only the authors. The peer reviewers of the journal and the editorial board must have also considered the report to be worthy of publication. They appear to have shared the authors' misconception despite a large number of studies that indicated that oxygen inhalation in the nonhypoxemic patient with PPH is not of value. That is to say, when searched for, beneficial responses to oxygen therapy were not found and it seems almost certain that oxygen is not an effective pulmonary vasodilator let alone an effective therapy in nonhypoxemic patients with PPH.

Five patients were made hypoxic by lowering their arterial PO_2 from 76 to 46 mmHg. There was a small increase in pulmonary vascular resistance in only two of the five patients. Two of the patients, when tested with isoproterenol showed brisk vasodilation.[8] Although these studies were employed in only a limited number of patients, they provide no support for the use of oxygen therapy in PPH.

There is overwhelming evidence that the use of supplemental oxygen increases longevity in patients with chronic obstructive lung disease. The NOTT study in the United States[51] and the MRC study in the United Kingdom[52] demonstrated increased survival with the use of oxygen on a daily basis. The latter study represented a prospective, randomized controlled clinical trial. This documentation has been available for at least 10 years.

It is not at all clear—in fact, it is dubious—that the increased survival is related to a reduction in pulmonary vascular resistance by oxygen administration. There are many mechanisms by which relief of hypoxemia improves survival.[53] Pulmonary hypertension in patients with COLD is multifactorial. There is anatomic loss of pulmonary vascular bed.[54] Increased alveolar pressures increase pulmonary vascular resistance.[55] Although alveolar hypoxia does result in pulmonary vasoconstriction, so does hypercapnia and reduced precapillary serum pH.[56]

Some studies have indicated that continuous inhalation of high oxygen reduces mean pulmonary artery pressure in chronic obstructive lung disease.[14] However, although statistically significant, the reductions in pulmonary artery pressure and pulmonary vascular resistance were small and did not result in normal values being achieved.[55] Long-term oxygen therapy has been reported to improve pulmonary hypertension in some studies and to have no effect in others.

Long-term oxygen administration clearly improves survival in COLD and no additional PRCCTs seem required to establish this intervention. Oxygen therapy is also useful in other hypoxemic lung diseases. This fact has been known for more than a decade. It is not clear, nor is it a therapeutically substantive question, whether a major mechanism of the improvement produced by oxygen inhalation is caused by decreased pulmonary vascular resistance. For example, it should not be considered acceptable to ask patients to accept the risks of cardiac catheterization merely to answer a physiologic question with little or no clinical relevance to their therapy.

It is puzzling that a discussion of the treatment of pulmonary hypertension in hypoxemic patients provides what certainly must be superfluous advice to most physicians to use chronic oxygen administration for this group of patients. If the use of oxygen for this purpose is not widely known among primary care physicians, patients with chronic obstructive lung disease are indeed in trouble.

Surgical Endarterectomy for Chronic Major Vessel Pulmonary Artery Thromboembolic Occlusion

The use of endarterectomy on segmental, lobar, main stem branches, or main pulmonary artery affected by thromboembolism dates back some 27 years to 1965.[57] The surgery is thus scarcely new. To be considered is the question of whether it represents a therapeutic breakthrough. Moser and his colleagues have provided the major impetus for the application of this form of surgical therapy for a highly specific and relatively uncommon cause of pulmonary hypertension, chronic large vessel thromboembolic occlusion.

The major clinical question implicit in any surgical approach is the prognosis of the untreated patients. It is necessary to compare the prognosis of treated versus untreated patients, to determine the clinical value of a given surgical procedure. An estimate of postoperative mortality following endarterectomy is available.[58,59] The postoperative mortality is 14%. It is not clear whether this value includes any deaths that occur during diagnostic procedures (perioperative mortality). At any rate the mortality is relatively high. What is known about the mortality of untreated disease? Little except that from the duration of symptoms until surgery there is an average of about 4.5 years and that 25% of patients have survival times of more than 5 years before surgery. As a result, it is almost certain that some of those dying perioperatively died prematurely because of the surgery. These should be taken into account in assessing the risk benefit ratio in the use of endarterectomy. To the best of our knowledge, this has not been done. The use of thromboendarterectomy thus represents an application of surgery to patients in whom neither the risks nor the prognostic benefits of the procedure are known. Obviously these questions could be answered by a careful PRCCT or by a study of a controlled group of patients carefully observed over a period of time, to determine accurately the prognosis of the untreated disease.

The use of thromboendarterectomy has yielded important physiologic data. For example, the presence of segmental or lobar disease is associated with generalized pulmonary hypertension.[58,59] It is established that complete acute loss of blood flow to an entire pulmonary artery does not cause resting pulmonary hypertension.[60] In general, pneumonectomy also does not result in resting pulmonary hypertension.[61] Why should a mechanical increase in lobar or segmental pulmonary vascular resistance cause generalized chronic pulmonary hypertension? The fact that it does points to some very interesting, and as yet unknown, physiologic mechanism. Whether, as the workers in this area suggest, it results from pressure spillover from the bronchial circulation[59] or whether there is

the release of some humoral agent (pulmonary arterial constrictor substance),[62] or whether there is some other mechanism is a fascinating question. But the answer to that question is of little help to the 14% of patients who have died as a result of pulmonary endarterectomy.

This in turn raises another issue. If relief of lobar or segmental obstruction reverses generalized pulmonary hypertension, why perform widespread endarterectomy? The mortality associated with lobectomy is apparently about one-third of that associated with regional endarterectomy.[63] Why not try that surgical approach in appropriate patients?

In addition to death and the usual complications of thoracic surgery, there have been three more or less specific complications: bilateral phrenic nerve paresis, reperfusion pulmonary edema, and acute postoperative psychiatric problems. How should these fit into a rational risk-benefit analysis?

The discrepancy between scientific interest and patient outcome is well illustrated by the occurrence of reperfusion pulmonary edema postoperatively in 90% of patients. The pulmonary circulation seems to resemble the coronary circulation and the cerebral circulation in the occurrence of reperfusion edema. When it became apparent in the first 25 patients that reperfusion pulmonary edema was exceedingly common, was this used as a signal to question the safety of the surgical procedure? It must be concluded that (1) the enthusiasm of those advising generalists to submit suitable patients to regional pulmonary endarterectomy is not based on acceptable data; and (2) there is a difference in objectives between those espousing a surgical procedure as a form of investigation and those seeking effective, relatively safe forms of treatment; and (3) after 26 years there is inadequate information about the prognosis of this group of patients, and (4) no PRCCT has been performed to document its risk-benefit ratio.

Megadoses of Diltiazem HCl (Cardizem) or Nifedipine

As previously noted, given an assumed, rapidly and universally fatal disease, three therapeutic strategies are commonly adopted: (1) the use of many different drugs, (2) the use of combinations of drugs, and (3) the use of high (mega)doses of drugs that seem to be ineffective over the usual dose range.

It is therefore not surprising that a new "breakthrough" is urged to be used on patients with PPH as follows:

Under direct hemodynamic monitoring (this can't be overemphasized) the patient is given 20 mg. of diltiazem HCl or 60 mg. of nifedipine (Procardia, Adalat) in consecutive hourly doses until reaching a 50 percent fall in pulmonary vascular resistance or a 33 percent fall in pulmonary artery pressure. Once the effective dose is determined, it can be maintained on an outpatient basis without hemodynamic monitoring.

(Rich and Rubin, unpublished observations.)

The titration procedure then depends on two surrogate criteria for efficacy: reduction in pulmonary vascular resistance and/or pulmonary artery pressure.

What is the nature of the evidence that patient outcome is improved? The following is provided:

> Patients whose death seemed imminent are now living normally after complete reversal of their pulmonary hypertension with total daily doses of 720-1000 mg diltiazem or 240 mg. nifedipine. Survival data are lacking and the number of patients studied is small but about 40 percent of patients in trials have benefited and the effects seem to be longlasting.

(Rich and Rubin, unpublished observations.)

This does sound somewhat like Galen in claiming efficacy for a recommended treatment.[64a]

> All who drink of this remedy recover in a short time, except those whom it does not help who all die. Therefore, it is obvious that it fails only in incurable cases.

Note the difference between the (above) description to the generalists and the report of the therapy provided in the medical scientific literature.

> The 2 responding patients who have been followed for less than a year have also reported a sustained (subjective) improvement in symptoms; of the non-responding (5) patients, the condition of 2 is unchanged, 2 have deteriorated and one has died.[65]

There is a report of symptomatic improvement in some of the long-term patients (over 1 year of treatment) and some evidence of right ventricular function improvement. How much improvement was related to placebo effect reported by Daukzter et al. in all patients being treated with routine doses of pulmonary vasodilators[35] is not known.

The use of high doses of calcium channel blockers then employs largely surrogate criteria to establish efficacy and ignores risks. There do not seem to be plans for an early PRCCT.

This review was made possible by an interesting historical accident, remotely analagous to having the opportunity of reviewing two different versions of the Dead Sea scrolls written some months apart. One of us received a prepublication copy of a paper projected for publication in March 1991. That served as the basis for the material provided above (Rich and Rubin, unpublished observations). Subsequently a modified version was published that differs in some respects from the original.[3] In general, the second (i.e., the published) version is more conservative in its interpretation and claims than the original. For example, we are told that in the first version that "But the past decade has seen two tremendous advances in therapy—high-dose calcium channel blockers for primary disease and surgical thromboendarterectomy for proximal throm-

boembolic disease." And further, "The most promising approach in primary pulmonary hypertension is the use of high-dose calcium channel blockers. For all practical purposes this has supplanted other vasodilator therapies."

In the printed version "tremendous advanced" has been converted to "encouraging advances" and no claims concerning the supplanting of other forms of vasodilator therapy are made.[3]

There are a number of other claims made and information provided that are extensively modified in the second printed version.[3] We have used the original paper as the focus of our analysis for two reasons. An analysis of it provides insight into the fragile, ephemeral nature of clinical information when it is based on data obtained in a nonrigorous manner. Analysis of the unpublished version provides a comparison with the published version—the latter being, of course, the only version available to the readers.

Secondary Pulmonary Hypertension

Secondary pulmonary hypertension is far more common than PPH. Approximately 9 to 11 million patients in the United States alone are said to suffer from chronic obstructive lung disease, and an unknown but significant percentage have associated pulmonary hypertension. In addition, millions of patients are suffering from pulmonary hypertension that is related to other lung or cardiac diseases. It would have been surprising if pulmonary vasodilator therapy had somehow not been tried on such patients.

There is no surprise. In 1986 seven patients with pulmonary hypertension secondary to chronic obstructive lung disease were treated with (ordinary dose) nifedipine. Three of the patients died within months following institution of potent pulmonary vasodilator therapy. The patients did have substantial improvement in hemodynamics but died nevertheless.[64] Therapy was successful, yet about one-half of these patients died.

Undaunted, new investigators proceeded. In a more recent study, 23 patients with pulmonary hypertension underwent right-sided cardiac catheterization and measurement of the response to pulmonary vasodilatation with prostacyclin.[31] In three of five patients with chronic obstructive lung disease, in two of two patients with pulmonary fibrosis due to sarcoidosis, and in one patient with pulmonary veno-occlusive disease there was a greater than 20% drop in pulmonary vascular resistance. There did not appear to be an institutional review of the project nor was informed consent even mentioned. But the authors propose that "short term testing for a vasodilator response, with a view to instituting long term therapy should not be restricted to patients with PPH. . . ."—this despite the failure of nifedipine, nitroglycerine, and oxygen to improve outcome in chronic obstructive lung disease with cor pulmonale.[66] This study raises some interesting issues. There are many causes of secondary pulmonary hypertension, which itself is a manifestation or stage affecting literally millions of patients in the United States alone.

In addition to chronic obstructive lung disease, other forms of lung disease, such as the interstitial diseases, may be associated with secondary pulmonary hypertension: persistent LV failure, collagen-vascular diseases, sleep apnea, environmental exposures, pulmonary embolic disease, systemic sclerosis, congenital heart disease, hepatic cirrhosis, and parasitic diseases, including kala-azar (leishmaniasis), shistosomiasis, filiarisis, and undoubtedly others. What role pulmonary hypertension plays in the mortality and prognosis of these diseases is largely unknown. Are we far from the day when it is proposed that most patients at risk of secondary pulmonary hypertension undergo cardiac catheterization, drug titration, and nonspecific treatment of secondary pulmonary hypertension, say, with pulmonary vasodilators? It may be predicted that such a development would be disastrous for the affected patients, not to mention for the economics of the delivery of medical care.

SUMMARY

PPH is a wastebasket diagnosis characterized by pulmonary hypertension and an absence of clear etiology. A pseudo-prognosis was established for the disorder that was accurate for only about 20% of patients. This pseudo-prognosis, based on inadequate data, suggested that PPH was rapidly and almost invariably fatal. This pseudo-prognosis was a potent driving force for aggressive management of these patients. This aggressive approach in turn has resulted in excess deaths and disability. Despite clear-cut evidence that the prognosis of PPH is substantially more favorable than previously believed, there has been little change in management. In fact, there is some opinion supporting the use of pulmonary vasodilators in secondary pulmonary hypertension also without any evidence of a favorable risk-benefit ratio in such patients. In particular, the requirement for PRCCTs to test any of the current diagnostic and therapeutic approaches rigorously seems to have been largely ignored. PPH thus provides an excellent model for the impact of an inaccurate prognosis (pseudo-prognosis) on physician practice and on patient outcome.

REFERENCES

1. Packer M: Is it ethical to administer vasodilator drugs to patients with primary pulmonary hypertension? (Editorial.) Chest 95:1173, 1989
2. Glanville AR, Burke CM, Theodore J, Robin ED: Primary pulmonary hypertension. Length of survival in patients referred for heart-lung transplantation. Chest 91:675, 1987
3. Rich S, Rubin LJ: New views on pulmonary hypertension. Patient Care 25:87, 1991
4. Hippocrates: Aphorisms. Edited by François Rabelais. Lyons, 1532
5. Burckhardt G: Brain Control. Wiley, New York, 1973, p 266
6. Fries JF: Systemic Lupus Erythematous in Prognosis Contemporary Outcomes of Disease. Edited by James F. Fries and George E. Ehrlich. The Charles Press Publishers, Bowie, Maryland. pp. 374–377, 1981
7. Fishberg AM: Heart Failure. Lea & Febiger, Philadelphia, 1940
8. Voelkel N, Reeves JT: Primary pulmonary hypertension. p. 573. In Moser KM (ed) Pulmonary Vascular Disease. Marcel Dekker, New York, 1979
9. Romberg E: Ueber sklerose der lungenarterien. Dtsch Arch Klin Med 48:197, 1891
10. Arillaga FC: Sclerose de l'artère pulmonaire secondaire à certaines états pulmonaires chroniques. Arch Mal Coeur 6:518, 1913
11. Dresdale D, Schultz TM, Michtom RJ: Primary pulmonary hypertension. I. Clinical and hemodynamic study. Am J Med 11:686, 1951
12. Wood P: Pulmonary hypertension with special reference to the vasoconstrictive factor. Br Heart J 21:557, 1959
13. Kay JM, Smith P, Heath D: Aminorex and the pulmonary circulation. Thorax 227:262, 1971
14. Heath D, Edwards JE: The pathology of pulmonary vascular hypertensive disease. Circulation 18:533, 1958
15. Wagenvoort CA, Wagenvoort CA: Pathology of Pulmonary Hypertension. Wiley, New York, 1977
16. Wood P: Diseases of the Heart and Circulation. J Lippincott, Philadelphia, 1956
17. Fuster V, Giulian ER, Brandenberg RO et al: The natural life history of idiopathic pulmonary hypertension. Am J Cardiol 47:422, 1981
18. Walcott G, Burchell HB, Brown AL, Jr: Primary pulmonary hypertension. Am J Med 49:70, 1970
19. Cherian G, Abraham MT, Ultman CB et al: Primary pulmonary hypertension. Arg Bras Cardiol 1:311, 1982
20. Wagenvoort VA, Wagenvoort N: Primary pulmonary hypertension: a pathological study of the lung vessels in 156 clinically diagnosed cases. Circulation 42:1163, 1970
21. Rozkovec A, Montanes R, Oakley CM: Factors that influence the outcome of primary pulmonary hypertension. Br Heart J 55:449, 1986
22. Editorial: A better outlook in primary pulmonary hypertension? Lancet 1:1420, 1986
23. Bourdillon PDV, Oakley CM: Regression of primary pulmonary hypertension. Br Heart J 38:264, 1976
24. Fujii A, Rabinowitz M, Matthews EC: A case of spontaneous resolution of idiopathic pulmonary hypertension. Br Heart J 46:574, 1981
25. Both A, Loogen F, Mauer W: Follow-up studies on patients with primary vascular pulmonary hypertension taking anorectics. Verh Dtsch Ges Inn Med 77:445, 1971
26. Shettigar UR, Hultgren HN, Specter M et al: Primary pulmonary hypertension: Favorable effect of isoproteranol. N Engl J Med 295:1414, 1976

27. Pietro DA, La Breshka KA, Shulman RM et al: Sustained improvement in primary pulmonary hypertension during six years of treatment with sublingual isoproteranol. N Engl J Med 310:1032, 1984

28. Chann NS, McLay J, Kenmard AC: Reversibility of primary pulmonary hypertension during six years of treatment with oral diazoxide. Br Heart J 57:207, 1987

29. Dantzer DR, D'Alonzo GE, Gianotti L et al: Vasodilators and primary pulmonary hypertension. Chest 95:1185, 1989

30. Packer M: Is it ethical to administer vasodilator drugs to patients with primary pulmonary hypertension? (Editorial.) Chest 95:1173, 1989

31. Jones K, Higenbottam T, Wallwork J: Pulmonary vasodilation with prostacyclin in primary and secondary pulmonary hypertension. Chest 96:784, 1989

32. Rubin LJ: Primary pulmonary hypertension. (Letter.) Chest 93:894, 1988

33. Packer M: Vasodilator therapy for primary pulmonary hypertension. Ann Intern Med 103:258, 1985

34. Rich S, Brundage BH, Levy PS: The effect of vasodilator therapy on the clinical outcome of patients with primary pulmonary hypertension. Circulation 71:1191, 1985

35. Osler W: Aequanimitas. Reprinted by Gryphon Editions, Birmingham, Alabama, 1985

36. Rinaldo JE, Rogers RW: Changing concepts of lung injury and repair. N Engl J Med 506:900, 1982

37. Pantoppidan H, Huttemeier, Quinn DA: p.1. In Zapol WM, Falke KJ (eds): Etiology, Demography and Outcome in Acute Respiratory Failure. Marcel Dekker, New York, 1985

38. Gaensler EA: p. 579. In Sackner MA (ed): Open and Closed Lung Biopsy in Diagnostic Techniques in Pulmonary Disease. Marcel Dekker, New York, 1981

39. Robin ED: The kingdom of the near dead: the shortened unnatural life history of primary pulmonary hypertension. Chest 92:330, 1987

40. Patient Registry for the Characterization of Primary Pulmonary Hypertension: Changes in registry policies concerning completeness and quality of data. PRPPH Newsl 1(3):1, 1983

41. Grossman W: Cardiac Catheterization and Angiography. Lea & Febiger, Philadelphia, 1974

42. Keane JF, Fyler DC: Hazards of cardiac catheterization in children with pulmonary hypertension due to primary pulmonary vascular obstruction. Lancet 1:863, 1977

43. Rich S, Dantzker DR, Ayers SM et al: National Prospective Study of Primary Pulmonary Hypertension. Ann Intern Med 107:216, 1987

44. Experiences from the National Institute of Health Registry on Primary Pulmonary Hypertension. The acute administration of vasodilators in primary pulmonary hypertension. Am Rev Respir Dis 140:1623, 1989

45. Gogol NV: Dead Souls. Translated by David Magarskack. Penguin-Viking, London, 1961

46. Atkins H: Radiopharmaceuticals in pulmonary medicine p. 29. In: Atkins HL (ed): Pulmonary Nuclear Medicine. Marcel Dekker, New York, 1984

47. PIOPED Investigators: Value of the ventilation/perfusion scan in acute pulmonary embolism: results of the prospective investigation of pulmonary embolism diagnosis (PIOPED). JAMA 263:2753, 1990

48. Goodman PC: Pulmonary angiography in clinics in chest medicine: Pulmonary embolism and hypertension. WB Saunders, Philadelphia, 1984 pp. 465–477

49. Bergofsky E: Active control of the normal pulmonary circulation. p. 233. In Moser KM (ed): Pulmonary Vascular Diseases. Edited by Kenneth M Moser. Marcel Dekker, New York, 1979

50. Nagasaka Y, Akutsu H, Lee YS et al: Long term favorable effect of oxygen administration on a patient with primary pulmonary hypertension. Chest 74:299, 1978

51. Nocturnal Oxygen Therapy Trial Group: Continuous or nocturnal oxygen therapy in hypoxemic chronic obstructive lung disease. Ann Intern Med 93:391, 1980

52. Medical Research Council Working Party: Long term domicillary oxygen therapy in chronic hypoxemic cor pulmonale complicating chronic bronchitis and emphysema. Lancet 1:681, 1981

53. Robin ED: Of men and mitochondria; coping with hypoxic dysoxia. Am Rev Respir Dis 122:517, 1980

54. Burrows B: Course and prognosis in advanced disease. p. 23. In Petty TL (ed): Chronic Obstructive Pulmonary Disease. Marcel Dekker, New York, 1978

55. Harris P, Heath D: The Human Pulmonary Circulation. Churchill Livingstone, Edinburgh, 1972

56. Fishman AP: Respiratory gases in the regulation of the pulmonary circulation. Physiol Rev 41:214, 1961

57. Moser KM, Houk N, Jones RC, Hufnagel CC: Chronic massive obstruction of the pulmonary arteries. Circulation 32:377, 1965

58. Moser KM, Daly PO, Petersen K et al: Thromboendarterectomy for chronic major-vessel thromboembolic disease. Ann Intern Med 107:560, 1987

59. Moser KM, Auger WR, Fedullo PF: Chronic major-vessel thromboembolic pulmonary hypertension. Circulation 81:1735, 1990

60. Okhuda K, Nakahara K, Weidner J et al: Lung fluid exchange after unequal pulmonary artery obstruction in sheep. Circ Res 43:152, 1978

61. Comroe JH, Forster RF, Dubois AB et al: The Lung Clinical Physiology and Pulmonary Function Tests. Yearbook Medical Publishers, Chicago, p. 86, 1970

62. Robin ED, Cross CE, Millen JE, Murdaugh HV, Jr: Humoral agent released from calf lung producing pulmonary arterial vasoconstriction. Science 156:827, 1967

63. Weiss W: Operative mortality and five year survival rates in men with bronchogenic carcinoma. Chest 66:483, 1974

64. Rubin LF, Moser KM: Long-term effects of nifedipine on hemodynamics and oxygen transport in patients with cor pulmonale. Chest 89:141, 1986

64a. Galen: Fourteen Books on Therapeutics (ARS Magna). Quoted in Silverman WA: Human Experimentation, a Guided Step into the Unknown. Oxford University Press, Oxford, 1985

65. Rich S, Brundage BH: High-dose calcium channel-blocking therapy for primary pulmonary hypertension: evidence for long-term reduction in pulmonary arterial pressure and regression of right ventricular hypertrophy. Circulation 76:135, 1987

66. Morley TF, Zappasodi SV, Belli A, Giudice JC: Pulmonary vasodilator therapy for chronic obstructive pulmonary disease and cor pulmonale. Treatment with nifedipine, nitroglycerine and oxygen. Chest 92:71, 1987

31

Aortic Aneurysm, Penetrating Ulcer of the Aorta, and Aortic Dissection

John A. Spittell, Jr.
Peter C. Spittell

AORTIC ANEURYSM

Aneurysm formation in both the thoracic and abdominal aorta is usually due to atherosclerosis and thus typically occurs after the age of 60 and more commonly in men than in women. With these points in mind, it is not surprising that coronary artery disease (CAD) is usually associated with, and must be a part of, the evaluation of the person with an aortic aneurysm.[1] Hypertension, common in this age group, seems to enhance aneurysm formation.[2] Less common than atherosclerosis as the etiology of aortic aneurysms are trauma, infections, including syphilis, arteritides, and hereditary connective tissue abnormalities.[3]

Thoracic Aortic Aneurysm

Most thoracic aortic aneurysms are asymptomatic until they become large enough to encroach on other structures in the mediastinum (e.g., the esophagus, trachea, or superior vena cava) or on the spine or chest wall. With effective antiluetic therapy, arteriosclerosis has become the most frequent etiology of thoracic aortic aneurysm; thus, their most common location is in the descending thoracic aorta.

Physical examination of the patient with a thoracic aortic aneurysm is often normal, unless pressure on the superior vena cava or left innominate vein leads to jugular venous distention, encroachment on the recurrent laryngeal nerve produces hoarseness, or dilation of the aortic root causes aortic valve regurgitation. Rarely, an aneurysm of the thoracic aorta is so large that it will cause palpable pulsatile expansion of the chest.

Unless there is calcification in the wall of the aneurysm, thoracic aortic aneurysm may simulate an intrathoracic neoplasm on plain chest radiographs,[4] so that another imaging procedure is needed to confirm the diagnosis. While aortography has been the classic method used in the past, computed tomography (CT) with intravenous contrast media enhancement (Fig. 31-1) is currently the preferred imaging procedure used to diagnose thoracic aortic aneurysm or to follow small aneurysms serially, at most centers. Magnetic resonance imaging (MRI), where available, is also an excellent means of imaging the thoracic aorta,[5] as is biplanar transesophageal echocardiography (TEE)[6] (Fig. 31-2).

The prognosis for untreated thoracic aortic aneurysm is poorer than that for untreated abdominal aortic aneurysm according to the most recent study in which the 1- and 3-year survival rates were 58.2% and

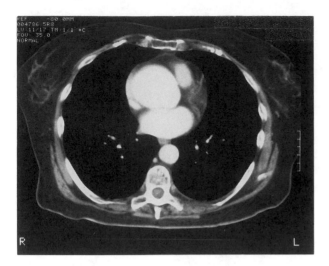

Fig. 31-1. CT scan of thoracic aortic aneurysm.

25.7%, respectively. Indeed, 51% of the nondissecting thoracic aortic aneurysms in this study ruptured and, significantly, all patients whose aneurysms ruptured had hypertension.[7]

For the patient with an atherosclerotic aneurysm of the thoracic aorta, surgical resection is indicated if the aneurysm is symptomatic, 6.0 cm in diameter or enlarging under observation, or in the case of significant or poorly controlled hypertension, provided associated conditions do not contraindicate surgery.[7,8] As in all patients with atherosclerotic disease of the aorta, associated coronary artery disease (CAD) must be carefully evaluated and taken into consideration in management decisions.

Several other etiologic types of thoracic aortic aneurysm have features that merit comment. Post-traumatic aneurysms that are typically located in the proximal descending thoracic aorta just beyond the origin of the left subclavian artery, even when asymptomatic, warrant surgical treatment because their stability is not predictable.[9] Surgical treatment of dilation of the ascending aorta measuring 6.0 cm in diameter in patients with Marfan syndrome, even if asymptomatic, is advisable to prevent the complications of aortic dissection and rupture.[10] Regardless of the etiology of a thoracic aortic aneurysm, any associated hypertension should be carefully controlled, both before and after surgical resection.[2]

Abdominal Aortic Aneurysm

Like other arterial aneurysms, those of the abdominal aorta are usually atherosclerotic in origin. With the increasing age of our population, abdominal aortic aneurysms are common, occurring in about 2% of persons over 60 years of age, about 10 times more fre-

quently in men than in women. Among the risk factors for atherosclerosis, smoking,[11] heredity,[12] and hypertension[2] appear to be particularly important in abdominal aortic aneurysm.

While most large abdominal aortic aneurysms (>6 cm in diameter) are symptomatic, it is important to remember that more than one-half the aneurysms smaller than 6 cm in diameter are asymptomatic. When symptomatic, the presenting symptoms in order of frequency are awareness of a pulsating abdominal mass with or without pain, abdominal and/or back pain, flank pain, and groin pain.[13] Thus, in more than one-half of patients with an abdominal aortic aneurysm, the diagnosis depends on careful physical examination of the abdominal aorta, which is remarkably reliable if the admonition of Sir William Olser is kept in mind:

> A mistake is not likely to occur if it is remembered that no pulsation, however forcible, no thrill, however intense, no bruit, however loud—singly or together—justify the diagnosis of an aneurysm of the abdominal aorta, only the presence of a palpable, expansile tumour.

Difficulties arise in obese patients, in elderly persons with a very tortuous aorta, and in persons with abdominal masses that transmit the pulsation of the aorta.

The most frequent complication of abdominal aortic aneurysm is rupture, but other complications that produce clinically interesting syndromes need to be kept in mind. Atheroembolism presenting as livedo reticularis and blue toes with associated hypertension and renal insufficiency must be recognized promptly, since the only effective therapy is resection of the abdominal aortic aneurysm to remove the source of the atheromatous debris.[14] Also, because of the proximity of the aorta to the ureters, in rare cases an abdominal aortic aneurysm can compress one or both ureters, producing hydronephrosis or even anuria.

Ultrasound is an accurate method used to diagnose and determine the size of an abdominal aortic aneurysm. CT with contrast enhancement is equally accurate and defines relationships of the aneurysm to other structures, but is more expensive than ultrasonography. Aortography is rarely necessary unless associated occlusive arterial disease is suspected.

The most frequent complication of abdominal aortic aneurysm is rupture, which bears an important relationship to the size of the aneurysm. In a population-based study, the risk of rupture over 5 years for aneurysms at least 5 cm in diameter was 25%, while for aneurysms smaller than 5 cm in diameter, the 5-year risk of rupture was 0%.[15] Accordingly, at most centers, an abdominal aortic aneurysm that is 5 cm in diameter or an aneurysm that is symptomatic is an indica-

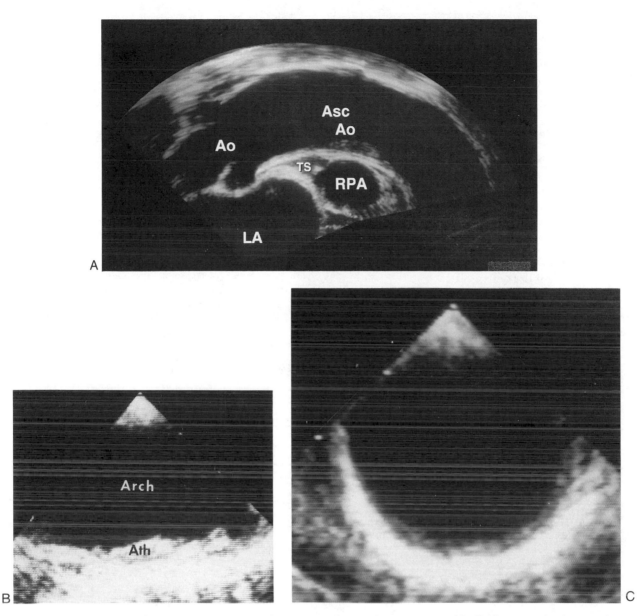

Fig. 31-2. Transesophageal echocardiographic imaging of thoracic aorta. **(A)** Wide-field composite image of the ascending aorta (Asc Ao) in longitudinal plane. **(B)** Aortic arch (arch). **(C)** Descending thoracic aorta. LA, left atrium; Ao, aorta; Ath, atheroma; RPA, right pulmonary artery; TS, transverse sinus. (From Seward et al.,[6] with permission.)

tion for surgical resection in a patient who is an acceptable surgical risk. In a patient with an abdominal aortic aneurysm smaller than 5 cm or in the patient who is a poor surgical risk, observation with ultrasound examination of the aneurysm every 3 to 4 months is indicated. While the rate of enlargement of an abdominal aortic aneurysm is variable,[16] there is some evidence that β-blockade may decrease the rate of growth of small abdominal aortic aneurysms.[17]

Since abdominal aortic aneurysms are atherosclerotic in origin, other manifestations of atherosclerosis, including CAD, cerebrovascular disease, occlusive peripheral arterial disease, and other arterial aneurysms, must be kept in mind and be a part of the evaluation of the person with an abdominal aortic aneurysm. Analysis of multiple series has shown that perioperative cardiac events are more than six times more likely in persons with clinically evident CAD than in those without;[18] accordingly, at some centers, coronary angiography is performed in all patients with an abdominal aortic aneurysm, to identify those in whom coronary artery surgery is considered appropriate prior to aneurysm surgery, to lessen the risk of a perioperative cardiac event. An alternative approach is to advise coronary angiography before aneurysm repair only if indicated by symptoms of or evidence of significant CAD on stress testing.[1,19]

In the aneurysm patient who is also hypertensive, associated occlusive renal artery disease should be considered, and if findings such as an upper abdominal bruit or a significant discrepancy in renal size on excretory urography are present, aortography is indicated to identify any renal artery lesion that can be corrected at aneurysm surgery.

PENETRATING ULCER OF THE AORTA

The symptom complex produced by the extension of atheromatous ulceration through the internal elastic lamina into the media of the aortic wall with hematoma formation has been distinguished from classic aortic dissection in recent years.[20–22] Along with the description of this lesion, which affects the descending thoracic aorta almost exclusively, the pathogenesis of the penetrating atherosclerotic aortic ulcer and its fate—medial hematoma, false aneurysm formation, or transmural rupture—have been documented[20] (Fig. 31-3).

The distinction of penetrating aortic ulcer from classic aortic dissection or a symptomatic thoracic aortic aneurysm seems justified by the clinical, pathologic, and angiographic differences (Table 31-1). When penetrating aortic ulcer is suspected, the first order of business is to select which imaging procedure to use (Fig. 31-4)—aortography, CT scan with contrast, TEE, or MRI—depending on availability and experience of the institution, since sufficient experience with penetrating aortic ulcer is still limited.

More experience with penetrating aortic ulcer is needed before the correct management, nonoperative or surgical resection, is clear. The experience of Hussain and colleagues suggests that transmural rupture of penetrating ulcers is uncommon; these investigators believe that nonoperative management with aggressive treatment of hypertension is appropriate initially, followed by serial CT and clinical evaluation.[22] The experience of Stanson and associates led to their recommendation of surgical resection and graft replacement of the involved portion of the thoracic aorta in addition to control of the hypertension.[20] When surgical treatment is considered, the occurrence of paraparesis in almost 30% of cases so managed must be kept in mind.[20]

AORTIC DISSECTION

Acute dissection of the thoracic aorta is the most common acute aortic lesion and, because of its protean manifestations, presents a diagnostic challenge. Accu-

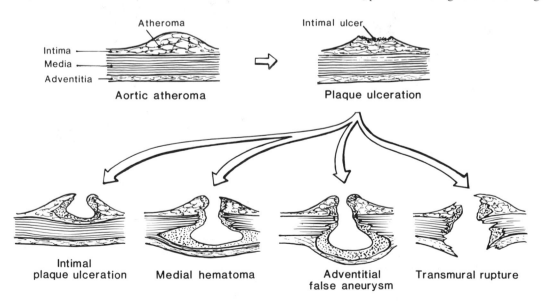

Fig. 31-3. Evolution of penetrating aortic atherosclerotic ulcer. Ulcerated atheroma may extend into the media and expose it to pulsatile aortic flow. Extension of ulcer into the media may precipitate a medial hematoma (localized dissection), pseudoaneurysm, or transmural rupture. Ulcer crater may become filled with thrombus and result in considerable underestimation of actual size of involved aortic segment. (From Stanson et al.,[20] with permission.)

TABLE 31-1. Features of Thoracic Aortic Lesions

	Penetrating Ulcer	Classic Dissection	Symptomatic Aneurysm
Age (yrs)	65+	40+	55+
Sex (M/F)	1/1	3/1	3/1
Predisposing conditions	Atherosclerosis Hyertension	Hypertension Congenital abnormality, aortic valve Marfan syndrome	Atherosclerosis ? Hypertension
Portion of thoracic aorta	Descending	Any	Any
Clinical features	Pain, chest, or upper back	Migating pain in chest, anterior or interscapular Aortic valve regurgitation Ischemia of various organ systems	Chest, any part Pressure on surrounding structures
Features on imaging	"Dimple" and/or medial hematoma on aortagram, CT scan, TEE and/or MRI False aneurysm	Intimal flap and/or distortion of true channel on aortagram, CT scan, TEE and/or MRI Aortic valve regurgitation on aortagram	Aneurysm on aortagram, CT scan, TEE and/or MRI

Abbreviations: CT, computed tomography; MRI, magnetic resonance imaging; TEE, transesophageal echocardiography.

rate diagnosis depends on a high degree of suspicion and an awareness of the clinical features and predisposing conditions. Hypertension is present in about 70% of patients who experience acute aortic dissection, particularly in those whose initial tear is beyond the origin of the left subclavian artery (i.e., type III or distal aortic dissection[23] (Fig. 31-5). Other risk factors for acute aortic dissection, particularly type I or proximal aortic dissection (Fig. 31-5), are congenital abnormalities of the aortic valve[24,25] and Marfan syndrome.[10]

In addition to the typical severe sudden pain in the anterior chest or interscapular area and its subsequent migration distally, the clinical features of acute aortic dissection may include neurologic findings, if the circulation to the brain or spinal cord has been compromised by the dissection and/or acute cardiac symptoms, if the aortic valve or pericardium are involved by the dissection.

Findings on examination of the patient with acute aortic dissection may include any or all of the following findings: hypertension, cardiac murmurs, friction rubs, neurologic findings, and/or changes in peripheral arterial pulses. If the dissection has extended into the abdominal aorta, there may be tenderness and increased diameter of the abdominal aorta. Combinations of certain clinical features strongly suggest the location of the initial tear and allow the alert clinician to suspect which type of acute aortic dissection has occurred:

Proximal (type I or II)
  Initial pain—anterior chest
  Pulse changes—right arm
  Pulse changes—right carotid

Aortic valve murmurs
Pericardial friction rub
Marfan syndrome
Distal (type III)
  Initial pain—interscapular
  Hypertension (more common than in proximal dissection)

Subsequent evaluation of the patient with suspected acute aortic dissection can be related to the conditions that have in the past been the erroneous diagnoses: acute myocardial infarction (AMI), cerebrovascular accident (CVA), acute peripheral arterial occlusion, and acute abdominal conditions.[26,27]

While a normal chest radiograph does not exclude acute aortic dissection, abnormalities of the supracardiac aortic shadow, particularly when previous films are available and when comparison with the current radiograph demonstrates an increase in the supracardiac aortic shadow[28] (Fig. 31-5). TEE has become the preferred screening procedure for acute aortic dissection at some centers,[29,30] while at other centers CT scanning with contrast enhancement, being generally available, is used to screen for acute aortic dissection, but it has the limitation of not being portable or demonstrating reentry in the distal aorta or aortic valve regurgitation. At still other centers, aortography has remained the diagnostic procedure of choice, but false-negative results can occur.[31] Early experience has shown that MRI is also an excellent method to diagnose acute aortic dissection.[32] Whichever diagnostic method is preferred, a cardinal maxim is to proceed with it promptly, after initiation of intensive pharmacologic therapy, whenever aortic dissection is a possibility.

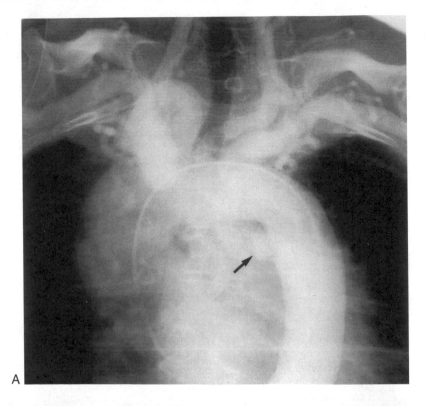

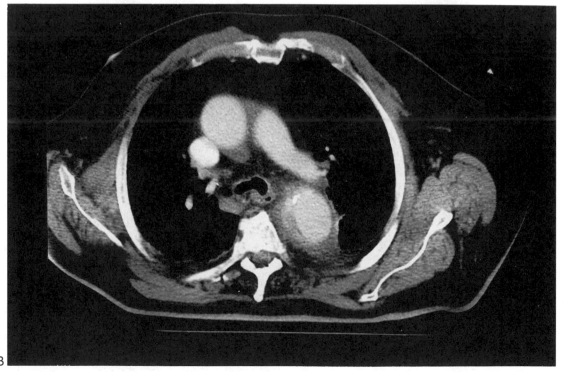

Fig. 31-4. Imaging of penetrating aortic ulcer. **(A)** Aortagram. **(B)** CT scan. (*Figure continues.*)

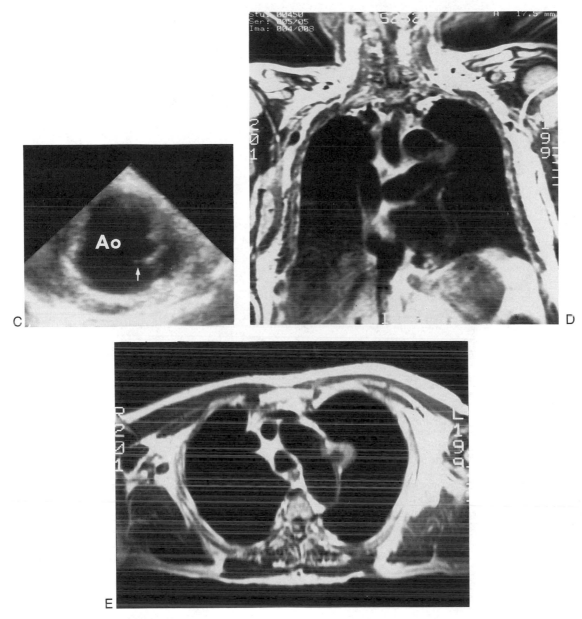

Fig. 31-4 (*continued*). (**C**) Transesophageal echocardiography demonstrates small intimal flap (large arrow), penetrating atheromatous ulcer, and small intimal hematoma in the descending thoracic aorta (Ao). (**D**) Magnetic resonance imaging scans of aorta of patient with penetrating aortic ulcer. Sagittal (D) and transverse (**E**) images reveal ulceration and penetration of wall of proximal descending thoracic aorta, with thickening of wall at site of ulceration. (From Cooke et al.,[21] with permission.)

The dismal prognosis of untreated acute aortic dissection is well documented by a number of studies[33–35]; about 70% die within 2 weeks of onset and, of those who do survive the acute phase, one-half or more will die within 1 year without treatment.[33,34] Rupture through the outer layer of the aorta is the most common cause of death, and reentry of the dissection (formerly considered "healing" of the dissection) is no protection against rupture.[34] Involvement of the ascending aorta (proximal dissection) has a worse

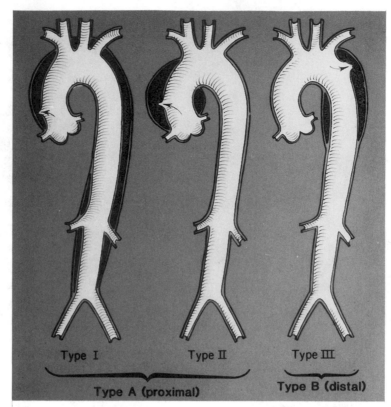

Fig. 31-5. Classification of aortic dissection. Type I, primary tear in ascending aorta and dissection involving aortic arch and distal aorta for a variable distance. Type II, dissection involving only ascending aorta. Type III, primary tear in subclavian artery, extending distally for a variable distance. (Modified from DeBakey et al.,[45] with permission.)

prognosis than does distal dissection. Associated CAD, cerebrovascular disease, and abdominal aortic aneurysm worsen the prognosis in acute aortic dissection.[35]

The initial management of suspected acute aortic dissection should include pharmacologic agents that decrease the force of ventricular contraction and control any hypertension. Intravenous sodium nitroprusside combined with β-blockade is preferred by many when the patient has hypertension,[36] while in the person with a normal blood pressure, β-blockade alone to decrease the force of ventricular ejection is indicated. Others have proposed the use of intravenous labetolol, with both α- and β-adrenoreceptor blocking action, for the emergent treatment of acute aortic dissection.[37] When β-blockers cannot be used, intravenous trimethapan can be used until other antihypertensive therapy can effect control of blood pressure.

Proximal aortic dissection is best treated by urgent surgical repair to prevent intrapericardial hemorrhage, aortic valve insufficiency, and/or rupture. Resection of the involved portion of the ascending aorta and replacement with a tubular graft is the usual surgical procedure[38,39]; if attachment of the aortic valve is disrupted, producing aortic valve insufficiency, resuspension of the valve is preferred, but if there is associated annuloaortic ectasia, a valved conduit may be used.[40] For those persons who for some reason do not undergo surgical treatment for their proximal aortic dissection, long-term pharmacologic therapy, ideally including β-blockade, is recommended.

In aortic dissection beginning distal to the origin of the left subclavian artery, management following the initial emergent pharmacologic stabilization is controversial.[41] Many recommend continuing pharmacologic therapy for stabilized, uncomplicated distal aortic dissection.[39,42,43] Others believe that surgical repair of distal dissections is warranted, given a patient without other life-threatening conditions, to prevent the development of dissection-related complications.[44] If long-term pharmacologic treatment is selected, close monitoring of the patient with regular CT scanning of the aorta for evidence of increasing aortic diameter, development of a saccular aneurysm, or symptoms related to the chronic dissection, all of which are indications for surgical treatment, is recommended.[39]

Regardless of the type of therapy used in the treatment of acute aortic dissection, long-term management with β-blockade, whether the patient is hypertensive or not, plus control of any hypertension is needed. Regular monitoring of the aorta with CT is recommended to evaluate any enlargement of the aorta, since subsequent rupture is size dependent; operative repair is recommended for symptomatic aortic enlargement (>5 cm) for patients who are acceptable surgical candidates otherwise.[39]

REFERENCES

1. Gersh BG, Rihal CS, Rooke TW et al: Evaluation and management of patients with both peripheral vascular and coronary artery disease. J Am Coll Cardiol 18:203, 1991
2. Spittell JA, Jr: Hypertension and arterial aneurysm. J Am Coll Cardiol 1:533, 1983
3. Glesby MJ, Pyeritz RE: Association of mitral valve prolapse and systemic abnormalities of connective tissue. JAMA 262:523, 1989
4. Shabian DM, Havid H, Faber LP et al: Lesions of the thoracic aorta and its arch simulating neoplasm. J Thorac Cardiovasc Surg 81:251, 1981
5. Lois JF, Gomes AS, Brown K et al: Magnetic resonance imaging of the thoracic aorta. Am J Cardiol 60:358, 1987
6. Seward JB, Khandheria BK, Edwards WD et al: Biplanar transesophageal echocardiography: anatomic correlations, image orientation, and clinical applications. Mayo Clin Proc 65:1193, 1990
7. Bickerstaff LK, Pairolero PC, Hollier LH et al: Thoracic aortic aneurysm: a population based study. Surgery 92:1103, 1982
8. Joyce JW, Fairbairn JF, Kincaid OW et al: Aneurysms of the thoracic aorta: a clinical study with reference to prognosis. Circulation 29:176, 1964
9. Quaini E, Colombo T, Donatelli F et al: Chronic traumatic aneurysms of the descending thoracic aorta. Texas Heart Inst J 12:143, 1989
10. Marsalese DL, Moodie DS, Vacante M et al: Marfan's syndrome: natural history and long-term follow-up of cardiovascular involvement. J Am Coll Cardiol 14:422, 1989
11. Auerbach O, Garfinkel L: Atherosclerosis and aneurysm of the aorta in relation to smoking habits and age. Chest 78:805, 1980
12. Darling RC III, Brewster DC, Darling RC et al: Are familial abdominal aortic aneurysms different? J Vasc Surg 10:39, 1989
13. Ryan EA, Kincaid OW, Spittell JA, Jr: Roentgenographic manifestations of abdominal aortic aneurysm. Postgrad Med 36:77, 1964
14. Spittell JA, Jr: Abdominal aortic aneurysms. Hosp Pract 21:105, 1986
15. Nevitt MP, Ballard DJ, Hallett JW: Prognosis of abdominal aortic aneurysms: a population based study. N Engl J Med 321:1009, 1989
16. Cronenwett JL, Sargent SK, Wall MH et al: Variables that affect the expansion rate and outcome of small abdominal aortic aneurysms. J Vasc Surg 11:260, 1990
17. Leach SD, Toole AL, Stern H et al: Effect of β-adrenergic blockade on the growth rate of abdominal aortic aneurysms. Arch Surg 123:606, 1988
18. Hertzer NR: Basic data concerning associated coronary disease in peripheral vascular patients. Ann Vasc Surg 1:616, 1987
19. Eagle KA, Coley CM, Newell JB et al: Combining clinical and thallium data optimizes preoperative assessment of cardiac risk before major vascular surgery. Ann Intern Med 110:859, 1989
20. Stanson AW, Kazmier FJ, Hollier LH et al: Penetrating atherosclerotic ulcers of the thoracic aorta: natural history and clinicopathologic correlations. Ann Vasc Surg 1:15, 1986
21. Cooke JP, Kazmier FJ, Orszulak TA: The penetrating aortic ulcer: pathologic manifestations, diagnosis and management. Mayo Clin Proc 63:718, 1988
22. Hussain S, Glover JL, Bree R et al: Penetrating atherosclerotic ulcers of the thoracic aorta. J Vasc Surg 9:710, 1989
23. Roberts WC: Aortic dissection: anatomy, consequences, and causes. Am Heart J 101:195, 1981
24. Larson EW, Edwards WD: Risk factors for aortic dissection: a necropsy study of 161 cases. Am J Cardiol 53:849, 1984
25. Roberts CS, Roberts WC: Dissection of the aorta with congenital malformation of the aortic valve. J Am Coll Cardiol 17:712, 1991
26. Spittell JA, Jr: Differential diagnosis of dissecting aneurysm. Prog Cardiovasc Dis 14:225, 1971
27. Cambria RP, Brewster DC, Gertler J: Vascular complications associated with spontaneous aortic dissection. J Vasc Surg 7:199, 1989
28. Earnest F IV, Mulim JR, Sheedy PF II: Roentgenographic findings in thoracic aortic dissection. Mayo Clin Proc 54:43, 1979
29. Erbel R, Daniel W, Visser C et al: Echocardiography in diagnosis of aortic dissection. Lancet 1:457, 1989
30. Hashimoto S, Kumada T, Osakada G et al: Assessment of transesophageal Doppler echocardiography in dissecting aortic aneurysm. J Am Coll Cardiol 14:1253, 1989
31. Eagle KA, Quertermous T, Kritzer GA et al: Spectrum of conditions initially suggesting acute aortic dissection but with negative aortagrams. Am J Cardiol 57:322, 1986
32. Lois JF, Gomes AS, Brown K et al: Magnetic resonance imaging of the thoracic aorta. Am J Cardiol 60:358, 1987
33. Hurst AE, Johns VJ Jr, Kime SW, Jr: Dissecting aneurysm of the aorta: a review of 505 cases. Medicine (Baltimore) 37:217, 1958
34. McCloy RM, Spittell JA, Jr, McGoon DC: The prognosis in aortic dissection. Circulation 31:665, 1965
35. Grondin C, David PR, Goor DA et al: Dissecting aneurysms of the thoracic aorta: a review of 52 cases with consideration of factors influencing prognosis. Ann Thorac Surg 4:29, 1967
36. Cooke JP, Safford RE: Progress in the diagnosis and management of aortic dissection. Mayo Clin Proc 61:147, 1986
37. Grubb BP, Sirio C, Zelis R: Intravenous labetolol in acute aortic dissection. JAMA 258:78, 1987
38. Miller DC: Acute dissection of the aorta—continuing need for earlier diagnosis and treatment. Mod Concepts Cardiovasc Dis 54:51, 1985

39. Crawford ES: The diagnosis and management of aortic dissection. JAMA 264:2537, 1990

40. Jex RK, Schaff HV, Peihler JM et al: Repair of ascending aorta dissection. J Thorac Cardiovasc Surg 93:375, 1987

41. Carrington G: Stronger case for early surgery in distal aortic dissections. Cardiology 8:21, 1991

42. DeSanctis RW, Doroghazi RM, Austen WG et al: Aortic dissection. N Engl J Med 317:1060, 1987

43. Glower DD, Fann JI, Speier RH et al: Comparison of medical and surgical therapy for uncomplicated descending aortic dissection. Circulation, suppl IV. 82:39, 1990

44. Roberts CS, Roberts WC: Frequency of healing of aortic dissection according to type of dissection and therapeutic significance. J Am Coll Cardiol 15:129A, 1990

45. DeBakey ME, Henly WS, Cooley DA et al: Surgical Management of dissecting aneurysms of the aorta. J Thorac Cardiovasc Surg 49:130, 1965

32
Peripheral Arterial Disease

John A. Spittell, Jr.
Peter C. Spittell

Peripheral arterial disease is common, since atherosclerosis is the most frequent cause of both occlusive and aneurysmal disease of the peripheral arteries. The lower-extremity arteries are much more frequently involved than those of the upper extremities. The etiologic spectrum of chronic occlusive peripheral arterial disease is quite broad (Table 32-1). A less common non-atherosclerotic type of occlusive peripheral arterial disease is suggested by its occurrence in a young person (under 40 years of age); by involvement of the upper extremity and/or digits, particularly when there is an associated systemic illness; and by the sudden occurrence of acute ischemia of an extremity without a prior history of occlusive arterial disease.

OCCLUSIVE PERIPHERAL ARTERY DISEASE

Arteriosclerosis Obliterans

Arteriosclerosis obliterans is usually seen in patients over 40 years of age and is more common in men. As in other forms of atherosclerosis, cigarette smoking, hyperlipidemia, and diabetes are predisposing factors. When arteriosclerosis obliterans (ASO) becomes symptomatic, the hallmark is intermittent claudication, but many persons with ASO are asymptomatic, and their identification depends on careful examination of the extremity arteries. Intermittent claudication characteristically occurs with walking and is relieved with rest, just as angina pectoris is related to

exertion or stress and is relieved by rest. Most of the disorders that may be confused with intermittent claudication are neurologic or musculoskeletal disorders (Table 32-2) that are easily differentiated by history or physical examination.

When ischemia becomes severe, the patient has pain at rest (ischemic rest pain) in addition to intermittent claudication. When traumatized, ischemic ulceration (most often on the toes, heel, over the malleoli, or on the dorsum of the foot) may occur (Fig. 32-1). Ischemic ulcers are readily differentiated from other common types of leg and foot ulcers by their severe pain, discrete edge, and pale base (Table 32-3). The frequent association of coronary artery disease (CAD) and ASO must always be kept in mind when planning management of ASO.[1]

Medical history and evaluation of the pulsations of the extremity arteries will localize the occlusive arterial disease. The degree of any ischemia can be reliably estimated by performance of elevation-dependency tests. The degree of any pallor of the skin and the time it takes to develop can be used to grade the elevation pallor (Table 32-4). After elevation, lowering the extremities to a dependent position permits observation of the time required for color to return to the skin and for the superficial veins to fill (Table 32-5) another index of the adequacy of the arterial circulation in the limb. Testing with noninvasive methodology, using the hand-held Doppler and a blood pressure cuff to determine the supine ankle and brachial systolic blood pressure before and 1 minute after standard exercise, is a most sensitive method of diagnosing occlusive ar-

TABLE 32-1. Classification of Occlusive Arterial Disease

Acute arterial occlusion
  Thrombotic arterial occlusion secondary to
    Atherosclerosis
      Arteriosclerosis obliterans
      Atherosclerotic aneurysm
    Thromboangiitis obliterans (Buerger's disease)
    Arteritis due to
      Connective tissue diseases
      Giant cell (temporal or cranial) arteritis
      Takayasu's arteritis
    Myeloproliferative disease
      Polycythemia vera
      Thrombocytosis
    Hypercoagulable states
      Complicating neoplastic disease
      Complicating ulcerative bowel disease
      Idiopathic ("simple") arterial thrombosis
    Trauma
      Arterial puncture and arteriotomy
      Secondary to fractures and bone dislocations
      Arterial entrapment
        Lower extremity
          Adductor tendon compression of superficial femoral artery
          Popliteal artery entrapment
        Upper extremity
          Thoracic outlet compression
          "Crutch" thrombosis
      Frostbite
Embolic arterial occlusion (arising from thrombi of)
  Cardiac origin
    Valvular heart disease, including valvular prostheses
    Acute myocardial infarction
    Myocardial aneurysm
    Atrial fibrillation
    Cardiomyopathy
    Infective endocarditis
  Proximal atherosclerotic plaques or arterial narrowing
  Proximal arterial aneurysms
    Atherosclerotic
    Poststenotic dilation
    Fibromuscular dysplasia
Miscellaneous causes
  Arterial spasm, secondary to
    Ergotism
    Trauma of blunt or penetrating type
    Intra-arterial injections
  Aortic dissection
    Luminal compression (by extension of the dissection into branch(es) of the aorta)
    Thrombotic occlusion at site of reentry
    Foreign bodies
      Bullet embolism
      Guide wires and catheters
Chronic arterial occlusive disease
  Arteriosclerosis obliterans
  Thromboangiitis obliterans (Buerger's disease)
  Arteritis
    Connective tissue disorders
    Giant cell (temporal or cranial) arteritis
    Takayasu's disease
  Trauma
    Blunt trauma
      Chronic occupational arterial occlusion in the hand
    Arterial entrapment
      Superficial femoral artery
      Popliteal artery
  Congenital arterial narrowing

(From Spittell,[15] with permission.)

TABLE 32-2. Symptomatic Conditions Misinterpreted as Intermittent Claudication

Level of Claudication	Misinterpretation
Foot	Foot strain
	Tight shoes
	Plantar neuroma
	Osteoporosis
Calf	Muscle strain
	Osteoarthritis of knee
	Flat feet
Thigh	Sciatica
	Lumbar spinal stenosis
Hip	Osteoarthritis of hip
	Lumbar spinal stenosis

(From Spittell,[15] with permission.)

terial disease in the lower extremities (Table 32-6) and provides an estimate of the degree of functional impairment imposed by it. While arteriography provides definitive information about the location of the occlusive arterial disease and the adequacy of the proximal and distal arterial circulation, it is not necessary to diagnose ASO and is needed only when a decision to restore pulsatile flow has been made (see below).

Knowledge of the natural history of ASO has been provided by several studies[2] and is helpful in planning therapy for the individual patient. Persons with ASO have a shortened life expectancy, mainly attributable to their CAD, with associated diabetes and continued smoking both having an additional adverse effect[2,3]; in the Framingham Study, the average annual mortality for men with symptomatic ASO was 39 per 1,000, while in men without ASO, the average annual mortality was 10 per 1,000 over a 14-year period.[4] As far as limb survival is concerned, the prognosis for the nondiabetic with only intermittent claudication is fairly good, on the order of 96% in 5 years.[2] Some early studies[5] suggested that persons with aortoiliac occlusive arterial disease are more likely to progress to limb-threatening ischemia than infrainguinal occlusive arterial disease, but more recent studies have shown that the level of disease is not a risk factor for progression. When the ischemia becomes more severe and ischemic rest pain or ischemic ulceration, or both, are present, the risk of limb loss increases to 10 to 20% in 5 years[6]; when diabetes is associated with symptomatic ASO, the limb loss increases fourfold to sixfold that in the nondiabetic with ASO.[2,3] One other important point about limb loss is that the available data indicate that limb loss is significantly increased when the person with ASO continues to use tobacco.[2] The importance of protection of the ischemic limb from all types of trauma is emphasized by the fact that more than 60% of amputations evolve from some type of trauma, much of it preventable.[7]

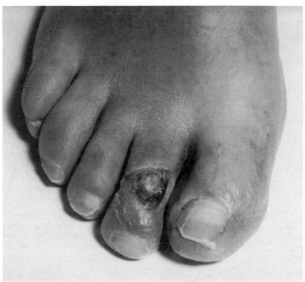

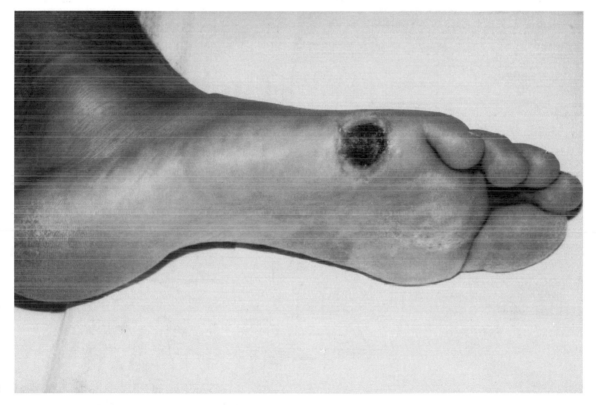

B

Fig. 32-1. (A) Ischemic ulcer of second toe of patient with arteriosclerosis obliterans. **(B)** Ischemic ulcer of distal lateral aspect of the foot of a patient with thromboangiitis obliterans. (From Spittell,[15] with permission.)

Prognostic data on intermittent claudication are important to decisions about management. The walking distance in nondiabetic persons with intermittent claudication remains stable over a 5-year period or increases in more than one-half if tobacco is interdicted.[2] The addition of a regular walking program can aid in increasing both the initial claudication distance and the maximum walking distance.[8] It bears repeating that continued use of tobacco has an impressive and unfavorable influence on mortality, amputation rate, and symptoms of the person with ASO. It is not yet clear what effect control of hyperlipidemia will

TABLE 32-3. Characteristics of Common Leg Ulcers

Characteristic	Ischemic Ulcer[a]	Venous Stasis Ulcer	Neurotrophic Ulcer
Onset	Trauma	Trauma (yes or no)	Spontaneous
Location	Toe, heel, foot	Medial distal leg	Sole of foot
Pain	Severe	Only with infection	Painless
Skin around ulcer	Atrophic—may be inflamed	Stasis changes—pigment	Callous
Ulcer edge	Discrete	Shaggy	Discrete
Ulcer base	Pale; eschar	Healthy	Healthy or pale

[a] Ischemic ulceration resulting from occlusive arterial disease. Ischemic ulceration from arteriolar disease has different characteristics.
(From Spittell,[15] with permission.)

have on the prognosis of the person with ASO, but current reports of slowing or regression of the atherosclerotic process in the aorta and femoral arteries are promising.

Drawing on the prognostic data, it is clear that all patients with ASO should stop tobacco use and protect their ischemic limb from all types of trauma: mechanical, chemical, and thermal. Walking regularly for 30 minutes, stopping as necessary, at least 5 days/week may improve the claudication distance over time. Pentoxifylline, a hemorrheologic agent, may further improve the walking distance, but recent studies indicate

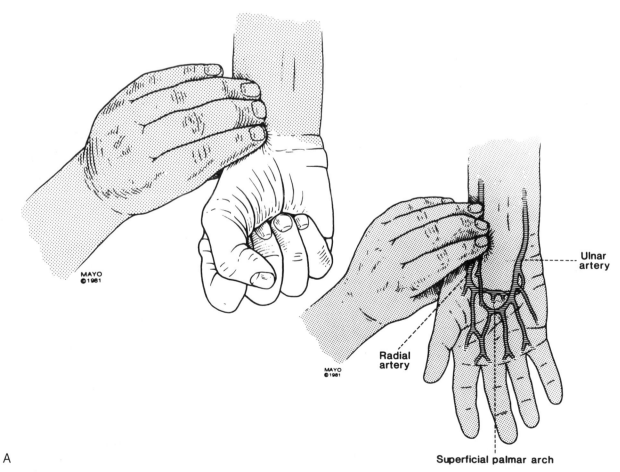

A

Fig. 32-2. Allen test. **(A)** Normal (negative) result, indicating patency of ulnar artery and superficia palmar arch. (*Figure continues.*)

TABLE 32-4. Grading of Elevation Pallor[a]

Grade of Pallor	Duration of Elevation
0	No pallor in 60 seconds
1	Definite pallor in 60 seconds
2	Definite pallor in less than 60 seconds
3	Definite pallor in less than 30 seconds
4	Pallor on the level

[a] Elevation of extremity at angle of 60 degrees above level. (From Spittell,[16] with permission.)

TABLE 32-5. Color Return and Venous Filling Time

Condition	Time for CR (sec)	VFT (sec)
Normal	10	15
Moderate ischemia	15–20	10–30
Severe ischemia	40+	40+

(From Spittell,[16] with permission.)

that a "target" population is most likely to benefit (e.g., those persons who have had their claudication for more than 1 year and who have an ankle systolic pressure of 80% or less that at the brachial level[9]).

As far as restoration of pulsative flow is concerned, for the nondiabetic person whose only symptom is intermittent claudication, its only goal is relief of the claudication and therefore should be offered as an elec-tive procedure, whether to be achieved by arterial sur-gery or percutaneous angioplasty. By contrast, in the diabetic person with symptomatic ASO and for all per-sons with ischemic rest pain or ischemic ulceration or both, restoration of pulsatile flow is indicated, as it may reduce the risk of limb loss. Arteriography is needed in the person with ASO only after the decision to restore pulsatile flow has been made.

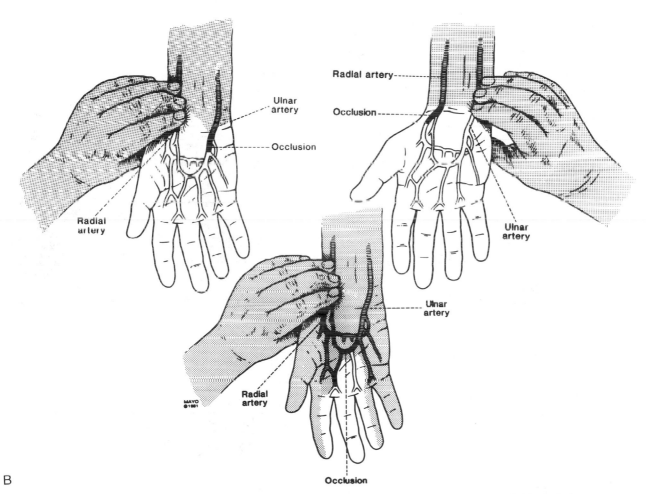

B

Fig. 32-2 (*continued*). **(B)** Abnormal (positive) results due to occlusion of ulnar artery (left), radial artery (right), and superficial palmar arch (bottom center). (From Spittell,[17] by permission of Mayo Foundation.)

TABLE 32-6. Noninvasive Laboratory Assessment of Arterial Insufficiency of the Legs

Degree of Arterial Insufficiency	Standard Exercise		Systolic Blood Pressure Index[a]	
	Claudication	Duration (min)	Before Exercise	After Exercise
Minimal	0	5	Normal to mildly abnormal	Abnormal
Mild	+	5	>0.8	>0.5
Moderate	+	<5	<0.8	<0.5
Severe[b]	+	<3	<0.5	<0.15

[a] Systolic pressure index is obtained by dividing the systolic ankle blood pressure by the systolic brachial blood pressure, both measured with the patient supine (normal, ≥0.95).

[b] Often the systolic ankle blood pressure is less than 50 mmHg.

(From Spittell et al.,[16] with permission.)

Thromboangiitis Obliterans (Buerger's Disease)

Thromboangiitis obliterans (TAO) is uncommon but not rare. It has distinctive clinical features (Table 32-7) that warrant its being considered an entity different from other types of occlusive peripheral arterial disease. Typically, the person with TAO is young, a regular user of tobacco, and more often a man, although with the increasing use of tobacco by women, the incidence of TAO in women can be expected to increase. Frequently the first symptom in TAO is intermittent claudication but, since the disease involves small and medium-sized arteries, the claudication is noted in the arch of the foot or lower calf. TAO also involves small and medium-sized veins, so about one-half of persons with TAO experience superficial thrombophlebitis when the disease is active (i.e., when they are using tobacco). When arterial insufficiency progresses, TAO ischemic rest pain develops and, with even minor trauma, ischemic ulceration of the toes or foot develops.

Examination of the person with TAO will reveal reduced or absent pulsation of one or both pedal arteries in most and reduced or absent pulsation of one or more of the arteries at the wrist in many. The Allen test (Fig. 32-2) is a particularly useful part of the physical examination of the patient with TAO, since it can con-

firm and localize occlusive arterial disease in the hand.[10] Pulsations of the larger arteries, such as the popliteal, femoral, and brachial, are normal; bruits over large arteries, so distinctive with ASO, are not heard in persons with TAO.

To confirm the occlusive arterial disease, noninvasive laboratory studies are useful. A 10-MHz Doppler flow detector is most useful in demonstrating occlusive disease in the digital arteries. Arteriography can

TABLE 32-7. Thromboangiitis Obliterans (Buerger's Disease): Criteria for Diagnosis

Age	<30 years
Sex	Males most often
Habits	Smoker
History	Superficial phlebitis
	Raynaud's phenomenon
	Claudication, arch or calf
Physical examination	Small arteries involved
	Upper extremity involved
Laboratory findings	Blood sugar normal
	Lipids normal
Radiography	No arterial calcification

(From Spittell,[15] with permission.)

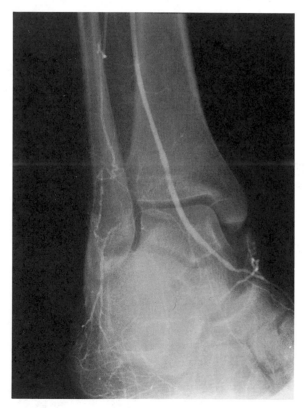

Fig. 32-3. Arteriogram showing typical segmental occlusions of arteries at the ankle level in a 19-year-old man with thromboangiitis obliterans. (From Spittell,[15] with permission.)

be helpful in diagnosis if the diagnosis of TAO is in doubt. Typically, there are multiple occluded segments of the small arteries of the distal part of the involved extremity (Fig. 32-3).

The prognosis of the person with TAO is quite different from that of persons with ASO. With TAO, survival is practically the same as for normal persons of the same age and sex. The risk of limb loss in TAO is, however, greater than for ASO; in a 10-year follow-up, 6% of persons with TAO lost toes, 6% lost fingers, and 13% lost a leg.[11] The activity of TAO and its progression are so closely related to tobacco use that the person with TAO can be advised that the disease will not progress if tobacco is never used again.

Management of TAO is similar to that of other types of occlusive peripheral arterial disease, except for the need to interdict the use of tobacco completely and permanently. Success in the management of TAO is directly related to permanent abstinence from tobacco. Restoration of pulsatile flow by surgery or an-

gioplasty is not a consideration because of the small arteries involved by TAO. If, after tobacco use has been discontinued, there is a need for vasodilation to assist in relief of rest pain or healing of ischemic ulceration, it is best achieved by regional sympathectomy.

Popliteal Artery Entrapment

Although much less common than ASO and TAO, popliteal artery entrapment deserves mention, since the repeated compression of the artery can result in thrombosis or poststenotic aneurysm with resultant ischemia of the foot.[12] Popliteal artery entrapment is typically seen in young men who complain of claudication of the calf or arch of the foot with walking but not with running. Sufficient numbers of cases have not been observed to define the natural history of popliteal artery entrapment but, when suspected, the diagnosis can be confirmed by arteriography. Management includes surgically freeing the artery of the muscular

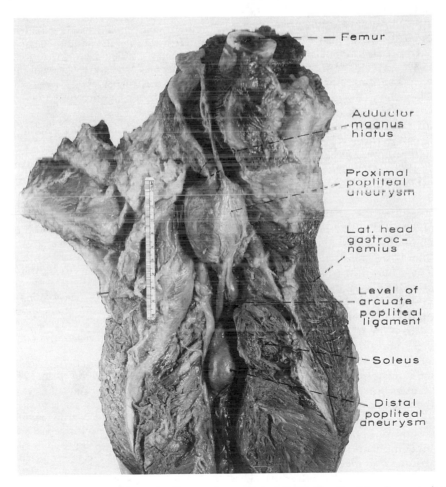

Fig. 32-4. Photograph of popliteal fossa in dissected amputated limb of patient having proximal and distal popliteal aneurysms. (From Gedge et al.,[18] with permission.)

entrapment and reconstruction or resection of an occluded or aneurysmal popliteal artery.

Arteritis

Any of the arteritides can involve the peripheral arteries.[12] In general, the connective tissue disorders involve digital arteries, while the giant cell arteritides (cranial arteritis and Takayasu's arteritis) involve the larger arteries, often at their origin from the aorta. The occlusive peripheral arterial disease is usually overshadowed by the other features of the arteritis.

Prognosis and treatment in these rare cases is basically that of the arteritis. If significant peripheral ischemia persists after the arteritis has been controlled, it can be managed appropriately.

PERIPHERAL ARTERY ANEURYSM

With the exception of femoral and popliteal artery aneurysm, aneurysms of extremity arteries are extremely rare and often of traumatic, infectious, or congenital origin. Femoral and popliteal artery aneurysms are usually arteriosclerotic, however, and most occur in men over 50 years of age.[13] Aneurysms of these two arteries occur in locations that suggest that frequent bending of the artery (the groin and the popliteal space) and poststenotic dilation (just distal to the tendinous hiatus of the adductor magnus muscle in the thigh and just below the level of the knee joint) play a role in their development (Fig. 32-4). Of note is the increasing frequency of false aneurysms of the femoral artery in the groin related to the numerous percutaneous transfemoral procedures and the frequency of aortofemoral arterial bypass grafts.

Unless care is taken to evaluate not only the presence of pulsation but the width and any expansile character of the femoral and popliteal arteries as well, aneurysms will be overlooked. It is important, in this respect, to remember the usual sites of aneurysm in these arteries as described above. One additional point that should evoke particular care in examining these arteries for aneurysm is their frequency in persons with aneurysms of the aorta.

While femoral and popliteal artery aneurysms may be seen as soft tissue masses of curvilinear calcification on plain radiographs, ultrasound is the most reliable diagnostic procedure, even if the aneurysm is thrombosed and, in the case of popliteal masses, will differentiate aneurysm from popliteal cyst.

The most frequent complications of femoropopliteal aneurysms are thromboembolic, producing various degrees of ischemia distally in the extremity. Less commonly, these aneurysms can compress adjacent veins, rupture, or become infected. Our experience is that about a third of these aneurysms will develop complications in 1 to 8 years, with resulting loss of limb in 3.5%.[14] Accordingly, surgical resection and replacement with a graft, preferably before any complications have occurred, is the treatment of choice if the person is a suitable surgical risk. In the latter context, the frequency of significant coronary artery disease in patients with atherosclerotic aneurysms must always be kept in mind in their evaluation.[1]

REFERENCES

1. Gersh BJ, Rihal CS, Rooke TW et al: Evaluation and management of patients with both peripherhal vascular and coronary artery disease. J Am Coll Cardiol 18:203, 1991
2. McDaniel MD, Cronwett JL: Basic data related to the natural history of intermittent claudication. Ann Vasc Surg 3:273, 1989
3. Schadt DC, Hines EA, Juergens JL: Chronic atherosclerotic occlusion of the femoral artery. JAMA 175:937, 1961
4. Kannel WB, Skinner JJ, Schwartz MJ et al: Intermittent claudication: incidence in the Framingham study. Circulation 41:875, 1970
5. Rosenbloom MS, Flanigan P, Schuler JJ et al: Risk factors affecting the natural history of intermittent claudication. Arch Surg 123:867, 1988
6. Juergens JL, Barker NW, Hines EA: Arteriosclerosis obliterans: review of 520 cases with special reference to pathogenic and prognostic factors. Circulation 21:188, 1960
7. Weis AJ, Fairbairn JF: Trauma, ischemic limbs, and amputation. Postgrad Med 43:111, 1968
8. Ernst EEW, Matria A: Exercise for intermittent claudication. Cardiol Board Rev 5:82, 1988
9. Lindegärde F, Jelnes R, Björkman H et al: Conservative drug treatment in patients with moderately severe chronic occlusive peripheral arterial disease. Circulation 80:1549, 1989
10. Allen EV: Thromboangiitis obliterans: methods of diagnosis of chronic occlusive arterial lesions distal to the wrist with illustrative cases. Am J Med Sci 178:237, 1929
11. McPherson JR, Juergens JL, Gifford RW: Thromboangiitis obliterans and arteriosclerosis obliterans: clinical and prognostic differences. Ann Intern Med 59:288, 1963
12. Spittell JA: Some uncommon types of occlusive peripheral arterial disease. Curr Probl Cardiol 8:6, 1983
13. Spittell JA: Clinical aspects of aneurysmal disease. Curr Probl Cardiol 5:6, 1980
14. Wychulis AR, Spittell JA, Wallace RB: Popliteal aneurysms. Surgery 68:942, 1970
15. Spittell JA, Jr: Diagnosis and management of occlusive peripheral arterial disease. Curr Probl Cardiol 15:7, 1990
16. Spittell JA, Jr: Recognition and management of chronic atherosclerotic occlusive peripheral arterial disease. Mod Concepts Cardiovasc Dis 50:19, 1981
17. Spittell JA, Jr: Occlusive peripheral arterial disease: guidelines for office management. Postgrad Med 71:137, 1982
18. Gedge SW et al: Aneurism of the distal popliteal artery ligament. Circulation 24:270, 1961

33

Risk Assessment for Noncardiac Surgery*

Dennis T. Mangano

Cardiovascular disease affects approximately one in four Americans (65/239 million),[1,2] accounting for approximately one million deaths per year, 1.5 million myocardial infarctions (MI), 0.6 million strokes, and 0.4 million cases of congestive heart failure (CHF). The health care cost exceeds $83 billion/year.[3] The problem will persist and likely worsen, since the prevalence of cardiovascular disease increases with age, and we are a rapidly aging population: 25 million Americans (10%) are now over the age of 65, including 2.7 million above age 85.[2,4]

IMPACT OF CARDIOVASCULAR DISEASE ON ANESTHESIA AND SURGERY

The presence of cardiovascular disease substantially affects the perioperative course of both cardiac and noncardiac surgery. The number of cardiac surgeries annually exceeds 400,000, including 285,000 coronary artery bypass graft (CABG) surgeries and 48,000 valve replacements,[5] with associated costs of more than $5 billion,[3] and is expected to increase, despite the introduction of angioplasty and laser surgery, as the prevalence of cardiovascular disease increases. Furthermore, it now appears that morbidity and mortality after cardiac surgery is increasing because of an increase in the severity of disease among patients pre-

senting for CABG surgery, who are often older and have extended courses of medical therapy, prior angioplasty, or revascularization.

For noncardiac surgical care, the impact of cardiovascular disease is even greater. Twenty-five million patients undergo noncardiac surgery annually,[5] approximately 1 million of these with diagnosed coronary artery disease (CAD), [that is, classic angina, Q waves on preoperative electrocardiogram (ECG)], another 2 to 3 million with two or more major risk factors for CAD, and 4 million more over 65 years of age. That is, 7 to 8 million noncardiac surgical patients annually are now at risk for cardiac morbidity or mortality (Fig. 33-1). In addition, older patients represent a 2.5-fold higher percentage of surgical patients than of the general population[5] and often require major intra-abdominal, thoracic, vascular, neurologic, or orthopaedic procedures that further stress existing cardiac risk factors. As the percentage of surgical patients over age 65 increases from 25 to 35% over the next 30 years, the number of noncardiac surgical procedures will increase by 50% (to 35 million),[1] and the number of older patients with cardiovascular disease will double, thereby increasing the number of noncardiac surgical patients at risk for adverse cardiac outcome. Perioperative cardiac morbidity is one of the leading causes of perioperative death. To preempt soaring surgical mortality rates, we must understand the perioperative risk factors associated with this morbidity well enough to define reliable predictors of adverse outcome that will optimize anesthetic and surgical management to benefit outcome.

---

* (Adapted from Mangano,[217] with permission.)

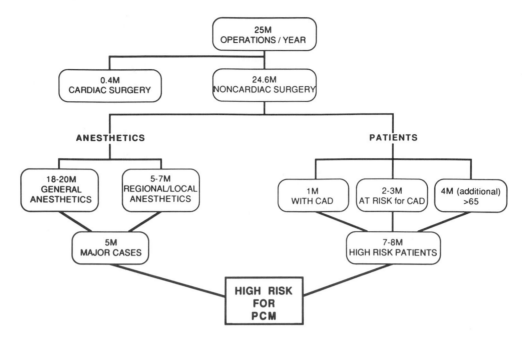

Fig. 33-1. Estimates of the numbers of surgeries and anesthetics, and the patients at risk of perioperative cardiac morbidity in the United States (1988). A total of 6 million (30%) surgical patients are over the age of 65. Two million of these patients are included in the coronary artery disease (CAD) and in the at-risk-of CAD groups, resulting in the 4 million over age 65 (and the 7 to 8 million total) represented. See text for further discussion. (Data from National Center for Health Statistics[1] and American Society of Anesthesiologists.[140])

Perioperative Cardiac Morbidity

Perioperative cardiac morbidity (PCM), including MI, unstable angina, CHF, serious arrhythmia, or cardiac death, is one of the leading causes of death after anesthesia and surgery.

Myocardial Infarction

The incidence of MI after noncardiac surgery in the general population is 0.0 to 0.7%[6-8] but increases to 1.1% in patients with CAD,[9] to 1.8% in those over age 40 with or without CAD,[10] to 5 to 8% in those with prior infarction[6,11-13] and 6 to 40% in those with recent MI,[6,11-15] and to 1 to 15% after vascular surgery[10,16-29] (Table 33-1). The mechanism(s) of perioperative MI is(are) generally unknown. Few MI occur intraoperatively; most occur postoperatively and are usually clinically silent,[6,10,14,15,17,30-36] making them difficult to detect and their precise onset difficult to determine. Altered pain perception due to residual anesthetic effects, administration of analgesics, or competing somatic stimuli (e.g., incisional pain) may be responsible for the predominant silence of perioperative MI, but

TABLE 33-1. Estimated Incidence of Perioperative Cardiac Morbidity: Noncardiac Surgery

Outcome	Incidence (%)	References
Myocardial ischemia		
Preoperative	24	79
Intraoperative	18–64	77–81,196,198,206–209
Postoperative	27–38	79,83
Myocardial infarction		
General population	0.1–0.7	6–8
Prior MI	1.9–7.7	6,11,12,14,15
Aortic Surgery	1–15	10,16–20,25–29
Recent MI	5.7–37	6,11,12,14,15,97
Unstable angina	Unknown	
Congestive heart failure		
Intraoperative	4.8	14
Postoperative	3.6	10
Serious arrhythmias		
Intraoperative	0.9–36	58–60
Postoperative	14–40.5	60
Cardiac death with PMI	36–70	7,30

Abbreviations: MI, myocardial infarction; PMI, perioperative myocardial infarction.
(From Mangano,[217] with permission.)

their etiology remains uncertain.[37-41] Atherosclerotic plaque rupture, intraluminal thrombosis, and coronary arterial wall spasm certainly can be exacerbated by perioperative events. First, increased coronary artery shear stresses may occur secondary to alterations in contractility, blood pressure, flow, and coronary tone.[37,39,42,43] Platelet aggregation may be enhanced because of increased catecholamines, changes in blood viscosity and coronary flow, and abnormal hemostasis[44-53] and vasospasm may be precipitated by release of humoral mediators during stress.[37-42,54] The mortality rate associated with perioperative MI ranges from 28 to 70%.[7,30] Mortality rates associated with other cardiac outcomes are unknown.

Postoperative Angina/Ischemia

Foster et al.[9] reported an 8.7% incidence of postoperative chest pain in patients with CAD undergoing noncardiac surgery, participating in the Coronary Artery Surgery Study (CASS) registry, versus 4.5% in patients without CAD, and 5.1% in those with previous CABG surgery (p = 0.004). Postoperative ischemia occurs significantly more often than chest pain and is predominantly silent. In fact, the incidence of postoperative ECG ST changes indicative of ischemia may be as high as 40% in patients with or at risk of CAD, with more than 85% of such episodes silent.[55] Moreover, there appears to be a strong association between the presence of postoperative ischemia and adverse outcome. The incidence of unstable angina following noncardiac surgery is unknown.

Congestive Heart Failure

The incidence of perioperative CHF is mild to moderate in at-risk patients.[10,14] Rao et al.[14] found a 4.8% (29/609) incidence of intraoperative "CHF" (pulmonary capillary wedge pressure [PCWP] >25 mmHg) in patients with previous MI. Goldman et al.[16] found a 3.6% incidence of postoperative CHF in patients older than 40 with or without CAD. A number of factors may play a role. In patients with CAD, isolated regional ischemia (producing papillary muscle dysfunction), global ischemia, or infarction may impair diastolic relaxation and systolic contraction and precipitate CHF. Perioperative increases in afterload or preload (secondary to catecholamine, temperature, fluid shift, or respiratory changes) will affect both diastolic and systolic function, and exacerbate CHF.[56,57] However, the relative contribution of these ischemic and mechanical effects remains uncertain, since few perioperative studies have used sufficiently sensitive detection techniques to permit discrimination.

Serious Arrhythmias

Of the studies investigating the incidence and characteristics of intraoperative arrhythmias,[58] only two have used continuous recording techniques,[59,60] and none has studied postoperative arrhythmias relative to the preoperative baseline pattern. Nevertheless, the incidence of detected intraoperative arrhythmias ranges from 13 to 84%, with ventricular arrhythmias ranging from 3 to 60%.[59-61] The incidence of serious intraoperative arrhythmias (e.g., persistent multifocal premature ventricular contractions, ventricular tachycardia, ventricular fibrillation) reportedly ranges from 0.9%[61] to 6.0%.[59] Postoperatively, there may be a 48% incidence of arrhythmias,[60] 28% of these ventricular, but how many are new or simply recapitulate the preoperative pattern is unknown. In addition, the relationship of perioperative serious arrhythmias to ischemia or other in-hospital or long-term adverse cardiac outcomes is unknown.

Cardiac Death

The cardiac mortality rates for patients with and without CAD in the CASS registry are reported to be 0.5% versus 2.4%, respectively.[9,10] A rate of 1.9% has been cited for patients over 40 years of age, independent of the presence of CAD.[10]

Conclusion

Since PCM is a primary cause of death after anesthesia and surgery, knowledge of its etiology and mechanisms is crucial. Approximately 50,000 patients per year sustain a perioperative MI and 20,000 of these die; in addition, the cost of treating in-hospital MI is approximately $12,000,[62] resulting in health-care costs of hundreds of millions of dollars for perioperative MI alone. Solution of this problem demands identification of the predictors of PCM, followed by therapeutic trials aimed at modifying such predictors and reducing PCM.

PREDICTORS OF PERIOPERATIVE CARDIAC MORBIDITY

More than 100 perioperative outcome studies have attempted to identify predictors of adverse cardiac outcome. Perioperative myocardial infarction (PMI) was first identified as a persistent problem in 1935,[63] but a decade passed before predictors of MI were explored, and two decades before investigators identified historical preoperative predictors of PCM readily obtainable from the routine history and physical examination.[6,11,12,17,31,32,63,64] Unfortunately, results differed, and the only historical predictor consistently identified as prognostic was recent MI, resulting in the commonly accepted practice of delaying surgery 6 months after an MI. Goldman et al.[10] attempted the first multifactorial approach to prioritizing predictors, assigning a relative value to a series of preoperative predictors to develop a cardiac risk index. Several studies have since challenged the usefulness of this index,[18,65,66] but the importance of this work remains unquestioned. Rao et al.[14] found that an assertive approach to perioperative monitoring and therapy was associated with substantially lower reinfarction rates/ substantially reduced reinfarction rates, but their findings have not been confirmed.

Studies of the prognostic value of specialized preoperative cardiac testing began in 1984. Exercise stress testing,[33,67–69] radionuclear imaging,[66,70,71] and dipyridamole thallium imaging[19,72–75] were studied over the next 5 years and advocated for use in patients undergoing noncardiac surgery.

In 1985, an important series of studies emerged.[76–82] Implicit in the preceding attempts to identify *preoperative* predictors was that the patient's preoperative chronic disease state was primarily responsible for PCM. However, the entire perioperative period is dynamic, suggesting that intra- and postoperative changes in hemodynamics, catecholamines, and myocardial oxygen balance may be equally important determinants of PCM. Outcome studies began to focus on the intraoperative "dynamic" predictors of PCM, particularly myocardial ischemia. Slogoff and Keats[82] and Smith et al.[78] demonstrated the importance of intraoperative ischemia, at least in patients undergoing CABG surgery. More recent studies[76,77,79,81,83] demonstrate that the postbypass and postoperative periods may be equally or more important periods of risk in patients undergoing noncardiac surgery.

THE PREOPERATIVE PREDICTORS

Historical Predictors

Age

Over the next 50 years, the population of the United States will grow by an estimated 49% (to 331 million)[84] the elderly population (over age 65) increasing approximately three times faster than other age groups (162%). Forty percent of all surgical procedures will be performed in patients over age 65, potentially compromised by CAD and MI, since these increase in incidence with age. Although age does not appear to affect resting ejection fraction, left ventricular (LV) volume, and regional wall motion,[85,86] it depresses cardiac response to different forms of stress, such as

exercise or exogenous catecholamines,[85,87,88] thereby contributing to greater surgical complications in aged patients[89–92] in whom perioperative MI is now the leading cause of postoperative death.[93] Nonetheless, investigators disagree on the predictive value of age[6,9,10,13,15,17,31,32,63,65,93] (Table 33-2). For example, Carliner et al.[65] report a 38% incidence of ischemia, MI, or cardiac death in patients older than 70% versus 7% in those aged 40 to 49, whereas Driscoll et al.[17] suggest that age is a significant predictor only when other factors are present. Age may not be as important as the patient's overall physiologic status.[94,95]

Previous Myocardial Infarction

Patients with prior MI have a higher risk of perioperative reinfarction (5 to 8%)[6,11,12,15,28] than do those without prior MI (0.1 to 0.7%)[6–8] and have a reinfarction mortality rate of 36 to 70%. The risk of reinfarction following a prior MI appears to decrease with time. That is, MI within 3 months results in a 30% (or higher) reinfarction rate, within 3 to 6 months, 15%, and thereafter, approximately 6%.[6,11,12,15,96] Investigators who challenge these data (Table 33-2) have found surgical mortality and cardiac morbidity to be independent of a previous MI within 3 to 6 months of surgery.[9,97] Rao et al.[14] found that perioperative reinfarction occurred in only 1.9% of 733 patients who had a previous MI, in only 5.7% of those with an MI that occurred less than 3 months earlier, and in only 2.3% of those with an MI that occurred 4 to 6 months earlier. The use by Rao et al. of preoperative optimization of the patient's status, aggressive invasive monitoring (radial and pulmonary arterial catheterization) and therapy, and prolonged stay in the intensive care unit (ICU) (3 to 4 days postoperatively) suggest that these studies may significantly reduce reinfarction rates and decrease PCM, but this has not been confirmed.[98] The cost of implementing such care for surgical patients with or at risk of CAD would be considerable.

Angina

A history of stable angina significantly increases the risk of MI and sudden death in ambulatory patients with CAD but is a controversial predictor in noncardiac surgical patients (Table 33-2). Some studies support angina as a predictor in this population,[6,17,28,64,99] while others find it a "conspicuously insignificant" predictor,[10] angina per se was not, or only the use of preoperative nitrates predictive.[9] One explanation for reports of low perioperative risk may be that patients with CAD have predominantly (75% or more) painless or silent ischemic episodes,[100,101] placing them at risk because of undetected *ischemia*, not the presence of such symptoms as angina.[102,103] The importance of

TABLE 33-2. Preoperative Risk Factors: Historical

Factor	Author, Reference, Year	
	Supported	**Refuted**
Age	Driscoll[17] (1961), Dack[63] (1963), Arkins[31] (1964), Goldman[10] (1977), Carliner[65] (1985), Foster[9] (1986)	Mauney[32] (1970), Tarhan[6] (1972), Steen[15] (1978), Djokovic[93] (1979), von Knorring[13] (1981)
Previous myocardial infarction (recent, <6 months)	Knapp[11] (1962), Topkins[12] (1964), Arkins[31] (1964), Frazer[215] (1967), Tarhan[6] (1972), Steen[15] (1978), Eerola[182] (1980), Hertzer[20] (1983), von Knorring[13] (1981); Schoeppel[29] (1983), Larsen[99] (1987)	Wells[97] (1981), Rao[14] (1983)
Previous myocardial infarction (old, undetermined)	Topkins[12] (1964), von Knorring[13] (1981), Sapala[64] (1975), Schoeppel[29] (1983), Cooperman[105] (1978), Larsen[99] (1987), Jamieson[28] (1982)	Manney[32] (1970), Goldman[10] (1977), Carliner[65] (1985), Foster[9] (1986)
Angina	Driscoll[17] (1961), Tarhan[6] (1972), Sapala[64] (1975), Larsen[99] (1987), Jamieson[28] (1982)	Goldman[10] (1977), Cooperman[105] (1978), Steen[15] (1978), Wells[97] (1981), von Knorring[13] (1981), Carliner[65] (1985), Rao[14] (1983), Foster[9] (1986)
Congestive heart failure	Goldman[10] (1977), Cooperman[105] (1978), Rao[14] (1983), Larsen[99] (1987), Foster[9] (1986)	
Hypertension	Driscoll[17] (1977), Mauney[32] (1970), Prys-Roberts[210] (1971), Tarhan[6] (1972), Steen[15] (1978), von Knorring[13] (1981), Schneider[108] (1983)	Goldman[10] (1977), Cooperman[105] (1978), Riles[119] (1979), Rao[14] (1983), Foster[9] (1986)
Diabetes mellitus	Driscoll[17] (1961), Tarhan[6] (1972), Hertzer[20] (1983), Foster[9] (1986), Larsen[99] (1987)	Mauney[32] (1970), Goldman[10] (1977), Steen[15] (1978)
Arrhythmia	Sapala[64] (1975), Goldman[10,148] (1977, 1978), Cooperman[105] (1978)	
Peripheral vascular disease	Driscoll[17] (1961), Jeffrey[18] (1983), Schoeppel[29] (1983), Boucher[19] (1985)	Goldman[10] (1977)
Valvular heart disease	Skinner[123] (1964), Goldman[10] (1977)	
Cholesterol		
Cigarette smoking		Foster[9] (1986)
Previous CABG surgery	Scher[128] (1976), McCollum[129] (1977), Mahar[125] (1978), Crawford[130] (1978), Read[127] (1978), Kimbris[131] (1981), Wells[97] (1981), Diehl[126] (1983), Schoeppel[29] (1983), Hertzer[16] (1984), Reul[124] (1986), Foster[9] (1986)	
Previous PTCA		
Cardiovascular therapy	Miller[116] (1975), Bruce[113] (1979), Foëx[212] (1983), Engelman[117] (1984), Cucchiara[144] (1986), Foster[9] (1986), Magnusson[133] (1986), Stone[209] (1988)	
Risk indices	Vacanti[180] (1970) ASA, Goldman[10] (1977), CRI, Djokovic[93] (1979) ASA, Cooperman[105] (1978) CRI, Zeldin[212] (1984) CRI, Detsky[213] (1986) modified CRI	Lewin[142] (1971) ASA, Jeffrey[18] (1983) CRI, Carliner[65] (1985) CRI, Gerson[66] (1985) CRI, Foster[9] (1986) CCS

Abbreviations: ASA, American Society of Anesthesiologists Classification; CRI, Cardiac Risk Index; CCS, Canadian Cardiovascular Society.
(From Mangano,[217] with permission.)

other angina-related factors, such as severity, character (e.g., Prinzmetal's), and instability, have not been studied.

Congestive Heart Failure

More than two million people in the United States have CHF[1]; in hospitalized patients aged 65 or older, CHF is the leading diagnosis-related group, according to data from the National Hospital Discharge Survey.[104]

Preoperative CHF is a predictor of PCM,[9,10,14,98,105] but the predictive value of specific signs is controversial. Goldman et al.[10] suggested that two signs of heart failure have predictive value—a third heart sound and jugular venous distention—but that others, like cardiomegaly, do not. Foster et al.[9] also found that a number of signs and symptoms, such as a third heart sound or orthopnea, were univariate predictors of outcome, but only the left ventricular wall-motion score was predictive, using multivariate analysis. The usefulness of other more quantified measures, such as ejection fraction, one of the best measures of global ventricular function,[106] has been investigated in several studies, whose results suggest that a depressed preoperative ejection fraction (<0.40, as determined by radionuclear imaging or ventriculography) is predictive of perioperative MI, reinfarction, and perioperative ventricular dysfunction.[56,70,71,99]

Whether preoperative hypertension is predictive of PCM also remains controversial (Table 33-2). Some investigators have shown that patients with untreated, poorly treated, or labile preoperative hypertension are at greater risk of perioperative blood pressure lability, arrhythmias, myocardial ischemia, and transient neurologic complications.[6,13,15,17,32,107–112] Withdrawal of preoperative hypertensive medications, such as β-blockers, calcium-channel blockers, or clonidine, is associated with greater perioperative blood pressure lability.[113–117] However, Foster et al.[9] found that preoperative hypertension was only a univariate predictor of PCM, and Goldman et al.,[118] Rao et al.,[14] and others[105,119] that mild-to-moderate preoperative hypertension did not predict irreversible cardiovascular outcomes. Rather, preoperative hypertension may predict several probable "intermediates" of outcome, such as intraoperative blood pressure lability and myocardial ischemia. The issue remains unresolved.

Diabetes Mellitus

Recent studies using sensitive techniques have reaffirmed earlier work[10,13,15,32] identifying diabetes as a potential predictor of PCM.[6,9,17,20,99] Altered autonomic versus normal tone in diabetics may indicate greater intraoperative risk of blood pressure lability.[120] The presence of diabetes in vascular surgery patients may identify a population in whom dipyridamole thallium imaging may be useful.[74] The relative risks of type I (insulin-dependent) versus type II diabetes, and treated versus untreated diabetes, and the effects of therapy and of controlling perioperative glucose levels, need to be analyzed.

Arrhythmias

The available data suggest that frequent premature ventricular contractions or rhythms other than normal-sinus on the preoperative electrocardiogram (ECG) are independent predictors of PCM in noncardiac surgical patients.[9,10,64,105] By contrast, the presence of bifascicular or trifascicular (complete or incomplete) block, right bundle-branch block, or left

anterior hemiblock does not appear to increase perioperative risk, unless these conditions are associated with a more serious condition, such as MI.[121,122]

Peripheral Vascular Disease

Patients with peripheral vascular disease undergoing vascular surgery have a high risk of PCM. MI occurs in as many as 15% of these patients and accounts for more than 50% of their perioperative mortality.[16,20] CAD also is prevalent; only 8% of these patients have normal preoperative angiograms.[16] Thus, their high perioperative and long-term morbidity and mortality may be related to the presence of CAD or the stresses of peripheral vascular surgery.[17–19,29] By contrast, Goldman et al.[10] found that peripheral vascular procedures convey no increased risk of perioperative MI or cardiac death, but that aortic surgery imparts a high risk of postoperative pulmonary edema. For nonvascular surgery, the perioperative risk associated with the presence of peripheral vascular disease is unknown.

Valvular Heart Disease

The perioperative risk associated with preoperative valvular heart disease in noncardiac surgical patients is difficult to assess because of other confounding factors commonly associated with valvular disease, including ventricular dysfunction, arrhythmias, pulmonary hypertension, and CAD. Limited data indicate that aortic stenosis is associated with increased perioperative mortality,[10,123] but other abnormalities may not be. Goldman et al.[10] found that mitral stenosis and insufficiency increased the risk of postoperative CHF, but that, in the absence of other predictors (e.g., an S_3 gallop or jugular venous distention), only aortic stenosis was a significant predictor, associated with a 14-fold increase in mortality. However, there are too few studies to assert the predictive value of either aortic or mitral valvular disease.

Cholesterol

The perioperative risk associated with hypercholesterolemia is unknown.

Cigarette Smoking

Foster et al.[9] found that cigarette smoking was neither a univariate or multivariate predictor of adverse cardiac outcome following noncardiac surgery, but theirs is the only data available.

Previous Coronary Artery Bypass Graft Surgery

Previous CABG surgery appears to confer protection against the development of PCM. At least 12 studies involving more than 2,000 patients report a significantly lower postoperative infarction rate and cardiac mortality in prior-CABG patients undergoing noncardiac surgery.[9,16,29,96,124–131] Data pooled from these studies show the postoperative incidence of MI in these patients to be 0 to 1.2% versus 1.1 to 6% in patients without prior CABG surgery, and mortality to be 0.5 to 0.9% versus 1 to 2.4%. Mortality rates in patients with previous CABG is 0.9%, patients without CAD 0.5% and in patients with CAD without prior CABG 2.4%.[9] By contrast, studies of simultaneous CABG and noncardiac surgery report higher mortalities (4 to 13%) attributed to the unstable nature of either coronary or vascular disease.[16,124]

Previous Percutaneous Transluminal Coronary Angioplasty

Coronary angioplasty is performed in more than 300,000 patients annually, equalling the number of CABG surgeries performed annually.[1] Newer adaptations of this technique, such as coronary atherectomy using mechanical and laser technologies, are being introduced. There are no data on the effects of angioplasty on patients undergoing subsequent noncardiac surgical procedures.

Cardiovascular Therapy

Preoperative withdrawal of cardiovascular medications is associated with a higher incidence of perioperative ischemia, dysrhythmias, MI, and cardiac death,[113–117] and the possible prophylactic benefit of pharmacologic therapies is being investigated. Several studies suggest that preoperative oral β-blocker therapy or pre-induction intravenous β-blocker therapy decreases the incidence of intraoperative ischemia in both cardiac and noncardiac surgical patients,[132–134] and that β-blocker therapy may be more effective prophylactically than preoperative calcium-channel blocker therapy.[135,136] Preoperative administration of clonidine has been shown to decrease anesthetic requirement,[137,138] catecholamines,[137] and blood pressure lability,[137,138] intraoperatively and postoperatively in CABG patients[138] and in hypertensive patients[137] undergoing noncardiac surgery. However, these studies were blinded and involved only a limited number of patients.[139] Thus, although a number of cardiovascular medications may be potentially useful, larger-scale outcome studies, particularly in patients undergoing noncardiac surgery, are necessary to identify those subgroups of patients who will benefit from prophylactic therapy.

Risk Indices

Multivariate risk indices proposed for quantifying preoperative predictors include the American Society of Anesthesiologists' (ASA) classification,[140] the car-

diac risk index,[10] the New York Heart Association (NYHA) classification,[141] and the Canadian Cardiovascular Society (CCS) classification.[141] The most widely used are the ASA classification and the cardiac risk index classifications. By multivariate analysis of 1,001 patients undergoing noncardiac surgery, Goldman et al.[10] identified, weighed, and summed nine significant predictors to form the cardiac risk index. On the basis of this index, four patient cohorts were classified according to progressively increased risk of morbid outcome. The general applicability of the cardiac risk index and other indices is being challenged,[9,18,65,66,142] with each index supported or refuted by an equal number of studies (Table 33-2). No consistently accurate and generally applicable risk index has been developed.

Diagnostic Testing Predictors

The diagnostic tests suggested for preoperative assessment of noncardiac surgical patients include exercise stress testing, echocardiography, radionuclear imaging, and, most recently, dipyridamole thallium imaging and ambulatory (Holter) ECG monitoring. Studies exploring their effectiveness as predictors are still few, and the results, at times, controversial (Table 33-3). Cost potentially limits their use. Individual tests range from $150 to $1,500; if applied routinely, even in a subgroup of the noncardiac surgical population at risk, the annual increase in national health-care costs would be in the tens to hundreds of millions of dollars. For example, preoperative use of dipyridamole thallium imaging in one-half the population requiring vascular procedures would increase the annual costs in excess of $100 million.

Routine Testing Modalities

Twelve-Lead Electrocardiography

Preoperative ECG abnormalities appear to be common, occurring in 40 to 70% of CAD patients undergoing noncardiac surgery and possibly related to age and the presence of known cardiac disease. The most frequent abnormality is ST-T wave changes (65 to 90%), followed by signs of LVH (10 to 20%), and Q waves (0.5 to 8%).[10,13,17,32,65,103,143–147]

The predictive value of preoperative ECG is controversial, despite its widespread use to obtain a baseline profile of patients with suspected or known heart disease. For example, Carliner et al.[65] report that an abnormal preoperative ECG (ST-T wave ischemic or nonspecific changes and intraventricular conduction delays) was the only statistically significant independent predictor of adverse cardiac outcome in noncardiac surgical patients over 40 years of age.[146] Goldman

TABLE 33-3. Preoperative Risk Factors: Diagnostic Tests

Factor	Author, Reference, Year	
	Supported	Refuted
12-lead ECG	Driscoll[17] (1961), Baers[144] (1965), Hunter[145] (1968), Cooperman[105] (1978), Mauney[32] (1970), von Knorring[13] (1981), Carliner[65,146] (1985, 1986)	Goldman[10] (1977)
Chest radiographic abnormalities	Goldman[10] (1977)	
Exercise-stress testing	Gage[67] (1977), Cutler[68,69] (1979, 1981), Gerson[66] (1985), von Knorring[33] (1986)	Carliner[65] (1985)
Ambulatory monitoring		
Precorial echocardiography		
Radionuclear imaging	Pasternack[70,71] (1984, 1985), Gerson[66] (1985)	
Dipyridamone-thallium imaging	Boucher[19] (1985), Brewster[75] (1985), Cutler[72] (1987), Leppo[73] (1987), Eagle[74] (1987)	London[214] (1988)
Magnetic resonance imaging/spectroscopy		
Cardiac catheterization	Herter[16,169] (1984, 1985)	

(From Mangano,[217] with permission.)

et al.[148] found that ECG abnormalities (including old Q waves, ST-T wave changes, or bundle-branch blocks) had no significant predictive value.

Chest Radiography

In patients with CAD, chest radiographic abnormalities predict ventricular function abnormalities detectable by ventriculography. The presence of cardiomegaly indicates a low ejection fraction (<0.40) in more than 70% of patients with CAD,[149] and the latter predicts PCM,[56,70,71,99] suggesting that preoperative radiographic cardiomegaly also might predict PCM.[9] However, Goldman et al.[10] support only the presence of a tortuous or calcified aorta, and not cardiomegaly.

Exercise Stress Testing

Preoperative exercise stress testing is yet another controversial predictor. Several studies have demonstrated that a positive ischemic response and a low exercise capacity predict adverse outcome (MI) following noncardiac surgery[33,66–69] and that preoperative exercise stress testing is a more sensitive indicator than the clinical history or preoperative ECG.[69] Cutler et al.[69] argued that asymptomatic patients would escape identification by risk-factor analysis and recommended routine use of preoperative exercise stress testing. By contrast, Carliner et al.[65] found that only the routine preoperative ECG, not preoperative exercise stress testing results, a statistically significant independent predictor of cardiac risk in noncardiac surgical patients over age 40. Thus, use of preoperative exercise stress testing for identification of at-risk patients remains controversial.

Ambulatory ECG Monitoring

Ambulatory ECG monitoring has proved successful in detecting ST-segment changes in patients with CAD and indicates that frequent episodes of ST depression,

indicative of subendocardial ischemia, occur during normal daily activities.[100,101,150–154] Typically, these episodes are asymptomatic (silent), probably unrelated to heart rate,[100,155,156] and potentially associated with myocardial perfusion abnormalities.[155] Whether these silent episodes represent myocardial ischemia remains to be determined, but they may be as indicative of the development of subsequent MI as angina-related episodes.[102,103]

Preoperative Holter monitoring,[76,79,157] indicates that 20 to 40% of surgical patients with, or at risk of, CAD have frequent ischemic episodes during the 48 hours preceding surgery, most (more than 75%) of which are clinically silent.[76,79,157] Raby et al.[158,159] found a relationship between preoperative ST episodes and adverse cardiac outcome in patients undergoing vascular surgery. The relative risk for in-hospital outcomes was 54, and that for longer-term outcomes was 5.4. These studies suggest that ambulatory Holter monitoring prior to surgery predicts short-term and long-term outcomes. By contrast, Fegert et al.[79] found that most adverse in-hospital outcomes were associated with postoperative, not preoperative, Holter ischemia. Until the discrepancy between these studies is resolved, the routine use of Holter monitoring in these patients preoperatively does not appear to be warranted.

Precordial Echocardiography

Precordial echocardiography is prognostic of both short-term and long-term outcomes in patients with acute MI,[160] but its preoperative prognostic value is unknown. However, radionuclear and angiographic studies have shown that preoperative ventricular dysfunction or segmental wall-motion abnormalities, detected using either technique, predict perioperative ventricular dysfunction.[56,70,71,99] Since echocardiography provides similar information less invasively and expensively, it is potentially more useful.

Transesophageal Echocardiography

Awake transesophageal echocardiography (TEE) is now used for characterizing left atrial thrombi, valvular vegetations, and prosthetic valvular function and for assessing dissecting aortic aneurysm.[161] [165] Its predictive value in noncardiac surgical patients has not been studied.

Radionuclear Imaging

The predictive value of preoperative radionuclear imaging has been studied primarily in vascular surgery patients. During lower-extremity revascularization or abdominal aortic aneurysm resection, the gated-pool-determined ejection fraction has been shown to be an independent predictor of PCM. Pasternack et al.[70,71] found that an ejection fraction of less than 0.35 was associated with a 75 to 85% incidence of perioperative MI, and an ejection fraction greater than 0.35 with a 19 to 20% incidence. Exercise radionuclear ventriculography has been studied in older patients scheduled for elective abdominal or thoracic surgery.[66] The inability to exercise for 2 minutes (with heart rate >99 beats/min) was found to be the best predictor of PCM. Neither resting ejection fraction nor historical predictors were as significant.

Preoperative dipyridamole thallium imaging recently has been studied in patients undergoing vascular surgery.[19,72–75,166] Although unblinded and uncontrolled, these studies demonstrated that preoperative dipyridamole thallium imaging is highly sensitive (89 to 100%), reasonably specific (53 to 80%), and superior to historical predictors or exercise stress testing. The negative predictive value (identifying the absence of abnormality) is nearly 100%. The positive predictive value (identifying the presence of abnormality) is low (17 to 50%), because of the large number of false-positive results, but increases when reperfusion criteria include two or more dysfunctional segments, or when high-risk subsets of patients are chosen for preoperative imaging.[72,74] For example, Eagle et al.[74] found that patients with a history of angina, prior MI, CHF, or diabetes mellitus had an outcome event rate of 37% versus 0% in patients without these predictors. More recently, Levinson et al.[167] used semiquantitative analysis of dipyridamole thallium 201 and demonstrated that perioperative risk in patients undergoing vascular surgery was related to the extend of thallium redistribution. Thus, dipyridamole thallium imaging may provide additional risk stratification in selected subgroups of patients.[166] In contrast to these data are recent data[168] that reexamine the predictive potential of thallium scintigraphy as a preoperative screening test. These investigators found that there was no association between redistribution defects and adverse cardiac outcomes, with more than 50% of adverse outcomes occurring in patients without redistribution defects. Similarly, no association was found between redistribution effects and perioperative ischemia; as well, more than 50% of all ischemic episodes occurred in patients without redistribution defects. Thus, until the discrepancy between these findings is resolved, the routine use of thallium 201 scintigraphy as a preoperative screening test in patients undergoing vascular surgery does not appear to be warranted.

Cardiac Catheterization

Studies of preoperative coronary angiography in patients undergoing vascular and general surgery[16,169] report a relatively high incidence of coronary stenosis in these patients, regardless of symptoms or other predictors, and lower early (1.5% versus 12%) and late mortality (12% versus 26%) rates accompanied by a higher cumulative 5-year survival rate (72% versus 43%) in those who have had CABG surgery before vascular surgery. Thus, angiography and ventriculography are useful for diagnosing patients who require CABG before noncardiac surgery. They also may be useful for predicting PCM. For example, a low ejection fraction (<0.40) determined by radionuclear imaging predicts PCM in patients undergoing vascular surgery, suggesting that ejection fraction information derived from preoperative ventriculography may be similarly predictive. However, the expense and morbidity associated with cardiac catheterization, and the existence of alternative less costly and risky techniques limit its application, even in high-risk patients.

Preoperative Predictors: Conclusions

Recent (<6 months) MI and current CHF are the only two consistently proven preoperative predictors of PCM. The value of other historical predictors, such as previous (old) MI, angina, previous CHF, hypertension, diabetes, and age, is still unresolved. Although selected populations may benefit by the use of specialized nonroutine testing, the efficacy and cost-effectiveness of these tests remain controversial.

INTRAOPERATIVE PREDICTORS

The "classic" intraoperative predictors studied for past two decades include choice of anesthetic, urgency of surgery, site of surgery, and duration of anesthesia and surgery. Recently recognized is that dynamic events occurring intraoperatively may affect outcome, independently of the preoperative cardiovascular disease state. That is, PCM can result from hypertension, hypotension, tachycardia, myocardial ischemia (ECG, TEE), ventricular dysfunction, and arrhythmias.

Classic Predictors

Choice of Anesthetic

No one anesthetic technique appears to offer unique benefits. Studies comparing the incidence of perioperative infarction, CHF, and arrhythmias in patients with cardiac disease during regional (spinal, epidural, upper extremity, local) versus general anesthesia[14,15,170,171] show no significant difference in the safety and outcome rates associated with either technique. For example, Rao et al.[14] report a 1.8% (12/659) reinfarction rate associated with general anesthesia versus 2.7% (2/74) with regional anesthesia. Other investigators suggest that regional anesthesia is superior to general anesthesia in containing MI, but small study populations and other methodologic limitations limit the accuracy of their findings.[64,171,172] Nonetheless, the regional technique does appear to benefit patients with prior MI undergoing transurethral prostatec-

tomy, whose reinfarction rate with spinal anesthesia is lower than 1% versus 2 to 8% with general anesthesia.[173,174] Regional anesthesia also may benefit patients with CHF, in whom spinal anesthesia is not associated with new or worsening heart failure, whereas general anesthesia results in relatively high rates of both.[148,175] The effect of the two techniques on arrhythmias (assessed using both continuing and intermittent ECG techniques) appears to be similar[59,148,174]; only the site of surgery is predictive in this population,[172] with the incidence of arrhythmias ranging from 53 to 100%, depending on the site.

Site of Surgery

Patients undergoing thoracic or upper abdominal surgery have a two- to threefold higher risk of perioperative cardiac complications[6,10,14,15,99] (Table 33-4). However, von Knorring et al.[13] found that neither the site nor the duration of surgery affected outcome in patients with CAD undergoing general orthopedic or trauma surgery; dynamic factors such as intraoperative hypotension were more important. The presence of such confounding variables complicates analysis.[9,12,13,17,105] Unquestionably, patients with CAD undergoing major vascular surgery are at increased risk of perioperative MI, CHF, and cardiac death. In-

TABLE 33-4. Intraoperative Risk Factors

Factor	Author, Reference, Year	
	Supported	**Refuted**
Classical risk factors		
Anesthetic	Rao[14] (1983)	Driscoll[17] (1961), Knapp[51] (1962), Topkins[12] (1964), Arkins[31] (1964), Mauney[32] (1970), Tarhan[6] (1972), Goldman[10] (1977), Steen[15] (1978), Djokovic[93] (1979), von Knorring[13] (1981)
Site of Surgery	Tarhan[6] (1972), Goldman[10] (1977), Rao[14] (1983), Larsen[99] (1987)	Driscoll[17] (1961), Cooperman[105] (1978), von Knorring[13] (1981)
Duration of anesthesia/ surgery	Arkins[31] (1961), Cogbill[179] (1967), Mauney[32] (1970), Goldman[10] (1977), Steen[15] (1978)	Driscoll[17] (1961), Topkins[12] (1964), Tarhan[6] (1972), Djokovic[93] (1979), von Knorring[13] (1981), Rao[14] (1983)
Emergency surgery	Arkins[31] (1964), Vacanti[180] (1970), Goldman[10] (1977), Djokovic[93] (1979), Larsen[99] (1987)	Rao[14] (1983)
Dynamic risk factors		
Hypertension	Plumlee[8] (1972), Steen[15] (1978)	Goldman[10] (1977), Riles[119] (1979), Schoeppel[29] (1983), Rao[14] (1983)
Hypotension	Wroblewski[181] (1952), Wasserman[34] (1955), Driscoll[17] (1961), Chamberlain[35] (1964), Mauney[32] (1970), Plumlee[8] (1972), Goldman[10,118] (1977, 1979), Steen[15] (1978), Mahar[125] (1978), Riles[119] (1979), Eerola[182] (1980), von Knorring[13] (1981), Schoeppel[29] (1983), Rao[14] (1983)	Nachlas[183] (1961)
Tachycardia	Rao[14] (1983)	
Myocardial ischemia	Smith[78] (1985)	
Ventricular dysfunction	Rao[14] (1983)	
Arrhythmias	Sapala[64] (1975), Steen[15] (1978)	Goldman[148] (1978), Rao[14] (1983)

(From Mangano,[217] with permission.)

farction rates as high as 15 to 40% have been reported during aortic-abdominal aneurysm repair and aorto-femoral bypass grafting.[16,20,21,25–28,176–178] The intraoperative stresses associated with vascular surgery, combined with underlying CAD, rather than surgical site, appear to be responsible for the high complication rate.[16,21–24]

Duration of Anesthesia and Surgery

Procedures lasting more than 3 hours are associated with a higher incidence of PCM[10,15,31,32,148,179] (Table 33-4), and, usually, major surgery involving greater hemodynamic changes and other stresses. Whether the duration of anesthesia and surgery per se has an independent effect on outcome is, therefore, unclear.[6,12–14,17,93]

Emergency Surgery

Most studies report that emergency surgery increases the risk of PCM by two- to fivefold[10,17,31,99,180] (Table 33-4); only one[14] suggests that no increased risk is associated with emergency procedures. Emergency surgery therefore does appear to be a risk factor for PCM.

Classic Predictors: Conclusions

Among the classic intraoperative predictors, emergency surgery, vascular surgery, and prolonged (>3 hours) thoracic or upper abdominal surgery appear to be independent predictors of perioperative morbidity, while choice of anesthetic does not.

Dynamic Predictors

Acute imbalances in myocardial oxygen supply and demand may produce ischemia which may, in turn, result in irreversible cardiac morbidity. Dynamic intraoperative changes may, therefore, predict PCM. However, most reports to date should be considered preliminary (Table 33-4).

Hypertension

The predictive value of intraoperative hypertension for PCM is unresolved (Table 33-4). Some investigators[8,15] suggest an independent relationship between hypertension and outcome, while others do not.[10,14,29,119] For example, Steen et al.[15] found a significantly higher perioperative reinfarction rate in patients with hypertension alone (9.2% versus 4.4% nonhypertensive patients), while Rao et al.[14] found a higher rate only in patients in whom hypertension with tachycardia developed.

Hypotension

Unlike hypertension, intraoperative hypotension appears to be an important independent predictor of PCM. The results of outcome studies conducted over the last 30 years (Table 33-4) are consistent with the physiologic findings,[8,10,13–15,17,29,32,34,35,119,125,181,182] with the exception of a retrospective study by Nachlas et al.[183] (Table 33-4), which reported finding no significant difference in mortality between patients with intraoperative hypotension (systolic blood pressure decrease >40 mmHg) versus those without (11.5% versus 8.1%, respectively, p = not significant).

Tachycardia

Slogoff and Keats[82] suggest a causal relationship between tachycardia and outcome in patients undergoing CABG surgery, and Rao et al.[14] a similar relationship in noncardiac surgical patients. The latter investigators found that perioperative MI occurred in two of 16 noncardiac surgical patients with tachycardia and in three of eight hypertensive patients with tachycardia; while not significant, these data do suggest a relationship between tachycardia and PCM.

Myocardial Ischemia

Among the technologies used to identify and characterize intraoperative ischemia in patients undergoing noncardiac surgery are ECG, transesophageal echocardiography, pulmonary artery monitoring, radionuclear imaging, cardiokymography, and biochemical assays.

ECG ST Abnormalities

It is unclear whether patients in whom ECG ST changes indicative of myocardial ischemia develop during noncardiac surgery are at greater risk of intraoperative and postoperative MI. Studies by Slogoff and Keats[82,182] in patients undergoing CABG support this hypothesis: prebypass ischemia increased the risk of MI by two- to threefold (2.5% to 6.9%). Pursuing this question further, Knight et al.[76,155] recently demonstrated that a chronic, often "silent" pattern of ischemia existed preoperatively in CABG patients (and may exist in noncardiac surgery patients[79]). Furthermore, the intraoperative pattern of ischemia was no worse than the preoperative pattern, implying that anesthesia and surgery may not be as stressful as previously assumed, and the intraoperative pattern may simply be a recapitulation of the chronic preoperative pattern. However, definitive outcome studies, contrasting the relative predictive value of preoperative, intraoperative, and even postoperative ischemia are unavailable, especially in noncardiac surgery patients.

TEE Wall-Motion/Thickening Abnormalities

Segmental wall-motion and wall-thickening abnormalities are more sensitive and earlier indices of myocardial ischemia than ECG changes in both animals and humans.[185–187] Preliminary data indicate that TEE wall-motion and wall-thickening changes indicative of myocardial ischemia, even when unaccompanied by ECG changes, are predictive of PCM.[78,80,188] Smith et al.[78] found that 4 of 50 major vascular or CABG patients in whom a perioperative MI developed had intraoperative wall-motion abnormalities, and only 1 of 4 had ECG abnormalities. Three of 4 had persistent intraoperative wall-motion abnormalities occurring in the same area as the infarct, and the fourth had a transient wall-motion abnormality. Recently, Leung et al.[80] found that the presence of immediate postbypass wall-motion abnormalities was the best predictor of PCM in patients undergoing CABG surgery. Fifty patients undergoing elective CABG surgery were studied using continuous TEE and ECG intraoperatively, and intermittently in the ICU. The incidence of wall-motion abnormalities exceeded the incidence of ST changes throughout all periods. Neither prebypass ECG abnormalities nor ECG abnormalities occurring at any time predicted adverse outcome. Only postbypass TEE abnormalities predicted outcome: 6 of 18 with postbypass wall-motion abnormalities had adverse outcome versus 0 of 32 without abnormalities. In noncardiac surgical patients, London et al.[81] reported a 33% incidence of intraoperative TEE wall-motion abnormalities in 95 patients with, or at risk of, CAD. Eight of the 9 patients in whom adverse cardiac outcomes developed had preceding intraoperative wall-motion abnormalities. Although suggestive, these data are only preliminary; the predictive value of TEE in noncardiac surgery patients remains unknown.

Pulmonary Artery Monitoring of Ischemia

Data from animal and human studies demonstrate that, during acute coronary occlusion, exercise precipitates ECG ST changes, and early and marked increases in LV end-diastolic pressure.[189–193] Thus, end-diastolic pressure appears to be an early and sensitive marker of ischemia. Whether PCWP is as sensitive a measure as end-diastolic pressure in either animals or humans is unknown. Studies in patients with acute MI challenge the possibility. Rahimtoola et al.[194] have shown that left ventricular end-diastolic pressure increases during ischemia, due to the effects of end-atrial

systolic emptying on the stiffened and ischemic left ventricle, but that these increases are not reflected in the mean diastolic pressure, the left-atrial pressure, or the PCWP. In vascular surgery patients, Häggmark et al.[195] reported that the sensitivity, specificity, and predictive value (positive and negative) of PCWP abnormalities (≥5 mmHg change from baseline, or the development of an abnormal waveform) for ischemia (ECG or cardiokymography abnormalities, or lactate production) ranged between 40 and 60%. In CABG patients, Lieberman et al.[196] also found a low positive predictive value (24%), but the negative predictive value was higher (85%); however, the PCWP was no better than central venous pressure measurement, except in patients with moderate to severe preoperative ventricular dysfunction. Leung et al.,[197] in CABG patients, found that 61% of TEE wall-motion abnormalities occurred without significant changes (more than 20% of control) in heart rate, systolic arterial pressure, or pulmonary artery pressure. Only 10% of episodes were accompanied by changes in pulmonary artery pressure of 5 mmHg or more. Roizen et al.[198] found that although 11 of 12 patients developed TEE wall-motion abnormalities when the aorta was cross-clamped above the supraceliac arteries, PCWP remained normal (≤12 mmHg) in 10 of 12, with only 2 of 12 patients having transient increases. These studies, therefore, call into question the value of pulmonary artery catheterization and monitoring for detection of intraoperative ischemia, except perhaps in patients with preoperative ventricular dysfunction. Further study is warranted.

Cardiokymographic Detection of Ischemia

Cardiokymography is a noninvasive technique that permits analogue representation of anterior wall motion. The probe is a capacitive plate placed over the chest wall emitting a low-energy, high-frequency (10-MHz) electromagnetic field. Motion within the field produces a change in capacitance, and therefore frequency of the oscillation, which is converted to the output voltage signal. Its limitations include the inability to detect wall motion that is not anterior, the presence of interfering noise produced by other artifactual motion, and the inability to maintain probe position during prolonged surgery or thoracic surgery. Previous studies in patients have demonstrated that cardiokymography is more sensitive and specific an indicator of CAD than the ECG.[195,199,200] Exercise cardiokymography has been shown to have similar sensitivity and specificity as exercise thallium and is significantly better than exercise ECG.[199] In surgical patients, Bellows et al.[199] demonstrated a 33% (8 of 24) incidence of cardiokymographic changes indicative of ischemia in patients with CAD (versus 4% [1 of 25] in patients without CAD), with 1 of 8 having ECG ST abnormalities, and 3/8 with increased PCWP (≥ 4 mmHg). Häggmark et al.[195] compared cardiokymography, single-lead (V_5) ECG, PCWP, and lactate extraction (left anterior descending artery [LAD]) in 53 vascular patients with CAD. In 74% of patients, one or more forms of ischemia developed, with 83% of the episodes detected by cardiokymography, 44% by ECG, 39% by PCWP, and 13% by lactate production. The relationship of cardiokymographic changes to TEE wall-motion abnormalities, or to adverse cardiac outcome, is unknown.

Ventricular Dysfunction

The increases in ventricular filling pressure associated with ventricular dysfunction deleteriously affect both myocardial oxygen supply (coronary artery backpressure) and demand (wall tension). In animals, the failing ventricle may not only precipitate ischemia but also exacerbate the effects of hypotension, hypertension, and tachycardia on the ischemic state of the ventricle.[202,203] Conversely, ischemia can precipitate ventricular dysfunction and increase end-diastolic pressure, particularly with severe stenosis in the presence of increased myocardial oxygen demand (e.g., exercise).[189-191]

Data from one large-scale study suggest a relationship between intraoperative dysfunction and outcome. Rao et al.[14] found that PCWP exceeded 25 mmHg in 29 of 607 patients monitored using pulmonary artery catheters. In 27% (8 of 29) of these patients with elevated PCWP, perioperative MI developed versus less than 1% of those with no increase in PCWP. Several other studies have suggested that operative mortality was decreased in patients undergoing aortic aneurysm repair, monitored with pulmonary artery catheters.[204,205] However, a number of limitations exist in these studies, and further investigation is necessary.

Arrhythmias

Of the four studies attempting to define the predictive value of intraoperative arrhythmias, two report that they are predictors of PCM,[15,64] and two that they are not.[14,148] Rao et al.[14] found no correlation between the incidence or type of dysrhythmias (other than tachycardia) and perioperative reinfarction. Goldman et al.[148] found a 4% incidence of new supraventricular tachycardias and a 7% incidence of intraoperative bradycardia, but both types of arrhythmia were unrelated to PCM. The results reported by Steen et al.[15] generally support the predictive value of arrhythmia,

but only indirectly: all eight of their patients who reinfarcted intraoperatively had clinical signs of either hypotension or dysrhythmia. None of these studies has rigorously measured intraoperative arrhythmias using continuously recorded ECG techniques.

Dynamic Intraoperative Predictors: Conclusions

Both intraoperative hypotension and tachycardia predict PCM. Hypertension remains a controversial predictor, and ventricular dysfunction and arrhythmias have not been adequately studied. Myocardial ischemia, as indicated by ECG, TEE, or cardiokymography, is a suggested predictor, but the data apply principally to patients undergoing CABG surgery. LV end-diastolic pressure is a sensitive measure of ischemia, but preliminary studies suggest that PCWP may be too insensitive. Finally, other measures, such as radionuclear imaging or lactate determination, used primarily in research studies, are impractical for routine clinical use.

POSTOPERATIVE PREDICTORS

Recent studies in both cardiac[76,80] and noncardiac[79,83] surgery have shown that postoperatively heart rate commonly increases by 25 to 50% over intraoperative values and that tachycardia (heart rate >100 bpm) occurs in 10 to 25% of patients. Whether postoperative tachycardia is related to ischemia remains unknown. However, these preliminary studies suggest that ischemia does occur most commonly during the postoperative period, and persists for 48 hours[79] or longer[83] after noncardiac surgery. Also, these postoperative ischemic episodes are usually unaccompanied by symptoms such as typical or atypical chest pain, symptoms of hypoperfusion, or ventricular failure. Thus, postoperative ischemia appears to be silent, and therefore difficult to detect.

CONCLUSIONS

Perioperative cardiac morbidity is and will continue to be an important health-care problem. Of the 25 million patients who undergo anesthesia and surgery in the United States annually, approximately 2 to 3 million have, or are at risk of, CAD; an additional 4 million are over the age of 65, and 5 million undergo major surgery. As the elderly population grows at three times the rate of other groups, the prevalence of cardiac disease will increase in our surgical population. The current incidence of PCM in this at-risk population remains unacceptably high, ranging from 2 to 15%.

Over the past 35 years, approximately 100 outcome studies have examined the problem of PCM in patients undergoing noncardiac surgery. Most have focused on preoperative historical predictors, of which only a recent MI or present CHF are proven predictors of PCM. The efficacy and cost-effectiveness of specialized preoperative cardiac testing, such as exercise stress testing or dipyridamole thallium imaging, remain controversial. Outcome studies of intraoperative predictors have shown that anesthetic choice does not affect outcome, but that emergency surgery, major vascular surgery, and prolonged thoracic or upper abdominal surgery are associated with increased risk. Among the dynamic intraoperative predictors, hypotension and tachycardia appear to predict outcome. Myocardial ischemia, although potentially important, has not been studied rigorously in patients undergoing noncardiac surgery. Studies of the postoperative period are few. Preliminary data suggest that the postoperative predictors for perioperative cardiac morbidity may be at least as critical as intraoperative factors.

MOST RECENT RESULTS

We recently published an article investigating the predictors of perioperative cardiac morbidity in at-risk patients undergoing noncardiac surgery.[216] Since this article has important applicability to the subject covered in this chapter, these findings are detailed. Four hundred seventy-four men with (243) or at high risk of (231) CAD who were undergoing elective noncardiac surgery were studied. Historical, clinical, laboratory, and physiologic data were collected during hospitalization and for 6 to 24 months after surgery. Myocardial ischemia was assessed by continuous ECG monitoring beginning two days before surgery and continuing for 2 days after.

Postoperative cardiac events in the hospital occurred in 83 patients (18%) and were classified as ischemic events (cardiac death, MI, or unstable angina), which occurred in 15 patients, CHF, which occurred in 30 patients, and ventricular tachycardia, which occurred in 38 patients. Postoperative myocardial ischemia occurred in 41% of patients monitored. Postop-

TABLE 33-5. Variables Associated With 83 Cardiac Outcomes Among 474 Patients Undergoing Noncardiac Surgery

Models	Odds Ratio	95% Confidence Interval	p-Value	N With Outcome and Variable/N With Variable
Univariable[a]				
Previous myocardial infarction	1.7	1.1–2.8	0.03	38/167
Definite coronary artery disease	1.9	1.2–3.1	0.01	54/248
History of arrhythmia	2.8	1.7–4.7	0.0001	37/123
History of congestive heart failure	2.9	1.6–5.0	0.0002	25/77
History of claudication	2.7	1.7–4.4	0.0001	42/150
Diabetes mellitus (treated with medication)	1.6	0.94–2.8	0.08	22/93
Preoperative use of nitrates	1.6	0.97–2.6	0.06	30/132
Preoperative use of digoxin for congestive heart failure	5.8	2.3–15	0.0001	10/19
Serum creatinine >0.023 μmol/L[b]	2.3	1.1–5.0	0.03	11/35
ASA score ≥3	2.5	1.3–5.0	0.007	72/354
Cardiac risk index (per 10 units)	1.8	1.2–2.7	0.002	
Vascular surgery	2.4	1.5–3.9	0.0003	44/168
Narcotic anesthesia	2.2	1.2–4.2	0.01	16/54
Preoperative Holter ischemia[c]	3.1	1.8–5.3	0.0001	28/84
Intraoperative Holter ischemia[d]	2.1	1.2–3.7	0.005	27/104
Postoperative Holter ischemia[e]	3.3	1.9–5.6	0.0001	46/167
Multivariable				
History of arrhythmia	2.2	1.3–3.9	0.006	—
Preoperative use of digoxin for congestive heart failure	3.3	1.1–1.1	0.04	—
Vascular surgery	1.8	1.1–3.2	0.03	—
Postoperative Holter ischemia	2.8	1.6–4.9	0.0002	—

[a] All variables are binary (yes or no) unless otherwise indicated. ASA denotes American Society of Anesthesiologists.
[b] Values in parentheses are 95% confidence intervals.
[c] Based on a denominator of 429 patients.
[d] Based on a denominator of 423 patients.
[e] Based on a denominator of 407 patients.
(From Mangano et al.,[218] with permission.)

TABLE 33-6. Variables Associated With 15 CAD Outcomes Among 474 Patients Undergoing Noncardiac Surgery

Models	Odds Ratio	95% Confidence Interval	p-Value	N With Outcome and Variable/N With Variable
Univariable[a]				
History of claudication	3.4	1.2–9.7	0.02	9/150
Activity level ≥ 5[b]	4.3	1.2–16	0.02	3/28
Preoperative use of nitrates	2.3	0.83–6.6	0.1	7/132
Serum creatinine ≥ 0.023 μmol/L[c]	5.0	1.5–17	0.004	4/35
Postoperative Holter ischemia[d]	9.2	2.0–42	0.004	12/167
Multivariable				
Postoperative Holter ischemia	9.2	2.0–42	0.004	—

Abbreviation: CAD, coronary disease.
[a] All variables are binary (yes/no) unless otherwise indicated.
[b] Severely limited (bed to chair) or medically restricted.
[c] Equivalent to 2 mg/dl.
[d] Based on denominator of n = 407 patients.
(From Mangano et al.,[218] with permission.)

erative myocardial ischemia was associated with a 2.8-fold increase in the odds of all adverse cardiac outcomes (95% confidence interval, 1.6 to 4.9; p <0.0002) and a 9.2-fold increase in the odds of an ischemic event (95% confidence interval, 2.0 to 42; p <0.004). Multivariate analysis disclosed no other clinical, historical, or perioperative variable to be independently associated with ischemic events, including cardiac risk index, history of previous MI or congestive heart failure, or the occurrence of ischemia before or during surgery (Tables 33-5 to 33-7).

These results demonstrate that postoperative myocardial ischemia during the first 48 hours after surgery confers a nearly threefold increase in the odds of having an adverse cardiac outcome and, more importantly, a ninefold increase in the odds of having an

ischemic event. These findings emphasize the importance of the postoperative period and extend the work of previous investigators who have demonstrated the importance of the patient's preoperative chronic disease state before surgery, as well as physiologic changes during the operation. They suggest that patients may warrant more intensive monitoring and intervention during the postoperative period.

Thus, these most recent data strongly suggest that increased attention and resources should be focused on the postoperative period. The ninefold increase in the risk of morbid ischemic events associated with the occurrence of myocardial ischemia after surgery suggests that prevention of (and possibly therapy for) postoperative ischemia may well hold the key to reducing perioperative cardiac morbidity.

TABLE 33-7. Results of Multivariable Analysis of Variables Associated With 30 CHF Outcomes Among 459 Patients Without CAD Outcomes, and 38 Ventricular Tachycardia Outcomes Among 430 Patients Without CAD or CHF Outcomes

Variables	Odds Ratio	95% Confidence Interval	p-Value
Associated with CHF[a]			
History of arrhythmia[b]	3.0	1.4–6.7	0.006
Diabetes mellitus (treated with medication)[b]	2.4	1.0 5.7	0.04
Duration of anesthesia and surgery (per hour)[c]	1.2	1.1–1.4	0.002
OR			
Vascular surgery[b]	3.5	1.6–7.9	0.002
Narcotic anesthesia[c]	2.5	1.0–6.5	0.05
OR			
Isoflurane/narcotic anesthesia[b]	0.35	0.16–0.76	0.008
Associated with ventricular tachycardia[a]			
Preoperative Holter ischemia	7.8	2.9–21	0.0001
Preoperative use of digoxin for congestive heart failure	12	2.8–50	0.0009

Abbreviation: CAD, coronary disease; CHF, congestive heart failure.
[a] All variables are binary (yes/no).
[b] Statistics for model containing history of arrhythmias, diabetes, vascular surgery, and isoflurane/narcotic anesthesia.
[c] Statistics for model containing history of arrhythmias, diabetes, duration of anesthesia and surgery, and narcotic anesthesia.
(From Mangano et al.,[218] with permission.)

ACKNOWLEDGMENTS

The author wishes to acknowledge and thank the investigators and staff of the Study of Perioperative Ischemia (S.P.I.) Research Group. This work was supported by grant R01-HL36744 from the National Institutes of Health.

REFERENCES

1. National Center for Health Statistics: Health, United States, 1988. p. 111. DHHS Publ. No. PHS 89–1232. Washington, D.C., US Public Health Service, 1989
2. Frye R, Higgins M, Beller G et al: Task Force III: major demographic and epidemiologic trends affecting adult cardiology. J Am Coll Cardiol 12:840, 1988
3. Weinstein M, Coxson P, Williams L et al: Forecasting coronary heart disease incidence, mortality, and cost: the coronary heart disease policy model. Am J Public Health 77:1417, 1987
4. Public Health Statistics: Current Population Reports. US Department of Commerce, Bureau of the Census, Washington, DC, 1988
5. National Center for Health Statistics: Vital Statistics of the United States, 1980. Vol II—Mortality. Part A. DHHS Publ. No. PHS 85–1101. US Public Health Service, Hyattsville, MD, 1985
6. Tarhan S, Moffitt E, Taylor W, Giuliani E: Myocardial infarction after general anesthesia. JAMA 220:1451, 1972
7. Roberts S, Tinker J: Cardiovascular disease. p. 33. *In* Brown D (ed): Risk and Outcome in Anesthesia. JB Lippincott, Philadelphia, 1988
8. Plumlee J, Boettner R: Myocardial infarction during and following anesthesia and operation. South Med J 65:886, 1972
9. Foster E, Davis K, Carpenter J et al: Risk of noncardiac operation in patients with defined coronary disease: the Coronary Artery Surgery Study (CASS) Registry Experience. Ann Thorac Surg 41:42, 1986
10. Goldman L, Caldera D, Nussbaum S et al: Multifactorial index of cardiac risk in noncardiac surgical procedures. N Engl J Med 297:845, 1977
11. Knapp R, Topkins M, Artusio JJ: The cerebrovascular accident and coronary occlusion in anesthesia. JAMA 182:332, 1962
12. Topkins M, Artusio J: Myocardial infarction and surgery: a five-year study. Anesth Analg 43:716, 1964
13. von Knorring J: Postoperative myocardial infarction: a prospective study in a risk group of surgical patients. Surgery 90:55, 1981
14. Rao T, Jacobs K, El-Etr A: Reinfarction following anesthesia in patients with myocardial infarction. Anesthesiology 59:499, 1983
15. Steen P, Tinker J, Tarhan S: Myocardial reinfarction after anesthesia and surgery. JAMA 239:2566, 1978
16. Hertzer N, Beven E, Young J et al: Coronary-artery disease in peripheral vascular patients. A classification of 1000 coronary angiograms and results of surgical management. Ann Surg 199:223, 1984
17. Driscoll A, Hobika J, Etsten B, Proger S: Clinically unrecognized myocardial infarction following surgery. N Engl J Med 264:633, 1961
18. Jeffrey C, Kunsman J, Cullen D, Brewster D: A prospective evaluation of cardiac risk index. Anesthesiology 58:462, 1983
19. Boucher C, Brewster D, Darling R et al: Determination of cardiac risk by dipyridamole-thallium imaging before peripheral vascular surgery. N Engl J Med 312:389, 1985
20. Hertzer N: Myocardial ischemia. Surgery 93:97, 1983
21. Crawford E, Bomberger R, Glaeser D et al: Aortoiliac occlusive disease: factors influencing survival and function following reconstructive operation over a twenty-five year period. Surgery 90:1055, 1981
22. Brown O, Hollier L, Pairolero P et al: Abdominal aortic aneurysm and coronary-artery disease. Arch Surg 116:1484, 1981
23. Rokey R, Rolak L, Harati Y et al: Coronary artery disease in patients with cerebrovascular disease: a prospective study. Ann Neurol 16:50, 1984
24. Tomatis L, Fierens E, Verbrugge G: Evaluation of surgical risk in peripheral vascular disease by coronary arteriography: a series of 100 cases. Surgery 71:429, 1972
25. Young A, Sandberg G, Couch N: The reduction of mortality of abdominal aortic aneurysm resection. Am J Surg 134:585, 1977
26. Hertzer N: Fatal myocardial infarction following lower extremity revascularization. Two hundred seventy-three patients followed six to eleven postoperative years. Ann Surg 193:492, 1981
27. Hertzer N: Fatal myocardial infarction following peripheral vascular operations. A study of 951 patients followed 6 to 11 years postoperatively. Cleve Clin Q 49:1, 1981
28. Jamieson W, Janusz M, Miyagishima R, Gerein A: Influence of ischemic heart disease on early and late mortality after surgery for peripheral occlusive vascular disease. Circulation, suppl I. 66:I–92
29. Schoeppel L, Wilkinson C, Waters J, Meyers N: Effects of myocardial infarction on perioperative cardiac complications. Anesth Analg 62:493, 1983
30. London M, Mangano D: Assessment of perioperative risk. p. 53. *In* Stoelting R, Barash P, Gallagher T (eds): Advances in Anesthesia. Year Book Medical Publishers, Chicago, 1988
31. Arkins R, Smessaert A, Hicks R: Mortality and morbidity in surgical patients with coronary-artery disease. JAMA 190:485, 1964
32. Mauney MJ, Ebert P, Sabiston DJ: Postoperative myocardial infarction: a study of predisposing factors, diagnosis and mortality in a high risk group of surgical patients. Ann Surg 172:497, 1970
33. von Knorring J, Lepäntalo M: Prediction of perioperative cardiac complications by electro-cardiographic monitoring during treadmill exercise testing before peripheral vascular surgery. Surgery 99:610, 1986
34. Wasserman F, Bellet S, Saichek R: Postoperative myocardial infarction: report of twenty-five cases. N Engl J Med 252:967, 1955

35. Chamberlain D, Seal-Edmonds J: Effects of surgery under general ansæthesia on the electrocardiogram in ischemic heart disease and hypertension. Br Med J 2: 784, 1964
36. Rosen M, Mushin W, Kilpatrick G et al: Study of myocardial ischa#ia in surgical patients. Br Med J 2:1415, 1966
37. Conti C, Mehta J: Acute myocardial ischemia: role of atherosclerosis, thrombosis, platelet activation, coronary vasospasm, and altered arachidonic acid metabolism. Circulation, suppl V. 75:V–84.
38. Willerson J, Hillis L, Winniford M, Buja L: Speculation regarding mechanisms responsible for acute ischemia heart disease syndromes. (Editorial.) J Am Coll Cardiol 8:245, 1986
39. Gorlin R, Fuster V, Ambrose J: Anatomic-physiologic links between acute coronary syndromes. (Editorial.) Circulation 74:6, 1986
40. Tomoike H, Egashira K, Yamamoto Y, Nakamura M: Enhanced responsiveness of smooth muscle, impaired endothelium-dependent relaxation and the genesis of coronary spasm. Am J Cardiol 63:33E, 1989
41. Yasue H, Ogawa H, Okumura K: Coronary artery spasm in the genesis of myocardial ischemia. Am J Cardiol 63: 29E, 1989
42. Falk E: Morphologic features of unstable atherothrombotic plaques underlying acute coronary syndromes. Am J Cardiol 63:114E, 1989
43. Werns S, Shea M, Lucchesi B: Free radicals and myocardial injury: pharmacologic implications. Circulation 74:1, 1986
44. Bush L, Campbell W, Buja L et al: Effects of the selective thromboxane synthetase inhibitor dazoxiben on variations in cyclic blood flow in stenosed canine coronary arteries. Circulation 69:1161, 1984
45. Bush L, Campbell W, Kern K et al: The effects of a 2-adrenergic and serotonergic receptor antagonists on cyclic blood flow alterations in stenosed canine coronary arteries. Circ Res 55:642, 1984
46. Willerson J, Campbell W, Winniford M et al: Conversion from chronic to acute coronary artery disease: speculation regarding mechanisms [editorial]. Am J Cardiol 54: 1349, 1984
47. Uchida Y, Yoshimoto N, Murao S: Cyclic fluctuations in coronary blood pressure and flow induced by coronary artery constriction. Jpn Heart J 16:454, 1975
48. Mansfield A: Alteration in fibrinolysis associated with surgery and venous thrombosis. Br J Surg 59:754, 1972
49. Britton B, Hawkey C, Wood W, Peele M: Stress—a significant factor in venous thrombosis? Br J Surg 61:814, 1974
50. Grabfield G: Factors affecting the coagulation time of blood. IX. The effect of adrenaline on the factors of coagulation. Am J Physiol 42:46, 1916
51. Hoffman B, Michel T, Brenneman T, Lefkowitz R: Interactions of agonists with platelet α-adrenergic receptors. Endocrinology 110:926, 1982
52. Zilla P, Fasol R, Groscurth P et al: Blood platelets in cardiopulmonary bypass operations. J Thorac Cardiovasc Surg 97:397, 1989
53. Folts J, Crowell E, Rowe L: Platelet aggregation in partially obstructed vessels and its elimination with aspirin. Circulation 54:365, 1976
54. Cowley M, DiSciascio G, Rehr R, Vetrovec G: Angiographic observations and clinical relevance of coronary thrombus in unstable angina pectoris. Am J Cardiol 63: 108E, 1989
55. Mangano D, Wong M, London M et al: Perioperative myocardial ischemia in patients undergoing noncardiac surgery. II. Incidence and severity during the first week following surgery. J Am Coll Cardiol 17:851, 1991
56. Mangano D: Biventricular function after myocardial revascularization in humans: deterioration and recovery patterns during the first 24 hours. Anesthesiology 62: 571, 1985
57. Mangano D: The effect of the pericardium on ventricular systolic function in man. Circulation 61:352, 1980
58. Atlee JI: Perioperative cardiac dysrhythmias. p. 3. *In* Atlee JI (ed): Cardiac Dysrhythmias and Anesthesia: Mechanisms, Recognition, Management. Year Book Medical Publishers, Chicago, 1985
59. Kuner J, Enescu V, Utsu F et al: Cardiac arrhythmias during anesthesia. Dis Chest 52:580, 1967
60. Bertrand C, Steiner N, Jameson A, Lopez M: Disturbances of cardiac rhythm during anesthesia and surgery. JAMA 216:1615, 1971
61. Vanik P, Davis H: Cardiac arrhythmias during halothane anesthesia. Anesth Analg 47:299, 1968
62. Harrison D: Cost containment in medicine: why cardiology? Am J Cardiol 56:10C, 1985
63. Dack S: Symposium on cardiovascular-pulmonary problems before and after surgery. postoperative problems. Am J Cardiol 12:423, 1963
64. Sapala J, Ponka J, Duvernoy W: Operative and nonoperative risks in the cardiac patient. J Am Geriatr Soc 23: 529, 1975
65. Carliner N, Fisher M, Plotnick G et al: Routine preoperative exercise testing in patients undergoing major noncardiac surgery. Am J Cardiol 56:51, 1985
66. Gerson M, Hurst J, Hertzberg V et al: Cardiac prognosis in noncardiac geriatric surgery. Ann Intern Med 103: 832, 1985
67. Gage A, Bhayana J, Balu V, Hook N: Assessment of cardiac risk in surgical patients. Arch Surg 112:1488, 1977
68. Cutler B, Wheeler H, Paraskos J, Cardullo P: Assessment of operative risk with electrocardiographic exercise testing in patients with peripheral vascular disease. Am J Surg 137:484, 1979
69. Cutler B, Wheeler H, Paraskos J, Cardullo P: Applicability and interpretation of electrocardiographic stress testing in patients with peripheral vascular disease. Am J Surg 141:501, 1981
70. Pasternack P, Imparato A, Bear G et al: The value of radionuclide angiography as a predictor of perioperative myocardial infarction in patients undergoing abdominal aortic aneurysm resection. J Vasc Surg 1:320, 1984
71. Pasternack P, Imparato A, Riles T et al: The value of the radionuclide angiogram in the prediction of perioperative myocardial infarction in patients undergoing lower extremity revascularization procedures. Circulation, Suppl II. 72:II–13, 1985

72. Cutler B, Leppo J: Dipyridamole thallium 201 scintigraphy to detect coronary artery disease before abdominal aortic surgery. J Vasc Surg 5:91, 1987

73. Leppo J, Plaja J, Gionet M et al: Noninvasive evaluation of cardiac risk before elective vascular surgery. J Am Coll Cardiol 9:269, 1987

74. Eagle K, Singer D, Brewster D et al: Dipyridamole-thallium scanning in patients undergoing vascular surgery. JAMA 257:2185, 1987

75. Brewster D, Okada R, Strauss H et al: Selection of patients for preoperative coronary angiography: use of dipyridamole-stress-thallium myocardial imaging. J Vasc Surg 2:504, 1985

76. Knight A, Hollenberg M, London M et al: Perioperative myocardial ischemia: importance of the preoperative ischemic pattern. Anesthesiology 68:681, 1988

77. London M, Hollenberg M, Wong M et al: Intraoperative myocardial ischemia: localization by continuous 12-lead electrocardiography. Anesthesiology 69:232, 1988

78. Smith J, Cahalan M, Benefiel D et al: Intraoperative detection of myocardial ischemia in high-risk patients: electrocardiography versus two-dimensional transesophageal echocardiography. Circulation 72:1015, 1985

79. Fegert G, Hollenberg M, Browner W et al: Perioperative myocardial ischemia in the noncardiac surgical patient, abstracted. Anesthesiology 69:A49, 1988

80. Leung J, O'Kelly B, Browner W et al: Prognostic importance of postbypass regional wall-motion abnormalities in patients undergoing coronary artery bypass graft surgery. Anesthesiology 71:16, 1989

81. London M, Tubau J, Wong M et al: The "natural history" of segmental wall motion abnormalities detected by intraoperative transesophageal echocardiography: a clinically blinded prospective approach, abstracted. Anesthesiology 69:A7, 1988

82. Slogoff S, Keats A: Does perioperative myocardial ischemia lead to postoperative myocardial infarction? Anesthesiology 62:107, 1985

83. Wong M, Wellington Y, London M et al: Prolonged postoperative myocardial ischemia in high-risk patients undergoing non-cardiac surgery, abstracted. Anesthesiology 69:A56, 1988

84. Anderson JM: National Institute on Aging Macroeconomic-Demographic Model. US DHHS Publ No. 84–2492. National Institute on Aging, Washington, DC, 1984

85. Port S, Cobb F, Coleman R, Jones R: Effect of age on the response of the left ventricular function to exercise. N Engl J Med 303:1133, 1980

86. Fleg H, Gerstenblidth G, Lakatta E: Pathophysiology of the aging in heart circulation. p. 11. In Messerli F (ed): Cardiovascular Disease in the Elderly. Martinus Nijhoff, Boston, 1984

87. Weisfeldt M: Aging of the cardiovascular system. (Editorial.) N Engl J Med 303:1172, 1980

88. Bertrand Y, Boelens D, Collin L et al: Preoperative assessment in geriatric patients for elective surgery. Acta Anaesthesiol Belg, suppl. 35:155, 1984

89. Drucker W, Gavett J, Kirshner R et al: Toward strategies for cost containment in surgical patients. Ann Surg 198:284, 1983

90. Harbrecht P, Garrison R, Fry D: The impact of demographic trends on hospital surgical care. Am J Surg 50:270, 1984

91. Cullen D, Ferrara L, Briggs B et al: Survival, hospitalization charges and follow-up results in critically ill patients. N Engl J Med 294:982, 1976

92. Roberts A, Woodhall D, Conti C et al: Mortality, morbidity, and cost-accounting related to coronary artery bypass graft surgery in the elderly. Ann Thorac Surg 39:426, 1985

93. Djokovic J, Hedley-Whyte J: Prediction of outcome of surgery and anesthesia in patients over 80. JAMA 242:2301, 1979

94. Greenberg A, Saik R, Pridham D: Influence of age on mortality of colon surgery. Am J Surg 150:65, 1985

95. Mohr D: Estimation of surgical risk in the elderly: a correlative review. J Am Geriatr Soc 31:99, 1983

96. Goldman L: Cardiac risks and complications of non-cardiac surgery. Ann Intern Med 98:504, 1983

97. Wells P, Kaplan J: Optimal management of patients with ischemic heart disease for noncardiac surgery by complementary anesthesiologist and cardiologist interaction. Am Heart J 102:1029, 1981

98. Lowenstein E, Yusuf S, Teplick R: Perioperative myocardial reinfarction: a glimmer of hope—a note of caution. (Editorial.) Anesthesiology 59:493, 1983

99. Larsen S, Olesen K, Jacobsen E et al: Prediction of cardiac risk in non-cardiac surgery. Eur Heart J 8:179, 1987

100. Deanfield J, Maseri A, Selwyn A et al: Myocardial ischmæia during daily life in patients with stable angina: its relation to symptoms and heart rate changes. Lancet 2:753, 1983

101. Cohn P: Silent myocardial ischemia: dimensions of the problem in patients with and without angina. Am J Med, suppl 4C. 80:1, 1986

102. Epstein S, Quyyumi A, Bonow R: Myocardial ischemia—silent or symptomatic. N Engl J Med 318:1038, 1988

103. Gottlieb S, Weisfeldt M, Ouyang P et al: Silent ischemia as a marker for early unfavorable outcomes in patients with unstable angina. N Engl J Med 314:1214, 1986

104. National Hospital Discharge Survey: United States, 1985. DHHS Publ No. (PHS) 87-Advance data no. 137, July 2, 1987). National Center for Health Statistics, Hyattsville, MD, 1987

105. Cooperman M, Pflug B, Martin EJ, Evans W: Cardiovascular risk factors in patients with peripheral vascular disease. Surgery 84:505, 1978

106. Moraski R, Russell RJ, Smith M, Rackley C: Left ventricular function in patients with and without myocardial infarction and one, two, or three vessel coronary artery disease. Am J Cardiol 35:1, 1975

107. Prys-Roberts C, Meloche R, Foëx P: Studies of anæthesia in relation to hypertension: I. Cardiovascular responses to treated and untreated patients. Br J Anæth 43:122, 1971

108. Schneider A: Assessment of risk factors and surgical outcome. Surg Clin North Am 63:1113, 1983

109. Smithwick R, Thompson J: Splanchnicectomy for essential hypertension. JAMA 152:1501, 1953

110. Prys-Roberts C: Hypertension and anesthesia—fifty years on. (Editorial.) Anesthesiology 50:281, 1979

111. Sprague H: The heart in surgery. An analysis of results of surgery on cardiac patients during the past ten years at the Massachusetts General Hospital. Surg Gynecol Obstet 49:54, 1929

112. Asiddao C, Donegan J, Whitesell R, Kalbfleisch J: Factors associated with perioperative complications during carotid endarterectomy. Anesth Analg 61:631, 1982

113. Bruce D, Croley T, Lee J: Preoperative clonidine withdrawal syndrome. Anesthesiology 51:90, 1979

114. Foëx P: Beta-blockade in ansæthesia. J Clin Hosp Pharm 8:183, 1983

115. Kaplan J, Dunbar R, Bland JJ et al: Propranolol and cardiac surgery: a problem for the anesthesiologist. Anesth Analg 54:571, 1975

116. Miller R, Olson H, Amsterdam E, Mason D: Propranolol-withdrawal rebound phenomenon. Exacerbation of coronary events after abrupt cessation of anti-anginal therapy. N Engl J Med 293:416, 1975

117. Engelman R, Hadji-Rousou I, Breyer R et al: Rebound vasospasm after coronary revascularization in association with calcium antagonist withdrawal. Ann Thorac Surg 37:469, 1984

118. Goldman L, Caldera D: Risks of general anesthesia and elective operation in the hypertensive patient. Anesthesiology 50:285, 1979

119. Riles T, Kopelman I, Imparato A: Myocardial infarction following carotid endarterectomy: a review of 683 operations. Surgery 85:249, 1979

120. Burgos L, Ebert T, Asiddao C et al: Increased intraoperative cardiovascular morbidity in diabetics with autonomic neuropathy. Anesthesiology 70:591, 1989

121. Venkataraman K, Madias J, Hood W: Indications for prophylactic preoperative insertion of pacemakers in patients with right bundle branch block and left anterior hemi-block. Chest 68:501, 1975

122. Rooney S, Goldiner P, Muss E: Relationship of right bundle-branch block and marked left axis deviation to complete heart block during general anesthesia. Anesthesiology 44:64, 1976

123. Skinner J, Pearce M: Surgical risk in the cardiac patient. J Chronic Dis 17:57, 1964

124. Reul GJ, Cooley D, Duncan J et al: The effect of coronary bypass on the outcome of peripheral vascular operations in 1,093 patients. J Vasc Surg 3:788, 1986

125. Mahar L, Steen P, Tinker J et al: Perioperative myocardial infarction in patients with coronary artery disease with and without aorta-coronary bypass grafts. J Thorac Cardiovasc Surg 76:533, 1978

126. Diehl J, Cali R, Hertzer N, Beven E: Complications of abdominal aortic reconstruction. An analysis of perioperative risk factors in 557 patients. Ann Surg 197:49, 1983

127. Read R, Murphy M, Hultgren H, Takaro T: Survival of men treated for chronic stable angina pectoris. A cooperative randomized study. J Thorac Cardiovasc Surg 75:1, 1978

128. Scher K, Tice D: Operative risk in patients with previous coronary artery bypass. Arch Surg 111:807, 1976

129. McCollum C, Garcia-Rinaldi R, Graham J, Debakey M: Myocardial revascularization prior to subsequent major surgery in patients with coronary artery disease. Surgery 81:302, 1977

130. Crawford E, Morris G, Howell J et al: Operative risk in patients with previous coronary artery bypass. Ann Thorac Surg 26:215, 1978

131. Kimbris D, Segal B: Coronary disease progression in patients with and without saphenous vein bypass surgery. Am Heart J 102:811, 1981

132. Slogoff S, Keats A, Ott E: Preoperative propranolol therapy and aortocoronary bypass operation. JAMA 240:1487, 1978

133. Magnusson J, Thulin T, Werner O et al: Hmæodynamic effects of pretreatment with metoprolol in hypertensive patients undergoing surgery. Br J Ansæth 58:251, 1986

134. Cucchiara R, Benefiel D, Matteo R et al: Evaluation of esmolol in controlling increases in heart rate and blood pressure during endotracheal intubation in patients undergoing carotid endarterectomy. Anesthesiology 65:528, 1986

135. Slogoff S, Keats A: Does chronic treatment with calcium entry blocking drugs reduce perioperative myocardial ischemia? Anesthesiology 68:676, 1988

136. Chung F, Houston P, Cheng D et al: Calcium channel blockade does not offer adequate protection from perioperative myocardial ischemia. Anesthesiology 69:343, 1988

137. Flacke J, Bloor B, Flacke W et al: Reduced narcotic requirement by clonidine with improved hemodynamic and adrenergic stability in patients undergoing coronary bypass surgery. Anesthesiology 67:11, 1987

138. Ghignone M, Calvillo, KL Q: Anesthesia and hypertension: the effect of clonidine on perioperative hemodynamics and isoflurane requirements. Anesthesiology 67:3, 1987

139. Longnecker D: Alpine anesthesia: can pretreatment with clonidine decrease the peaks and valleys? (Editorial.) Anesthesiology 67:1, 1987

140. American Society of Anesthesiologists: New classification of physical status. Anesthesiology 24:111, 1963

141. Braunwald E, The history, p. 1. In Braunwald E (ed): Heart Disease: A Textbook of Cardiovascular Medicine. WB Saunders, Philadelphia, 1984

142. Lewin I, Lerner A, Green S et al: Physical class and physiological status in the prediction of operative mortality in the aged sick. Ann Surg 174:217, 1971

143. Rabkin S, Horne J: Preoperative electrocardiography: its cost-effectiveness in detecting abnormalities when a previous tracing exists. Can Med Assoc J 121:301, 1979

144. Baers S, Nakhjavan F, Kajani M: Postoperative myocardial infarction. Surg Gynecol Obstet 120:315, 1965

145. Hunter P, Endrey-Waler P, Bauer G, Stephen F: Myocardial infarction following surgical operations. Br Med J 4:725, 1968

146. Carliner N, Fisher M, Plotnick G et al: The preoperative electrocardiogram as an indicator of risk in major noncardiac surgery. Can J Cardiol 2:134, 1986

147. Goldberger A, O'Konski M: Utility of routine electrocardiogram before surgery and on general hospital admission: critical review and guidelines. Ann Intern Med 105:552, 1986

148. Goldman L, Caldera D, Southwick F et al: Cardiac risk factors and complications in noncardiac surgery. Medicine (Baltimore) 57:357, 1978

149. Mangano D: Preoperative assessment. p. 341. In Kaplan J (ed): Cardiac Anesthesia. Grune & Stratton, Orlando, FL, 1987

150. Cohn P, Lawson W: Characteristics of silent myocardial ischemia during out-of-hospital activities in asymptomatic angiographically documented coronary-artery disease. Am J Cardiol 59:746, 1987

151. Coy K, Imperi G, Lambert C, Pepine C: Silent myocardial ischemia during daily activities in asymptomatic men with positive exercise test responses. Am J Cardiol 59:45, 1987

152. Rocco M, Barry J, Campbell S et al: Circadian variation of transient myocardial ischemia in patients with coronary artery disease. Circulation 75:395, 1987

153. Shea M, Deanfield J, Wilson R et al: Transient ischemia in angina pectoris: frequent silent events with everyday activities. Am J Cardiol 56:34E, 1985

154. Cecchi A, Dovellini E, Marchi F et al: Silent myocardial ischemia during ambulatory electrocardiographic monitoring in patients with effort angina. J Am Coll Cardiol 11:934, 1983

155. Chierchia S, Lazzari M, Freedman B et al: Impairment of myocardial perfusion and function during painless myocardial ischemia. J Am Coll Cardiol 1:924, 1983

156. Campbell S, Barry J, Rebecca G et al: Active transient myocardial ischemia during daily life in asymptomatic patients with positive exercise tests and coronary-artery disease. Am J Cardiol 57:1010, 1986

157. Knight A, Hollenberg M, London M et al: Myocardial ischemia in patients awaiting coronary artery bypass grafting. Am Heart J 117:1189, 1989

158. Raby K, Goldman L, Ma C et al: Correlation between preoperative ischemia and major cardiac events after peripheral vascular surgery. N Engl J Med 321:1296, 1989

159. Raby K, Goldman L, Cook E et al: Long-term prognosis of myocardial ischemia detected by Holter monitoring in peripheral vascular disease. Am J Cardiol 66:1309, 1990

160. Nishimura R, Reeder G, Miller FJ et al: Prognostic value of predischarge 2-dimensional echocardiogram after acute myocardial infarction. Am J Cardiol 53:429, 1984

161. Erbel R, Borner N, Steller D et al: Detection of aortic dissection by transesophageal echocardiography. Br Heart J 58:45, 1987

162. Koenig K, Kasper W, Hofmann T et al: Transesophageal echocardiography for diagnosis of rupture of the ventricular septum or left ventricular papillary muscle during acute myocardial infarction. Am J Cardiol 59:362, 1987

163. Erbel R, Rohmann S, Drexler M et al: Improved diagnostic value of echocardiography in patients with infective endocarditis by transesophageal approach: a prospective study. Eur Heart J 9:43, 1988

164. Gussenhoven E, Taams M, Roelandt J et al: Transesophageal two-dimensional echocardiography: its role in solving clinical problems. J Am Coll Cardiol 8:975, 1986

165. Seward J, Khandheria B, Oh J et al: Transesophageal echocardiography: technique, anatomic correlations, implementation, and clinical applications. Mayo Clin Proc 63:649, 1988

166. Eagle K, Coley C, Newell J et al: Combining clinical and thallium data optimizes preoperative assessment of cardiac risk before major vascular surgery. Ann Intern Med 110:859, 1989

167. Levinson J, Boucher C, Coley C et al: Usefulness of semi-quantitative analysis of dipyridamole thallium-201 redistribution for improving risk stratification before vascular surgery. Am J Cardiol 66:406, 1990

168. Mangano D, London M, Tubau J et al: Dipyridamole thallium-201 scintigraphy as a preoperative screening test. A reexamination of its predictive potential. Circulation 84:493, 1991

169. Hertzer N: Clinical experience with preoperative coronary angiography. J Vasc Surg 2:510, 1985

170. Backer C, Tinker J, Robertson D, Vlietstra R: Myocardial reinfarction following local anesthesia for ophthalmic surgery. Anesth Analg 59:257, 1980

171. Prough D, Scuderi P, Stullken E, Davis CJ: Myocardial infarction following regional anesthesia for carotid endarterectomy. Can Ansæth Soc J 31:192, 1984

172. McAuley C, Watson C: Elective inguinal herniorraphy after myocardial infarction. Surg Gynecol Obstet 159:36, 1984

173. Erlik D, Valero A, Birkhan J, Gersh I: Prostatic surgery and the cardiovascular patient. Br J Urol 40:53, 1968

174. McGowen S, Smith G: Anesthesia for transurethral prostatectomy: a comparison of spinal intradural analgesia with two methods of general ansæthesia. Ansæthesia 35:847, 1980

175. Yeager M, Glass D, Neff R, Brinck-Johnsen T: Epidural anesthesia and analgesia in high-risk surgical patients. Anesthesiology 66:729, 1987

176. Thompson J, Hollier L, Patman R, Persson A: Surgical management of abdominal aortic aneurysms: factors influencing mortality and morbidity—a 20-year experience. Ann Surg 181:654, 1975

177. Hicks G, Eastland M, DeWeese J et al: Survival improvement following aortic aneurysm resection. Ann Surg 181:863, 1975

178. Roizen M, Sohn Y, Stoney R: Intraoperative management of the patient requiring supraceliac aortic occlusion. p. 312. *In* Wilson S, Veith F, Hobson RJ, Williams R (eds): Vascular Surgery: Principles and Practice. McGraw-Hill Book Co, New York, 1987

179. Cogbill C: Operation in the aged. Arch Surg 94:2202, 1967

180. Vacanti C, VanHouten R, Hill R: A statistical analysis of the relationship of physical status to postoperative mortality in 68,388 cases. Anesth Analg 49:565, 1970

181. Wroblewski F, La Due J: Myocardial infarction adds a postoperative complication of major surgery. JAMA 150:1212, 1952

182. Eerola M Eerola, R, Kaukinen, S, Kaukinen L: Risk factors in surgical patients with verified preoperative myocardial infarction. Acta Ansæthesiol Scand 24:219, 1980

183. Nachlas M, Abrams S, Goldberg M: The influence of arteriosclerotic heart disease on surgical risk. Am J Surg 101:447, 1961

184. Slogoff S, Keats A: Further observations on perioperative myocardial ischemia. Anesthesiology 65:539, 1986

185. Tennant R, Wiggers C: The effect of coronary occlusion on myocardial contraction. Am J Physiol 112:351, 1935

186. Hauser A, Gangadharan V, Ramos R et al: Sequence of mechanical, electrocardiographic and clinical effects of repeated coronary artery occlusion in human beings: echocardiographic observations during coronary angioplasty. J Am Coll Cardiol 5:193, 1985

187. Wohlgelernter D, Cleman M, Highman H et al: Regional myocardial dysfunction during coronary angioplasty: evaluation by two-dimensional echocardiography and 12 lead electrocardiography. J Am Coll Cardiol 7:1245, 1986

188. Topol E, Weiss J, Guzman P et al: Immediate improvement of dysfunctional myocardial segments after coronary revascularization: detection by intraoperative transesophageal echocardiography. J Am Coll Cardiol 4:1123, 1984

189. Malmborg R: A clinical hemodynamic analysis of factors limiting the cardiac performance in patients with coronary heart disease. Acta Med Scand, suppl 426. 177: 1, 1965

190. Martin C, McConahay D: Maximal treadmill exercise electrocardiography. Correlations with coronary arteriography and cardiac hemodynamics. Circulation 46: 956, 1972

191. Moir T, DeBra D: Effect of left ventricular hypertension, ischemia and vasoactive drugs on the myocardial distribution of coronary flow. Circ Res 21:65, 1967

192. Benchimol A, Maroko P, Pedraza A et al: Left ventricular end diastolic pressure and cardiac output at rest and during exercise in patients with angina pectoris. Cardiology 53:261, 1968

193. Parker J, Chiong M, West R, Case R: Sequential alterations in myocardial lactate metabolism, ST-segments and left ventricular function during angina induced by atrial pacing. Circulation 40:113, 1969

194. Rahimtoola S, Loeb H, Ehsani et al: Relationship of pulmonary artery to left ventricular diastolic pressures in acute myocardial infarction. Circulation 46:283, 1972

195. Häggmark S, Hohner P, Ostman M et al: Comparison of hemodynamic, electrocardiographic, mechanical and metabolic indicators of intraoperative myocardial ischemia in vascular surgical patients with coronary artery disease. Anesthesiology 70:19, 1989

196. Lieberman R, Orkin F, Jobes D, Schwartz A: Hemodynamic predictors of myocardial ischemia during halothane anesthesia for coronary-artery revascularization. Anesthesiology 59:36, 1983

197. Leung J, O'Kelly J, Browner W et al: Are regional wall motion abnormalities detected by transesophageal echocardiography triggered by acute changes in supply and demand?, abstracted. Anesthesiology 69:A801, 1988

198. Roizen M, Beaupre P, Alpert R et al: Monitoring with two-dimensional transesophageal echocardiography: comparison of myocardial function in patients undergoing supraceliac, suprarenal-infraceliac, or infrarenal aortic occlusion. J Vasc Surg 1:300, 1984

199. Bellows W, Bode RJ, Levy J et al: Noninvasive detection of periinduction ischemic ventricular dysfunction by cardiokymography in humans: preliminary experience. Anesthesiology 60:155, 1984

200. Silverberg R, Diamond G, Vas R et al: Noninvasive diagnosis of coronary artery disease: the cardiokymographic stress test. Circulation 61:579, 1980

201. Weiner D, Investigators P: Accuracy of cardiokymography during exercise testing: results of a multicenter study. J Am Coll Cardiol 6:502, 1985

202. Dunn R, Griggs DJ: Ventricular filling pressure as a determinant of coronary blood flow during ischemia. Am J Physiol 244:H429, 1983

203. Hillis L, Izquierdo C, Davis C et al: Effect of various degrees of systemic arterial hypertension on acute canine myocardial ischemia. Am J Physiol 240:H855, 1981

204. Whittemore A, Clowes A, Hechtman H, Mannick J: Aortic aneurysm repair: reduced operative mortality associated with maintenance of optimal cardiac performance. Ann Surg 192:414, 1980

205. Crawford E, Walker H, Saleh S, Normann N: Graft replacement in descending thoracic aorta: results without bypass of shunting. Surgery 89:73, 1981

206. Roy W, Edelist G, Gilbert B: Myocardial ischemia during non-cardiac surgical procedures in patients with coronary-artery disease. Anesthesiology 51:393, 1979

207. Reiz S, Balfor E, Sorensen V et al: Isoflurane—a powerful coronary vasodilator in patients with coronary artery disease. Anesthesiology 59:91, 1983

208. Coriat P, Harari A, Daloz M, Viars P: Clinical predictors of intraoperative myocardial ischemia in patients with coronary artery disease undergoing non-cardiac surgery. Acta Anæsthesiol Scand 26:287, 1982

209. Stone J, Foëx P, Sear J et al: Myocardial ischemia in untreated hypertensive patients: effect of a single small oral dose of a beta-adrenergic blocking agent. Anesthesiology 68:495, 1988

210. Prys-Roberts C, Meloche R, Foëx P: Studies of anæsthesia in relation to hypertension. I. Cardiovascular responses to treated and untreated patients. Br J Anæsth 43:122, 1971

211. Foëx P: Beta-blockade in anæsthesia. J Clin Hosp Pharm 8:183, 1983

212. Zeldin R: Assessing cardiac risk in patients who undergo noncardiac surgical procedures. Can J Surg 27: 402, 1984

213. Detsky A, Abrams H, Forbath N et al: Cardiac assessment for patients undergoing noncardiac surgery: a multifactorial clinical risk index. Arch Intern Med 146: 2131, 1986

214. London M, Tubau J, Harris D et al: Dipyridamole thallium imaging predicts intraoperative ischemia in patients undergoing major vascular surgery. J Am Coll Cardiol 11:162A, 1988

215. Frazer JG, Ramachandran MB, Davis HS: Anesthesia and recent myocardial infarction. JAMA 199:96, 1967

216. Mangano D, Browner W, Hollenberg M et al, SPI Research Group: Association of perioperative myocardial ischemia with cardiac morbidity and mortality in men undergoing noncardiac surgery. N Engl J Med 323:1781, 1990

217. Mangano DT: Perioperative cardiac morbidity. Anesthesia 72:153, 1990

218. Mangano DT, Browner WS, Hollenberg M et al: Association of perioperative myocardial ischemia with cardiac morbidity in men undergoing noncardiac surgery. New Engl J Med 323:178, 1990

Section VII

PROGNOSIS AS RELATED TO CARDIAC SURGERY

34

Risk Assessment and Prognosis Related to Coronary Artery Bypass Grafting

Lucien Campeau

This chapter discusses risk assessment with respect to the operative mortality and morbidity, and the prognosis concerning clinical outcome, quality of life, and survival following coronary artery bypass graft (CABG) surgery. The results of this operation have changed over time since its introduction some 25 years ago, influenced by patient selection, and improved surgical technology, anesthesiology, and postoperative care.

The first coronary artery bypass operation in a human being using a saphenous vein graft (SVG) was performed in November 1964 by Garrett, Dennis, and DeBakey, but it was reported only in 1973.[1] Favaloro, who performed his first CABG case in May 1967, reported his experience of 15 cases in 1968 and received most of the credit for this new procedure. Subsequently, Johnson and Lepley also began to employ this technique and championed the use of multiple bypasses. Although Spencer and associates in 1964 performed 16 end-to-side anastomoses between the left internal mammary artery (IMA) and the circumflex artery (CX) in dogs, it was Kolessov from Leningrad who in 1966 did the first IMA anastomosis to the left anterior descending coronary artery (LAD) in humans. Green and Spencer performed the first IMA anastomo-sis in a human being in the United States in 1968.[1] IMA grafts were shown during the early 1980s to remain patent much longer than SVG and became the conduit of choice, used alone or in combination with saphenous veins.[2]

Most information regarding risk assessment and prognosis concerns surgery using an inverted autogenous saphenous vein as the bypass conduit. Nonetheless, more recent studies have shown a definite superiority of IMA grafts concerning their long-term patency, their lack of atherosclerotic degeneration, hence their much better postoperative clinical course and survival.

RISK ASSESSMENT

Perioperative Mortality (First 30 days)

Perioperative mortality rates have changed constantly since this surgery was introduced in 1967[3–5] (Table 34-1). It decreased progressively from 5 to 6% at the outset to about 1% during the early 1980s, coinciding with improved patient selection, greater expertise in surgical technology, routine hypothermic cardi-

TABLE 34-1. Perioperative Mortality Rates of Coronary Artery Bypass Surgery

Population	Range (%)	Average (%)
All patients		
1968–1975	4–12	6
1976–1983	0–4	2
1984–1991	3–8	6
Elective <70 yr old	0–3	1
Emergent	10–50	20
Poor LV function	5–20	12
Women	3–9	6
≥70 years	5–12	7
Reoperation early	1–6	3
Reoperation late	3–16	8
Left main coronary artery stenosis	3–13	8

oplegia protection of the myocardium, and optimal postoperative care. However, the operative risk has returned to about 6% in recent years because of the changing profile of patients undergoing bypass surgery. Patients are now older, are more frequently operated on an emergency basis, and have more extensive disease and poorer left ventricular (LV) function—all conditions associated with a higher operative risk. Also, patients operated because of failed coronary angioplasty and patients undergoing a second operation are subjected to a higher risk: 5 to 15%. Furthermore, patients with single and double vessel disease who previously had a lower operative risk are now frequently managed successfully either by medical therapy or by percutaneous balloon catheter angioplasty. At our institution, the perioperative mortality during 1987 and 1988 was 4.5%, a rate substantially higher than the 0.9% rate in patients operated on during the early 1980s.[6]

Age and Early Mortality

Older patients, above 65 years, generally have a higher perioperative mortality. In the Coronary Artery Surgery Study (CASS) registry, it was 5.2% in 1,086 patients 65 years and older, compared with 1.9% in the 7,827 younger patients.[7] At the Cleveland Clinic Foundation, from January 1976 through June 1982, the early mortality was 4.7% in patients 75 years or older, compared with 2% in patients aged 65 to 74 years.[8] According to Naunheim et al.,[9] emergency operation in octogenarians is associated with an unacceptably high mortality (75%), whereas no death occurred in 19 elective cases. Although several studies based on multivariate analysis have reported that old age is an independent correlate of operative mortality, the data suggest that advanced age is a marker rather for severity of both the cardiac and associated noncardiac diseases and that age per se may not be an added

risk factor. Dorros et al.[10] concluded that the higher mortality was probably unrelated to the extent of coronary artery disease (CAD), but rather to the severity of LV wall contraction abnormalities. The risk has decreased appreciably during the past decade because of improved myocardial preservation and particularly as a result of optimal postoperative medical management.[11] The prevalence of patients over 75 years of age is increasing steadily. Age per se is not considered a contraindication, but the selection of patients is critical and must include, in particular, a thorough evaluation of potential associated diseases. On the other hand, few deaths are reported in patients under 40 years of age: none in six series.[12–17]

Gender and Early Mortality

Most series report a perioperative death rate higher in women than in men, ranging from 2.9 to 8.8%.[18–20] In patients operated on from 1969 to 1973 Bolooki et al.[18] observed a mortality of 8.8% in women, compared with 2% in men, for a relative risk ratio of 4.8. In patients operated on later, between 1973 and 1979, Douglas et al.[21] reported a mortality of 2.2% versus 1%, a relative risk of 2.2. Others have found that it was not significantly greater than that observed in male patients.[22] However, the higher mortality observed in women does not appear to be related to the female gender per se, but more to their smaller physical size and hence smaller vessels.[20,23] Nonetheless, women tend to be older, to have more extensive CAD, and are more likely to have diabetes and hypertension, conditions that may be associated with a higher operative risk.

Women now represent 15 to 25% of operated patients. They are operated on more frequently on an emergency basis for unstable angina and for postinfarction angina; elective surgery for effort angina occurs less frequently than in men. These considerations may also explain the apparent higher operative mortality.

Reoperation and Early Mortality

Reoperation for recurrence of clinical manifestations of CAD is being performed with an increasing frequency, varying from 10% to 18% of CABG cases.[24,25] The perioperative mortality rate for reoperation in the CASS registry was 5.3%, compared with 3.1% for the initial operation.[26] Laird-Meeter et al.[27] had a 5.6% early mortality in reoperated patients and only 1.2% at the first CABG. At the Cleveland Foundation Clinic, the 4.8% operative mortality at reoperation during the early years decreased to 2% in 1982, but it was still higher than the below 1% level for first bypass grafting during that period.[28] The early mortality varies markedly from one reported series to another, depending primarily on the interval between both operations. It is not as high for reoperation within 5 to 6 years of the first operation. In such cases, progression of the disease in the native circulation and obstructive changes in the grafts associated with hyperplasia of the intima are responsible for these clinical failures. By contrast, perioperative mortality is much higher for reoperation 7 to more years after the first because it is more frequently performed because of late graft changes caused by atherosclerosis and thrombosis. Embolization of clots and atherosclerotic debris from partially obstructed grafts into the distal coronary bed during surgical manipulations is a constant threat and frequently results in perioperative myocardial infarction (MI).[28-30] Furthermore, at second operation, patients are older and have more associated noncardiac disease, and the bypassed arteries are frequently of poorer quality. Marshall et al.[31] had a 6% early mortality in patients reoperated on for atherosclerotic grafts 6 to 13 years after the initial operation. At our institution, during a 5-year period from 1984 to 1989, 331 patients had a reoperation more than 1 year after the initial one, for a mean interval of 106 ± 40 months.[29] Saphenous graft atherosclerotic disease was present in 73%. The early mortality was 12% compared with 2% for patients who had a first operation during the same period. Brenowitz et al.[32] reported a 12% in-hospital mortality in 150 patients who had bypass grafting for the third time or more.

Predictors of Early Mortality

Predictors of surgical mortality most frequently identified by multivariate discriminant analysis are as follow: age above 70 years, urgency (as opposed to elective surgery), poor LV function, severe and diffuse CAD, left main CAD, and incomplete revascularization.[25,28,33-35]

Perioperative Myocardial Infarction

The incidence of MI has been reported within the range of 4 to 30%, depending on the diagnostic criteria.[36] The diagnosis of perioperative MI is not easily ascertained. A new pathologic Q wave is quite specific, but it lacks sensitivity. Q waves are absent in 30% of autopsy-proven cases of infarction.[37] ST-T wave changes are not helpful because they are frequently caused by postsurgical pericarditis. Measuring creatinine kinase-MB isoenzyme improves the sensitivity as well as technetium 99m pyrophosphate scintigraphy.[38] However, the significance of a single abnormal test is still debated, particularly when the results of several tests are discordant. Chaitman et al.[39] found Q-wave infarction in 4.6% of the CASS registry. A Na-

tional Institutes of Health Consensus meeting postulated an incidence of perioperative MI of 5% for patients with stable angina and of 10% for those having unstable angina before surgery.[40] At our institution, the incidence of perioperative MI was 13% in 1980 to 1981 when two of the following three findings were present: new abnormal Q wave, creatinine-kinase-MB above 100 IU/l, and a positive pyrophosphate scintigraphy.[41] It is now close to 6%.[6]

It is generally agreed that the incidence of perioperative MI has decreased appreciably during the past decade mainly because of improvements in myocardial protection and surgical techniques, as well as more complete revascularization.[42] The hospital mortality is greater among patients who sustain a perioperative infarction. Chaitman et al.[39] report an early mortality 10 times greater in patients with a Q-wave infarction (9.7% versus 1.3%). The 3-year cumulative survival was also shortened, 85% in patients who had a transmural infarction as compared with 95% in those who did not. Langou et al.[36] reported an early mortality of 15.4% in patients with perioperative MI and only 1.6% in patients without MI. In the study by Force et al.,[43] it was found that during the subsequent 30 months, patients with perioperative MI were more likely than patients who did not to experience a cardiac event, death, nonfatal MI, unstable angina, or (CHF). However, patients with an MI who were adequately revascularized and who had a postoperative ejection fraction greater than 40% had an event-free survival rate similar to that of patients without MI.

Arrhythmias

At our institution, among 1,567 patients who had myocardial revascularization in 1987 and 1989, 13.6% had arrhythmias during the immediate postoperative period, but malignant rhythm disturbances were the apparent cause of death in only 3% of cases.[6] Complete heart block occurred in about 5% of patients, was most always transient, and led to insertion of a permanent pacemaker in less than 1% of cases.

Rubin et al.[44] documented ventricular arrhythmia by predischarge 24-hour ambulatory electrocardiographic (ECG) monitoring in 92 patients with normal LV function who underwent elective surgery and found that 57% had one or several of the following complex rhythm disturbances: couplets (32%) nonsustained ventricular tachycardias (21%), and R-on-T phenomenon (4%). No risk factor identified patients at higher risk, and these patients, over a period of 6 to 24 months, did not have a higher incidence of sudden death, cardiac death, syncope, MI, or cerebrovascular accident (CVA).

Congestive Heart Failure

CHF was observed in only 2.4% of cases at our institution,[6] but it was the second most frequent cause of death, i.e. in 33 percent of the cases. Cardiac complications are most frequently observed in older patients, patients with an ejection fraction less than 30%, a greater number of inserted grafts, and following prolonged cardiopulmonary bypass and aortic cross-clamping. It was most common among patients after reoperation (7.8%) than following a first procedure (1.6%). It may be related to poor preoperative LV function, suboptimal myocardial perioperative preservation, or perioperative MI.

Neurologic Complications

Stroke has been estimated to occur in .9 to 5.2% of cases. It was the cause of death in 5.7% at our institution during 1987 to 1988, and almost always in older patients.[6] Previous atrial fibrillation and history of stroke have been implicated as risk factors. It appears that the presence of carotid bruits also increases the risk of stroke, but it is comparable to the reported risk of stroke from endarterectomy.[45] Minor neuropsychological dysfunction is common and is usually transient.[46] Very few patients of working age do not return to work because of neurologic deficit related to the surgery.[47]

PROGNOSIS

Improvement and Recurrence of Angina

Nonrandomized studies report improvement rates of effort angina varying from 70 to 90% of patients 1 year after surgery,[50] of whom about 75% are symptom free.[49] This early improvement appears related to the completeness of revascularization. However, there is a failure rate of 3 to 13% per year, recurrences being rather rare during the first 5 to 6 years and more frequent during the subsequent years.[50] Early recurrences appear related mainly to progression of the disease in the native coronary arteries, whereas late loss of improvement appears also caused by SVG atherosclerosis. In our experience, angina was improved in 88% of survivors and was totally relieved in 69% about 1 year after surgery.[50] At 12 years, only 47% of survivors remained improved and 37% were angina free (Fig. 34-1). The attrition rate was 41% overall, giving a yearly attrition rate of 3.7%; it was only 1.6% during the first 6 years and 6.6% during the last 6 years.

In the randomized European Coronary Surgery

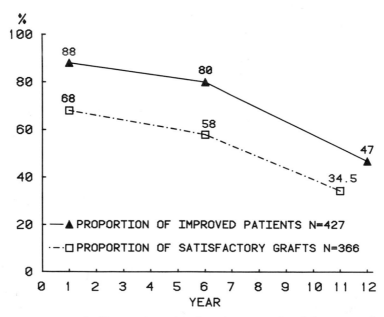

Fig. 34-1. Improvement rates of effort angina related to the rates of satisfactory grafts. The proportion of improved patients parallels closely the proportion of opened grafts without narrowing ≥50%, suggesting that improvement is greatly dependent on the integrity of the grafts. (From Campeau,[109] with permission.)

TABLE 34-2. Complete Improvement of Effort Angina in the Randomized Clinical Trials

	Follow-up (yr)	Treatment Assigned (% of Patients)	
		Surgical	Medical
ECSG[a]	1	58	14
	5	46	28
CASS[b]	1	66	30
	5	63	38
	10	47	42

[a] ECSG, European Coronary Surgery Group. This study included patients with angina class 2 to 3 at entry.

[b] CASS, Coronary Artery Surgery Study. This trial included asymptomatic postmyocardial infarction (22% in each group) and grade 1 to 2 effort angina at baseline.

Study (ECSS) of patients who had moderately severe effort angina, partial and complete improvement at 1 year was noted in 83%, and at 5 years in 75% of surgically assigned patients compared with 45% and 60%, of medically assigned patients, respectively.[51] Also, 58% of surgically assigned patients were angina free 1 year after surgery, and 46% at 5 years compared with 14% and 28% of medically assigned patients, respectively (Table 34-2). In the U.S. National Heart, Lung, and Blood Institute Coronary Artery Surgery Study (CASS), 78% had mild effort angina and 22% were symptom free in both groups at baseline.[52] At 1 and 5 years after randomization, a significantly larger proportion of surgical patients were symptom free (66% at 1 year and 63% at 5 years), compared with the medically assigned patients (30% at 1 year and 38% at 5 years). However, at 10 years, this favorable influence observed in patients with two and three vessel disease was no longer present at 10 years. This late loss of the favorable influence of surgery concerning relief of angina was also noted concerning survival in the VA Study.[53] It was attributed to the late graft changes produced by atherosclerosis, which in our experience involves at least two-thirds of grafts at 10 to 12 years.[54]

The improvement of angina has been objectively documented by an improvement in the exercise capacity and disappearance of exercise-induced myocardial ischemia.[55–57] In the randomized CASS, the proportion of surgically assigned patients with a positive ECG stress test at 5 years was significantly less from that in the medically assigned patients.[52]

Survival

All three large randomized clinical trials with follow-up from 10 to 12 years show a prolonged survival only in certain subsets of surgical patients compared to that of medically assigned patients (Table 34-3). No trial has demonstrated that survival is increased in all patients, regardless of the number of involved vessels

and of the quality of the LV function. Two trials, the Veterans Administration Cooperative Study (VA study) and the CASS included patients having one to three vessel disease and patients with and without LV function impairment.[53,58] The European study included patients with two to three vessel disease and left ventricular ejection fraction (LVEF) greater or equal to 50%.[51] In this trial, surgery was found superior both at 5 to 7 years and at 10 to 12 years in all their patients. The VA and the European studies comprised patients having moderate to severe effort angina, whereas the CASS included patients who had either mild angina or were symptom free after MI.

The VA study was the first trial to show increased survival after CABG in patients having a left main coronary artery stenosis (LMCAS) greater or equal to 50%,[59] but mostly when associated with a significant right coronary artery stenosis or some abnormality of LV function. As an isolated lesion, the difference between surgery and medical therapy was statistically significant only at 18 to 30 months. The ECSS also showed improved survival in this subset of symptomatic patients,[60] but the difference was not statistically significant presumably because of the small number of patients studied (Table 34-3). The CASS excluded left main coronary stenosis. However, in reviewing the CASS registry, Chaitman et al.[61] compared 1,183 patients with LMCAS operated on with 309 who were not. They found that LMCAS equal to or greater than 65% had a longer 3-year survival following surgery and that only patients with associated significant right coronary artery obstruction appeared to benefit. We have also observed in a retrospective study that only patients having both LMCAS and right coronary artery narrowing equal or greater than 70% had a more favorable survival after surgery.[62] It is generally accepted, however, that surgery is indicated for LMCAS equal to or greater than 65% whether or not there is associated right CAD or LV dysfunction, in asymptomatic as well as in symptomatic patients.

Both the CASS and VA studies showed a longer survival following surgery in patients with triple vessel disease and impaired LV function.[53,58] Survival was prolonged in the VA Study only at 5 years, whereas it was significantly better in CASS only at 10 years. In the CASS, the subset had an ejection fraction of 35 to 49%. In these two trials, triple vessel disease with normal LV function did not appear to be beneficial. By contrast, in the European subset with three vessel disease, longer survival rates at 5 to 7 years and at 10 to 12 years were found for surgical patients in both groups, those with mild segmental abnormalities of LV contraction and those without (the ejection fraction was greater than or equal to 50% in all patients).[63] Double vessel disease was shown to benefit from surgery only in the European Study and also only when

TABLE 34-3. Long-Term Survival Rates in Randomized Trials of Coronary Bypass Surgery

Population Studied	Study[a]	Interval After Surgery					
		5–7 yr			10–12 yr		
		MED	Surg	p-Value	MED	Surg	p-Value
All patients	VA	78%	83%	NS	57%	58%	NS
	CASS	90%	92%	NS	79%	82%	NS
With 2–3 vessel disease[b]	European	81%	91%	0.0002	70%	76%	0.02
With 2 vessel disease (anyone)	European	86%	89%	NS	70%	76%	NS
	VA	85%	79%	NS	69%	55%	0.04
	CASS	94%	95%	NS	79%	83%	NS
With 2 vessel disease (LAD included)	European	80%	90%	0.0004	65%	76%	0.007
With 3 vessel disease (all patients)	VA	75%	81%	NS	50%	50%	NS
	European	82%	94%	0.0003	69%	78%	0.01
	CASS	89%	93%	NS	75%	76%	NS
and abnormal LV function	VA	52%	76%	0.05	38%	50%	NS
	CASS	80%	90%	NS	58%	75%	0.05
With left main coronary artery stenosis[c]	VA	64%	80%	NS			
	European	58%	82%	NS			

Abbreviations: CASS, Coronary Artery Surgery Study; MED, medical therapy; NS, not significant; VA, Veterans Administration Cooperative Study.
[a] See text for study identification.
[b] Single vessel excluded and EF ≥50%.
[c] Excluded in CASS.

a LAD stenosis was present (Table 34-3). In the CASS and VA studies, patients with single or with double vessel disease, regardless of LV function or involvement of the LAD, did not live longer following CABG. In fact, survival at 10 to 12 years in the VA Study was better in the medically assigned patients.

It also appears from these randomized trials that patients with one to several of the following features are most likely to have a prolonged survival after CABG: moderately severe angina and a positive ECG stress test (ST depression ≥1.5 mm). Other clinical features were more frequently found in patients who had an improved survival: history of MI, history of hypertension, resting ST-segment abnormalities, peripheral arterial disease, and older age.[53,63]

In nonrandomized studies, the preoperative predictors of late death were age, LV dysfunction, previous MI, prior cardiac surgery and diffuse CAD.[64] Schaff et al.[65] found that only the presence of diseased ungrafted arteries significantly influenced event-free survival and concluded that survival and late functional results 10 years after surgery were related to the adequacy of revascularization. Lawrie et al.[66] also concluded that the 5-year survival was related to the residual disease (incomplete revascularization) but also to age and left ventricular function. Using stepwise multivariate analysis, Laird-Meeter et al.,[67] who studied survival at 5 to 10 years after CABG in 1,041 consecutive patients, established an association between late death and impaired LV function and extent of vascular disease. Using a multivariate Cox model analysis in a study of 2,000 patients, Adler et al.[68] identified emergent operation with cardiogenic shock, ejection fraction less than 50%, preoperative history of CHF, left main coronary artery narrowing, and diabetes, as independent correlates of shortened survival.

The improved long-term survival following surgery is similar in women and men in spite of the higher perioperative mortality in the former.[20–22,69]

From the CASS registry, 1,491 patients 65 years of age or older who had angina as their primary symptom were studied concerning survival.[70] The mean follow-up period was 4.4 years. The cumulative 6-year survival was 80% in the 861 operated patients as compared with 63% in the 630 medically treated patients. The differences in favor of surgery were statistically significant in the group aged 65 to 69 years and 70 to 74 years. Operated patients 75 years and older had a 75% survival rate compared with 56% for the medically treated patients, a nonsignificant difference, perhaps because this group included only 42 patients. When survival curves were adjusted for all the major significant variables, such as LV function, CHF, number of diseased arteries, number of associated disease, and age, the 6-year survival, as in the CASS randomized series in younger patients, was not better following CABG in patients with single vessel disease and in patients with normal LV wall motion regardless of the number of vessels involved.

Late Cardiac Events

The following late complications are frequently observed: recurrence of effort angina, unstable angina, acute myocardial infarction (AMI), and heart failure.

TABLE 34-4. Cardiac Events in 145 patients 2 to 14 Years After Bypass Surgery (Mean Follow-up of 8.4 ± 5 Years)

Event	No. of Patients	%
Recurrent or worsened angina	55	37
Unstable angina	31	21
Myocardial infarction	25	17
Heart failure	12	8
Any single event	81	56

(From Lambert et al.,[71] with permission.)

We have identified the predictive variables of these late events in a series of 145 patients who had routine serial control angiographic examinations 2 to 14 years after CABG[71] (Table 34-4). Univariate analysis showed that unstable angina and AMI correlated with preoperative unstable angina. Heart failure was related to the preoperative LV contraction score and also inversely to the number of grafted arteries. The number of inserted grafts was the only variable selected by stepwise logistic regression analysis showing an inverse relationship with any of the cardiac events, suggesting that the incompleteness of revascularization was the best predictor of these unfavorable late events. It is also of interest that preoperative unstable angina was frequently present in patients in whom either AMI or unstable angina developed years after grafting. The tendency for thrombus formation that was responsible for the preoperative instability may continue to operate after surgery. Graft failure and progression of atherosclerosis in the native coronary arteries may be promoted by the same platelet dysfunction that existed prior to surgery. In the randomized trials, the rates of nonfatal MI during the first 5 years after randomization were similar: 11 to 14% of the medically assigned patients and 14 to 15% of the surgically assigned patients. At our institution, patients with previous bypass surgery had smaller MIs with fewer complications, most likely because of the presence of less jeopardized myocardium distal to the infarct-producing lesion.[72] In fact, post-CABG patients tend to occlude smaller arteries, such as diagonal branches or marginal branches, which have not been bypassed. On the other hand, unstable angina after CABG appears to have a poor long-term prognosis because they are less amenable to revascularization compared to the unoperated patients with unstable angina, although their clinical features and hospital course are not different.[73]

Quality of Life

The most important consideration is the relief of angina, discussed earlier. Also of concern are return to work and subsequent hospitalization. Retrospective

studies have reported a return to work in 51 to 90% of patients who were 65 years old or younger. There appears, however, to be no significant gain compared with preoperative status.[74–76] Previous strenuous work, lower level of education, and duration of employment before surgery seemed more frequently related to postoperative unemployment.[77] In the 60- to 70-year-old patients, surgery seems to accelerate the rate of retirement; the reason given by most patients is a desire to relax.[75] Employment status was not different in both treatment groups in three randomized trials.[52,78,79] This lack of gain in the employment status is not related to physical disability, since excellent relief of angina, improvement of objectively demonstrated exercise tolerance, and decreased use of antianginal drugs were observed in all three clinical trials.

The frequency of subsequent hospitalizations is significantly less in post-CABG patients. Hamilton et al.[80] showed that the rates of hospitalization during a mean follow-up of 6 years for a matched pair cohort of medically and surgically treated patients were significantly lower in post-CABG patients: 19% year versus 26% year. This was due to a significant reduction rate of myocardial infarction. In the CASS, however, there was no significant difference in the number of hospitalizations during the 10-year follow-up between medically and surgically assigned patients.[52]

CHANGES IN SAPHENOUS VEIN GRAFTS

Changes in SVGs may occur early or late. The early modifications consist of endothelial denudation, thrombosis, and intimal fibromuscular hyperplasia. The late changes are also thrombosis, and atherosclerotic degeneration.

Early Thrombosis

Endothelial denudation of various degree occurs during harvesting and storage of the vein.[81] It is presumably caused by mechanical trauma related to removal and preparation of the vein, by ischemia resulting from the removal of the blood supply, and by inappropriate storage before it is implanted.[81]

This endothelial injury favours platelet adhesion and aggregation that results in thrombus formation. Thrombosis is the most frequent cause of early graft occlusion.[82] It may occur in grafts without technical imperfections, although it develops more frequently whenever the blood flow is decreased because of technical imperfections, such as kinks, inappropriately tight anastomosis, or in grafts to arteries having a poor distal runoff. Platelet-inhibitor therapy reduces early graft thrombotic occlusions by 30 to 50%.[83]

Intimal Fibrous Hyperplasia

Intimal fibrous hyperplasia (IFH) is observed on pathologic examination in all grafts within the first month.[82,84–86] It is a consequence of reparative and adaptive processes. Endothelial injury leads to smooth muscle cell proliferation and migration from the media to the intima, resulting in fibromuscular thickening of the tunica intima. In addition to this healing process, progression of this IFH is enhanced by the high pressure and pulsatile flow of the arterial system. Similar lesions are present in veins of arteriovenous fistulae. Also, Bulkley and Hutchins[87] consider that early developing concentric thrombus associated with the endothelial injury is transformed in fibrous hyperplasia plaques. This IFH develops in all grafts, but its magnitude is variable. It generally produces a diffuse reduction of the graft lumen by 25%, on average (Fig. 34-2). However, in about 20% of grafts, minimal IFH occurs, and the lumen appears unchanged on serial cineangiograms at 2 to 3 weeks after grafting and 1 year. Focal IFH develops rarely on the body of the graft, and more frequently near anastomotic sites.[84,88]

Diffuse or focal IFH, when severe, may cause early graft occlusion, usually associated with a superimposed thrombus.[84] The improved graft patency at one year associated with platelet-inhibitor drugs is most likely due to the prevention of thrombosis. In fact, FIH does not appear to be prevented or diminished in man by currently available platelet-inhibitor drugs.[83]

Both focal and diffuse IFH may be lessened by improved handling and storage of the vein specimen.[89–92] We have observed a significantly lower incidence of focal lesions and less severe diffuse IFH after modifica-tion of surgical techniques and particularly in patients who received veins of smaller diameter, harvested from below the knee, and who also had larger grafted arteries.[93] It appears that in general the magnitude of IFH is directly proportional to the initial diameter of the graft and inversely proportional to the capacity of the distal runoff of the grafted artery, as if the diameter of the conduit tended to approximate that of the grafted artery (Fig. 34-2).

Diffuse IFH does not appear to progress after the first postoperative year[94] and, as an isolated lesion, it rarely leads to late graft occlusion (Fig. 34-2). However, the incidence of late graft failure in our experience is closely related to the magnitude of IFH, in both our serial cineangiographic and pathologic studies.[95,96] This relationship suggests that IFH predisposes to thrombosis, perhaps because of endothelial dysfunction, and above all to atherosclerotic degeneration. Indeed, FIH has been considered by many pathologists as an early manifestation of atherosclerosis.[87,97]

Graft Atherosclerosis

Atherosclerosis is seldom observed on pathologic examination before the third postoperative year,[96] and it rarely produces wall irregularities and occlusion on cineangiograms before the fifth year.[54] By the tenth year, two-thirds of the grafts are diseased, with occlusion in half and wall irregularities in the other half[54] (Fig. 34-3). Around 10 to 12 years after surgery, in patients with cineangiographic evidence of graft disease, one-half the grafts show lesions compatible with atherosclerosis, and the other grafts that are apparently

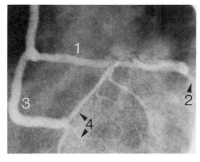
10 days

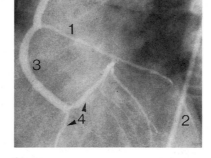
1 year

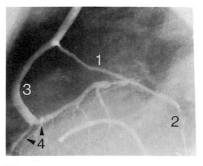
12 years

Fig. 34-2. Cineangiograms of a saphenous vein Y graft to the left coronary artery system at 10 days, 1 year, and 12 years after surgery, showing diffuse reduction of the lumen by fibrous hyperplasia of the intima. By 1 year, the lumen of the graft limb (1) to the small marginal branch of the circumflex artery (2) has decreased by 60%, whereas only a 10% decrease in the internal diameter is observed in the limb (3) to the left anterior descending coronary artery (4), which has a much greater distal runoff, as compared with the circumflex branch. This diffuse narrowing of the graft occurs between 10 days and 1 year and shows no subsequent progression.

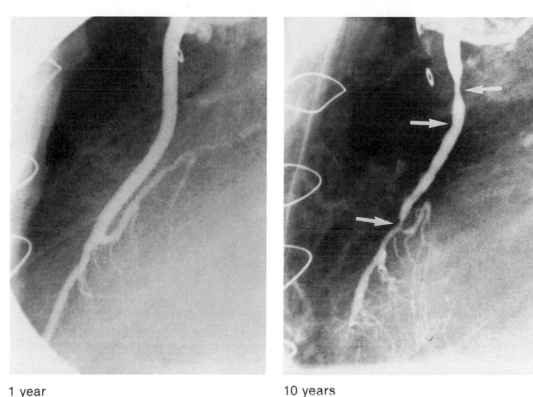

1 year   10 years

Fig. 34-3. Cineangiograms of a saphenous vein graft to the left anterior coronary artery at 1 year and 10 years after surgery. At 1 year, the graft appears intact, but at 10 years, numerous wall irregularities have developed, producing narrowings of various degrees (shown by the arrows), and attributed to atherosclerosis.

intact on the cineangiograms almost always show disease on pathologic examination.[31]

Graft Patency

Close to 1 year after surgery, the patency rate is 70 to 85%.[83] It appears that antiplatelet drugs improves early patency by preventing thrombosis, particularly in vein grafts connected to small arteries.[98] Patency to the LAD may be as high as 90% in vein grafts 1 year after grafting, irrespective of treatment (i.e., with or without antiplatelet drugs).[99] In our experience, the cumulative patency was 92% at 1 year in grafts without significant anastomotic narrowings related to inappropriate surgical techniques noted at the 2- to 3-week angiographic examination and connected to arteries having a good distal runoff (≥ 50 ml/min), as determined by a graft flow measured at the time of surgery (Fig. 34-4). No occlusion was observed at 1 to 5 to 7 years in these 97 "perfect grafts." A marked attrition followed between 6 and 11 years, with a cumulative patency at 11 years of only 69%. The 1-year patency is usually 75 to 85% when all grafts are included, and attrition close to 1 to 2% per year at 1 to 5 years after

surgery, resulting in a 5- to 6-year patency of 70 to 80%. The failure rate is greater during the subsequent 5 to 6 years, averaging between 3 and 5 percent, leading to a 10- to 12-year patency rate of 45 to 65%.[54,83,100–104]

Risk Factors and Graft Disease

Risk factors of CAD appear to be related to these late SVG changes, particularly diabetes, elevated lipids, and smoking.[105] It is postulated that optimal control of these risk factors may retard graft atherosclerosis. One clinical trial has shown that lowering LDL-cholesterol and raising HDL-cholesterol blood levels decreases significantly the incidence of new lesions in grafts.[106] Graft occlusion, however, has not been less frequent presumably because the correction of lipid abnormalities does not prevent thrombus formation, which is so frequent in these grafts with and without atherosclerosis.[96,107] Aspirin and low-intensity oral anticoagulation in addition to lipid-lowering therapy are now being tested as means of preventing late graft occlusion (NHI-NHLBI-Post-CABG Clinical Trial).

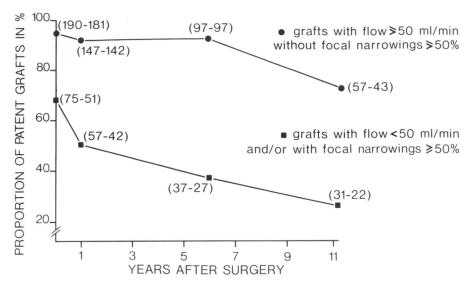

Fig. 34-4. Cumulative graft patency at 2 weeks, 1 year, 6 years, and 11 years shown for two groups of saphenous vein grafts. Group 1 (●) grafts with flow of ≥50 ml/min measured at surgery suggesting a good distal runoff, and/or absence of focal narrowings ≥50%, particularly at anastomotic sites caused by inappropriate surgical techniques. Group 2 (■) grafts with flows of <50 ml/min and/or focal narrowings ≥50%. The cumulative patency was 92% at 1 and 6 years, and 69% at 11 years for grafts of group 1 and 50% at 1 year, 37% at 6 years and 26% at 11 years for grafts in group 2.

Clinical Outcome and Saphenous Vein Graft Changes

Clinical outcome depends on the fate of the grafts and changes in the unbypassed native coronary arteries.[3,50,108] In our experience, the proportion of patients whose angina remains improved parallels closely the proportion of hemodynamically satisfactory grafts (i.e., without narrowing greater than or equal to 50%[109]) (Fig. 34-1). Similarly, an unfavorable postoperative clinical course, manifested by either recurrent or worsened effort angina, unstable angina, MI, and heart failure, was significantly more frequent in patients whose grafts showed late changes 10 to 12 years after CABG, either wall irregularities or closure, compared with those whose grafts appeared intact: 69% versus 31% (Table 34-5). In patients whose grafts showed late changes at 5 to 7 years after grafting, death or unfavorable cardiac events occurred more frequently during the ensuing 5 years, in comparison with patients whose grafts appeared intact (Table 34-6). In the former group, death or complications were observed in 68.6% as compared with an incidence of 40.5% in the latter group.[109]

INTERNAL MAMMARY ARTERY GRAFTS

IMA grafts have been widely used during the past 5 to 10 years because of their higher long-term patency; 82 to 94% of IMA grafts to the LAD are patent 5 to 12

TABLE 34-5. Clinical Course 10 to 12 Years After Grafting Related to Graft Status at That Time

Clinical Course	No. of Patients	Without Late Graft Changes	With Late Graft Changes[b]	p-Value
Favorable	58	33–57%	25–43%	<0.01
Unfavorable[a]	80	25–31%	55–69%	

[a] One or more cardiac events: acute MI, unstable angina, recurrent or worsened effort angina, or heart failure.

[b] Wall irregularities or closure developing between 1 and 10 to 12 years.

TABLE 34-6. Cardiac Events Occurring Between 5–7 Years and 12 Years After Grafting Related to Graft Status at 5–7 Years

Cardiac Events[a]	No. of Patients	All Grafts Intact	With Narrowing or Closure	p-Value
Absent	44	22–59%	22–31%	<0.02
Present	63	15–41%	48–69%	

[a] Recurrent or worsened effort angina, unstable angina, acute MI, or heart failure.

years after CABG, a much better long-term patency than that reported for vein grafts (45 to 65%).[100-104] The left IMA is generally accepted to be the best conduit for the LAD. The use of both IMA grafts to bypass the left coronary system is now common; in more than one-half of cases, they are placed in combination with SVGs in order to bypass the right coronary artery and marginal Cx branches whenever needed for optimal revascularization. However, the long-term patency of IMA grafts to vessels other than the LAD is unknown. In contrast with SVGs, IMA grafts seldom develop atherosclerosis, at least during the first 10 to 12 years after surgery.[86,100-104]

Because IMA grafts remain functional much longer than SVGs, unfavorable cardiac events, such as unstable angina and MI are less frequent.[110,111] Relief of angina remains longer and survival is better in patients who receive IMA grafts, as compared with those in whom only SVGs are placed. This more favorable clinical outcome in patients receiving IMA grafts as compared with those having only SVGs is not evident, however, during the first 5 to 6 years.[112,113] The lower incidence of atherosclerotic disease in IMA grafts as compared with SVGs explains the superior long-term clinical results (i.e., 10 to 12 years after surgery), and most likely for much longer.

SUMMARY

With improved surgical technologies, anesthesia, and postoperative medical management, the perioperative mortality of coronary bypass surgery is now close to 1% in patients below 70 years of age who are operated on an elective basis. However, it is still high, at 3 to 16% in certain subsets of patients and in certain conditions: women, older patients, emergent operations, poor LV function, certain anatomic patterns such as left main coronary artery stenosis, particularly with a left dominant coronary artery distribution, and reoperation because of atherosclerotic graft disease. The most frequent serious complication is perioperative AMI, which occurs in 5 to 10% of cases. It is the most frequent cause of early death.

Improvement of effort angina, frequently associated with objective evidence of the absence or lessening of myocardial ischemia, is generally observed up to 5 to 10 years after surgery. Survival has also been shown to increase following surgery in patients with two to three vessel disease, particularly when the left anterior descending artery is involved, and also when associated with an abnormal LV function and objective evidence of ischemia.

Atherosclerosis and clot formation associated with fibrous hyperplasia of the intima are observed in two-thirds of grafts 10 to 12 years after surgery. These late graft changes and the progression of the disease in the native coronary arteries are responsible for the deterioration of clinical results which may be observed as early as the fifth postoperative year. They also explain why many subsets of operated patients have a longer survival only up to 10 years.

The long-term results concerning quality of life and survival appear much superior in patients who had one to several internal mammary artery grafts as compared to those whose grafts were all saphenous veins. In fact, the internal mammary artery seldom develops atherosclerosis and remains opened much longer. It is likely that current indications of bypass surgery are based on the results obtained following saphenous vein grafting are too conservative, particularly as it pertains to long-term survival. All patients with multiple vessel disease, including the LAD and objective evidence of ischemia, may well have a prolonged survival for 10 to 20 years when IMA grafts are used.

REFERENCES

1. Connolly JE: The history of coronary artery surgery. J Thorac Cardiovasc Surg 76:733, 1978
2. Spencer FC: The internal mammary artery: the ideal coronary bypass graft? N Engl J Med 314:50, 1986
3. Naunheim KS, Fiore AC, Wadley JJ et al: The changing profile of the patient undergoing coronary artery bypass surgery. J Am Coll Cardiol 11:494, 1988
4. Christakis GT, Ivanov J, Weisel RD et al: The changing pattern of coronary artery bypass surgery. Circulation, suppl I. 80:I-151, 1989
5. Morin JE, Symes JF, Guerraty A1 et al: Coronary artery bypass profile in Canada and the United States. Can J Cardiol 6:319, 1990
6. Pelletier LC, Carrier M: Early postoperative care and complications. p. 3. In Waters D, Bourassa MG, Brest AN (eds): Care of the Patient with Previous Coronary Bypass Surgery. FA Davis, Philadelphia, 1991
7. Gersh BJ, Kronmal RA, Frye RL et al: Coronary arteriography and coronary artery bypass surgery: morbidity and mortality in patients ages 65 years or older. A report of the Coronary Artery Surgery Study. Circulation 67:483, 1983
8. Loop FD, Lytle BW, Cosgrove DM et al: Coronary artery bypass graft surgery in the elderly. Indications and outcome. Cleve Clin J Med 55:23, 1988
9. Naunheim KS, Kern MJ, McBride LR et al: Coronary artery bypass surgery in patients aged 80 years or older. Am J Cardiol 59:804, 1987
10. Dorros G, Lewin RF, Daley P, Assa J: Coronary artery bypass surgery in patients over age 70 years: report from the Milwaukee cardiovascular data registry. Clin Cardiol 10:377, 1987
11. Ennabli K, Pelletier LC: Morbidity and mortality of coronary artery surgery after the age of 70 years. Ann Thorac Surg 42:197, 1986
12. Kelly TF, Craver JM, Jones EL, Hatcher CR: Coronary revascularization in patients 40 years and younger: sur-

gical experience and long term follow-up. Am Surg 44: 675, 1978

13. Laks H, Kaiser GC, Barner HB et al: Coronary revascularization under age 40 years: risk factors and results of surgery. Am J Cardiol 41:584, 1978

14. de Mozzi P, Bortolotti U, Corbara F et al: Obstructive coronary disease in young subjects: results of the surgical treatment by aortocoronary bypass. G Ital Cardiol 9:465, 1979

15. De Olivera SA, Santana GP, Barchi CA et al: Direct myocardial revascularization in young patients: analysis of 100 consecutive cases without operative mortality. J Cardiovasc Surg 18:9, 1977

16. FitzGibbon GM, Hamilton MG, Leach AJ et al: Coronary artery disease and coronary bypass grafting in young men: experience with 138 subjects 39 years of age and younger. J Am Coll Cardiol 9:977, 1987

17. Sanoudos GM, Moggio RA, McClung JA et al: Coronary revascularization in young patients. Texas Heart Inst J 13:131, 1986

18. Bolooki H, Vargas A, Green R et al: Results of direct coronary artery surgery in women. J Thorac Cardiovasc Surg 69:271, 1975

19. Kennedy JW, Kaiser GC, Fisher LD et al: Clinical and angiographic predictors of operative mortality from the Collaborative Study in Coronary Artery Surgery (CASS). Circulation 63:793, 1981

20. Loop FD, Golding LR, MacMillan JP et al: Coronary artery surgery in women compared with men: analyses of risks and long-term results. J Am Coll Cardiol 1:383, 1983

21. Douglas JS Jr, King SB III, Jones EL et al: Reduced efficacy of coronary bypass surgery in women. Circulation, suppl II. 64:II–11, 1981

22. Killen DA, Reed WA, Arnold M et al: Coronary artery bypass in women: long-term survival. Ann Thorac Surg 34:559, 1982

23. Fisher LD, Kennedy JW, Davis KB et al: Association of sex, physical size, and operative mortality after coronary artery bypass in the Coronary Artery Surgery Study (CASS). J Thorac Cardiovasc Surg 84:334, 1982

24. Foster ED: Reoperation for coronary artery disease. Circulation, suppl V. 72:V–59, 1985

25. Lytle BW, Loop FD, Cosgrove DM et al: Fifteen hundred coronary reoperations. J Thorac Cardiovasc Surg 93: 847, 1987

26. Foster ED, Fisher LD, Kaiser GC, Myers WO: Principal investigators of CASS and their associates: Comparison of operative mortality and morbidity for initial and repeat coronary artery grafting: the coronary artery study (CASS) registry experience. Ann Thorac Surg 38:563, 1984

27. Laird-Meeter K, Van Domburg R, Van Den Brand MJBM et al: Incidence, risk, and outcome of reintervention after aortocoronary bypass surgery. Br Heart J 57: 427, 1987

28. Loop FD, Lytle BW, Gill CC et al: Trends in selection and results of coronary artery reoperations. Ann Thorac Surg 36:380, 1983

29. Grondin CM, Pomar JL, Hébert Y et al: Reoperation in patients with patent atherosclerotic coronary vein grafts. J Thorac Cardiovasc Surg 87:379, 1984

30. FitzGibbon GM, Keon WJ: Atheroembolic perioperative infarction during repeat coronary bypass surgery: angiographic documentation in a survivor. Ann Thorac Surg 43:218, 1987

31. Marshall WG, Jr, Saffitz J, Kouchoukos NT: Management during reoperation of aortocoronary saphenous vein grafts with minimal atherosclerosis by angiography. Ann Thorac Surg 42:163, 1986

32. Brenowitz JB, Johnson WD, Kayser KL et al: Coronary artery bypass grafting for the third time or more. Results of 150 consecutive cases. Circulation, suppl I. 78: I–166, 1988

33. Wright JG, Pifarré R, Sullivan HJ et al: Multivariate discriminant analysis of risk factors for operative mortality following isolated coronary artery bypass graft. Chest 91:394, 1987

34. Teoh KH, Christakis GT, Weisel RD et al: Increased risk of urgent revascularization. J Thorac Cardiovasc Surg 93:291, 1987

35. Kennedy JW, Kaiser GC, Fisher LD et al: Multivariate discriminant analysis of the clinical and angiographic predictors of operative mortality from the collaborative study in coronary artery surgery (CASS). J Thorac Cardiovasc Surg 80:873, 1980

36. Langou RA, Wiles JC, Peduzzi PN et al: Incidence and mortality of perioperative myocardial infarction in patients undergoing coronary artery bypass grafting. Circulation, suppl II. 56:II–54, 1977

37. Johnson WJ, Achor RWP, Burchell HB, Edwards JE: Unrecognized myocardial infarction. Arch Intern Med 103:253, 1959

38. Brindis RG, Brundage BH, Ullyot DJ et al: Graft patency in patients with coronary artery bypass operation complicated by perioperative myocardial infarction. J Am Coll Cardiol 3:55, 1984

39. Chaitman BR, Alderman EL, Sheffield LT et al: Use of survival analysis to determine the clinical significance of new Q waves after coronary bypass surgery. Circulation 67:302, 1983

40. National Institutes of Health Consensus Development Conference Statement on Coronary Bypass Surgery: Scientific and clinical aspects. Circulation, suppl II. 65: II–126, 1982

41. Guiteras Val P, Pelletier LC, Hernandez MG et al: Diagnostic criteria and prognosis of perioperative myocardial infarction following coronary bypass. J Thorac Cardiovasc Surg 86:878, 1983

42. Burton JR, Fitzgibbon GM, Keon WJ, Leach AJ: Perioperative myocardial infarction complicating coronary bypass. J Thorac Cardiovasc Surg 82:758, 1981

43. Force T, Hibberd P, Weeks G et al: Perioperative myocardial infarction after coronary artery bypass surgery. Clinical significance and approach to risk stratification. Circulation 82:903, 1990

44. Rubin DA, Nieminski KE, Monteferrante JC et al: Ventricular arrhythmias after coronary artery bypass graft surgery: incidence, risk factors and long-term prognosis. J Am Coll Cardiol 6:307, 1985

45. Reed GL III, Singer DE, Picard EH, DeSanctis RW: Stroke following coronary-artery bypass surgery. A case-control estimate of the risk from carotid bruits. N Engl J Med 319:1246, 1988

46. Smith PLC, Newman SP, Ell PJ et al: Cerebral consequences of cardiopulmonary bypass. Lancet 1:823, 1986

47. Shaw PJ, Bates D, Cartlidge NEF et al: Neurological complications of coronary artery bypass graft surgery: six month follow-up study. Br Med J 293:165, 1986

48. Taylor GJ, Malik SA, Colliver JA et al: Usefulness of atrial fibrillation as a predictor of stroke after isolated coronary artery bypass grafting. Am J Cardiol 60:905, 1987

49. Campeau L, Lespérance J, Hermann J et al: Loss of the improvement of angina between 1 and 7 years after aortocoronary bypass surgery. Correlations with changes in vein grafts and in coronary arteries. Circulation, suppl I. 60:I–1, 1979

50. Campeau L, Enjalbert M, Lespérance J, Bourassa MG: Course of angina 1 to 12 years after aortocoronary bypass surgery related to changes in grafts and native coronary arteries. Can J Surg 28:496, 1985

51. European Coronary Surgery Study Group: Long-term results of prospective randomized study of coronary artery bypass surgery in stable angina pectoris. Lancet 2: 1173, 1982

52. CASS Principal Investigators and their Associates: Coronary Artery Surgery Study (CASS): a randomized trial of coronary artery bypass surgery. Quality of life in patients randomly assigned to treatment groups. Circulation 68:951, 1983

53. The Veterans Administration Coronary Artery Bypass Surgery Cooperative Study Group: Eleven-year survival in the Veterans Administration randomized trial of coronary bypass surgery for stable angina. N Engl J Med 311:1333, 1984

54. Campeau L, Enjalbert M, Lespérance J et al: Atherosclerosis and late closure of aortocoronary saphenous vein grafts: sequential angiographic studies at 2 weeks, 1 year, 5 to 7 years, and 10 to 12 years after surgery. Circulation, suppl II. 68:II–1, 1983

55. Rahimtoola SH: Postoperative exercise response in the evaluation of the physiologic status after coronary bypass surgery. Circulation, suppl II. 65:II–106, 1982

56. Weiner DA, McCabe CH, Roth RL et al: Serial exercise testing after coronary artery bypass surgery. Am Heart J 101:149, 1981

57. Gohlke H, Gohlke-Bärwolf C, Samek L et al: Serial exercise testing up to 6 years after coronary bypass surgery: behavior of exercise parameters in groups with different degrees of revascularization determined by postoperative angiography. Am J Cardiol 51:1301, 1983

58. CASS Principal Investigators and their associates: Coronary Artery Surgery Study (CASS): a randomized trial of coronary artery bypass surgery. Survival data. Circulation 68:939, 1983

59. Takaro T, Hultgren HN, Lipton MJ et al: The VA cooperative randomized study of surgery for coronary arterial occlusive disease. II. Subgroup with significant left main lesions. Circulation, suppl III. 54:III–108, 1975

60. European Coronary Surgery Study Group: Prospective randomized study of coronary artery bypass surgery in stable angina pectoris: a progress report on survival. Circulation, suppl II. 65:II–67, 1982

61. Chaitman BR, Fisher LD, Bourassa MG et al: Effect of coronary bypass surgery on survival patterns in subsets of patients with left main coronary artery disease. Am J Cardiol 48:765, 1981

62. Campeau L, Corbara F, Crochet D et al: Left main coronary artery stenosis. The influence of aortocoronary bypass surgery on survival. Circulation 57:1111, 1978

63. Varnauskas E and the European Coronary Surgery Study Group: Twelve-year follow-up of survival in the randomized european coronary surgery study. N Engl J Med 319:332, 1988

64. Rutherford JD, Whitlock RML, McDonald BW et al: Multivariate analysis of the long-term results of coronary artery bypass grafting performed during 1976 and 1977. Am J Cardiol 57:1264, 1986

65. Schaff HV, Gersh BJ, Pluth JR et al: Survival and functional status after coronary artery bypass grafting: results 10 to 12 years after surgery in 500 patients. Circulation, suppl II. 68:II–200, 1983

66. Lawrie GM, Morris GC, Jr, Silvers A et al: The influence of residual disease after coronary bypass on the 5-year survival rate of 1274 men with coronary artery disease. Circulation 66:717, 1982

67. Laird-Meeter K, van Domburg R, Bos E, Hugenholtz PG: Survival at 5 to 10 years after aorto-coronary bypass operations in 1041 consecutive patients. Eur Heart J 8:449, 1987

68. Adler DS, Goldman L, O'Neil A et al: Long-term survival of more than 2,000 patients after coronary artery bypass grafting. Am J Cardiol 58:195, 1986

69. Hall RJ, Elayda MA, Gray A et al: Coronary artery bypass: long term follow-up of 22,284 consecutive patients. Circulation, suppl II. 68:II–20, 1983

70. Gersh BJ, Kronmal RA, Schaff HV et al: Comparison of coronary artery bypass surgery and medical therapy in patients 65 years of age or older. A nonrandomized study from the Coronary Artery Surgery Study (CASS) registry. N Engl J Med 313:217, 1985

71. Lambert M, Kouz S, Campeau L: Preoperative and operative predictive variables of late clinical events following saphenous vein coronary artery bypass graft surgery. Can J Cardiol 5:87, 1989

72. Waters DD, Pelletier GB, Haché M et al: Myocardial infarction in patients with previous coronary artery bypass surgery. J Am Coll Cardiol 3:909, 1984

73. Waters DD, Walling A, Roy D, Théroux P: Previous coronary artery bypass grafting as an adverse prognostic factor in unstable angina pectoris. Am J Cardiol 58:465, 1986

74. Guvendik L, Rahan M, Yacoub M: Symptomatic status and pattern of employment during a five-year period following myocardial revascularization for angina. Ann Thorac Surg 34:383, 1982

75. Johnson WD, Kayser KL, Pedraza PM, Shore RT: Employment patterns in males before and after myocardial revascularization surgery. A study of 2229 consecutive male patients followed for as long as 10 years. Circulation 65:1086, 1982

76. Almeida D, Bradford JM, Wenger NK et al: Return to work after coronary bypass surgery. Circulation, suppl II. 68:II–205, 1983

77. Boulay FM, David PP, Bourassa MG: Strategies for improving the work status of patients after coronary artery bypass surgery. Circulation, suppl III. 66:III–43, 1982

78. Booth DC, Deupree RH, Hultgren HN et al: Quality of life after bypass surgery for unstable angina. 5-year follow-up results of a Veterans Affairs Cooperative Study. Circulation 83:87, 1991

79. Varnauskas E and the European Coronary Surgery Study Group: Survival, myocardial infarction, and employment status in a prospective randomized study of coronary bypass surgery. Circulation, suppl V. 72:V–90, 1985

80. Hamilton WM, Hammermeister KE, DeRouen TA et al: Effect of coronary artery bypass grafting on subsequent hospitalization. Am J Cardiol 51:353, 1983

81. Unni KK, Kottke BA, Titus JL et al: Pathologic changes in aortocoronary saphenous vein grafts. Am J Cardiol 34:526, 1974

82. Vlodaver Z, Edwards JE: Pathologic analysis in fatal cases following saphenous vein coronary arterial bypass. Chest 64:555, 1973

83. Verstraete M, Brown BG, Chesebro JH et al: Evaluation of antiplatelet agents in the prevention of aorto-coronary bypass occlusion. Eur Heart J 7:4, 1986

84. Lawrie GM, Lie JT, Morris GC et al: Vein graft patency and intimal proliferation after aortocoronary bypass. Early and long term angio-pathologic correlations. Am J Cardiol 38:856, 1976

85. Barboriak J, Batayias GE, Pintar K et al: Pathological changes in surgically removed aortocoronary vein grafts. Ann Thorac Surg 21:524, 1976

86. Atkinson JB, Forman MB, Vaughn WK et al: Morphologic changes in long-term saphenous vein bypass gifts. Chest 88:341, 1985

87. Bulkley BH, Hutchins GM: Accelerated atherosclerosis. A morphologic study of 97 saphenous vein coronary artery bypass grafts. Circulation 55:163, 1977

88. Grondin CM, Meere C, Castonguay Y et al: Progressive and late obstruction of an aortocoronary bypass graft. Circulation 43:698, 1971

89. Leung DY, Glagov S, Mathews MB: Cyclic stretching stimulates synthesis of matrix components by arterial smooth muscle cells in vitro. Science 191:475, 1976

90. Ip JH, Fuster V, Badimon L et al: Syndromes of accelerated atherosclerosis: role of vascular injury and smooth muscle cell proliferation. J Am Coll Cardiol 1:1667, 1990

91. Bonchek LI: Prevention of endothelial damage during preparation of saphenous veins for bypass grafting. J Thorac Cardiovasc Surg 79:911, 1980

92. Brody WR, Kosek JC, Angell WW: Changes in vein grafts following aorto-coronary bypass induced by pressure and ischemia. J Thorac Cardiovasc Surg 64:847, 1972

93. Campeau L, Crochet D, Lespérance J et al: Postoperative changes in aortocoronary saphenous vein grafts revisited. Angiographic studies at 2 weeks and at one year in two series of consecutive patients. Circulation 52:369, 1975

94. Lespérance J, Bourassa MG, Saltiel J et al: Angiographic changes in aortocoronary vein grafts: lack of progression beyond the first year. Circulation 48:633, 1973

95. Kouz S, Campeau L, Lespérance J et al: The role of early graft changes in late aortocoronary saphenous vein graft closure. J Am Coll Cardiol 7:34A, 1985

96. Solymoss BC, Leung TK, Pelletier LC, Campeau L: Pathologic changes in coronary artery saphenous vein grafts and related etiologic factors. p. 45. In Waters D, Bourassa MG, Brest AN (eds): Care of the Patient with Previous Coronary Bypass Surgery. FA Davis, Philadelphia, 1991

97. Lie JT, Lawrie GM, Morris GC, Jr: Aortocoronary bypass saphenous vein graft atherosclerosis: anatomic study of 99 vein grafts from normal and hyperlipoproteinemic patients up to 75 months postoperatively. Am J Cardiol 40:906, 1977

98. Buring JE, Hennekens CH: Antiplatelet therapy to prevent coronary artery bypass graft occlusion. Circulation 82:1044, 1990

99. Goldman S, Copeland J, Moritz T et al: Internal mammary artery and saphenous vein graft patency. Effects of aspirin. Circulation, suppl IV. 82:IV–237, 1990

100. Tector AJ, Schmahl TM, Janson B et al: The internal mammary artery graft. JAMA 246:2181, 1981

101. Okies JE, Page US, Bigelow JC et al: The left internal mammary artery: the graft of choice. Circulation, suppl I. 70:I–213, 1984

102. Grondin CM, Campeau L, Lespérance J et al: Comparison of late changes in internal mammary artery and saphenous vein grafts in two consecutive series of patients 10 years after operation. Circulation, suppl I. 70: I–208, 1984

103. Lytle BW, Loop FD, Cosgrove DM et al: Long-term (5 to 12 years) serial studies of internal mammary artery and saphenous vein coronary bypass grafts. J Thorac Cardiovasc Surg 89:248, 1985

104. Ivert T, Huttunen K, Landou C, Björk VO: Angiographic studies of internal mammary artery grafts 11 years after coronary artery bypass grafting. J Thorac Cardiovasc Surg 96:1, 1988

105. Campeau L: Coronary risk factors and the postbypass patients. p. 123. In Waters D, Bourassa MG, Brest AN (eds): Care of the Patient with Previous Coronary Bypass Surgery. FA Davis, Philadelphia, 1991

106. Blankenhorn DH, Nessim SA, Johnson RL et al: Beneficial effects of combined colestipol-niacin therapy on coronary atherosclerosis and coronary venous bypass grafts. JAMA 257:3233, 1987

107. Neitzel GF, Barboriak JJ, Pintar K et al: Atherosclerosis in aortocoronary bypass grafts. Morphologic study and risk factor analysis 6 to 12 years after surgery. Arteriosclerosis 6:594, 1986

108. Loop FD, Cosgrove DM, Kramer JR et al: Late clinical and arteriographic results in 500 coronary artery reoperations. J Thorac Cardiovasc Surg 81:675, 1981

109. Campeau L: Late changes in saphenous vein coronary artery bypass grafts and their implications in clinical practice. Can J Cardiol, suppl A. 3:23A, 1987

110. Loop FD, Lytle BW, Cosgrove DM et al: Influence of the internal-mammary-artery graft on 10-year survival and other cardiac events. N Engl J Med 314:1, 1986

111. Cameron A, Kemp HG, Jr, Green GE: Bypass surgery with the internal mammary artery graft: 15 year follow-up. Circulation, suppl III. 74:III–30, 1986

112. Jones JW, Ochsner JL, Mills NL, Hughes L: Clinical comparison between patients with saphenous vein and internal mammary artery as a coronary graft. J Thorac Cardiovasc Surg 80:334, 1980

113. Tyras DH, Barner HB, Kaiser GC et al: Bypass grafts to the left anterior descending coronary artery. J Thorac Cardiovasc Surg 80:327, 1980

35

Risk Assessment and Prognosis of Coronary Artery Bypass Grafting in Patients With Left Ventricular Dysfunction

R. Sudhir Sundaresan
Nicholas T. Kouchoukos

Coronary artery bypass grafting (CABG) is an established and highly effective therapy for coronary arterial occlusive disease. In large randomized trials, CABG has been consistently shown to be more effective than medical therapy for the relief of angina pectoris. The results of randomized trials comparing CABG with percutaneous transluminal coronary artery angioplasty (PTCA) are not currently available. The comparative benefit of CABG on other unfavorable outcome events, such as acute myocardial infarction (AMI) and cardiac-related death, is less certain.

In the early experience with CABG, it became apparent that severe preoperative left ventricular (LV) dysfunction was associated with a high operative mortality rate.[1,2] It also appeared that LV function was not consistently improved by CABG.[3] More recently, randomized trials and observational studies have demonstrated a benefit in survival from CABG over medical therapy in patients with substantial impairment of LV function.[4-7] This benefit has resulted in part from reduction in the early mortality following CABG.

This chapter presents the criteria for defining LV dysfunction and for selection of patients with substantial impairment of LV function for CABG. The results of medical and surgical treatment from randomized trials and large observational studies are also described.

DEFINITION OF LEFT VENTRICULAR DYSFUNCTION

Numerous techniques to quantitate the severity of LV dysfunction have been proposed and evaluated, and their description is beyond the scope of this chap-

TABLE 35-1. Assessment of Resting Global Left Ventricular Function

Left Ventricular Function	Ejection Fraction	Left Ventricular Wall Motion Score (CASS)
Normal	≥0.55	5
Mild dysfunction	0.45–0.54	6–10
Moderate dysfunction	0.35–0.44	11–15
Severe dysfunction	0.25–0.34	16–20
Very severe dysfunction	<0.25	>20

Abbreviation: CASS, Coronary Artery Surgery Study.

ter. A useful and widely used index of LV function is the resting LV ejection fraction (LVEF). This measurement provides an estimate of global LV systolic function. It is most frequently obtained by qualitative estimation or by quantitative measurements from the LV angiogram in the peak systolic and end-diastolic frames obtained at the time of cardiac catheterization. It can also be determined by noninvasive methods, such as echocardiography and radioisotope imaging. A resting LVEF of 0.55 or above is generally considered normal. A classification of LV dysfunction based on the resting LVEF is shown in Table 35-1.

The Coronary Artery Surgery Study (CASS) assessed global LV function by calculating a *wall motion score*, based on the sum of five segmental wall-motion scores, using the following grading system: 1, normal; 2, moderate hypokinesis; 3, severe hypokinesis; 4, akinesis; 5, dyskinesis; and 6, aneurysm. Segmental wall motion was assessed in the right anterior oblique (RAO) projection of the LV cineangiogram.[8] A score of 5 (5 segmental wall-motion scores each equal to 1) denotes normal LV function. A score of 16 or above denotes severe dysfunction. The relationship between EF and the CASS LV wall-motion score is shown in Table 35-1. This discussion considers only patients with severe or very severe LV dysfunction (resting EF <0.35, CASS wall-motion score >15).

PREVALENCE OF LEFT VENTRICULAR DYSFUNCTION AMONG PATIENTS UNDERGOING CORONARY ARTERY BYPASS GRAFTING

In the CASS study, 160 of 780 patients (20%) with one, two, or three vessel disease randomized to either medical or surgical therapy had ejection fractions of 0.35 to 0.49.[4] In a study from the University of Alabama, 192 of 1,500 patients (13%) undergoing biplane left ventriculography had a LVEF of 0.35 or less and were considered candidates for CABG.[6]

PREOPERATIVE EVALUATION OF PATIENTS WITH SEVERE LEFT VENTRICULAR DYSFUNCTION

When global LV dysfunction is severe, myocardial scarring is usually extensive. This extensive scarring often limits the recovery of LV function after CABG. However, segments of the LV wall that are hypokinetic or even akinetic at rest preoperatively often demonstrate improved systolic function after CABG.[9,10] This finding suggests that viable myocardial cells, which may be stunned or hibernating, exist in hypokinetic or akinetic segments and that their function can be enhanced by CABG. Demonstration of important areas of reversible ischemia preoperatively is therefore desirable. Selection of patients for CABG in whom substantial areas of reversible ischemia exist (usually in the distribution of at least two of the three major coronary arteries) will likely improve the resting LV function and enhance survival.

METHODS TO DETECT MYOCARDIAL ISCHEMIA

Angina Pectoris

The presence of angina pectoris strongly suggests the presence of ischemic but viable myocardium, even in the presence of severely or very severely depressed resting ejection fraction.[1,5–7,11]

Noninvasive Studies

Thallium 201 Scintigraphy

Injection of thallium during an exercise test or after injection of dipyridamole will often permit differentiation of ischemic, hypokinetic, or akinetic myocardium from scar tissue. After a time delay (usually above 3 hours), thallium will be distributed in areas of myocardium that contain viable cells, whereas it will not be distributed in areas of scar.

Exercise Radionuclide Ventriculography

Technetium 99m is injected to evaluate LV ejection and wall motion immediately after exercise. The normal response to exercise is an increase in ejection fraction of at least 5%. If the ejection fraction falls, or if wall-motion abnormalities are observed, ischemic LV dysfunction is usually present. Improvement in regional wall motion has been observed after CABG and is associated with increased regional myocardial perfusion.[10] This has been noted even in areas of scarring from previous myocardial infarction (MI). These findings support the concept that viable, but stunned or hibernating myocardial cells are distributed throughout hypokinetic or even akinetic segments and that their function can be improved by revascularization.

INDICATIONS FOR CORONARY ARTERY BYPASS GRAFTING

In general, patients with severe LV dysfunction who have coronary arterial occlusive disease suitable for CABG in at least two of the three major coronary arterial systems, and who have evidence for reversible myocardial ischemia (angina pectoris and/or positive thallium scintigraphic or radionuclide ventriculographic studies), should be considered candidates for CABG. Patients with profound LV dysfunction (EF 0.15 to 0.20), no angina, and evidence for little or no reversibly ischemic myocardium are not likely to benefit from surgical revascularization.

Severe coexisting conditions that limit life expectancy are relative contraindications to the CABG operation in this subgroup of patients. These include severe debility, pronounced mental deterioration, and severe pulmonary, renal, and other organ system disease. Older age in itself is not a contraindication for operation, but hospital mortality and morbidity will be increased in patients over the age of 75 years.

NATURAL HISTORY

Limited information exists about the natural history of patients with coronary arterial occlusive disease, including those with LV dysfunction. Since the withholding of either medical or interventional treatment is not currently justifiable, the best information comes from data obtained early in the era of coronary arteriography and left ventriculography before the widespread use of CABG. After the introduction of CABG and the implementation of clinical trials comparing medical with surgical therapy, patients initially receiving medical treatment were permitted to "cross over" to surgical treatment. The resulting "nonsurgical" group does not accurately reflect the true natural history of the disease.

The extent of coronary arterial occlusive disease as defined by coronary arteriography and the severity of LV dysfunction, most commonly defined by left ventriculography, are the most powerful determinants of survival. Oberman et al.[12] in 1972 analyzed the survival of 246 patients who had coronary arteriography between 1965 and 1970 and who did not undergo CABG during the follow-up interval, which extended to 50 months. Mortality was directly related to the number of diseased coronary arteries (Table 35-2). Since left ventriculography was not routinely performed in these patients, symptoms of congestive heart failure, (CHF) were used as a surrogate for LV dysfunction (patients with cardiomyopathy and valvular heart disease were excluded). The presence of symptoms of congestive failure was associated with a substantially higher mortality then when those symptoms were not present (Table 35-2).

In an analysis of more than 14,000 patients from the CASS registry who received medical treatment, the severity of LV dysfunction as determined by LVEF or wall-motion score, was a stronger determinant of survival than the extent of coronary arterial occlusive disease[13] (Fig. 35-1).

RESULTS OF CORONARY ARTERY BYPASS GRAFTING IN PATIENTS WITH SEVERE LEFT VENTRICULAR DYSFUNCTION

In general, the CABG operation is indicated for relief of symptoms (usually angina pectoris) that are unresponsive to medical treatment (or coronary artery angioplasty) and when the duration of freedom from unfavorable events (death, MI, return of symptoms) can be predicted with reasonable confidence to be appreciably longer than with other forms of treatment.[14]

Comparisons of outcome after CABG with that of alternate forms of therapy are most appropriately made by comparing the time-related comparative benefit of the CABG operation.[14] Endpoints that can be examined include death and freedom from symptoms

TABLE 35-2. Mortality by Symptoms of Congestive Heart Failure and Number of Vessels Diseased

No. of Vessels Diseased	Symptoms of CHF			No Symptoms of CHF		
	Dead	Alive	Mortality Rate (%)	Dead	Alive	Mortality Rate (%)
0	1	8	11.1	2	87	2.2
1	1	5	16.7	1	39	2.5
2	9	5	64.3	4	32	11.1
3	7	9	43.8	8	28	22.2
Total:	18	27	40.0	15	186	8.1

Abbreviatiion: CHF, congestive heart failure.
(From Oberman et al.,[12] with permission.)

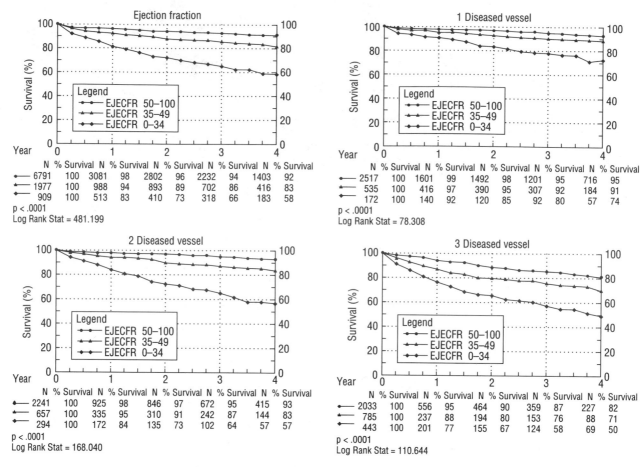

Fig. 35-1. Four-year survival data for patients with at least one vessel disease, less than 50% left main coronary artery obstruction, and a measured ejection fraction (EJEC FR). (From Mock et al.,[13] with permission.)

(angina pectoris, cardiac failure), from fatal or nonfatal MI, or from additional interventional therapy (angioplasty or repeat CABG). Prospective randomized trials provide the most useful information about the relative efficacy of surgical and nonsurgical therapy. Unfortunately, randomized trials in patients with severe LV dysfunction have not been performed. The randomized portion of the CASS study did show a significant difference in survival at 7 years in favor of surgical treatment in patients with mild or moderate LV dysfunction (LFEF of 0.35 to 0.49) and three vessel disease.[4]

In the absence of randomized trials, useful information can be obtained from observational studies, provided that the relevant clinical and angiographic variables of the groups under study are documented.

Survival

A study from the CASS nonrandomized registry of patients with an EF of 0.35 or less treated medically and surgically, demonstrated a significantly higher

overall survival rate among the surgically treated patients when the survival curves were adjusted for all other significant prognostic variables.[5] When survival of these patients was analyzed according to tertiles of EF at or below 0.35 (upper, middle, and lower), the difference in survival was statistically significant only for those patients in the lower tertile (EF of ≤0.25).

In this study, which included 420 medically treated patients, all patients who underwent initial medical therapy were considered suitable candidates for CABG. Patients with ventricular aneurysms, some of which were resected at operation, were included. During the follow-up interval, which extended to 7 years, 9% of patients originally treated by medical therapy crossed over to surgical treatment. These patients usually underwent CABG because of failure of medical therapy or worsening symptoms. Withdrawal from the medically treated group of substantial numbers of patients whose symptoms worsen may yield more favorable survival curves for the remaining patients. The survival curves may then not accurately reflect the

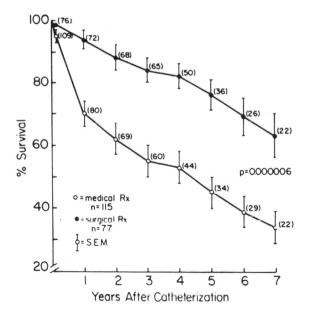

Fig. 35-2. Cumulative survival of the 77 surgically treated and 115 medically treated (Rx) patients. Numbers in parentheses are the patients alive at the end of that interval. Seven-year survival rates were 63 and 34%, respectively. S.E.M., standard error of the mean. (From Pigott et al.,[6] with permission.)

"true" natural history of the patients originally under study. Thus, survival curves of medically and surgically treated patients treated nonrandomly or by randomization must be interpreted with caution if patients cross over from medical to surgical therapy.

In a study from the University of Alabama of patients with coronary arterial occlusive disease and with ejection fractions of 0.35 or less determined by biplane angiography, survival at 7 years for 77 surgically treated patients was 63% and for 115 medically treated patients was 34%[6] (Fig. 35-2). The baseline characteristics of the medically and surgically treated groups were comparable, except for a significantly higher prevalence of angina, unstable angina, and triple vessel disease in the surgically treated group. Patients with LV aneurysms were excluded. All the medically treated patients were considered suitable candidates for CABG. During the follow-up interval, only 3 (2.6%) of the medically treated patients crossed over to surgical treatment at 25, 31, and 35 months after cardiac catheterization (the date of initial exposure).

The severity of LV dysfunction had an adverse effect on survival in both the medically and surgically treated groups (Fig. 35-3A and B). However, survival of the surgically treated patients with an EF of 0.26 to 0.35, and 0.25 or less was significantly greater than that of the corresponding medically treated patients

(Fig. 35-3A and B). When the proportional hazards model of Cox was used to adjust for other important prognostic variables, the type of treatment (medical or surgical) remained statistically significant (p < 0.03) in predicting relative risk of death at 5 and 7 years (relative risk medical to surgical of 2.58 and 2.12, respectively).

A study from Duke University of 710 patients with a LVEF of 0.40 or less, treated medically and surgically, showed a higher survival rate among the surgically treated patients[7] (Fig. 35-4). The survival curves were adjusted for known prognostic factors. In this study, ventricular resection was performed in 69 of the 301 surgically treated patients. Twenty-six (6%) of the 409 patients initially treated medically crossed over to surgical treatment more than 6 months after catheterization.

When the patients were subgrouped according to tertiles of EF, surgical survival benefit was apparent in each third of the study group (Fig. 35-5). Survival benefit was greater in those patients with moderate to severe LV dysfunction than in those with only modest dysfunction. The adverse effect of worsening LV dysfunction for both medically and surgically treated patients is again demonstrated. Survival in this group of patients was also affected by the severity of the coronary arterial occlusive disease (Fig. 35-6). Surgical treatment provided substantial benefit in patients with two or three vessel coronary artery disease (CAD).

All the above observational studies demonstrate a benefit from surgical treatment on survival in patients with substantial impairment of LV function. They also consistently demonstrate that for subgroups defined by clinical and coronary artery anatomic characteristics, the patients with the more severe degrees of LV dysfunction are likely to experience the largest absolute benefit in survival. Although operative risk will be higher in patients with severe LV dysfunction, this risk appears justified in view of the poor prognosis without surgical treatment.

Freedom from Nonfatal Myocardial Infarction

The study from the University of Alabama determined the incidence of nonfatal MI in the follow-up interval.[6] Data were available for 178 (93%) of the 192 patients. The incidence was significantly lower among the surgically treated patients (Fig. 35-7).

Relief of Symptoms

The nonrandomized CASS registry study comparing patients with poor LV function treated medically and surgically showed that patients with angina as the predominant symptom were relieved of this symptom to a greater extent with surgical therapy.[5] There was no

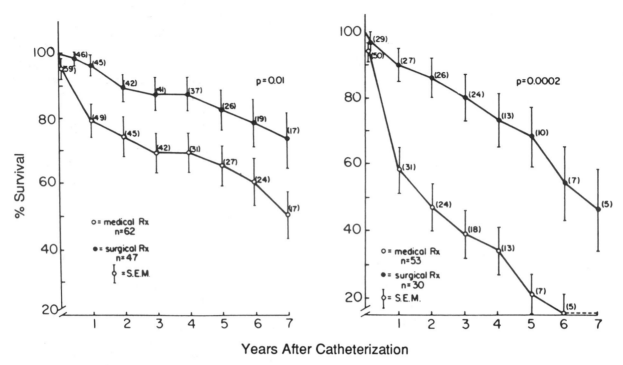

Years After Catheterization

Fig. 35-3. (**A**) Cumulative survival of 47 surgically treated and 62 medically treated patients with an EF of 0.26 to 0.35. Seven-year survival rates were 73% and 50%, respectively. (**B**) Cumulative survival of 30 surgically treated and 53 medically treated patients with an EF of ≤ 0.25. Seven-year survival rates were 46% and 15%, respectively. S.E.M., standard error of the mean. (From Pigott et al.,[6] with permission.)

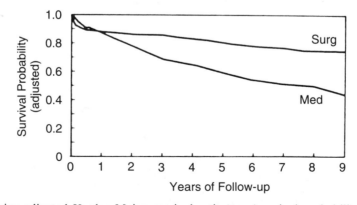

Fig. 35-4. Plot showing adjusted Kaplan-Meier survival estimates (survival probability) and time (years of follow-up) for patients with LVEF of ≤ 0.40 at baseline cardiac catheterization, treated medically (Med) and surgically (Surg) at Duke University Medical Center. These survival curves are adjusted for known prognostic factors. (From Bounous et al.,[7] with permission.)

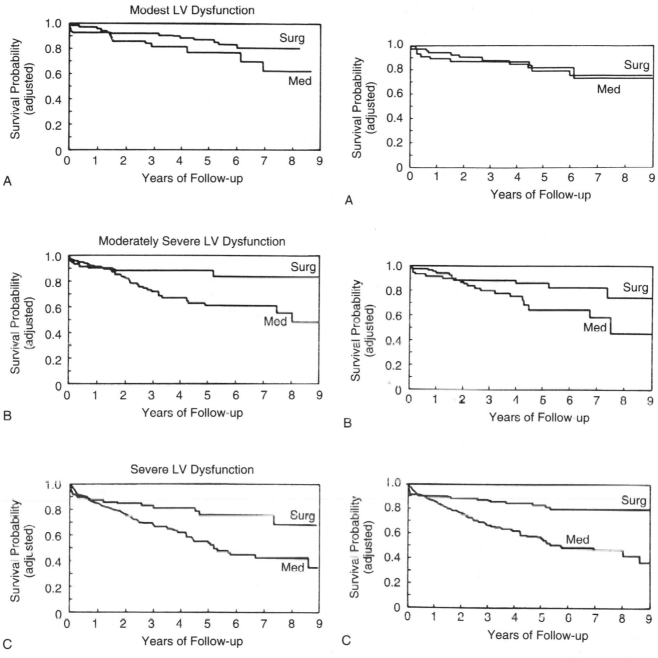

Fig. 35-5. Plot showing adjusted Kaplan-Meier survival estimates (survival probability) and time (years of follow-up) of the study population divided according to baseline LVEF. Med, medically treated; Surg, surgically treated. **(A)** Upper tertile of EF (median ejection fraction of 0.38). **(B)** Mid-tertile of EF (median EF of 0.32). **(C)** Lower tertile of EF (median EF of 0.24). (From Bounous et al.,[7] with permission.)

Fig. 35-6. Plot showing adjusted Kaplan-Meier survival estimates (survival probability) and time (years of follow-up) of the study population divided according to baseline number of diseased coronary arteries. Med, medically treated; Surg, surgically treated. **(A)** Patients with one vessel disease. **(B)** Patients with two vessel disease. **(C)** Patients with three vessel disease. (From Bounous et al.,[7] with permission.)

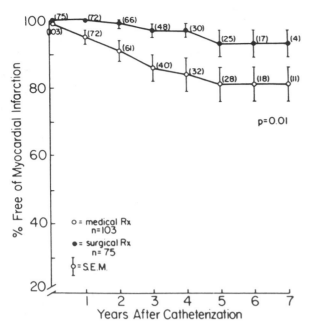

Fig. 35-7. Cumulative incidence of freedom from nonfatal myocardial infarction for 75 surgically treated and 103 medically treated patients with available follow-up information. Seven-year rates were 93% and 81%, respectively. S.E.M., standard error of the mean. (From Pigott et al.,[6] with permission.)

greater relief of symptoms of heart failure with surgical therapy than with medical therapy. In general, relief of symptoms of CHF and improvement in LVEF (at rest and after exercise) have been less consistently observed in patients with substantial impairment of LV function than in patients with normal or near normal ventricular function.

CONCLUSIONS

The data presented, obtained primarily from observational studies, demonstrate that substantial benefit can be derived from CABG in patients with coronary arterial occlusive disease and LV dysfunction. Selection of patients for CABG is critically important; documentation of the presence of reversibly ischemic myocardium is essential for an optimal outcome. In addition to the relief of angina pectoris, improvement in global and regional LV function has been documented in the majority of patients. Although symptoms of cardiac failure are not consistently improved after operation, a significant benefit in terms of increased survival following CABG as compared with

medical treatment has been observed, with the greatest comparative benefit occurring in those patients with the most severe impairment of LV function. Operative risk is higher than that for patients with normal or minimally impaired ventricular function, but this risk is appropriate in view of the poor prognosis with nonoperative treatment. With current operative techniques, this mortality does not exceed 5 to 7% for most patients.

REFERENCES

1. Spencer FC, Green GE, Tice DA et al: Coronary artery bypass grafts for congestive heart failure. J Thorac Cardiovasc Surg 62:529, 1971
2. Zubiate P, Kay JH, Mendez AM: Myocardial revascularization for the patient with drastic impairment of function of the left ventricle. J Thorac Cardiovasc Surg 73:84, 1977
3. Hammermeister KE, Kennedy JW, Hamilton GW et al: Aorto-coronary saphenous vein bypasses: failure of successful grafting to improve resting left ventricular function in chronic angina. N Engl J Med 290:186, 1974
4. Passamani E, Davis KB, Gillespie MJ et al: A randomized trial of coronary artery bypass surgery: survival of patients with a low ejection fraction. N Engl J Med 312:1665, 1985
5. Alderman EL, Fisher LD, Litwin P et al: Results of coronary artery surgery in patients with poor left ventricular function (CASS). Circulation 68:785, 1983
6. Pigott JD, Kouchoukos NT, Oberman A et al: Late results of surgical and medical therapy for patients with coronary artery disease and depressed left ventricular function. J Am Coll Cardiol 5:1036, 1985
7. Bounous EP, Mark DB, Pollock BG et al: Surgical survival benefits for coronary disease patients with left ventricular dysfunction. Circulation, suppl I. 78:1–151, 1988
8. Killip T (ed): The National Heart, Lung, and Blood Institute Coronary Artery Surgery Study (CASS). Circulation, suppl I. 63:I–1, 1981
9. Shearn DL, Brent BN: Coronary artery bypass surgery in patients with left ventricular dysfunction. Am J Med 80:405, 1986
10. Brundage BH, Massie BM, Botvinick EH: Improved regional ventricular function after successful surgical revascularization. J Am Coll Cardiol 3:902, 1984
11. Goenen M, Jacquemart JL, Galvez S et al: Preoperative left ventricular dysfunction and operative risks in coronary bypass surgery. Chest 92:804, 1987
12. Oberman A, Jones WB, Riley CP et al: Natural history of coronary artery disease. Bull NY Acad Med 48:1109, 1972
13. Mock MB, Ringqvist I, Fisher LD et al: Survival of medically treated patients in the Coronary Artery Surgery Study (CASS) Registry. Circulation 66:562, 1982
14. Kirklin JW, Akins CW, Blackstone EH et al: Guidelines and indications for coronary artery bypass graft surgery: A report of the ACC/AHA Task Force. J Am Coll Cardiol 17:543, 1991

36
Postinfarction Angina

William E. Curtis
Timothy J. Gardner

Although the morbidity and mortality from an acute myocardial infarction (AMI) have been reduced substantially over the past two decades,[1,2] AMI complicated by postinfarction angina still represents an extremely high-risk condition that requires aggressive medical and possible surgical intervention. Historically, medical management of this complication has been attended by a poor prognosis with a high rate of reinfarction and cardiac death. Likewise, initial reports of a high early surgical mortality generally distinguished operative intervention as carrying a prohibitive risk.[3] Progress in the standard pharmacologic management, the addition of percutaneous transluminal coronary angioplasty (PTCA), the judicious use of the intra-aortic balloon pump, and improved myocardial preservation during cardiac surgery are some of the recent advances that have had a favorable impact on this high-risk population over the past decade. This chapter reviews the definition, incidence, prognosis and pathophysiology of postinfarction angina, then proposes a treatment strategy based on the current risk stratification for this subset of patients.

DEFINITION AND INCIDENCE

Postinfarction angina can be defined as recurrent or persistent chest pain occurring at rest or with minimal exertion, usually accompanied by electrocardiographic (ECG) ischemic changes, 24 hours to 30 days after AMI. The chest pain that occurs during AMI is thought to arise from nerve fibers in ischemic, but still viable, myocardium.[4] Experimental studies have demonstrated that, despite complete coronary occlusion, myocardial tissue can remain viable in the region at risk for up to 6 hours.[5] Patients who survive AMI, therefore, frequently endure chest pain for several hours following the event, particularly if reperfusion of the affected myocardium was not accomplished. Thus, chest pain occurring within the first 6 to 12 hours can usually be attributed to the initial injury but, after 24 hours, these symptoms probably represent recurrent ischemia to viable but jeopardized myocardium. Such findings generally herald the onset of ventricular arrhythmias and infarct extension, thereby increasing the size of the infarct and further impairing left ventricular (LV) function. The surgical literature makes further distinction of this population by reporting typically on those patients with "unstable" postinfarction angina, including patients refractory to medical therapy and those who are not suitable candidates for, or not responsive to, PTCA.

The concomitant presence of ischemic ECG changes in patients with postinfarction chest pain contributes significantly to the specificity of identifying patients who actually have recurrent ischemia. In a study of patients with non-Q wave infarction, Gibson et al.[6] reported that, compared with patients with angina alone, patients with angina associated with ECG changes were nearly four times more likely to suffer reinfarction or death. Recently, several studies have even advocated the wider use of Holter monitoring in clinically suspicious patients on the basis that it enhances detection of recurrent ischemia, particularly in those with "silent," or asymptomatic ischemia.[7–10]

The incidence of postinfarction angina is reported to be 20 to 60%, depending on the specific criteria and patient population studied.[11-16] Studies from large referral centers generally reflect an inflated incidence compared with the general population. Patients with non-Q wave infarctions[15-17] and those with preinfarction angina[16,18] may also have a higher incidence of postinfarction angina. Interestingly, the early use of thrombolytic therapy, which has been shown to reduce early mortality after AMI, has not been shown to reduce the incidence of either postinfarction angina or reinfarction compared with placebo.[19,20]

PROGNOSIS

Patients who clinically exhibit signs and symptoms of recurrent ischemia are at high risk of infarct extension and cardiac death (Fig. 36-1). In one of the earlier studies conducted to identify patients with postinfarction angina as a high-risk subset of patients, Stenson and colleagues[21] reported that six of nine patients with postinfarction chest pain and transient ST-segment changes sustained reinfarction and that three of these nine patients subsequently died.[21] Following this study, Schuster and Bulkley[14] reported an overall 56% mortality among 70 patients with postinfarction angina treated medically over a 6-month follow-up period. More than one-half of the survivors were classified as having had unstable angina, and nearly one-third ultimately underwent coronary revascularization. In another study of patients with non-Q wave infarction, Gibson et al.[6] reported that postinfarction angina developed in 43% of 576 patients within the first 2 weeks after the event. Compared with patients without postinfarction angina, reinfarction (12.2% versus 3.6%) and death (6.1% versus 1.5%) occurred more frequently during the first 2 weeks after infarction in patients with postinfarction angina.

Comparisons between patients with transmural versus nontransmural infarctions suggest that recurrent infarction is more common among the latter. Hutter and associates[17] correlated nontransmural infarctions with a lower risk of early mortality than transmural infarction (9% versus 20%) but a higher risk of reinfarction over a 57-month follow-up period (57% versus 17%). Similarly, Marmor and associates[13] reported that 43% of patients with an initial subendocardial infarction sustained an early recurrent infarction compared with only 8% of those with a transmural infarction. In addition, the early mortality rate for patients with a subendocardial infarction and extension was more than two times that of patients without extension (16% versus 7%). They concluded that nontransmural myocardial infarction is an unstable ischemic event associated with a greater risk of reinfarction and late mortality.

Recurrent ischemia may produce arrhythmias and transient impairment of myocardial function that can result in sudden death. Recurrent ischemia that leads to infarct extension or reinfarction is likewise a poor prognostic sign. In-hospital mortality rates following reinfarction have been shown to be as high as 43% for patients with a non-Q-wave infarction.[22] Similarly, Fraker and associates[23] reported that the risk of mortality in patients with infarct extension compared with those without extension was significantly higher when determined for in-hospital (36% versus 9%) (Fig. 36-2) and 1-year (24% versus 9%) mortality. More recently, Gilpin et al., reported that the 1-year mortality rate for patients with reinfarction is twice as high as that of patients without evidence of reinfarction (16.4% versus 8.4%).[24]

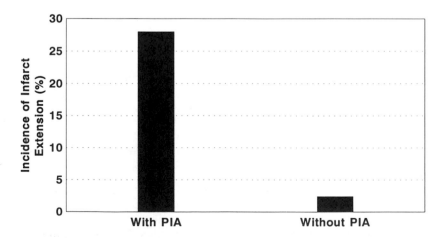

Fig. 36-1. Incidence of infarct extension. (From Bosch et al.,[16] with permission.)

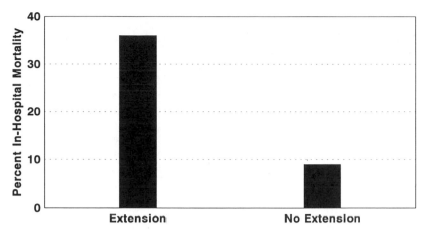

Fig. 36-2. In-hospital mortality related to infarct extension. (From Fraker et al.,[23] with permission.)

PATHOPHYSIOLOGY

Postinfarction angina is caused by recurrent ischemia to residual viable myocardium. Clinicopathologic studies have identified two types of postinfarction ischemia: ischemia at the border zone of the infarct and ischemia at a distance from the infarct.[25] Compared with patients who have ischemia in the infarct zone, patients with ischemia at a distance have a lower final Killip class, more deaths attributable to ventricular arrhythmias, significantly smaller infarcts at autopsy, and a significantly higher 6-month mortality (72% versus 33%).[14,25] Schuster and Bulkley[14] concluded from one study that death in patients with ischemia at a distance appears to be related more to the ischemic events than the actual mass of myocardium lost. Interestingly, both the pathophysiology and natural history of patients with ECG evidence of ischemia at a distance are similar to that of patients with non-Q-wave infarctions, who generally have less myocardial necrosis compared with patients with Q-wave infarctions, but a higher long-term case fatality rate.[26]

Anatomically, high-grade coronary artery obstructive disease is a distinct feature of patients with postinfarction angina. Bosch and colleagues[16] have been able to correlate early recurrent ischemia to a higher number of diseased vessels, a higher number of diseased coronary artery segments, less collateral circulation to the myocardium at risk, and fewer collateral vessels distal to a tight stenosis. Both pathologic and angiographic studies confirm that patients with postinfarction angina have two vessel and three vessel disease more frequently than do patients without recurrent ischemia.[14,16,27–29] Morphologically, compared with patients without postinfarction angina, the stenoses associated with postinfarction angina are longer[30] and more frequently type 2 eccentric lesions[29,31] (asym-metric with a narrow neck and/or irregular borders), suggesting that an unstable plaque with mural thrombus may be involved in postinfarction unstable angina.[32]

The importance of intraluminal coronary thrombus has also been established in the pathophysiology of postinfarction angina. In a prospective study of 268 consecutive coronary angiograms, Bresnahan et al.[33] reported that not only do patients with unstable angina have intracoronary thrombus more frequently than do those with stable angina (35% versus 2.5%) but that patients with intracoronary thrombus sustain subsequent AMI with postinfarction angina more frequently than do those without thrombus.[33]

Coronary artery spasm has also been implicated as a precipitant of postinfarction angina, albeit its true prevalence as a significant contributor to this syndrome has never been documented.[34,35] Recent experimental and clinical studies have demonstrated, however, that endothelial cell dysfunction, associated with stenotic coronary vessels and possibly reperfusion injury, can potentiate coronary artery spasm in a postinfarction setting.[36–42] Endothelial cells are known to participate in the function of maintaining coronary arterial tone by release of endothelium-derived relaxing and constricting factors. Several animal studies have shown abnormal endothelial cell function following coronary occlusion and reperfusion.[40,42,43] VanBenthuysen and associates[42] demonstrated that coronary arteries reperfused after 60 minutes of occlusion sustain a nondenuding endothelial cell injury that results in increased vasomotor reactivity to vasoconstrictor agents. Mehta et al.[40] also demonstrated impaired coronary vasodilator reserve in a canine model of coronary reperfusion. In addition, several human studies suggest that the abnormal endothelial-cell-mediated vasomotor responses of atherosclerotic coronary arteries could promote coronary vasospasm.[37,38] This may have therapeutic implications regarding pharmacologic means of reducing the activity or presence of certain known mediators of vasoconstriction or endothelial injury, such as platelets, and possibly leukocytes.

TREATMENT

Initial Management

The initial management of postinfarction angina is essentially the same as that for classic angina pectoris and includes rest and the use of nitroglycerin, β-adrenergic blockade,[44,45] heparin,[46,47] aspirin,[46,47] and calcium antagonist therapy.[48] Failure to relieve persistent or recurrent angina with these measures requires urgent coronary angiography to establish suitability for revascularization.[49] In addition, it is not uncommon for these patients to require an intra-aortic balloon pump for hemodynamic instability.

Most patients with unstable postinfarction angina will have high-grade two vessel or three vessel coronary obstructions associated with intracoronary thrombus in the infarct-related artery.[14,16,27–29] In this setting, the clinician must determine the feasibility and risks of coronary artery bypass grafting (CABG) versus PTCA.

Currently, there does not appear to be a role for thrombolytic therapy in the treatment strategy for postinfarction angina. Although two large studies of thrombolytic therapy have demonstrated as much as a 20% reduction in the early mortality for patients treated within 12 hours of AMI,[19,20] a recent randomized placebo-controlled study, using intracoronary streptokinase and recombinant tissue-type plasminogen activator in patients with postinfarction angina, failed to demonstrate a reduction in either clinical or ECG evidence of ischemic events despite successful lysis of the clots.[26] Studies comparing thrombolytic and antiplatelet therapy for postinfarction angina have not yet been performed.

PTCA

Conversely, PTCA, initially confined to patients with stable angina pectoris, has emerged over the past decade as a practical addition to current therapeutic options for patients with postinfarction angina, good function, and single vessel disease.[50] Although patients with single vessel disease and good ventricular function would be expected to have an overall good prognosis, Gleckel et al.[43] have reported that 20% of patients with single vessel disease and postinfarction angina suffered reinfarction or cardiac death within 39 months of follow-up.

PTCA in patients with postinfarction angina, most of whom had single vessel disease, has proved technically successful in 80 to 91% of patients initially, depending on the morphology and location of the lesion.[51–56] In addition, both Sabbah[57] and de Feyter[58] have demonstrated that global and regional myocardial function improve after PTCA in this setting.

The excellent technical success and functional improvement observed in these high-risk patients, however, have been accompanied by a high incidence of complications compared with elective coronary angioplasty.[59,60] Gottlieb et al.[53] reported complications in 19% of patients in whom PTCA was attempted. In the Mayo Clinic's report on 70 patients with postinfarction angina, the initial technical success rate was 80%, but the procedure-related mortality was 2%, and emergent coronary artery bypass was required in 11% of patients.[51] Safian and colleagues,[55] from Beth Israel Hospital in Boston, similarly reported an excellent initial PTCA success rate in patients with non-Q-wave postinfarction angina, but also noted procedure-related complications in 10% of the patients studied. Procedure-related MI is reported to be as high as 8%, and emergent CABG is required in 2 to 15% of patients with postinfarction angina undergoing PTCA, as shown in Table 36-1. In addition, long-term follow-up reveals a high rate of recurrent angina and restenosis that ultimately results in repeat PTCA in 7% to 19% of patients and coronary artery bypass in 5 to 13% of patients treated initially with PTCA.[51–56]

Application of PTCA to patients with postinfarction angina and multivessel disease has not been studied adequately; however, current evidence suggests that, although the rate of technical success is comparable to that achieved in patients with single vessel disease, the rate of complications and recurrent angina are significantly higher in patients with multivessel disease.[56,61,62] In summary, angioplasty can be performed with a high degree of technical success in selected patients with a low early and late mortality but is associated with a relatively high complication rate and recurrence of symptoms that will culminate in a second revascularization procedure in approximately one-third of patients in whom it is performed under these circumstances.

CABG

The role of CABG in patients with unstable postinfarction angina has always been controversial. Despite its clear effectiveness in reducing recurrent symptoms, infarct extension, and long-term mortality, it has historically been associated with high early mortality rates. An early study by Dawson et al.,[62a] in 1974, reported an operative mortality of 38% in patients who had undergone CABG within 1 week of AMI. The mor-

TABLE 36-1. Early and Late Results Following PTCA

Investigators	Year	n	Technical Success (%)	MI (%)	Procedure-Related Mortality (%)	Emergent CABG (%)	Long-term Follow-up				
							Mean Follow-up (mo)	Mortality (%)	MI (%)	Angina (%)	PTCA (%)	CABG (%)
Gottlieb et al.[53]	1987	47	91	4.7	2.3	2.3	16	0	3	19	13	5
Safian et al.[a55]	1987	68	87	1.5	0	2	17	0	2	41	24	7
Suryapranata et al.[54]	1988	114	91	5	0	7.1	20	0	6	32	18	6
Hopkins et al.[52]	1988	54	81	0	0	3.7	11	0	2.3	25	19	7
Holt et al.[51]	1988	69	80	NA	2	14.5	21	0	3.6	24	13	9
de Feyter, et al.[50]	1991	53	87	8	0	9	6	0	2	26	6.5	13

Abbreviations: NA, not available; MI, myocardial infarction; PTCA, percutaneous transluminal angioplasty; CABG, coronary artery bypass grafting.
[a] Includes only non-Q wave AMI.

tality decreased by one-half (16%) when surgery was performed during weeks 2 through 4 and by one-half again (5.8%) if surgical intervention could be delayed into the second month after AMI.[3] Other studies supported these findings. As Hill et al.[3] concluded, "In patients with recent infarction and impending extension, the risk of surgery appears to be prohibitively high." During the 20 years since that report, the expectations from surgical intervention in this high-risk subset of patients has improved in conjunction with advancements in operative techniques, myocardial preservation, anesthesia, and perioperative care.

Although operative mortality for early surgical intervention in postinfarction patients is still excessive, it now approaches that for elective coronary artery bypass surgery. Recent studies demonstrate that operative mortality for patients with unstable postinfarction angina, operated on within the first 30 days following AMI, ranges between 5% and 9% (Table 36-2). Long-term mortality in these patient series ranged

from 0% to 7.5%, and the incidence of recurrent angina was 4 to 28% in studies with mean follow-ups of 13 to 69 months. Actuarial survival at 1 year is reported to be 96% and ranges from 83% to 88% at 5 years[63-66] (Fig. 36-3)

Risk Factors in CABG

Timing

Probably the most difficult clinical decision to make when contemplating CABG for these patients is optimal timing of the operation. This decision continues to be an ongoing dilemma for cardiologists and surgeons because it is difficult to study; patients requiring emergent operative intervention are those with the greatest hemodynamic instability, hence the highest operative risk. Naturally, those who can be sustained medically, and for whom operative intervention is delayed, are better surgical candidates. Even in the pa-

TABLE 36-2. Early and Late Results of CABG

Investigators	Year	n	Mean Age	Interval AMI-CABG (days)	Mean EF (%)	OM (%)	Long-term Follow-up		
							Mean Follow-up (Months)	Late Mortality (%)	Angina (%)
Levine et al.[77]	1979	80	52	<30	NA	8.8	33	1	20
Jones et al.[66]	1981	116	53	<30	55	0	14	4.3	28
Molina et al.[78]	1983	38	61	<14	34	10.5	36	5.2	NA
Williams et al.[70]	1983	103	58	<30	NA	1.9	15.4	1	4
Rankin et al.[79]	1984	52	NA	<30	45	3.8	24	8	NA
Baumgartner et al.[80]	1984	34	59	<30	52	9	13.7	3	4
Singh et al.[81]	1985	108	59	<30	NA	1.8	35	7.5	27
Breyer et al.[46]	1985	75	61	<30	54	8	13	0	7.4
DiSesa et al.[65]	1985	110	57	<42	19	12.7	NA	NA	NA
Jones et al.[48]	1987	107	NA	<30	NA	8.4	29.4	2.2	14
Naunheim et al.[74]	1988	185	NA	<30	NA	6.5	NA	NA	NA
Connolly et al.[64]	1988	96	65	<42	48	7.3	21	2.3	5
Kouchoukos et al.[69]	1989	240	63	<30	NA	3.3	NA	NA	NA
Gardner et al.[63]	1989	300	62	<30	47	5	22.3	5.5	NA
Curtis et al.[71]	1991	993	61	<84	NA	4.9	NA	NA	NA

Abbreviations: EF, ejection fraction; OM, operative mortality.

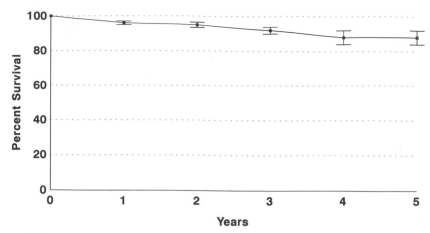

Fig. 36-3. Actuarial survival. (From Gardner et al.,[63] with permission.)

tient who is hemodynamically stable, however, evidence of recurrent ischemia despite maximal medical therapy identifies an unstable patient. In a study reported by Fraker et al.,[23] recurrent infarction occurred an average of only 3.4 days after an AMI in patients with postinfarction angina and carried a 36% mortality. In a similar study, by Singer and associates,[67] the mortality for patients readmitted to the coronary care unit (CCU) for evidence of recurrent postinfarction ischemia was 26%. It is therefore important to distinguish those patients with stable postinfarction angina from those with unstable postinfarction angina, and not to delay surgical intervention in the latter for fear of the operative mortality alone. Even in a classic study recommending a "concerted effort at preoperative medical stabilization prior to CABG surgery in patients with persistent refractory myocardial ischemia soon after acute myocardial necrosis," Roberts and co-workers[68] were able to achieve "medical stabilization" in only 12 of the 20 patients.

The surgical literature has continued to address the issue of the most appropriate timing for revascularization in this population. In a study of 240 patients, Kouchoukos et al.[69] reported a 30-day mortality of 3.3% for patients who underwent bypass surgery for persistent or recurrent ischemia and did not find any relationship between the timing of surgery after infarction and operative mortality. Breyer et al.[46] reported an overall operative mortality of 8% in 75 patients who underwent CABG within 30 days of AMI. Only the presence of decreased ejection fraction was associated with an increased risk of mortality. Williams et al.[70] reported on 103 patients under similar circumstances and noted that, despite the increased need for inotropic agents and intra-aortic balloon pumping (IABP) and the increased occurrence of arrhythmias and perioperative infarctions in those operated on earlier after infarction, there was no association between the time

of operation after infarct and early or late mortality. In a series of 300 consecutive patients reported by Gardner et al.,[63] the location of the infarct and the need for a preoperative IABP, but not the timing of revascularization, were determined independent predictors of operative mortality. Finally, the largest and most recent report to address this question was a retrospective study by Curtis et al.,[71] which discussed 993 patients who underwent isolated CABG for postinfarction angina. The time from AMI to CABG was divided into five intervals (Fig. 36-4). Although the operative mortality was three times higher in patients operated on within the first 24 hours of AMI compared with those whose surgery was undertaken between 1 and 3 weeks, stepwise logistic regression analysis did not demonstrate the interval from AMI to be a significant operative risk variable. Unstable angina was the strongest predictor of mortality. Curtis and colleagues concluded that, in patients with stable postinfarction angina, operative mortality with CABG is not increased despite a recent AMI.

Cardiogenic Shock

The presence of cardiogenic shock after an MI is associated with a high mortality.[72,73] Patients with postinfarction angina accompanied by cardiogenic shock continue to represent a formidable therapeutic challenge. Naunheim et al.[74] reported, that, compared with postinfarction patients operated on for indications of unstable angina, the operative mortality for patients with postinfarction angina complicated by cardiogenic shock is nearly eight times higher (6.1% versus 47.8%). In another report, DiSesa and colleagues[65] reviewed their experience with 110 patients with postinfarction angina and noted that the operative mortality for patients who underwent CABG within the first 2 weeks after AMI dropped from 20% to

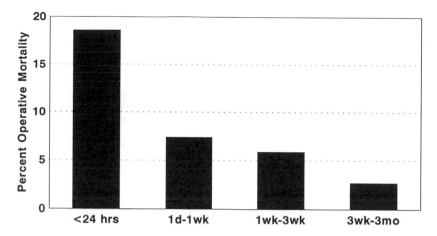

Fig. 36-4. Mortality versus recency of surgery for acute myocardial infarction. (From Curtis et al.,[71] with permission.)

0%, when patients in cardiogenic shock were excluded. The overall operative mortality for patients in cardiogenic shock operated on within the first 6 weeks of AMI was 61%. Other indicators of severe LV dysfunction, including low preoperative ejection fractions and the need for a preoperative IABP, have also been shown to be predictors of operative mortality.[46,63]

There is still no consensus on the appropriate timing of surgery in this specific group either. The use of more effective pharmacologic treatment, ventricular assist devices, and the IABP has improved the overall outcome of patients with cardiogenic shock, but only when combined with subsequent revascularization.[72] In a review of 75 patients who had surgical revascularization for postinfarction angina within 4 weeks of AMI, Breyer and co-workers[46] demonstrated that decreased ejection fraction was a statistically significant risk factor for operative mortality. However, in this same population, the interval between operative intervention and AMI was not associated with increased risk of mortality. Similarly, Katz et al.[75] reported that in 26% of patients undergoing CABG within 4 weeks of AMI, postoperative cardiac failure had developed. Preoperative failure (defined as the need for inotropic support), ejection fraction less than 45%, and preoperative ischemia were determined to be significant risk factors of postoperative cardiac failure. Again, the time interval between AMI and the operation was not found to be an important predictor of cardiac failure. One study that supports postponement of surgery in these patients, although not by any statistical measure, is reported by Jones et al.[48] These investigators simply noted that the only patients who died with postinfarction angina complicated by shock were those who underwent CABG within 7 days of AMI. The study by Hochberg and colleagues[76] which advocated delay of surgical revascularization by at least 4 weeks for patients with an ejection fraction of less than 50%,

was confined to those patients in whom operative timing was considered elective. Hochberg's group acknowledged that more critically ill patients may require emergent revascularization.

Other risk factors that have been shown repeatedly, but not consistently, to affect the outcome of operative intervention in patients with postinfarction angina include female gender, older age, anterior or transmural infarction, and previous surgical revascularization.[46,63,64,71,74,75] In the first large study, in which it is known to have been evaluated in this population, failed PTCA was reported to be a potential risk factor for operative mortality.[71]

CONCLUSIONS

On the basis of these studies, we advise that patients with postinfarction angina receive aggressive medical management, including the pharmacologic treatment proved effective for patients with unstable angina and the use of an IABP for hemodynamic instability. In patients refractory to these measures, urgent angiography is indicated. Coronary angioplasty should be considered in the patient with good function and proximal single vessel disease (other than the left main coronary artery) that is morphologically suitable for this procedure. For patients with significant left main, two vessel, or three vessel coronary artery disease, CABG should be considered.

REFERENCES

1. Pell S, Fayerweather WE: Trends in the incidence of myocardial infarction and in the associated mortality and morbidity in a large employed population, 1957–1983. N Engl J Med 312:1005, 1985

2. Pryor DB, Harrell FE, Jr, Lee KL et al: An improving prognosis over time in medically treated patients with coronary artery disease. Am J Cardiol 52:444, 1983

3. Hill JD, Kerth WJ, Kelly JJ et al: Emergency aortocoronary bypass for impending or extendind myocardial infarction. Circulation 44:I–105, 1971

4. Malliani A, Lombardi F: Consideration of the fundamental mechanisms eliciting cardiac pain. Am Heart J 103: 575, 1982

5. Laffel GI, Braunwald E: Thrombolytic therapy. A new strategy for the treatment of acute myocardial infarction. N Engl J Med 311:710, 1984

6. Gibson RS, Young PM, Boden WE et al: Prognostic significance and beneficial effect of diltiazem on the incidence of early recurrent ischemia after non-Q-wave myocardial infarction: results from the Multicenter Diltiazem Reinfarction Study. Am J Cardiol 60:203, 1987

7. Ouyang P, Chandra NC, Gottlieb SO: Frequency and importance of silent myocardial ischemia with ambulatory electrocardiographic monitoring in the early in-hospital period after acute myocardial infarction. Am J Cardiol 65:267, 1990

8. Gottlieb SO, Weisfeldt ML, Ouyang P et al: Silent ischemia as a marker for early unfavorable outcomes in patients with unstable angina. N Engl J Med 314:1214, 1986

9. Nademanee K, Intarachot V, Josephson MA et al: Prognostic significance of silent myocardial ischemia in patients with unstable angina. J Am Coll Cardiol 10:1, 1987

10. Biagini A, Testa R, Carpeggiani C et al: Detection of spontaneous episodes in post-infarction angina. Comparison between CCU and Holter monitoring. Eur Heart J 7:43, 1986

11. Brower RW, Fioretti P, Simoons M et al: Surgical versus non-surgical management of patients soon after acute myocardial infarction. Br Heart J 54:460, 1985

12. Lofmark R: T wave changes and postinfarction angina pectoris predictive of recurrent myocardial infarction. Br Heart J 45:512, 1981

13. Marmor A, Sobel BE, Roberts R: Factors presaging early recurrent myocardial infarction ("extension"). Am J Cardiol 48:603, 1981

14. Schuster EH, Bulkley BH: Early post-infarction angina. Ischemia at a distance and the infarct zone. N Engl J Med 305:1101, 1981

15. Madigan NP, Rutherford BD, Frye RL: The clinical course, early prognosis and coronary anatomy of subendocardial infarction. Am J Med 60:634, 1976

16. Bosch X, Theroux P, Waters DD et al: Early postinfarction ischemia: clinical, angiographic, and significance. Circulation 75:988, 1987

17. Hutter AM, DeScanctis RW, Flynn T et al: Nontransmural myocardial infarction: a comparison of hospital and late clinical course of patients with that of matched patients with transmural anterior and transmural inferior myocardial infarction. Am J Cardiol 48:595, 1981

18. Matthews E, Amsterdam EA, Lee G et al: Occurence of angina pectoris in relation to history of myocardial infarction: lack of abolition of angina by infarction, abstracted. Circulation, suppl 3. 55/56:III-5, 1977

19. Gruppo Italiano per lo Studio della Streptochinasi nell'Infarto Miocardico (GISSI): Effectiveness of intravenous thrombolytic treatment in acute myocardial infarction. Lancet 1:397, 1986

20. ISIS-2 (Second International Study of Infarct Survival) Collaborative Group: Randomised trial of intravenous streptokinase, oral aspirin, both, or neither among 17187 cases of suspected acute myocardial infarction: ISIS-2. Lancet 2:349, 1988

21. Stenson RE, Flamm MD, Zaret BL et al: Transient ST-segment elevation with postmyocardial infarction angina: prognostic significance. Am Heart J 89:449, 1975

22. Maisel AS, Ahnve S, Gilpin E et al: Prognosis after extension of myocardial infarct: the role of Q or non-Q wave infarction. Circulation 71:211, 1985

23. Fraker TD, Jr, Wagner GS, Rosati RA: Extension of myocardial infarction: incidence and prognosis. Circulation 60:1126, 1979

24. Gilpin E, Ricou F, Dittrich H et al: Factors associated with recurrent myocardial infarction within year after acute myocardial infarction. Am Heart J 121:457, 1991

25. Schuster EH, Bulkley BH: Ischemia at a distance after acute myocardial infarction: a cause of early postinfarction angina. Circulation 62:509, 1980

26. Ouyang P, Shapiro EP, Gottlieb SO: Thrombolysis in postinfarction angina. Am J Cardiol 68:119B, 1991

27. DeServi S, Vaccari L, Graziano G et al: Clinical and angiographic data in early post-infarction angina. Eur Heart J, suppl C. 7:69, 1986

28. Midwall J, Ambrose J, Pichard A et al: Angina pectoris before and after myocardial infarction. Angiographic correlations. Chest 81:681, 1982

29. Lo YS, Abi Mansour P, Kaplan KJ et al: Angiographic coronary morphology in postinfarction angina. Cathet Cardiovasc Diagn 16:155, 1989

30. Lange RA, Cigarroa RG, Hillis LD: Angiographic characteristics of the infarct-related coronary artery in patients with angina pectoris after myocardial infarction. Am J Cardiol 64:257, 1989

31. Ambrose JA, Winters S, Stern A et al: Angiographic morphology and the pathogenesis of unstable angina pectoris. J Am Coll Cardiol 5:609, 1985

32. Levin DC, Fallon JT: Significance of the angiographic morphology of localized stenoses: histopathologic correlations. Circulation 66:316, 1982

33. Bresnahan DR, Davis JL, Holmes DR, Jr et al: Angiographic occurrence and clinical correlates of intraluminal coronary artery thrombus: role of unstable angina. J Am Coll Cardiol 6:285, 1985

34. Hamada Y, Matsuda Y, Takashiba K et al: Multivessel coronary artery spasm causing myocardial infarction and postinfarction angina. Am Heart J 113:1024, 1987

35. Moran TJ, French WJ, Abrams HF et al: Postmyocardial infarction angina and coronary spasm. Am J Cardiol 50: 197, 1982

36. Furchgott RF: Role of endothelium in responses of vascular smooth muscle. Circ Res 53:557, 1983

37. Ginsburg R, Bristow MR, Davis K et al: Quantitative pharmacologic responses of normal and isolated human epicardial coronary arteries. Circulation 69:430, 1984

38. Ludmer PL, Selwyn AP, Shook TL et al: Paradoxical vasoconstriction induced by acetylcholine in atherosclerotic coronary arteries. N Engl J Med 315:1046, 1986

39. Forstermann U, Mugge A, Alheid U et al: Selective attenuation of endothelium-mediated vasodilation in atherosclerotic human coronary arteries. Circ Res 62:185, 1988

40. Mehta JL, Nichols WW, Donnelly WH et al: Impaired canine coronary vasodilator response to acetylcholine bradykinin after occlusion-reperfusion. Circ Res 64:43, 1989

41. Hodgson JM, Marshall JJ: Direct vasoconstriction and endothelium-dependent vasodilation. Mechanisms of acetylcholine effects on coronary flow and diameter in patients with nonstenotic coronary arteries. Circulation 79:1043, 1989

42. VanBenthuysen KM, McMurtry IF, Horwitz, LD: Reperfusion after acute coronary occlusion in dogs impairs endothelium-dependent relaxation to acetylcholine and augments contractile reactivity in vitro. J Clin Invest 79:265, 1987

43. Gleckel L, Wulkan S, Koss JH et al: Significance of postinfarction angina in patients with single vessel disease, abstracted. J Am Coll Cardiol 7:208A, 1986

44. A report of the Holland Interuniversity Nifedipin/Metoprolol trial (HINT) research group: Early treatment of unstable angina in the coronary care unit: a randomised, double blind, placebo controlled comparison of ischaemia in patients treated with nifedipine or metoprolol or Report of the Holland Interuniversity Nifedipine/Metoprolol (HINT) Research Group. Br Heart J 56:400, 1986

45. Gottlieb SO, Weisfeldt ML, Ouyang P et al: Effect of the addition of propranolol to therapy with nifedipine unstable angina pectoris: a randomized, double-blind, placebo-controlled trial. Circulation 73:331, 1986

46. Breyer RH, Engelman RM, Rousou JA et al: Postinfarction angina: an expanding subset of patients undergoing coronary artery bypass. J Thorac Cardiovasc Surg 90:532, 1985

47. Theroux P, Quimet H, McCans J et al: Aspirin, heparin or both to treat acute unstable angina. N Engl J Med 319:1105, 1988

48. Jones RN, Pifarre R, Sullivan HJ et al: Early myocardial revascularization for postinfarction angina. Ann Thorac Surg 44:159, 1987

49. Epstein SE, Palmeri ST, Patterson RE: Evaluation of patients after acute myocardial infarction. Indications for cardiac catheterizations and surgical intervention. N Engl J Med 307:1467, 1982

50. de Feyter PJ, Serruys PW, Brand M et al: Percutaneous transluminal coronary angioplasty for unstable postinfarction angina. Am J Cardiol 68:125B, 1991

51. Holt GW, Gersh BJ, Holmes DR, Jr et al: Results of percutaneous transluminal coronary angioplasty for pectoris early after acute myocardial infarction. Am J Cardiol 61:1238, 1988

52. Hopkins J, Savage M, Zalewski A et al: Recurrent ischemia in the zone of prior myocardial infarction: results of coronary angioplasty of the infarct-related artery. Am Heart J 115:14, 1988

53. Gottlieb SO, Walford GD, Ouyang P: Initial and late results of coronary angioplasty for early postinfarction angina. Cathet Cardiovasc Diagn 13:93, 1987

54. Suryapranata H, Beatt K, de Feyter PJ et al: Percutaneous transluminal coronary angioplasty for angina after a

non-Q-wave acute myocardial infarction. Am J Cardiol 61:240, 1988

55. Safian RD, Snyder LD, Snyder BA et al: Usefulness of percutaneous transluminal coronary angioplasty for unstable angina pectoris after non-Q-wave acute myocardial infarction. Am J Cardiol 59:263, 1987

56. de Feyter PJ, Serruys PW, Arnold A et al: Coronary angioplasty of the unstable angina related vessel in patients with multivessel coronary artery disease. Eur Heart J 7:460, 1986

57. Sabbah HN, Brymer JF, Gheorghiade M et al: Left ventricular function after successful percutaneous transluminal coronary angioplasty for postinfarction angina pectoris. Am J Cardiol 62:358, 1988

58. de Feyter PJ, Suryapranata H, Serruys PW et al: Effects of successful percutaneous transluminal coronary on global and regional left ventricular function in unstable pectoris. Am J Cardiol 60:993, 1987

59. Hurley DV, Bresnahan DR, Holmes DR, Jr: Staged thrombolysis and percutaneous transluminal coronary angioplasty for unstable and postinfarction angina. Cathet Cardiovasc Diagn 18:67, 1989

60. Cameron J, Buchbinder M, Wexler L et al: Thromboembolic complications of percutaneous transluminal angioplasty for myocardial infarction. Cathet Cardiovasc Diagn 13:100, 1987

61. Wohlgelernter D, Cleman M, Highman HA et al: Percutaneous transluminal coronary angioplasty of the "culprit lesion" for management of unstable angina pectoris in patients multivessel coronary artery disease. Am J Cardiol 58:460, 1986

62. Cowley MJ, Vetrovec GW, DiSciascio G et al: Coronary angioplasty of multiple vessels: short and long term results. Circulation 72:1314, 1985

62a. Dawson, JT, Hall RJ, Hallman GL et al: Mortality in patients undergoing coronary artery bypass surgery after myocardial infarction. Am J Cardiol 33:483, 1974

63. Gardner TJ, Stuart RS, Greene PS et al: The risk of coronary bypass surgery for patients with postinfarction angina. Circulation 79:179, 1989

64. Connolly MW, Gelbfish JS, Rose DM et al: Early coronary artery bypass grafting for complicated acute myocardial infarction. J Cardiovasc Surg (Torino) 29:375, 1988

65. DiSesa VJ, O'Neil AC, Bitran D et al: Aggressive surgical management of postinfarction angina: results of myocardial revascularization early after transmural infarction (predictors of mortality). Ann Thorac Surg 48:757, 1989

66. Jones EL, Waites TF, Craver JM et al: Coronary bypass for relief of persistent pain following acute myocardial infarction. Ann Thorac Surg 32:33, 1981

67. Singer DE, Mulley AG, Thibault GE et al: Unexpected readmissions to the coronary-care unit during from acute myocardial infarction. N Engl J Med 304:625, 1981

68. Roberts AJ, Sanders JH, Jr, Moran JH et al: The efficacy of medical stabilization prior to myocardial revascularization in early refractory postinfarction angina. Ann Surg 197:91, 1983

69. Kouchoukos NT, Murphy S, Philpott T et al: Coronary artery bypass grafting for postinfarction angina pectoris. Circulation 79:168, 1989

70. Williams DB, Ivey TD, Bailey WW et al: Postinfarction

angina: results of early revascularization. J Am Coll Cardiol 2:859, 1983

71. Curtis JJ, Walls JT, Salam NH et al: Impact of unstable angina on operative mortality with coronary revascularization at varying time intervals after myocardial infarction. J Thorac Cardiovasc Surg 102:867, 1991

72. Johnson SA, Scanlon PJ, Loeb HS et al: Treatment of cardiogenic shock in myocardial infarction by intraaortic balloon counterpulsation surgery. Am J Med 62:687, 1977

73. Alonso DR, Scheidt S, Post M et al: Pathophysiology of cardiogenic shock. Quantification of necrosis, clinical, pathologic and electrocardiographic. Circulation 48:588, 1973

74. Naunheim KS, Kesler KA, Kanter KR et al: Coronary artery bypass for recent infarction. Predictors of mortality. Circulation 78:I122, 1988

75. Katz NM, Kubanick TE, Ahmed SW et al: Determinants of cardiac failure after coronary bypass surgery 30 days of acute myocardial infarction. Ann Thorac Surg 42:658, 1986

76. Hochberg MS, Parsonnet V, Gielchinsky I et al: Timing of coronary revascularization after acute myocardial infarction. Early and late results in patients revascularized seven weeks. J Thorac Cardiovasc Surg 88:914, 1984

77. Levine FH, Gold HK, Leinbach RC et al: Safe early revascularization for continuing ischemia after acute myocardial infarction. Circulation 60:I5, 1979

78. Molina JE, Dorsey JS, Emanuel DA et al: Coronary bypass operation for early postinfarction angina. Surg Gynecol Obstet 157:455, 1983

79. Rankin JS, Newton JR, Jr, Califf RM et al: Clinical characteristics and current management of medically refractory unstable angina. Ann Surg 200:457, 1984

80. Baumgartner WA, Borkon AM, Zibulewsky J et al: Operative intervention for postinfarction angina. Ann Thorac Surg 38:265, 1984

81. Singh AK, Rivera R, Cooper GN, Jr et al: Early myocardial revascularization for postinfarction angina: results and long-term follow-up. J Am Coll Cardiol 6:1121, 1985

37

Preoperative Risk Assessment, Operative Risk, and Survival After Valve Replacement for Aortic Stenosis

Ole Lund

EPIDEMIOLOGIC FEATURES AND TREATMENT OF CHOICE

The prospect for patients with significant and symptomatic aortic stenosis has changed completely since the introduction of aortic valve replacement some 30 years ago. By contrast, the prognostic outlook for patients on optimal medical treatment has not changed from the 1940s[1] until today,[2] the average survival time being 4.5 years after the onset of angina, 3 years after the first episode of syncope, and less than 1 year after the onset of congestive heart failure (CHF). At the present stage of open heart surgery, an operative mortality of less than 1% and a normal sex- and age-specific long-term survival after valve replacement for aortic stenosis are achievable goals.[3–6]

The actual incidence of aortic stenosis in the Western world is not known but is apparently rising, despite the massive reduction in the incidence of rheumatic fever during this century.[7] At Aarhus University Hospital in Denmark, we performed valve replacement for aortic stenosis in 8, 20, 30, and 50 patients per one million inhabitants in our well-defined catchment area in 1970, 1980, 1985, and 1989, respectively.[3] In addition, aortic stenosis has surpassed mitral disease as the most common single cause of heart valve surgery in Western centers[2,3,8]; of 1,001 patients who had primary heart valve replacement performed at our center during 1976 to 1986, 49% had isolated aortic stenosis, 13% had aortic regurgitation (including patients with endocarditis or associated stenosis), 28% had mitral valve replacement (or reconstruction), and 10% had double (or triple) valve replacement.[3] In high-risk areas for rheumatic fever, such as India, 65% had isolated mitral valve disease and 16% had combined mitral and aortic disease.[9] An etiologic shift from rheumatic valvulitis to acquired stenosis in bicuspid aortic valves and an increasing fraction of elderly patients with dystrophic calcification of a tricuspid valve in the Western world are part of the explanation.[10]

This increase in the incidence of patients with acquired aortic stenosis who were operated on could have several explanations, of which increasing longevity of the population is one. In particular, the increase during the 1970s is without doubt to a large extent related to an increasing willingness to operate before end-stage disease was prevalent,[4,5] as well as to a decreasing reluctance to refer patient to heart centers for presurgical investigation. The increase through the 1980s is probably explained in part by the spread of echocardiography either alone or in combination with the Doppler technique, which has made a reliable diagnosis readily available outside heart centers. The gradual upward displacement of an age limit for aortic valve replacement[4,5,11] also played a role, as did the renewed interest in aortic stenosis in the elderly spurred by the introduction in 1986 of balloon valvuloplasty as a possible alternative to valve replacement in elderly patients.[12]

The enthusiasm surrounding this new and appealing treatment modality for calcific aortic stenosis in the elderly, percutaneous balloon valvuloplasty, has already faded 5 years after its introduction. As long-term follow-up studies became available, a significant problem of early restenosis materialized.[13,14] The failure rate now closely resembles that of open heart, direct-vision debridement of calcium combined with commisurotomy performed in the late 1950s and early 1960s: the failure rate (death, restenosis) approached 100% within 3 to 5 years after the procedure.[15–17] At the 1990 Annual Meeting of the European Society of Cardiology, it was concluded that balloon valvuloplasty was not an alternative to aortic valve replacement.[18–20] The key results were 2- and 3-year cumulative freedoms from failure of 25%[18] and 7%,[19] respectively, and a 3-year survival rate of no more than 28%.[19] In contrast to such results stand those obtained after valve replacement for calcific aortic stenosis in patients aged 70 years or more at our institution: the early mortality (≤30 days after the operation) was reduced to 3% by consistently performing concomitant coronary artery bypass grafting (CABG) in case of associated significant coronary artery disease (CAD) (47% of patients), and the patients surviving 30 days had a normal sex- and age-specific long-term survival (5-year survival of 75%); 1 year after the operation, 63% of the surviving patients were asymptomatic and another 30% had only minor functional disability; more than 60% of the linearized rate of prosthesis-related cerebral events (embolism, hemorrhage) of 2.7% per patient-year could be accounted for by the normal stroke rate in the background population of this age group.[6] Aortic valve replacement in octogenarians has been performed with good results.[21]

The appalling prognosis for patients on medical treatment and the failure of balloon valvuloplasty to give lasting palliation thus leave aortic valve replacement almost supremely reigning in the treatment of aortic stenosis in adult patients.

CONTROVERSY IN TIMING OF OPERATION

Today, timing of valve replacement for aortic stenosis is largely determined by three conventions. The first of these is that aortic stenosis is characterized by slow anatomic progression over decades with a gradual and discrete onset of symptoms[2]; this offers ample time for surgical intervention. Turina and associates[22] found it advisable to postpone operation in patients with significant aortic stenosis and functional class 2 symptoms until marked symptomatic deterioration.

The second convention has as an integral part the afterload mismatch theory was proposed by Ross.[23] It is an old observation that patients with aortic stenosis and severely reduced left ventricular ejection fraction (LVEF) may recover completely after a successful valve replacement, with the ejection fraction returning to normal.[24] There is a strong inverse relationship between afterload (systolic wall stress) and ejection fraction and other systolic function indices,[23,25] and the primary impact of valve replacement is a reduction of the systolic pressure load and thus the afterload on the left ventricle. The afterload mismatch theory states that, in spite of normal intrinsic myocardial function, reduced ejection fraction may result from excessive wall stress and inadequate hypertrophy when the preload and inotropic reserve are used; the ejection fraction can be extrapolated back to a normal value, provided the afterload can be reduced.[23,26] Urgent operation in patients with reduced LV systolic function should thus in many cases be unnecessary.[26]

As the cornerstone of the third convention, "prosthetic valve disease" fits beautifully into the former two. The risk of prosthetic valve-related complications (e.g., thromboembolism, anticoagulant related bleeding) is an argument for postponing the operation. The prevailing attitude is that late results after aortic valve replacement depend on the prosthesis.[10,22,26–29] Quoting Selzer's words from 1987: "The prognosis and natural history in patients with prosthetic aortic valves become those of the prosthesis rather than those of the underlying disease in terms of morbidity and mortality."[10]

Most investigators thus find little or no place for operative intervention early during the course of aortic stenosis.[10,22,26,27,29,30] Recent reports from large American and European centers accordingly show that 80 to 94% of patients were in functional classes 3 to 4 before aortic valve replacement.[8,31–33]

However, recent results contradict the role of afterload mismatch in more than a few patients with aortic stenosis. Those with severe CHF symptoms prior to valve replacement have the most dilated hearts (increased pre- and afterload, reduced ventricular function) and the highest left ventricular end-diastolic pressure (i.e., increased preload).[3] Patients with afterload mismatch should be looked for in this group, and the pronounced and almost obligatory functional and objective recovery early after the operation is in good agreement with the afterload mismatch theory.[34] However, this early improvement of the patients has proved to be only of short duration. Recurrence of CHF and cardiac dilation was determined by their preoperative state, thus indicating irreversible myocardial disease.[34] Using a preload independent measure of intrinsic LV function, Wiesenbaugh and associates[35] also questioned the quantitative importance of the afterload mismatch theory. They found that rather than afterload mismatch and inadequate hypertrophy, impaired contractability secondary to extensive hypertrophy in patients with normal systolic wall stress was the predominant cause of reduced pump function in aortic stenosis.

Recent reports from our institution clearly show that "prosthetic valve disease" is a problem that can be differentiated in patients who have been operated on both for aortic stenosis and for aortic regurgitation.[36,37] Factors underlying advanced preoperative heart failure and coronary artery disease (CAD) (as well as the use of porcine bioprostheses, because of late tissue failure, and the obsolete Lillehei-Kaster valve) independently determined the long-term rate of these complications. The 10-year freedom from thromboembolism was as high as 98% in the absence of risk factors.[36] By using the risk of "prosthetic valve disease" to postpone operation, in essence one achieves nothing more than producing or intensifying the problem.

The timing of operation for aortic stenosis is thus controversial. Operative intervention earlier in the course of the disease than is customary today becomes desirable, however, if it can be demonstrated that the result is an overall normal sex- and age-specific long-term survival.[3]

THE 1965 TO 1986 AARHUS SERIES

The Aarhus series consists of 690 consecutive patients operated on at our institution during 1965 to 1986. The 690 patients (male-to-female ratio 2.4:1; age 14 to 78, mean 59 years) had an average peak-to-peak systolic aortic valve gradient of 96 mmHg. Functional class 3 or 4 symptoms were prevalent in 71% of patients, and 38% had had LV failure (pulmonary edema or auscultatory and radiographically verified pulmonary congestion) within 1 year before the operation.[4] A Starr-Edwards caged ball valve was implanted in 78% of patients, a disk valve in 20% (St. Jude valve in 15%), and a porcine bioprosthesis in 2%.[4] All patients

except 8 of 15 who received a bioprosthesis were started on lifelong coumadin treatment 1 day after the operation. We previously showed that the old Starr-Edwards valve, and, not least, the Silastic ball valve, which is still in use, have long-term performance rates comparable to those of the St. Jude bileaflet disk valve.[38,39]

All operations were performed during complete cold crystalloid cardioplegic cardiac arrest. Bretschneider's acalcemic and hyponatremic cardioplegic principle[40-43] has been used consistently at our center since 1964.[44] This is an important consideration in studies dealing with predictability of early and late prognosis after valve replacement: the prognostic information of a preoperative risk factor is preserved through the operation to a far higher degree than is the case with operations without crystalloid cardioplegia.[3] Intraoperative anoxic damage is significantly minimized by crystalloid cardioplegic heart arrest.[45-48] This was demonstrated by Kirklin,[49] who found that an incremental risk factor for early mortality after aortic valve replacement, such as ischemic (aortic cross-clamp) time, lost its importance after the introduction of crystalloid cardioplegia: only the functional class (i.e., a measure of degree of preoperatively deranged heart status) still had prognostic value. Some studies have shown Bretschneider's principle and the hyperkalemic principle to be equally protective in terms of intraoperative anoxic myocardial damage,[46,50] while Schnabel and associates[51] found the former method advantageous. The value of crystalloid cardioplegia received no general worldwide acceptance until the late 1970s or early 1980s.

Evaluation and Stratification of Operative Risk

The hazard rate (instantaneous death rate) dropped by a factor of 6 from the first to second postoperative month in our series. Hereafter it remained at a low and primarily constant level during the more than 20 years of follow-up. *Thirty days was consequently chosen as the cutoff point in the analysis of early mortality after the operation.*[4]

Thirty-day mortality rate was 8.7 in the total 22-year series.[4] Early mortality was 20% for the first 100 consecutive operations (until October 1972), 7.8% for the ensuing 490 (until June 1985), and 2% for the last 100.[4] These time-specific mortality rates are in good agreement with results from numerous studies; the reduction over time is in part related to a trend toward earlier operation.[4]

A total of 45 of 60 (75%) early deaths had cardiogenic causes, while none was related to the prosthetic valve. Autopsy in 57 of these deaths revealed significant stenotic or occlusive CAD in 36 (63%); CABG concomitant with valve replacement had been performed in only two of these patients.[4] Unrevascularized CAD thus seemed to be a significant risk factor, but preoperative coronary arteriography was performed in only 205 patients (mainly with angina pectoris as limiting symptom) since 1975.

Aortic stenosis is characterized by concentric LV hypertrophy, which by itself has a significant ischemic potential, especially in the endocardial half of the myocardium.[52-55] Associated CAD thus results in "double ischemic jeopardy." It is therefore reasonable to expect a detailed multivariate stratification of operative risk to turn out successful only if an estimate of (preoperatively undiagnosed) CAD is included as a potential risk factor. For this purpose, we developed a CAD score by logistic regression analysis on the 205 patients with angiography[56] (Table 37-1). In agreement with the results of other investigators,[57,58] a low aortic valve gradient, high age, angina, male gender, and previous MI increased the probability of CAD. By using a cutoff point of 4.37, the score had a positive predictive value of 66% with 16% false-negative results. The score was calculated for all 690 patients and, by using the above cutoff point, the series was divided into 460 patients with a low CAD score (presumed low risk of CAD) and 230 with a high score (presumed high risk of CAD).[4] Autopsy revealed CAD in 93% of 27 early deaths in patients with a high CAD score and in 37% of 30 deaths in patients with a low score.[4] The latter relatively high fraction may be explained by the low sensitivity of the score, but also by simple selection, since CAD in numerous studies, including one by the present group,[56] is a significant risk factor for early mortality.

A simple bivariate risk stratification of the patients indicated that early operative intervention is warranted in aortic stenosis.[4] Early mortality rate was zero in functional class 1 patients (N = 8) with no preoperative digitalis or diuretic treatment and comparable to a rate of 0.9% in 112 functional class 2 patients who also did not receive modifying treatment. Conversely, early mortality rate was 9.1% in 77 class 2 patients who did receive digitalis and/or diuretic treatment and 8.9% in 406 class 3 patients in whom treatment for CHF had no modifying influence. Early mortality was 18.4% in 87 class 4 patients, all of whom received failure treatment. Preoperative digitalis and/or diuretic treatment thus probably served to mask symptoms in functional class 2 patients thereby delaying operation to a prognostically unfavorable point.[4] Long-term survival of 30-day survivors was similarly significantly influenced by preoperative symptom-masking treatment.[5] We found the same influence of preoperative heart failure treatment in our patients who were operated for aortic regurgitation.[59] These findings strongly contradict the above recommendation by Turina and associates,[22] that is, to postpone operation in mildly symptomatic patients until marked symptomatic aggravation is prevalent.

In the multivariate (logistic regression) analysis of the early mortality rate, the early operative period from 1965 to 1971 (N = 79, early mortality rate 21.5%) was an independent risk factor.[4] Thus, some of the deaths occurring during this early era were not explained by patient-related factors (41% of 17 deaths had causes other than cardiogenic, including surgical bleeding, respiratory problems, and infection). Other investigators have noted dependence of time frame in more recent series, but the reduction in the mortality rate of these investigations coincided with the introduction of crystalloid cardioplegia.[60]

Because of the adverse influence of early operative

TABLE 37-1. Prediction (Logistic Regression Model) of Coronary Artery Disease in 205 Patients With Coronary Arteriography, 1975 to 1986[a]

Predictor Variable	b	SE	p
Aortic valve (peak-to-peak systolic) gradient	−0.023	0.005	<0.0001
Patient age	0.093	0.024	<0.001
Angina	1.129	0.409	0.001
Male gender	0.484	0.199	0.01
Previous myocardial infarction	0.525	0.247	0.03
CAD score = $b_1z_1 + b_2z_2 + \ldots + b_iz_i$ = 4.29 ± 1.44, −1.10 to 7.82 (mean ± SD, range)	No. of patients with CAD		
−1.10–4.37 (N = 105)	17 (16%)		
4.38–7.82 (N = 100)	66 (66%)		p <0.0001

Abbreviations: b, regression coefficient; CAD, coronary artery disease; SE, standard error.

[a] The z-value equaled the discrete value for peak-to-peak systolic gradient and age; z for the other variables equaled 1 if the risk factor was present, and −1 if not. The negative regression coefficient of peak-to-peak systolic gradient indicates drecreasing probability of CAD with increasing gradient. Note that the CAD score with 4.38 as point of division had a positive predictive value for CAD of 66% with 16% false-negative results.

(From Lund et al.,[56] with permission.)

era on the early mortality rate, further multivariate analysis was performed on the 611 patients operated on during 1972 to 1986. A large battery of pre- and intraoperative variables were entered into the analysis.[4] The final risk model is shown in Table 37-2. LV failure completely neutralized the influence of age; mortality rate did not differ between age groups in patients with LV failure but rose linearly with age in those without.[4] The problem was circumvented by making a design variable, age X, having the discrete value of age for patients without LV failure and a value of zero (thus neutralizing age), for patients with LV failure; with this modification, age had an independent prognostic value (Table 37-2).

As judged by the regression coefficients of the independent risk factors of the model, LV failure, as full-blown pulmonary edema as well as discrete pulmonary stasis, had by far the strongest predictive value. Reduced LVEF had a rather low, inconsistent value as a mortality predictor after valve replacement for aortic stenosis.[24,61] In agreement with the shortcomings of the afterload mismatch theory, it is therefore tempting to direct an explanation of the present strong role of LV failure as a risk factor for irreversible myocardial disease that primarily affects diastolic function. Severely deranged LV diastolic function is an early key mark in the pathophysiologic changes associated with any form of pressure overload hypertrophy[62-64] and CHF,[65] and even acute pulmonary edema[66] in the presence of normal systolic function are consistent findings.

A high ECG hypertrophy score (calculated from Romhilt and Estes[67]; specificity of greater than 93% for LV hypertrophy[67-69]) also was an incremental risk factor for early mortality[4] (Table 37-2). This is proba-

bly explained by the ischemic potential of hypertrophy. Furthermore, LV systolic[27] and diastolic[70] function are both inversely related to degree of hypertrophy.

Not unexpectedly, a high CAD score was independently related to death rate (Table 37-2). This score emphasized the well-known detrimental influence of associated CAD and the "double ischemic impact" on the myocardium; the influence of a high CAD score was predominantly related to unrevascularized CAD.[4]

The risk stratification of Table 37-2 was highly significant. No deaths occurred in the six low-risk groups, while mortality rose exponentially with risk estimate in the last four groups. The mortality rate (average 2%) was acceptable in groups I-VIII. A main conclusion may be drawn at this point: operative intervention in aortic stenosis in the minimally symptomatic state, before medical (symptom masking) treatment becomes necessary, before episodes of LV failure have occurred, and before pronounced LV hypertrophy is prevalent, results in an early mortality rate approaching zero. One may also tentatively assume that consistent CABG in case of associated CAD may further reduce early mortality rate in the high-risk groups.

Influence of Associated Coronary Artery Disease

Our findings strongly indicate that the prevalence of associated CAD increased through the 22 year operative period.[4] The fraction of patients with a high CAD score increased from below 20% during 1965 to 1969 to almost 40% during 1980 to 1986,[4] while angina as a limiting symptom tripled from 11% to 32%.[3] An increasing fraction of elderly patients is part of the ex-

TABLE 37-2. Multivariate Prediction (Logistic Regression Model) of Early Mortality (≤30 days) in 611 Patients in the 1972 to 1986 Series[a]

Risk Factor[b]	b	SE	p
1. LV failure	5.50	1.72	0.00003
2. Age X	0.15	0.05	0.00004
3. ECG hypertrophy score ≥9	0.56	0.17	0.0007
4. High CAD score	0.42	0.17	0.01

Risk score = $b_1z_1 + b_2z_2 + b_3z_3 + b_4z_4$: mean 3.77 ± 1.97 (standard deviation), range −3.78–6.88; 10 equidistant risk score groups (cutoff points: −2.71, −1.65, . . . , 4.75, 5.81):

	I	II	III	IV	V	VI	VII	VIII	IX	X	Total
No. of patients	4	4	18	24	39	53	88	175	164	42	611
No. of deaths	0	0	0	0	0	0	2	7	21	13	43
Rate (%)[c]	0	0	0	0	0	0	2.3	4.0	12.8	31.0	7.0

Abbreviations: CAD, coronary artery disease; ECG, electrocardiogram; LV, left ventricular.
[a] See Table 37-1 for explanations. Age X had the discrete value of age for patients without and a value of 0 for those with LV failure.
[b] See text.
[c] p <0.0001.
(From Lund et al.,[4] with permission.)

planation.[4] The prevalence of CAD in adult patients with aortic stenosis was 42 to 43% in contemporary series in which no lower age limit for angiography was applied.[3,71]

The expectation of a beneficial influence of CABG concomitant with valve replacement is rational given the "double ischemic jeopardy" of patients with aortic stenosis and associated CAD. Furthermore, most early deaths after open heart surgery in general,[72] and after aortic valve replacement in particular,[3] are related to myocardial ischemia and low cardiac output. However, double operation (i.e., valve replacement and CABG) is still regarded by many as a dangerous procedure. This assumption stems from observations that combined operation carried a considerably higher operative mortality than did isolated valve replacement.[57,58] On the other hand, these results were obtained in series in which crystalloid cardioplegia was not used. Apart from CABG, cardioplegia is the measure that may limit intraoperative and early postoperative anoxic myocardial damage. In series with consistent use of cardioplegia, double operation resulted in early mortality rates of only 2 to 5%.[56,73,74] Nevertheless, omission of coronary angiography and even CABG in cases of proven CAD in patients with aortic stenosis is still advocated,[75–77] and no study has previously shown an independent mortality reducing influence of concomitant CABG.

The influence of a high CAD score, as shown in Table 37-2, was to some extent modified by the coexistence of patients who actually had CABG performed.[4] In order to circumvent this problem and to provide a solution to the above controversy, we analyzed separately 205 patients with preoperative coronary angiography (angio group) and 307 patients without (no-angio group) who were operated on during 1975 to 1986.[56] In the angio group, 122 patients did not have CAD, 55 with CAD underwent valve replacement with

concomitant CABG, while the remaining 28 patients with CAD did not have CABG performed. The patients of the no-angio group were divided into one group of 73 with a high CAD score (Table 37-1; high probability of CAD) and one of 234 with a low score (low probability of CAD).[56]

In the angio group, the patients with CAD were older (mean 65 versus 60 years), comprised more men (83% versus 69%), and had more functional disability (functional classes III-IV in 84% versus 63%) than did those without CAD. The 55 patients with bypassed CAD and the 28 with unbypassed CAD differed in some important aspects: those who underwent CABG had more functional disability and worse and more pronounced CAD (triple vessel or left main stem CAD in 47% versus 14%) than did those without CABG.[56] The patients who underwent CABG thus a priori had a higher operative risk than was true for both patients with unbypassed CAD and those without CAD.

Despite these differences in a priori risk assessment 30-day mortality rate was 4.1% in the 122 patients without CAD, 3.6% in the 55 with CABG, and 17.9% in the 28 with unrevascularized CAD.[56] The results of multivariate analysis are shown in Table 37-3.[56] The relative risk (exp[regression coefficient]) was 0.5 (a decrease as compared with overall risk) in patients with CAD and CABG and 0.6 for those without CAD, while CAD without CABG increased the operative risk by a factor of 3.2 despite the fact that these patients had less pronounced CAD than did those with CABG. Multivariate analysis of the 83 patients with CAD clearly underlined that *omission of CABG was the decisive incremental risk factor.*[56] In patients with CABG, early mortality was 3.4% in case of single or double vessel CAD (N = 29) and 3.8% in case of triple vessel or left main stem CAD (N = 26); in patients without CABG, the figures were 8.3% (N = 24) and 75% (N = 4), respectively.

TABLE 37-3. Multivariate Prediction (Logistic Regression Analysis) of Early Mortality ($\leq$30 Days) in 205 Patients With Preoperative Coronary Angiography, 1975 to 1986[a]

Risk Factor[b]	Regression Coefficient	p	Combination of Risk Factors					
DV level								
1. CAD and CABG	-0.659		x	—	x	—	—	—
2. No CAD	-0.505	0.04	—	x	—	x	—	—
3. CAD, no CABG	1.164		—	—	—	—	x	x
Right ventricular failure	0.796	0.01	—	—	x	x	—	x
No. of patients with combination			44	99	11	23	22	6
No. of early deaths			1	1	1	4	4	1
Rate (%)			2	1	9	17	18	17

Abbreviations: CABG, coronary artery bypass grafting; CAD, coronary artery disease; DV, design variable; x, risk factor present.

[a] The combinations of risk factors were arranged from left to right in order of increasing risk, as indicated by the sum of the regression coefficients of the risk factors included in each combination.

[b] See text.

[c] p <0.01.

(From Lund et al.,[56] with permission.)

In the no-angio group early mortality was 6.4% in the 234 patients with a low CAD score and 16.4% in the 73 with a high score.[56] The results of the multivariate risk analysis in this group (Table 37-4) showed that a high CAD score indicating unrevascularized CAD increased the risk by a factor of 1.5. It is important to realize that angina had no predictive value in any of the risk models.

The overall long-term survivals of the various patient groups are shown in Figure 37-1. CABG did not modify survival after the first 30 postoperative days; the curves for CAD patients with and without CABG ran almost in parallel. For our 30-day survivors, 5-year cumulative survival was 90% in the absence of CAD (N − 117), 71% in single or double vessel CAD, both with (N = 28) and without (N = 22) CABG, and 70% in triple vessel or left main stem CAD with CABG (N = 25). Multivariate (Cox regression) analysis confirmed these observations: CAD was an independent incremental risk factor (relative risk of 2.6) in the 193 patients of the angio group who were alive after 30 days, while CABG had no modifying influence.[56] Also Czer and co-workers[78] were unable to show any beneficial influence of CABG on late survival. Since CABG in isolated CAD prolongs life predominantly in patients with triple vessel or left main stem disease,[79] it is, however, reasonable to assume that our patients with associated triple vessel or left main stem CAD would have been worse off also as regards late survival had they not undergone CABG.

The long-term survival of patients in the no-angio group with a low CAD score (5-year survival in 30-day survivors of 92%) did not differ from that of patients in the angio group without CAD. The patients with a high CAD score had the same overall survival characteristics as patients with CAD and no CABG (Fig. 37-1). Cox analysis in the 280 30-day survivors in the no-angio group showed that a high CAD score was an independent risk factor giving a risk increase of 2.2 comparable to that of CAD in the angio group.[56]

These results prompted our conclusion that coronary arteriography should be performed in all adult patients (at least 20 years of age) with aortic stenosis and that all patients with significant CAD (luminal diameter reduction of 50% or greater), should have CABG performed concomitantly with valve replacement.[56] This has been done consistently at our center since January 1, 1988. Analysis of our surgical series from the following 24 months (1988 + 1989 series) was used for validation of this conclusion.[3]

The 1988 and 1989 series comprised a total of 122 consecutive patients with isolated aortic stenosis. As regards the preoperative risk profile, these patients were comparable to the 1975 to 1986 angio group. Only 2 patients did not have angiography performed; both patients underwent operation on an emergency basis for severe intractable heart failure (1 died). In the remaining 120 patients, angiography showed single or double vessel CAD in 38 (32%) and triple vessel or left main stem CAD in 13 (11%). Early mortality was 2.9% in 69 patients without CAD and 3.9% in 51 with combined valve replacement and CABG.[3] One of the two deaths in the latter group occurred on the operating table in a 59-year-old man with functional class 4 symptoms and central occlusion of both the left anterior descending (LAD) and left circumflex artery (CX); postmortem autopsy revealed a Teflon pledget lodged 3 cm down his dominant right coronary artery obstructing the vessel. Nevertheless, the rationale of a policy of consistent CABG in all patients with CAD, irrespective of the presence of angina pectoris, was unambiguously underscored.

LATE RETURN OF CONGESTIVE HEART FAILURE

In spite of an almost obligatory functional and objective improvement early after valve replacement,[24,34,80] a distressing and enigmatic recurrence of CHF has long been known to occur several years later,[81–84] and also in patients with no functional limitations 1 year after the operation.[34] Apart from mal-

TABLE 37-4. Multivariate Prediction (Logistic Regression Analysis) of Early Mortality (≤30 Days) in 307 Patients Without Preoperative Coronary Angiography, 1975 to 1986[a]

Risk Factor[b]	Regression Coefficient	p	Combination of Risk Factors			
Left ventricular failure	0.706	0.002	—	—	x	x
High CAD score	0.428	0.04	—	x	—	x
No. of patients with combination			136	29	98	44
No. of early death			4	2	11	10
Rate (%)[c]			3	7	11	23

[a] See Table 37-3 for explanations.
[b] See text.
[c] p <0.001.
(From Lund et al.,[56] with permission.)

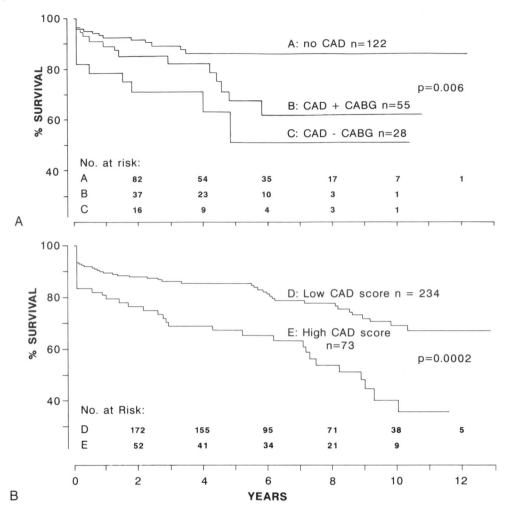

Fig. 37-1. (**A**) Cumulative survival (early deaths included) in patients with preoperative coronary arteriography, 1975–1986. Group A consisted of patients without CAD. Group B were patients with CAD who had CABG performed. Group C were patients with CAD who did not have CABG performed. The 5-/10-year survival rates ±SE were 86 ± 4%/86 ± 4% in group A, 68 ± 8%/62 ± 9% in group B, and 51 ± 13%/51 ± 13% in group C. Numbers above the abscissa indicate patients at risk during follow-up. (**B**) Cumulative survival (early deaths included) in patients without preoperative coronary arteriography, 1975–1986. Group D included patients with a low CAD score (low probability of CAD, see text). Group E were patients with a high CAD score (high probability of CAD). The 5-/10-year survival rates ±SE were 86 ± 2%/69 ± 4% in group D and 67 ± 6%/41 ± 8% in group E. Numbers above the abscissa indicate patients at risk during follow-up. (From Lund et al.,[56] with permission.)

function of the prosthetic valve or of the native mitral valve in a few patients,[82] no explanation of the phenomenon has been given, and no specific therapy is available.

Macroscopic scattered streaky fibrosis, often to a marked degree, has been noted in most patients who died from native aortic stenosis[85] but also in as many as 90% of patients dying up to 14 years after valve replacement.[86] CHF late after operation can thus represent exhaustion of the remaining myocardium as

also proposed by Buckberg.[83] Another part of the explanation could be the general inability of LV hypertrophy to dwindle completely after valve replacement with a well-performing non-obstructive prosthesis[34,86–88]: residual hypertrophy may suggest some degree of sustained ischemic jeopardy. Our results[34,86,87] supported these speculations and provided an answer to the enigma. Scattered streaky fibrosis and hypertrophy of the left ventricle even late after valve replacement for aortic stenosis were predicted by preoperative deranged heart status and not by type or size of the prosthetic valve.[86] The fibrosis was also associated with residual hypertrophy and not with CAD.[86] Furthermore, in patients who had no functional disability 1 year after the operation, recurrence of CHF noted at 10-year control was related exclusively to the preoperative starting point, to advanced disease before the operation.[34] Finally, preoperative data were significantly predictive of LV function recorded at a mean of 12 years after the operation, and impaired function in turn depended on residual hypertrophy.[34] Diastolic performance was the only independent correlate of death from CHF (65% of all deaths) occurring during an ensuing 3-year observation period.[87]

These connections also significantly contradict both the afterload mismatch theory and the view that there is ample time for surgical intervention in aortic stenosis associated with minor symptoms. In addition to early mortality, postponed operation and worsened heart status predict residual hypertrophy, streaky myocardial fibrosis, and impaired systolic and diastolic LV function, all of which result in late recurrence of, and death from, CHF. The explanation must be preoperatively established irreversible myocardial disease that, in most patients, does not prevent early improvement but, nevertheless, determines late outcome. Lund and Væth[89] termed the above predictabili-

ties a "biological memory" of the heart, which was later rephrased "prognostic memory" by Lund.[5]

Figure 37-2 shows the long-term survival of the 630 patients in our 1965 to 1986 series who were alive 30 days after the operation, compared with the survival of a general Danish background population matched with the patients for sex and age (using the published Danish life-tables for each specific operative year). Also, the relative survival is shown (ratio of conditional survival probability for a given operative year of patients and of background population; a value close to 1.0 thus indicates normal patient survival, while a lower value indicates excess mortality). The patients showed a slight excess mortality during the first and third postoperative year; thereafter, patient and background curves ran almost in parallel. Excess mortality seemed to recur after the twelfth year, especially during the thirteenth and nineteenth years.[5] A total of 54% of all late deaths were cardiogenic (30% caused by CHF), 18% were prosthesis related, and 28% had other causes.[5] Of 151 deaths occurring during the first 12 postoperative years, 52% were cardiogenic compared with 68% of 25 later deaths; 25% and 64%, respectively, were caused by CHF.[5] At this point, the diverging survival curves of patients and background population seem to indicate a palliative nature of aortic valve replacement, as is the view of Lindblom and associates[90] and Abdelnoor and co-workers.[91] How-

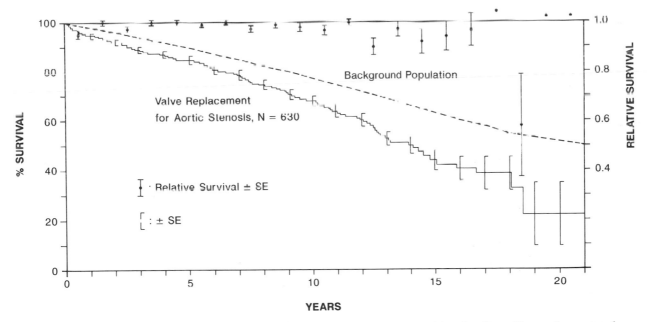

Fig. 37-2. Cumulative survival ± SE in the 30-day survivors of the 1965–1986 series ("step" curve) compared with the survival of a general Danish background population (dashed curve) matched for sex, age, and operative year. Also, relative survival rates ± SE (upper data points) for each year of follow-up are given (SE of the relative survival is 0 for years when no patients died). The 5-, 10-, and 15-year patient survivals ± SE were 85 ± 2%, 68 ± 2%, and 44 ± 4%, respectively. (From Lund,[5] with permission.)

ever, further analysis of our series indicated that this view should be modified.[5]

The survival characteristics shown in Figure 37-2 confirmed a previous suspicion[89] and quantified the late excess mortality after valve replacement for aortic stenosis primarily caused by CHF. Instantaneous rate of death from CHF accordingly rose significantly after the twelfth postoperative year, after a period of low and constant risk.[3] In order to secure normal (sex- and age-specific) survival after valve replacement for patients with aortic stenosis, late excess mortality must be eliminated. From the above speculations, it is reasonable to suspect that earlier operation than has until now been customary may bring about the change.

Preoperative Risk Assessment and Stratification of Long-term Survival

Table 37-5 shows some pertinent preoperative variables of the 630 patients who were alive 30 days after the operation in relationship to four succeeding operative periods, while Figure 37-3 gives the long-term survival for the same four periods. The improvement in long-term survival rates during the first three periods was probably explained by successive improvements in preoperative patient status, as evidenced by descreasing cardiothoracic index and decreasing prevalence of functional class 3 to 4 symptoms, LV failure, and ventricular ectopic beats in the electrocardiogram (ECG), since these variables had strong prognostic influence by univariate testing.[5] Earlier operative intervention rather than time frame thus determined the

prognostic improvements. This was underlined by the multivariate Cox analysis (see below): operative year had no independent predictive value.[5] Operative year independently influenced long-term survival in the studies by Cormier and co-workers[92] and by Mitchell and associates[93] covering operative periods comparable to the present one. Introduction of crystalloid cardioplegia in the late 1970s,[92,93] however, presumably explained the influence of operative year.

No further prognostic improvement took place from the third to fourth operative period (Fig. 37-3) in spite of continued improvement of preoperative patient profile (Table 37-5). However, the 22-year period also witnessed increasing patient age, increasing prevalence of secondary kidney failure and of angina pectoris as limiting symptom, and decreasing aortic valve gradient (Table 37-5). The latter can be interpreted as decreasing severity of aortic stenosis, but the direction of the prognostic influence of aortic valve gradient (the lower the gradient, the worse the prognosis; see below) speaks otherwise. In any respect, old age, angina, and low gradient were related to increasing probability of CAD in the angio group (Table 37-1) as was kidney failure.[5] This is in good agreement with the previously mentioned steady increase in the number of patients with a high CAD score, pointing toward an increasing prevalence of associated CAD. The adverse influence of CAD can thus finally have "broken through" the general improvements in patient status and so explain the lack of a further prognostic improvement in the last of the four operative periods.

Multivariate Cox regression analysis of long-term

TABLE 37-5. Preoperative Data in Relationship to Year of Operation in 30-Day Survivors of 1965 to 1986 Series[a]

Preoperative Data	1965–1971 (N = 62)	1972–1976 (N = 164)	1977–1981 (N = 158)	1982–1986 (N = 246)
Age[b] (year)	56 ± 9	57 ± 11	59 ± 10	61 ± 11
NYHA functional classes 3 and 4[c]	87% (54)	76% (126)	68% (108)	63% (153)
Angina pectoris as limiting symptom[b]	10% (6)	23% (37)	27% (43)	33% (81)
Left ventricular failure[d,e]	50% (31)	39% (64)	36% (57)	30% (74)
Kidney failure[c,f]	3% (2)	7% (11)	21% (33)	26% (65)
ECG ventricular ectopic beats[b]	11% (7)	5% (9)	3% (5)	2% (5)
ECG hypertrophy score[c,d]	8.8 ± 1.5	7.7 ± 2.4	7.4 ± 2.6	7.0 ± 2.7
Cardiothoracic index[c]	0.56 ± 0.06	0.53 ± 0.06	0.52 ± 0.06	0.51 ± 0.06
Systemic pulse pressure (mmHg)[b,g]	44 ± 13	48 ± 16	50 ± 17	52 ± 17
Peak-to-peak systolic pressure gradient (mmHg)[e]	100 ± 23	99 ± 29	97 ± 32	91 ± 32
Left ventricular end-diastolic pressure (mmHg)[e]	14 ± 10	17 ± 9	18 ± 9	18 ± 10

Abbreviations: ECG, electrocardiography; NYHA, New York Heart Association.
[a] Values are mean ± SD or % (N of patients).
[b] p <0.01.
[c] p <0.0001.
[d] See text.
[e] p <0.05.
[f] Serum creatinine >100 μmol·L^{-1}
[g] Systolic minus diastolic blood pressure (sphygmomanometry).
(From Lund,[5] with permission.)

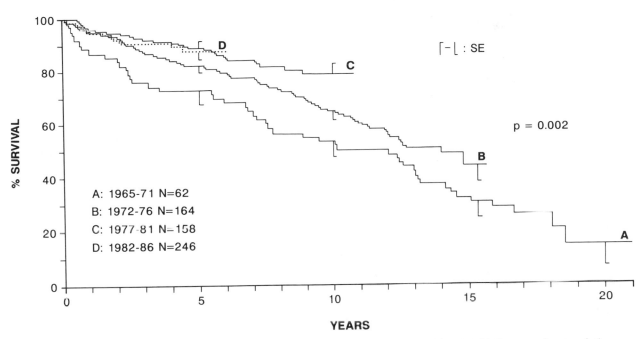

Fig. 37-3. Cumulative survival rates in relationship to year of operation in the 30-day survivors of the 1965–1986 series. Standard error (SE) is given for every fifth year. The 5- and 10-year survival rates ±SE for the four operative periods were A, 73 ± 6%/53 ± 6%; B, 82 ± 3%/65 ± 4%; C, 89 ± 3%/79 ± 4%; and D, 87 ± 3%/-. (From Lund,[5] with permission.)

survival gave the results shown in Table 37-6.[5] *Aortic valve* (peak-to-peak systolic) *gradient* was the strongest independent risk factor; its negative regression coefficient indicates that gradient and death rate were inversely related. A simple explanation is that only a "good ventricle" is able to produce the high blood flow that determines a high gradient of a narrow stenotic valve, whereas the gradient drops synchronously with decompensation of the ventricle.[24] Moreover, a high preoperative gradient has been related to normal systolic and diastolic left ventricular function recorded at an average of 12 years after valve replacement.[34]

Cardiothoracic index was directly related to death rate, and *LV failure* was an equally significant independent risk factor (Table 37-6). Dilation and decreasing ejection fraction are end-stage phenomena in the LV decompensation process.[26] High cardiothoracic index and LV failure were the chief predictors of scattered streaky fibrosis of the left ventricle noted at autopsy up to 14 years after the operation.[86]

The adverse prognostic influence of a *prosthetic orifice diameter of 15 mm or less* is probably explained by maintenance to some degree of pressure load on the left ventricle, given the inborn pressure gradients of available small prostheses.[94–96] Small prosthesis size was related to female gender and small body size and thus to a small aortic annulus.[3] Given the better proportion between orifice and outer diameter of a St.

Jude valve as compared with, for example, a Starr-Edwards valve,[3] one should prefer the former in patients with a narrow aortic annulus. Annulus diameter did not have independent prognostic value, but the result may indicate that a diameter so small as to fit only one of the smallest St. Jude valves should lead to enlargement of the annulus, to accommodate a larger prosthesis. This has been done with acceptable results.[97,98]

The strong independent value of patient age may be easily comprehended, given an average starting age of 59 years and a follow-up period of more than 20 years. Ventricular ectopic beats also independently increase late mortality rate. Laky and co-workers[99] have shown that rising occurrence of myocardial scarring late in the evolution of secondary pressure overload hypertrophy was paralleled by increasing incidence of ventricular ectopic beats. The adverse influence of *male gender* was probably explained by a higher incidence in middle-aged men than in women of ischemic heart disease and cancer.[100] Finally, the prognostic influence of *antianginal or antiarrhythmic treatment* might be related to CAD, to an arrhythmic potential attributable to myocardial microscarring, and to the same type of symptom masking and operation-postponing effects observed for digitalis or diuretic treatment.

A further rationale has emerged for separating risk analysis into an early high-risk phase and a later phase

TABLE 37-6. Independent Predictors of Long-Term Survival in 30-Day Survivors of 1965 to 1986 Series: Results of Cox Regression Analysis

Predictor Variable/Risk Factor[a]	b	SE	p
Aortic valve (peak-to-peak systolic) gradient	−0.012	0.003	0.0001
Cardiothoracic index	5.075	1.398	0.0003
LV failure	0.585	0.167	0.0005
Prosthetic orifice diameter of ≤15 mm	0.726	0.226	0.001
Patient age	0.026	0.009	0.003
Ventricular ectopic beats	0.760	0.266	0.004
Male gender	0.415	0.196	0.03
Antianginal or antiarrhythmic treatment	0.342	0.162	0.03
Global χ^2		99.1 (p < 0.000001)	

Prognostic index[b] = $z_1b_1 + z_2b_2 + \ldots + z_pb_p$. Mean, 3.785 ± 0.782 (SD); range, 1.478–6.332.
Cutoff points[c] for 10 equidistant prognostic index intervals: (1.963), 2.448, 2.933, 3.418, 3.903, 4.388, 4.873, 5.358, (5.843).

Abbreviations: SD, standard deviation; SE, standard error of regression coefficient; LV, left ventricular.

[a] See text.

[b] Calculated for each patient from Cox model.

[c] The 10 prognostic index intervals identified 10 groups of patients; the two low index groups were joined, as were the two high index groups, because of a limited number of patients with extreme prognostic index values. Thus, eight risk groups were created (see Fig. 37-4). Note that b, b_1, b_2, . . . , b_p are the regression coefficients; z_1, z_2, . . . , z_p are the values of risk factors for each patient (equals 1 if risk factor present and 0 if not; equals discrete value for peak-to-peak systolic gradient, cardiothoracic index, and age).

(From Lund,[5] with permission.)

of low and primarily constant risk[3]: risk factors may considerably change their significance between phases (cf. Tables 37-2 and 37-6). Analysis of early and late deaths as one continuum may therefore be erroneous, since construction of parametric regression models that take into account phase-dependent changes in significance of risk factors and their multitude of mutual interactions may be extremely difficult or even impossible, especially when a large battery of potential risk factors is at hand, as in our studies.[3]

Apart from the author's group,[5,89] only three groups of investigators,[73,92,101] have previously performed multivariate analysis of long-term survival in patients with valve replacement for aortic stenosis. The results as regards independent risk factors differed widely, probably because of several pertinent factors. In none of the latter three studies was crystalloid cardioplegia used consistently.[73,92,101] One study dealt with combined valve replacement and CABG exclusively[73] and one included early mortality,[92] while the others did not,[73,101] and two studies included patients with associated operative procedures other than CABG.[92,101] No previous attempt has been made to stratify patients according to the identified multivariate risk model and to compare observed survivals in the resulting risk groups.

A prognostic index was calculated for each patient from the final Cox model of Table 37-6. By cutting the index into equidistant intervals, eight risk groups were identified. Their observed survival rates are shown in Figure 37-4. Also, their survivals predicted from the Cox model were calculated. Observed (standard error)/predicted 15-year cumulative survival rates from risk groups 1 to 8 were 90% (7)/86%, 84% (6)/78%, 62% (10)/67%, 57% (6)/53%, 37% (8)/37%, 20% (10)/19%, 12% (8)/8%, and 4% (4)/1%, respectively; the percentages of deaths from cardiac causes were 0%, 17%, 36%, 45%, 55%, 59%, 71%, and 75%, respectively.[5] Furthermore, each risk group had a general Danish background population specifically matched for sex and age. The survival of each of these background populations, b1 to b8, is compared with that of the patient risk group depicted in Figure 37-4A; Figure 37-4B depicts the relative survivals of the risk groups. It may be concluded that a normal sex- and age-specific long-term survival was obtained in risk groups I to III, that there was a slight late excess mortality in group IV, and that significantly increasing excess mortalities prevailed in groups V to VIII.[5] Clearly, patients comparable to those in risk group VIII should still be offered urgent operation; at best, the 3-year survival rate during optimal medical treatment in severely symptomatic patient is no more than 20%[102] (5-year survival was 36% in group VIII[5]). The decreasing survival probability of background populations b1 to b8 is explained by the influence of age in the Cox model; mean ages of patients in groups I to VIII and of their corresponding background population were 41, 52, 53, 60, 62, 64, 66, and 67 years, respectively.

The highly significant prognostic influence of the prognostic index together with the composition of the Cox model from which it was calculated strongly underline the existence of the prognostic memory of the hearts of patients with aortic stenosis. It should be noted that neither the risk models for early mortality (Tables 37-2 to 37-4) nor the Cox model (Table 37-6) included intraoperative variables; none of the latter had independent prognostic value. Apart from small prosthetic orifice and male gender, the independent risk factors were related to preoperatively deranged heart status. The prognostic index is thus predominantly related to preoperatively established irreversible myocardial disease. Finally, it was likely that the prognostic index had universal validity for patients with aortic stenosis.[5]

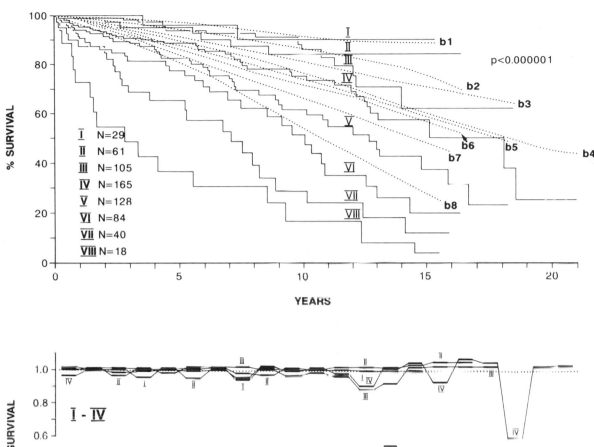

Fig. 37-4. Cumulative and relative survival rates. **(A)** Cumulative (observed) survival rate in risk groups I-VIII. Risk groups were identified by dividing the prognostic index calculated for each patient from the Cox model into equidistant intervals (see Table 37-6). Survival rate of each risk group is compared with the survival rate of a general Danish background population selectively matched for sex, age, and operative year (b1 to b8). **(B)** Relative survival rate in risk groups I-IV (upper) and V-VIII (lower). Relative survival rate ±1 SE (approximately 70% confidence limit) was <1.0 for the ensuing years of follow-up (*, if relative survival +2 SE, i.e., approximative 95% confidence limit, was <1.0). Groups I and II: none; group III: 13 years; group IV: 1, 13, and 19* years; group V: 1,* 8, 11, 14, and 17 years; group VI: 1,* 6, 10, 11,* 13, and 15 years; group 7: 1,* 3,* 6, 8,* 9, 13, and 15 years; group VIII: 1,* 2,* 10, and 13 years. (From Lund,[5] with permission.)

Curative Potential of Early Operative Intervention

The prognostic index calculated for all 690 patients of our 1965 to 1986 series identified eight risk groups by using the same points of division as for the 630 patients who were alive after 30 days (Table 37-6); the 30-day mortality rates from low- to high-risk estimate were 0% (of 29 patients), 1.6% (of 62), 3.7% (of 109), 5.2% (of 174), 9.2% (of 141), 17.6% (of 102), 20.0% (of 50), and 21.7% (of 23).[3] The prognostic index calculated from the Cox model (Table 37-6) and the risk score for early mortality (Table 37-2) of the 611 patients operated during 1972 to 1986 were strongly correlated (r = 0.77).[3] These results joined thus tied up the connection between the highly detailed and significant preoperative risk stratification for early mortality and the prognostic index for long-term survival. It has also been shown that patients who obtained a normal long-term survival rate (risk groups I to III, Fig. 37-4) had a normal rate (equal to that of background population) of stroke and myocardial infarction in particular, and probably of the dominant long-term complications, thromboembolism and (anticoagulant-related) hemorrhage, in general.

CONCLUSION

As an overall conclusion, it can be stated that operative intervention in patients with aortic stenosis, as soon as even discrete symptoms appear, before medical treatment becomes necessary, and before any of the risk factors make their appearance, should be strongly advocated. Early operative intervention, equivalent to a low prognostic index, results in an early mortality rate approaching zero and a normal sex- and age-specific long-term survival.[3]

Coronary arteriography in all adult patients with aortic stenosis and CABG concomitant with valve replacement in case of significant CAD should be regarded as mandatory; CABG reduces early mortality rate to a level comparable to that of patients without CAD. Given the progressive nature of CAD and the fact that CABG probably modifies late survival only in triple vessel or left main stem CAD, a true normal long-term survival can probably not be expected in patients with associated CAD.

REFERENCES

1. Olesen KH, Warburg E: Isolated aortic stenosis—the late prognosis. Acta Med Scand 160:437, 1958
2. Horstkotte D, Loogen F: The natural history of aortic valve stenosis. Eur Heart J, suppl E. 9:57, 1988
3. Lund O: Valve replacement for aortic stenosis: the curative potential of early operation. Aarhus, Denmark: Aarhus University; Thesis. 1992
4. Lund O, Pilegaard H, Nielsen TT et al: Thirty-day mortality after valve replacement for aortic stenosis over the last 22 years. A multivariate risk stratification. Eur Heart J 12:322, 1991
5. Lund O: Preoperative risk evaluation and stratification of long-term survival after valve replacement for aortic stenosis. Reasons for earlier operative intervention. Circulation 82:124, 1990
6. Lund O, Nielsen TT, Magnussen K et al: Valve replacement for calcified aortic stenosis in septuagenarians infers normal life-length. Scand J Thorac Cardiovasc Surg 25:37, 1991
7. Crawford MH: Valvular heart disease: overview. Curr Opinion Cardiol 4:189, 1989
8. Czer LSC, Chaux A, Matloff JM et al: Ten-year experience with the St. Jude Medical valve for primary valve replacement. J Thorac Cardiovasc Surg 100:44, 1990
9. John S, Ravikumar E, Jairaj PS et al: Valve replacement in the young patient with rheumatic heart disease. J Thorac Cardiovasc Surg 99:631, 1990
10. Selzer A: Changing aspects of the natural history of valvular aortic stenosis. N Engl J Med 317:91, 1987
11. Lytle BW, Cosgrove DM, Taylor PC et al: Primary isolated aortic valve replacement. Early and late results. J Thorac Cardiovasc Surg 97:675, 1989
12. Cribier A, Savin T, Saoudi N et al: Percutaneous transluminal valvuloplasty of acquired aortic stenosis in elderly patients: an alternative to valve replacement? Lancet 1:63, 1986
13. Block PC, Palacios IF: Clinical and hemodynamic follow-up after percutaneous aortic valvuloplasty in the elderly. Am J Cardiol 62:760, 1988
14. Desnoyers MR, Isner JM, Pandian NG et al: Clinical and noninvasive hemodynamic results after aortic balloon valvuloplasty for aortic stenosis. Am J Cardiol 62:1078, 1988
15. Baird RJ, Lipton IH, Labrosse CJ et al: An evaluation of the late results of aortic valve repair. J Thorac Cardiovasc Surg 49:562, 1965
16. Hurley PJ, Lowe JB, Barratt-Boyes BG: Debridement valvotomy for aortic stenosis in adults. Thorax 22:314, 1967
17. Crosby IK, Muller WH, Jr: Acquired disease of the aortic valve. p. 1280. In Sabiston DC, Jr, Spencer FC (eds): Surgery of the Chest. 4th Ed. W.B. Saunders Company, Philadelphia, 1983
18. Rodriguez AR, Minor ST, West MS et al: Balloon aortic valvuloplasty is not an effective long term therapy for calcific aortic stenosis with left ventricular dysfunction, abstracted. Eur Heart J, suppl. 11:74, 1990
19. Chevalier B, Lancelin B, Dapelo A, Dormagen V: Long term survival rate after percutaneous aortic valvuloplasty in the elderly, abstracted. Eur Heart J, suppl. 11:74, 1990
20. Bernard Y, Bassand JP, Schiele F et al: Comparative results of percutaneous aortic valvuloplasty and aortic valve replacement in elderly patients, abstracted. Eur Heart J, suppl. 11:74, 1990

21. Levinson JR, Akins CW, Buckley MJ et al: Octogenarians with aortic stenosis. Outcome after aortic valve replacement. Circulation, suppl I. 80:49, 1989
22. Turina J, Hess O, Sepulci F, Krayenbuehl HP: Spontaneous course of aortic valve disease. Eur Heart J 8:471, 1987
23. Ross J, Jr: Afterload mismatch and preload reserve: A conceptual framework for the analysis of ventricular function. Prog Cardiovasc Dis 18:255, 1976
24. Carabello BA, Green LH, Grossman W et al: Hemodynamic determinants of prognosis of aortic valve replacement in critical aortic stenosis and advanced congestive heart failure. Circulation 62:42, 1980
25. Gunther S, Grossman W: Determinants of ventricular function in pressure-overload hypertrophy in man. Circulation 59:679, 1979
26. Ross J, Jr: Afterload mismatch in aortic and mitral valve disease: implications for surgical therapy. J Am Coll Cardiol 5:811, 1985
27. Krayenbuehl HP, Hess OM, Ritter M et al: Left ventricular systolic function in aortic stenosis. Eur Heart J, suppl E. 9:19, 1988
28. Rose AG: Pathology of Heart Valve Replacement. MTP Press, Lancaster, 1987
29. Carabello BA: Prognosis of aortic valve disease. Curr Opinion Cardiol 4:223, 1989
30. Braunwald E: Valvular heart disease. p. 1023. In Braunwald E (ed): Heart Disease. A Textbook of Cardiovascular Medicine. 3rd Ed. WB Saunders, Philadelphia, 1988
31. Keenan RJ, Armitage JM, Trento A et al: Clinical experience with the Medtronic-Hall valve prosthesis. Ann Thorac Surg 50:748, 1990
32. Hackett D, Fessatidis I, Sapsford R, Oakley C: Ten year clinical evaluation of Starr-Edwards 2400 and 1260 aortic valve prostheses. Br Heart J 57:356, 1987
33. Montalescot G, Thomas D, Drobinski G et al: Clinical and ultrasound results after aortic valve replacement: Intermediate-term follow-up with the St. Jude Medical prosthesis. Am Heart J 118:104, 1989
34. Lund O, Jensen FT: Functional status and left ventricular performance late after valve replacement for aortic stenosis. Relation to preoperative data. Eur Heart J 9: 1234, 1988
35. Wiesenbaugh T, Booth D, DeMaria A et al: Relationship of contractile state to ejection performance in patients with chronic aortic valve disease. Circulation 73:47, 1986
36. Lund O, Pilegaard HK, Magnussen K et al: Long-term prosthesis-related and sudden cardiac-related complications after valve replacement for aortic stenosis. Ann Thorac Surg 50:396, 1990
37. Magnussen K, Lund O, Knudsen MA et al: Valve replacement for aortic regurgitation: earlier operation may reduce the rate of late complications related to the prostheses. Thorac Cardiovasc Surg 38:295, 1990
38. Lund O, Knudsen MA, Pilegaard HK et al: Long-term performance of Starr-Edwards silastic ball valves and St. Jude Medical bi-leaflet valves. A comparative analysis of implantations during 1980–86 for aortic stenosis. Eur Heart J 11:108, 1990
39. Pilegaard HK, Lund O, Nielsen TT et al: Twenty-two-year experience with aortic valve replacement. Starr-Edwards ball valves versus disc valves. Texas Heart Inst J 18:24, 1991
40. Bretschneider HJ, Hübner G, Knoll D et al: Myocardial resistance and tolerance to ischemia: physiological and biochemical basis. J Cardiovasc Surg 16:241, 1975
41. Bretschneider HJ, Gebhard MM, Preusse CJ: Reviewing the pros and cons of myocardial preservation within cardiac surgery. p 21. In Longmore DB (ed): Towards Safer Cardiac Surgery. MTP Press, Lancaster, 1981
42. Bretschneider HJ: Myocardial protection. Thorac Cardiovasc Surg 28:295, 1980
43. Preusse CJ, Gebhard MM, Bretschneider HJ: Myocardial "equilibration processes" and myocardial energy turnover during initiation of artificial cardiac arrest with cardioplegic solution—reasons for a sufficiently long cardioplegic perfusion. Thorac Cardiovasc Surg 29:71, 1981
44. Søndergaard T, Senn A: Klinische Erfahrungen mit der Kardioplegie nach Bretschneider. Langenbecks Arch Chir 319:661, 1967
45. Beyersdorf F, Krause E, Sarai K et al: Clinical evaluation of hypothermic ventricular fibrillation, multi-dose blood cardioplegia, and single-dose Bretschneider cardioplegia in coronary surgery. Thorac Cardiovasc Surg 38:20, 1990
46. Schaper J, Scheld HH, Schmidt U, Hehrlein F: Ultrastructural study comparing the efficacy of five different methods of intraoperative myocardial protection in the human heart. J Thorac Cardiovasc Surg 92:47, 1986
47. Hjelms E, Vejlsted H: Myocardial protection during aortic valve replacement. Scand J Thorac Cardiovasc Surg 16:29, 1982
48. Conti VR, Bertranou EG, Blackstone EH et al: Cold cardioplegia versus hypothermia for myocardial protection. J Thorac Cardiovasc Surg 76:577, 1978
49. Kirklin JW: A letter to Helen. J Thorac Cardiovasc Surg 78:643, 1979
50. Scheld HH, Görlach G, Mulch J et al: Protection of the hypertrophied human heart by adjusting regional myocardial temperature to a safe level. Thorac Cardiovasc Surg 33:235, 1985
51. Schnabel PhA, Gebhard MM, Pomykay Th et al: Myocardial protection: left ventricular ultrastructure after different forms of cardiac arrest. Thorac Cardiovasc Surg 35:148, 1987
52. Alyono D, Anderson RW, Parrish DG et al: Alterations of myocardial flow associated with experimental canine left ventricular hypertrophy secondary to valvular aortic stenosis. Circ Res 58:47, 1986
53. Vincent WR, Buckberg GD, Hoffman JIE: Left ventricular subendocardial ischemia in severe valvar and supravalvar aortic stenosis. A common mechanism. Circulation 49:326, 1974
54. Trenouth RS, Phelps NC, Neill WA: Determinants of left ventricular hypertrophy and oxygen supply in chronic aortic valve disease. Circulation 53:644, 1976
55. Marcus ML, Doty DB, Hiratzka LF et al: Decreased coronary reserve. A mechanism for angina pectoris in patients with aortic stenosis and normal coronary arteries. N Engl J Med 307:1362, 1982

56. Lund O, Nielsen TT, Pilegaard HK et al: The influence of coronary artery disease and bypass grafting on early and late survival after valve replacement for aortic stenosis. J Thorac Cardiovasc Surg 100:327, 1990

57. Miller DC, Stinson EB, Oyer PE et al: Surgical implications and results of combined aortic valve replacement and myocardial revascularization. Am J Cardiol 43:494, 1979

58. Hancock EW: Aortic stenosis, angina pectoris, and coronary artery disease. Am Heart J 93:382, 1977

59. Pilegaard HK, Lund O, Nielsen TT et al: Early and late prognosis after valve replacement in aortic regurgitation. Preoperative risk stratification and reasons for a more aggressive surgical approach. Thorac Cardiovasc Surg 37:231, 1989

60. DiLello F, Flemma RJ, Anderson AJ et al: Improved early results after aortic valve replacement: analysis by surgical time frame. Ann Thorac Surg 47:51, 1989

61. Croke RP, Pifarre R, Sullivan H et al: Reversal of left ventricular dysfunction following aortic valve replacement for aortic stenosis. Ann Thorac Surg 24:38, 1977

62. Lavine SJ, Follansbee WP, Shreiner DP, Amidi M: Left ventricular diastolic filling in valvular aortic stenosis. Am J Cardiol 57:1349, 1986

63. Topol EJ, Traill TA, Fortuin NJ: Hypertensive hypertrophic cardio- myopathy of the elderly. N Engl J Med 312: 277, 1983

64. Oldershaw PJ, Dawkins KD, Ward DE, Gibson DG: Diastolic mechanisms of impaired exercise tolerance in aortic valve disease. Br Heart J 49:568, 1983

65. Dougherty AH, Naccarelli GV, Gray EL et al: Congestive heart failure with normal systolic function. Am J Cardiol 54:778, 1984

66. Bier AJ, Eichacker PQ, Sinoway LI et al: Acute cardiogenic pulmonary edema: clinical and noninvasive evaluation. Angiology 39:211, 1988

67. Romhilt DW, Estes EH, Jr: A point-score system for the ECG diagnosis of left ventricular hypertrophy. Am Heart J 75:752, 1968

68. Romhilt DW, Bove KE, Norris RJ et al: A critical appraisal of the electrocardiographic criteria for the diagnosis of left ventricular hypertrophy. Circulation 40: 185, 1969

69. Casale PN, Devereux RB, Kligfield P et al: Electrocardiographic detection of left ventricular hypertrophy: development and prospective validation of improved criteria. J Am Coll Cardiol 6:572, 1985

70. Inouye I, Massie B, Loge D et al: Abnormal left ventricular filling: an early finding in mild to moderate systemic hypertension. Am J Cardiol 53:120, 1984

71. Magovern JA, Pennock JL, Campbell DB et al: Aortic valve replacement and combined aortic valve replacement and coronary artery bypass grafting: predicting high risk groups. J Am Coll Cardiol 9:38, 1987

72. Lund O, Johansen G, Allermand H et al: Intraaortic balloon pumping in the treatment of low cardiac output following open heart surgery—immediate results and long-term prognosis. Thorac Cardiovasc Surg 36:332, 1988

73. Lytle BW, Cosgrove DM, Goormastic M, Loop FD: Aortic valve replacement and coronary bypass grafting for pa-

tients with aortic stenosis and coronary artery disease: early and late results. Eur Heart J, suppl E. 9:143, 1988

74. Cohn LH, Allred EN, DiSesa VJ et al: Early and late risk of aortic valve replacement. A 12 year concomitant comparison of the porcine bioprosthetic and tilting disc prosthetic aortic valves. J Thorac Cardiovasc Surg 88: 695, 1984

75. Borow KM, Wynne J, Sloss LJ et al: Noninvasive assessment of valvular heart disease: Surgery without catheterization. Am Heart J 106:443, 1983

76. Sutton MG St. John, Sutton M St. John, Oldershaw P et al: Valve replacement without preoperative cardiac catheterization. N Engl J Med 305:1233, 1981

77. Delaye J, Chevalier P, Delahaye F, Didier B: Valvular aortic stenosis and coronary atherosclerosis: pathophysiology and clinical consequences. Eur Heart J, suppl E. 9:83, 1988

78. Czer LSC, Gray RJ, Stewart ME et al: Reduction in sudden late death by concomitant revascularization with aortic valve replacement. J Thorac Cardiovasc Surg 95: 390, 1988

79. European Coronary Surgery Study Group: Long-term results of prospective randomised study of coronary artery bypass surgery in stable angina pectoris. Lancet 2: 1173, 1982

80. Smith N, McAnulty JH, Rahimtoola SH: Severe aortic stenosis with impaired left ventricular function and clinical heart failure: results of valve replacement. Circulation 58:255, 1978

81. Bristow JD, Kremkau EL: Hemodynamic changes after valve replacement with Starr-Edwards prosthesis. Am J Cardiol 35:716, 1975

82. Goldman MR, Boucher CA, Block PC et al: Spectrum of congestive heart failure late after aortic valve or mitral replacement: differentiation of valvular versus myocardial cause by radionuclide ventriculogram-ejection fraction. Am Heart J 102:751, 1981

83. Buckberg GD: Left ventricular subendocardial necrosis. Ann Thorac Surg 24:379, 1977

84. Hancock EW: Timing of valve replacement for aortic stenosis. Circulation 82:310, 1990

85. Wigle ED: Myocardial fibrosis and calcereous emboli in valvular heart disease. Br Heart J 19:539, 1957

86. Lund O, Larsen KE: Cardiac pathology after isolated valve replacement for aortic stenosis in relation to preoperative patient status. Early and late autopsy findings. Scand J Thorac Cardiovasc Surg 23:263, 1989

87. Lund O, Jensen FT: Late cardiac deaths after isolated valve replacement for aortic stebosis. Relation to impaired left ventricular diastolic performance. Angiology 40:199, 1989

88. Pantely G, Morton M, Rahimtoola SH: Effects of successful, uncomplicated valve replacement on ventricular hypertrophy, volume, and performance in aortic stenosis and in aortic incompetence. J Thorac Cardiovasc Surg 75:383, 1978

89. Lund O, Væth M: Prediction of late results following valve replacement in aortic valve stenosis. Seventeen years of follow-up examined with the Cox regression analysis. Thorac Cardiovasc Surg 35:295, 1987

90. Lindblom D: Long-term clinical results after aortic

valve replacement with the Björk-Shiley prosthesis. J Thorac Cardiovasc Surg 95:658, 1988

91. Abdelnoor M, Hall KV, Nitter-Hauge S et al: Risk factors of morbidity and mortality in surgically treated chronic aortic valvular heart disease. Rev Epidemiol Sante Publ 36:89, 1988

92. Cormier B, Luxereau P, Bloch C et al: Prognosis and long-term results of surgically treated aortic stenosis. Eur Heart J, suppl E. 9:113, 1988

93. Mitchell RS, Miller DC, Stinson EB et al: Significant patient-related determinants of prosthetic valve performance. J Thorac Cardiovasc Surg 91:807, 1986

94. Foster AH, Tracy CM, Greenberg GJ et al: Valve replacement in narrow aortic roots: serial hemodynamics and long-term clinical outcome. Ann Thorac Surg 42:506, 1986

95. Henze A: The Bjork-Shiley tilting disc valve in aortic valve disease (Diss.). Scand J Thorac Cardiovasc Surg, suppl. 14:1, 1974

96. Pyle RB, Mayer JE, Jr, Lindsay WG et al: Hemodynamic evaluation of Lillehei-Kaster and Starr-Edwards prostheses. Ann Thorac Surg 26:336, 1978

97. David TE, Uden DE: Aortic valve replacement in adult patients with small aortic annuli. Ann Thorac Surg 36:577, 1983

98. Manouguian S, Seybold-Epting W: Patch enlargement of the aortic valve ring by extending the aortic incision into the anterior mitral leaflet. New operative technique. J Thorac Cardiovasc Surg 78:402, 1979

99. Laky D, Constantinescu S, Filipescu G et al: The biology of the myocardium in chronic hypoxia. Note I. Myocardial lesions in experimental chronic heart failure. Morphol Embryol 31:295, 1985

100. National Board of Health: Causes of death in Denmark 1982. Vital Statistics 1:8, 1984. J.H. Schultz, Copenhagen, 1984

101. Acar J, Luxereau Ph, Ducimetiere P et al: Prognosis of surgically treated chronic aortic valve disease. Predictive indicators of early postoperative risk and long-term survival, based on 439 cases. J Thorac Cardiovasc Surg 82:114, 1981

102. Schwarz F, Baumann P, Manthey J et al: The effect of aortic valve replacement on survival. Circulation 66:1105, 1982

38

Risk Assessment and Prognosis of Patients With Heart and Heart-Lung Transplantation

Jolene M. Kriett
Stuart W. Jamieson

During the past decade, transplantation has become an established option in the treatment of patients with end-stage cardiac and pulmonary disease. Currently, about 2,500 heart and 200 combined heart-lung transplant procedures are performed annually.[1] However, while the number of potential recipients has continued to increase, further application of this therapy is limited by the availability of suitable donor organs. Therefore, selection of those recipients most likely to benefit from transplantation remains essential.

As of October 1990, more than 14,000 heart and 850 combined heart-lung transplant procedures had been reported to the Registry of the International Society for Heart Transplantation (ISHT) from more than 200 transplant centers worldwide.[2] More than 85% of these cases were performed since 1985, and information on the long-term outlook with transplantation continues to accumulate. This chapter reviews the recent literature as well as data from the ISHT Registry that relate to risk assessment and prognosis in heart and combined heart-lung transplantation.

PROGNOSIS WITHOUT TRANSPLANTATION

End-Stage Cardiac Disease

The natural history of patients with severe left ventricular (LV) dysfunction without surgical intervention has been examined in a number of studies. The Framingham data indicate a 5-year survival of less than 50% if symptoms of congestive heart failure (CHF) are present.[4] Almost one-half of patients with idiopathic cardiomyopathy die within 2 years.[5] Factors associated with a worse prognosis are age over 55 years, marked cardiomegaly, a cardiac index less than 3 L/min/m^2, and a left ventricular end-diastolic pressure (LVEDP) of more than 20 mmHg. More than 85% of patients with these findings died during the 2-year follow-up period. Other factors affecting survival are the presence of complex ventricular arrhythmias[6] and poor clinical status despite medical therapy.[7]

521

CHF secondary to ischemic heart disease (ISH) has been associated with an even worse prognosis than that for idiopathic cardiomyopathy.[7,8] Franciosa et al.[7] reported one and two year mortality rates of 46 and 69% in patients with ischemic cardiomyopathy compared with 23 and 48% in patients with dilated idiopathic cardiomyopathy.

In children, survival with congenital heart disease (CHD) is dependent on the type and complexity of the defects. In most cases, conventional repairs or palliative procedures with delayed total correction are possible. Neonates with hypoplastic left heart syndrome have a minimal prospect of survival beyond 1 month without staged palliation or transplantation.[9,10] Survival in children with dilated cardiomyopathy has been correlated with age at presentation and with the development of significant ventricular arrhythmias.[11]

Further information on survival with continued medical therapy, rather than operative intervention, is furnished by the subgroup of patients with end-stage heart disease considered for heart transplantation who do not receive grafts. The outcome of these patients prior to 1984 was examined in a multicenter survey.[12] Of referred patients, 24% died before completion of the pretransplant evaluation, and an additional 18% died while waiting for a suitable donor organ. More than 1,700 patients are currently on heart transplantation waiting lists in the United States; the average waiting period has increased to more than 5 months. Recent studies have indicated that approximately one in three of these patients will die before a suitable donor organ becomes available.[13–16] Results in children appear to be similar, and Mayer et al.[17] reported 37% of children died while waiting for a donor organ.

End-Stage Pulmonary Disease

As the natural history of end-stage pulmonary disease is largely dependent on the etiology of pulmonary failure, length of survival without transplantation is even more difficult to predict than in heart disease alone. Patients with primary pulmonary hypertension have an expected survival from onset of symptoms of 2 to 3 years.[18,19] The level of pulmonary hypertension, a low cardiac index, oxygen desaturation, and right heart failure have all been associated with poor prognosis. Eisenmenger's syndrome, which develops in up to 20% of patients with uncorrected congenital heart defects, follows a progressive downhill course during the second and third decades. Survival beyond the age of 50 is rare. The prognosis of patients with chronic obstructive pulmonary disease has been related to deterioration in pulmonary function studies and to the development of cor pulmonale.[20,21] Pulmonary fibrosis

has been associated with a 50% mortality within 5 years of diagnosis.[22]

Medical therapy for end-stage pulmonary disease remains limited. Vasodilator and continuous oxygen therapy may improve pulmonary hemodynamics and alleviate symptoms in some patients, but little improvement in survival has been demonstrated.[18,20]

In patients with cystic fibrosis, the most common fatal hereditary disease, the limited life span is related to progressive destruction of pulmonary tissue by repeated infections and the subsequent development of cor pulmonale. Improvements in medical and nutritional therapy during the past 25 years have enabled more patients with cystic fibrosis to survive to adulthood.[23] A clinical scoring system based on general activity level, physical and chest radiography findings, and nutritional status correlates with prognosis.[24] For those patients with the highest clinical scores, the median survival beyond 18 years of age is 12 years, while a low clinical score has been associated with a median survival of only 5 years. Low clinical score, low weight percentile, and colonization with *Pseudomonas cepacia* indicate a very poor prognosis.

Of those patients accepted for transplantation, reports indicate that 30 to 56% of candidates awaiting combined heart-lung transplantation will die before donor organs become available.[19,25] Currently the waiting time for combined heart-lung candidates is several times that for heart transplantation. In only 10% of donors are the lungs suitable for transplantation. In addition, the large number of heart transplant candidates further limits the availability of combined heart-lung blocks.

HEART TRANSPLANTATION

Heart transplantation techniques were developed to provide treatment for patients with end-stage cardiac disease in whom other conventional medical or surgical therapies were either not effective or not applicable. It has been estimated that more than 16,000 adults and 2,000 children per year in the United States could potentially benefit from heart transplantation.[3] Candidates considered appropriate for heart transplantation are those patients with symptomatic medically refractory heart failure and limited survival expectancy without major contraindications to transplantation.

Currently, more than 80% of heart recipients will survive more than 1 year after heart transplantation, and the 5-year actuarial survival from all centers reporting to the registry is 71%.[2] As results with heart transplantation have improved over the past decade, patient selection criteria have been extended on many fronts. Factors that may affect early and late results

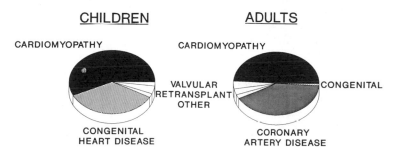

Fig. 38-1. Indications for heart transplantation in children and adults.

with heart transplantation, including recipient selection, tissue matching, transplantation technique, and immunosuppressive regimens, are reviewed in the following discussion.

Recipient Diagnosis

The types of cardiac disease that have led to heart transplantation, as reported to the ISHT Registry,[2] are shown in Figure 38-1. End-stage cardiac failure caused by cardiomyopathy has been the most common indication for heart transplantation in both children and adults. The second most common indication has been coronary artery disease (CAD) in adults (41% of cases), and congenital heart disease in children (35% of recipients). During the past few years, as the number of young recipients has increased, the percentage with congenital heart disease has continued to rise, exceeding, in 1989 for the first time, cardiomyopathy as the primary indication for heart transplantation in children. Valvular heart disease and retransplantation have each accounted for an additional 4% of recipients. Other less common indications for heart transplantation have included myocarditis, refractory arrhythmias, cardiac amyloidosis, Chagas disease, and cardiac tumors.

The original heart disease leading to heart trans-

plantation appears to have little effect on outcome.[1,26] The ISHT Registry data grouped by indication for transplantation are shown in Table 38-1. Cardiomyopathy, CAD, valvular heart disease, and myocarditis are associated with similar operative risk and late survival. Recipients with congenital heart disease have been found to have a higher operative risk. However, almost one-half of this group have been under 5 years of age, and other risk factors in these patients include a higher incidence of pulmonary hypertension and pretransplant hemodynamic instability and increased complexity of the procedure, because of the cardiac anomalies or prior palliative procedures.[27-32] If operative deaths are excluded, there is no difference in late survival for any of the major indications for heart transplantation.

In patients with cardiac amyloidosis, however, recurrence of amyloid deposits in the transplanted heart has been reported within 4 months.[33,34] While hemodynamically significant cardiac amyloidosis occurred in only one patient, a multicenter survey[35] found that three of six patients who survived the perioperative period subsequently died of progressive systemic amyloidosis, 13 to 46 months after transplantation. The ISHT Registry has received data on 22 recipients with cardiac amyloidosis ranging in age from 33 to 66 years. Two recipients died within 30 days, and actuarial sur-

TABLE 38-1. Effect of Type of Heart Disease on Orthotopic Transplantation Results Since 1980

			Survival Data (%)		
		Operative Deaths	1 Yr		5 Yr
Indication	n	(%)	(%)	(%)[a]	(%)
Cardiomyopathy	6,790	9.3	81.7	(89.8)	71.7
Coronary artery disease	5,065	10.0	80.2	(88.8)	70.6
Valvular heart disease	580	12.1	81.8	(93.0)	75.0
Congenital heart disease	497	21.3[b]	73.5[b]	(93.3)	62.1[b]
Myocarditis	126	9.5	81.5	(87.4)	—

[a] Excluding operative deaths.
[b] p <0.01 by chi-square.
(Date from Kaye MP: personal communication.)

vival is 71% at 1 year and 50% at 3 years. Three of seven late deaths were related to amyloidosis.

Many systemic illnesses that previously excluded patients from acceptance for heart transplantation are now considered "relative" contraindications. For example, an increasing number of patients with diabetes mellitus have undergone transplantation, without an observed difference in survival or infectious episodes.[36] The ISHT Registry data on more than 350 diabetic heart transplant recipients show an operative mortality of 9.6% with a 1-year actuarial survival of 79%, comparable to results in nondiabetic recipients.

Patients with a history of malignancy and chemotherapy or radiotherapy-induced cardiomyopathy have also received heart transplants.[37] Forty-three recipients ranging in age from 10 to 59 years with chemotherapy- or radiation-induced cardiomyopathy have been reported to the ISHT Registry. Only one operative death has been reported, and survival at 1 year is 80%. Recurrence of prior malignancy or increased risk of post-transplant lymphoproliferative disease has not been reported. Any active malignancy, however, would remain a contraindication to transplantation.

A number of patients with renal or hepatic failure have had combined heart plus kidney transplantation or liver transplantation, or both. Forty-three heart recipients with simultaneous multiple organ transplantation (kidney, 38; liver, 7; pancreas, 2) have been reported to the ISHT Registry.[2] Three patients had combined heart-liver-kidney transplantation. Of patients with combined heart-kidney transplantation, 4 of 35 (11.4%) died within 30 days, the 1-year survival is 79% (n = 20 at 1 year). Two of 7 (28.6%) combined heart-liver recipients died within 30 days, one died at 6 years, and four are living 3 months to 2 years after transplantation. There appears to be no substantially increased risk associated with combined heart-kidney operations. The number of patients with other types of multiple organ transplantation is too small to draw reasonable conclusions, although it would be reasonably anticipated for survival to be somewhat lower.

Recipient Gender

It has been suggested that recipient gender relates to survival. Some centers have reported a higher survival rate in men,[26] while others have found no difference.[38] Women have also been reported to have a higher incidence of rejection during the first 4 months, with more men successfully weaned off steroids, while no difference was found in operative mortality, incidence of infection, or long-term survival.[39] The ISHT Registry data, shown in Table 38-2, indicates a slight but statistically significant higher operative mortality for

women. If operative deaths are excluded, 1-year survival is similar for male and female heart recipients.

Recipient Age

Age restrictions have been extended to include both younger and older recipients. The ISHT Registry has received data on recipients ranging in age from newborns to 70 years with a mean age of 45 years.[2] During the 1980s, heart transplantation in children was the most rapidly developing field, and this now accounts for more than 9% of transplants annually.[1] Transplantation in infants and young children has been responsible for the major increases in annual numbers of pediatric transplants. In 1989, more than one-half of pediatric recipients were under the age of 5 years, and of these, most were younger than 1 year. While most heart transplant recipients have been 30 to 55 years of age, most programs have extended the upper age limit to 65 years.

The operative mortality and survival data grouped by recipient age are shown in Table 38-2. Although the overall results for heart transplantation have been similar for children and adults,[1,27] the operative risk has been higher in young children. The early mortality for orthotopic heart transplantation in adults since 1980 has been 10% and is 24% for young children. Late survival is similar in both groups.

The results with heart transplantation in recipients over the age of 55 years have been excellent. No difference has been reported in length of hospital stay, operative mortality, incidence of infection or rejection, or long-term survival.[26,40] However, as may be antici-

TABLE 38-2. Effect of Recipient Gender and Age on Orthotopic Heart Transplantation Results Since 1980

Sex	n	Operative Deaths (%)	Survival Data		5 Yr (%)
			1 Yr		
			(%)	(%)[a]	
Male	10,877	9.7	80.8	(89.6)	71.5
Female	2,453	12.5[b]	78.6[b]	(89.5)	68.7[b]

Age (yr)	n	Operative Deaths (%)	Survival Data		5 Yr (%)
			1 Yr		
			(%)	(%)[a]	
0–4	356	23.9[b]	69.6	(91.5)	—
5–9	113	15.0	73.8	(86.0)	66.5
10–18	548	11.5	77.9	(87.8)	67.1
19–54	9,170	10.0	80.9	(89.9)	71.4
55–70	3,320	9.8	80.5	(89.2)	72.4

[a] Excluding operative deaths.
[b] p <0.01 by chi-square.
(Data from Kaye MP: personal communication.)

pated, the risk of steroid-induced diabetes and osteoporosis is higher in the older recipients.[40]

Preoperative State and Assist Devices

The ISHT Registry has received data on the pretransplant clinical status of more than 5,000 heart recipients from U.S. centers. Almost all these recipients have been in New York Heart Association (NYHA) class 3 (21%) or class 4 (78%). Slightly more than one-half required hospitalization during the period immediately preceding transplantation. Of those hospitalized, 79% required intensive care unit (ICU) monitoring and inotropic or other additional support. Prior to transplantation, 4.9% of recipients required ventilatory support, 8.4% underwent placement of intra-aortic balloon pumps, and 3.9% had cardiac assist devices inserted.

Since 1985, ventricular assist devices and the total artificial heart have been used as a "bridge to transplantation" in patients with hemodynamic decompensation. Of patients who require mechanical cardiac assistance, 20 to 47% will become unsuitable for transplantation because of sepsis, multisystem organ failure, or neurologic complications.[15,41,42] Cabrol et al.[15] reported that in patients with chronic CHF, the use of the total artificial heart fails to reverse other organ dysfunction, although in young patients with acute cardiac decompensation, mechanical support may reverse organ failure and permit subsequent transplantation.

The 1989 report of the Combined Registry for the Clinical Use of Mechanical Ventricular Assist Pumps and the Total Artificial Heart[41] reported 363 patients on mechanical support. Of 272 patients (75%) subsequently transplanted, the operative mortality was 28%. Actuarial 2-year survival for all types of mechanical assist was 65%; however, the subgroup of recipients with pretransplant univentricular assist devices had a higher survival (83%).

The ISHT Registry operative mortality and survival data associated with recipient clinical status prior to transplantation are shown in Table 38-3. In hemodynamically stable recipients, the operative risk is less than 10%. The need for additional support more than doubles the early mortality rate. Also, patients who required either a biventricular assist device or total artificial heart had a significantly higher operative mortality than did patients with a LV assist device. The higher operative risk appears to be the major factor accounting for the lower survival in recipients who require mechanical cardiac support prior to transplantation. Of those recipients that survive the perioperative period, 1-year survival is more than 80%.

TABLE 38-3. Effect of Recipient Clinical Status on Orthotopic Heart Transplantation Results Since 1980

Recipient Status	n	Operative Deaths (%)	Survival Data 1 Yr (%)	Survival Data 1 Yr (%)[a]
Not hospitalized	2,559	6.1	86.6	(92.0)
In-hospital	615	6.0	84.0	(89.2)
In ICU	1,276	7.8	85.4	(92.4)
In ICU on support	997	14.2[b]	78.1	(90.7)
Ventilator	268	21.6[b]	71.0	(90.2)
IABP	457	10.7	80.3	(89.6)
LVAD	94	11.7	81.4	(92.1)
BIVAD	61	27.1[b]	63.6[b]	(83.6)
TAH	61	24.6[b]	63.6[b]	(84.3)

Abbreviations: ICU, intensive care unit; IABP, intraaortic balloon pump; LVAD, left ventricular assist device; BIVAD, biventricular assist device; TAH, total artificial heart.
[a] Excluding operative deaths.
[b] $p < 0.01$ by chi-square.
(Data from Kaye MP: personal communication.)

Tissue Matching

Because of the limitations of organ preservation, allocation of donor hearts, in contrast to kidneys, has been based only on ABO blood group compatibility, and not on HLA typing. Inadvertent transplantation of ABO-incompatible hearts has been associated with extremely poor results. A worldwide survey of eight cases described hyperacute rejection in five patients (63%) and a 50% mortality in less than 2 months.[43]

The effect of ABO compatibility compared with ABO identity on recipient outcome is less clear. Nakatani et al.[44] reported a higher 1 year survival rate for ABO-identical hearts (80% versus 62%) with a lower incidence of fatal rejection in the ABO-identical group. However, others have found no difference in survival based on ABO blood group donor-recipient identity.[45]

The effect of HLA mismatch as related to rejection and survival in heart transplant recipients has been examined retrospectively in a limited number of patients.[26,45–47] The number of HLA mismatches has been associated with a higher incidence of rejection,[45,46] but no effect on late survival was evident.[46] Another study indicated a significantly better 4-year survival with one or less mismatches at AB loci, compared with recipients with four mismatches (88% versus 54%).[47] In addition, the group with fewer mismatches had fewer infectious complications, possibly related to lower immuno-suppressive requirements. Yacoub et al.[26] reported HLA-DR mismatching to have the greatest effect on survival. Those recipients with one DR mismatch had a 2-year survival of 84% versus 68% for those with two DR mismatches. It would thus seem prudent to match donor hearts as well as possible, but the current shortage of donors internationally makes this an academic matter.

Transplantation Procedure

Of the two techniques of heart transplantation, orthotopic and heterotopic, orthotopic procedures have been performed in the vast majority of cases (98%).[1] The heterotopic technique has generally been reserved for patients with markedly elevated and fixed pulmonary vascular resistance (>6 Wood units) or in cases of significant recipient-donor size mismatch (more than 20% of cases).[48] As shown in Table 38-4, the ISHT Registry data indicate a significantly lower operative risk, as well as a higher late survival for orthotopic transplantation. While a major factor is the higher early mortality, if operative deaths are excluded, late mortality also remains higher after heterotopic transplantation. Of those recipients who survive the first year, the risk of death is 1.4%/year for orthotopic transplantation, and 2.7%/year for heterotopic procedures. Few centers still perform this technique.

It is clear that the presence of pulmonary hypertension is a major factor in early mortality with orthotopic heart transplantation.[49–51] Ten percent of operative deaths have been related to elevated pulmonary vascular resistance (PVR) with donor right heart failure.[2] Pretransplant evaluation of the response to vasodilators or the use of the PVR index (PVRI) has been suggested for better identification of those patients at significant risk of donor right heart failure.[49,50] Addonizio et al.[50] reported that 33% of patients with a PVRI higher than 6 Wood units/m^2 developed significant right heart failure and five of these six patients (83%) died perioperatively. The use of larger donors, short donor ischemic times, and pharmacologic manipulation of pulmonary hypertension (e.g., isoproterenol, nitroprusside, and PGE1), for patients with elevated PVR has been suggested. Also, the use of the explanted heart from heart-lung recipients with pulmonary hypertension as the donor organ for heart transplantation ("domino operation") provides a "conditioned" right ventricle for recipients with significant pulmonary hypertension.

TABLE 38-4. Effect of Transplant Technique on Heart Transplantation Results Since 1980

Technique	n	Operative Deaths (%)	Survival Data		
			1 Yr		5 Yr
			(%)	(%)^a	(%)
Orthotopic	13,616	10.4	80.3	(89.3)	71.1
Heterotopic	272	24.6^b	59.7^b	(78.1)^b	46.1^b

^{a} Excluding operative deaths.
^{b} p <0.01 by chi-square.
(Data from Kaye MP: personal communication.)

Immunosuppressive Regimens

A decrease in the morbidity and mortality associated with infection and rejection has been observed with the use of cyclosporine-based immunosuppression. This has been a major factor related to the improved survival with heart transplantation during the past decade.[38,45,51,52] An increase in 1-year survival from 63 to 81%, and 5-year survival from 36 to 60% with the use of cyclosporine was reported in the Stanford series.[38] Almost all units currently use a combination of cyclosporine, azathioprine, and steroids (triple therapy), and analysis of the results from the Registry demonstrates that improved survival is obtained with the three drugs used together.[1,51]

More recently, the addition of OKT3, a murine monoclonal T-cell antibody, has been reported to be highly effective for rejection prophylaxis as well as the reversal of refractory acute rejection.[53] The reported advantage of OKT3 is its lack of renal, hepatic, or hematopoietic toxicity, although serious side effects, including hypotension, pulmonary edema, bronchospasm, and aseptic meningitis, are not uncommon.[53,54] The use of OKT3 has not been associated with an increase in bacterial infections, although the risk of cytomegalovirus (CMV) infection may be higher.[55] However, the ISHT Registry data indicate that the addition of OKT3 to a triple drug regimen appears to have no appreciable effect on survival.[1]

PROGNOSIS OF HEART TRANSPLANTATION

Survival following heart transplantation has improved markedly during the past two decades, as shown in Figure 38-2. In a review of 206 Stanford heart recipients prior to the introduction of cyclosporine, the 1-year survival rate did increase from 22% (1968) to 67% (1979).[56] This improvement was attributed to careful recipient selection and increased experience in early postoperative management, including the use of rabbit antithymocyte globulin and immunologic monitoring with T-cell counts, the liberal use of endomyocardial biopsy, and retransplantation for resistant rejection.

During the 1980s, further improvements in the morbidity and mortality associated with heart transplantation have continued. Of more than 14,000 heart transplants reported to the ISHT Registry since 1980, more than 10,000 patients are alive. Operative mortality has fallen to less than 10%, and the 5-year survival has risen to 70%. Better than 1,500 recipients have lived more than 5 years, and 91 have now survived more than 10 years after transplantation.

Although many factors affect prognosis in heart

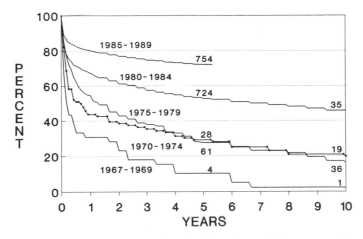

Fig. 38-2. Actuarial survival associated with orthotopic heart transplantation.

transplantation, most patients can expect improved length of survival and quality of life with transplantation compared with medical therapy for heart failure. However, the ideal immunosuppressive regimen has not yet been developed, and all transplant patients continue to be faced with increased susceptibility to infection, and the risks of acute and chronic rejection, as well as side effects of chronic immunosuppression.

The causes of early (<30 days) and late death in heart recipients since 1980, as reported to the ISHT Registry, and the cause of death related to survival interval are shown in Figures 38-3 and 38-4. While infection and rejection continue to be the primary causes of death in heart transplant recipients, one half of deaths within the first month have been due to technical or cardiac complications, including primary graft

failure (30%), right heart failure associated with pulmonary hypertension (10%), cardiac arrest (5%), and hemorrhage (5%). The even greater risk of such complications in children may be related to the higher incidence of elevated pulmonary vascular resistance, worse pretransplant clinical status, and complex congenital heart defects.[28,29]

The outlook for patients with early graft failure attributable to inadequate organ preservation, pulmonary hypertension, or refractory acute rejection is not encouraging. Miller et al.[41] reported on 45 patients who required mechanical support (ventricular assist device; VAD) for early donor organ failure. Only 14 recipients (31%) recovered adequate cardiac function, and only 8 patients (18%) were discharged from hospital. The option of retransplantation for early graft fail-

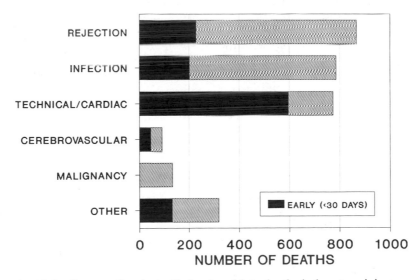

Fig. 38-3. Causes of early (<30 days) and late deaths in heart recipients.

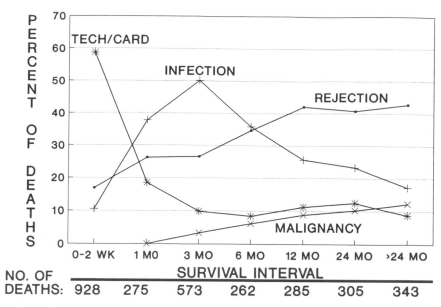

Fig. 38-4. Causes of death in heart recipients relative to survival interval.

ure has not proved very successful, largely because by the time it becomes obvious that this strategy is essential and a second donor is found, recipients have sustained secondary organ damage or infection.

Advances in immunosuppression, diagnostic techniques, and antimicrobial therapy have decreased the incidence of infectious complications following heart transplantation.[57] However, infections continue to be a major cause of morbidity and mortality in heart recipients. Approximately one-third of recipients sustain one or more major infections, with the risk of infection highest after any period of augmented immunosuppression.[58] Prior to 1981, 58% of deaths in the Stanford heart recipients were due to infection, most commonly bacterial.[56] More recently, infections, usually viral or fungal, have been reported to cause 17 to 36% of deaths among heart recipients.[2,38,58] As shown in Figure 38-4, from 1 to 3 months after transplantation, infections account for 50% of deaths. After 3 months, the risk of death from infection continues to decrease, possibly related to lowered steroid requirements.

Acute and chronic rejection remain important factors in survival after heart transplantation. The use of cyclosporine-based immunosuppression has been associated with decreased morbidity and mortality from rejection.[52] However, various reports indicate that 50 to 87% of recipients will still have one or more episodes of acute rejection within the first year after heart transplantation.[27,38,58] The incidence of acute rejection appears to be similar in children and adults,[27] although infants have been reported to require less immunosuppression.[30] Acute rejection has been the re-

ported cause in 16 to 24% of deaths after heart transplantation.[2,38,58]

The development of accelerated atherosclerosis in the transplanted heart remains the major impediment to long-term survival. In the earliest series from Stanford, all nine recipients who survived at least 3 years developed graft atherosclerosis.[59] In more recent reports from Stanford, graft disease was present in 27% of 1-year survivors[60] and was the primary cause in 14% of deaths. In a prospective angiographic study of patients on cyclosporine, Uretsky et al.[61] reported evidence of coronary graft atherosclerosis in 18% of recipients at 1 year, 27% at 2 years, and 44% at 3 years after transplantation.

In support of graft atherosclerosis as a type of chronic rejection, Uretsky and co-workers found that 64% of recipients with disease at 1 year and 83% with disease at 2 years had a history of recurrent rejection episodes. However, others have reported no correlation with the number of rejection episodes experienced during the first year or with the use of cyclosporine-based immunosuppressive therapy.[62] The development of graft atherosclerosis has not been related to the original disease of the recipient, recipient or donor age, HLA mismatch, smoking, dosage of steroids, or cholesterol subfractions.[38,61,62] Some centers have reported a lower incidence in children.[27,30] CMV infection and elevated triglyceride levels do appear to be related to this condition, however.[62,63] Despite an early report by Griepp et al.[59] indicating a beneficial effect of the use of antiplatelet therapy, others have not shown a decrease in the risk of graft atherosclerosis.[61,62]

Because of chronic immunosuppression, heart transplant recipients are also at increased risk of malignancy, most commonly lymphoproliferative disease. Lymphoma was reported in 4.6% of patients from 67 to 853 days after heart transplantation in the Stanford series,[38] although the risk was lower (1.3%) after the introduction of lower-dose cyclosporine protocols. Trento et al.[29] found the diffuse form of lymphoproliferative disease to be more common in children with response to a decrease in immunosuppressive therapy and the use of Acyclovir in one-half of cases. As shown in Figure 38-4, the risk continues to increase with survival interval, and malignancy accounts for 12% of deaths in recipients who survive more than 2 years.

Rehabilitation in heart transplant recipients has been excellent.[27,38,40] In the Stanford series,[38] 97% of 1-year survivors were in NYHA class 1. Olivari and colleagues[40] reported that 94% of young adult and 83% of older patients (above 55 years of age) returned to work, living normal life-styles, within 3 months of heart transplantation. Results in the pediatric transplant population have also been excellent.[27,30]

The major chronic side effects of current immunosuppressive regimens include hypertension, renal dysfunction, and diabetes. The incidence of post-transplantation hypertension has ranged from 52 to 92% of recipients with cyclosporine-based therapy.[27,38,40,64,65] Ozdogan et al.[65] found a lower risk in patients under 20 years of age, while others have reported no difference with recipient age.[27,64] Olivari et al.[64] reported that 92% of recipients on triple drug immunosuppression required medical therapy for hypertension within the first 6 months after transplantation. While this did not correlate with serum creatinine or cyclosporine levels, weight gain was greater in patients with hypertension. The nephrotoxic effect of cyclosporine does result in mild renal dysfunction, but this appears to remain stable over the long term.[27,64]

The incidence of post-transplant diabetes appears to be lower using cyclosporine-based immunosuppression; this is probably because of the decreased need for steroid therapy. Rhenman et al.[36] reported the development of diabetes after transplantation in 22% of patients during the precyclosporine era, compared with the current rate of 8%. Ladowski,[66] who also found an 8% rate, reported that the development of post-transplant diabetes could not be predicted from recipient age, sex, race, HLA typing, or steroid dose. In addition, the presence of post-transplant diabetes was not found to be associated with a difference in incidence of infection, graft atherosclerosis, or survival.

Heart Retransplantation

The ISHT Registry entries as of October 1990 included 388 heart recipients who had undergone retransplantation, including 13 recipients who had undergone a third heart transplantation. Time to retransplantation ranged from 1 day to 12 years. Early retransplantation was required for primary graft failure and/or technical problems in 25% of cases and for early rejection in an additional 19% of cases. The major indication for retransplantation has been chronic rejection.[1,52,62] During the 1980s, operative mortality for cardiac retransplantation has been 34%, with similar results in both children and adults.[2]

The risk of early or late death has been related to the indication for retransplantation, the clinical status of the patient at the time of reoperation, and the time interval to retransplantation. Dein et al.[52] reported the 1980 to 1988 Stanford experience in 23 patients. Retransplantation was performed for graft atherosclerosis in 14 patients and for acute rejection in 9 patients. Those with graft atherosclerosis had similar survival and infection rates as for the primary transplant, while more patients with refractory acute rejection were hemodynamically unstable at retransplantation and had a much lower 1-year survival (44% versus 85%). Miller et al.[41] reported 37 recipients requiring mechanical support for acute rejection. Of 22 retransplants, only 7 patients (32%) were discharged from hospital.

The ISHT Registry data confirm that recipients requiring early retransplantation have a much higher operative mortality (63% if <1 month and 42% if 1 to 6 months).[1] If heart retransplantation is performed more than 6 months after the initial operation, the operative risk (14%) and late survival are improved, although not equal to the primary transplant procedure. ISHT Registry survival data for orthotopic retransplantation compared with the primary procedure are shown in Figure 38-5. Of the 13 patients receiving a third heart transplant, only one patient has survived more than 4 years.

HEART-LUNG TRANSPLANTATION

The application of pulmonary transplantation as realistic therapy for end-stage pulmonary failure required the development of immunosuppressive agents that would permit normal tissue healing. The use of cyclosporine immunosuppression in the animal laboratory in 1978[67] and in clinical heart transplantation in 1980,[68] led to the first successful human combined heart-lung procedure at Stanford in 1981.[69] Because of the encouraging early heart-lung results, single lung transplantation was reintroduced in 1983,[70] followed by the development of the double lung transplant technique in 1985.[71] With three options now available for patients with end-stage pulmonary disease, the indications for each procedure continue to evolve. Many factors, including patient age, degree of other organ involvement, previous thoracic operations, recipient

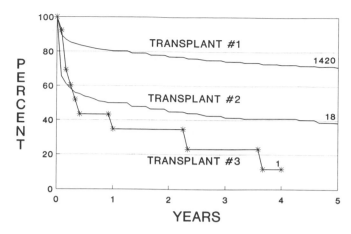

Fig. 38-5. Actuarial survival associated with retransplantation in heart recipients.

cardiac function, and type of pulmonary disease influence the selection of the optimal procedure for each candidate.

As a result of the extended waiting period for combined heart-lung candidates and recent expansion in single lung transplantation, combined heart-lung transplantation is currently reserved for patients with bilateral septic conditions (i.e., cystic fibrosis and bronchiectasis) and for patients with irreparable or irreversible cardiac dysfunction associated with end-stage pulmonary disease. Experience in pulmonary thromboendarterectomy patients has shown that normalization of pulmonary arterial pressure permits rapid recovery of right ventricular function.[72] As similar results occur with single lung transplantation, this technique can be used in many patients with primary pulmonary hypertension (PPH) and Eisenmenger syndrome. If necessary, congenital heart defects can be simultaneously corrected at the time of lung transplantation.[73] Single lung transplantation is also an option in patients with emphysema as, perhaps unexpectedly, a clinically significant ventilation-perfusion mismatch does not occur.[74]

As in heart transplantation, candidates for pulmonary transplantation have severely restricted exercise tolerance and limited life expectancy. Selection criteria for combined heart-lung transplantation have remained more strict than for heart or even single lung transplantation. Major organ dysfunction must be limited to the heart and lungs. Prior chest surgery is also a significant concern, as the risk of hemorrhage from extensive pleural and pericardial adhesions is increased.

As of October 1990, the ISHT Registry has received information on more than 1,100 pulmonary transplant procedures, including more than 860 combined heart-lung transplantations, from more than 60 centers worldwide.[2] More than 200 combined heart-lung

transplants were performed in 1989, but the use of this technique now appears to be decreasing. This decrease is related both to limitations in donor availability and to the recent growth in single and double lung transplantation. Including all recipients reported to the ISHT Registry since 1981, operative mortality for combined heart-lung transplantation has been 23%. Actuarial survival data indicate 1- and 5-year survival rates of 60% and 45% (n = 47 at 5 years). Less information is available on risk factors for combined heart-lung transplantation than for heart transplantation because of both the smaller number of recipients and the shorter period of follow-up.

The indications for combined heart-lung transplantation reported to the ISHT Registry are shown in Figure 38-6. During the early 1980s, most recipients fell into two main groups: those with PPH and those with Eisenmenger's syndrome.[1] During the past few years, a shift has occurred in the indications for combined heart-lung replacement. Experience in patients with cystic fibrosis has increased rapidly. In 1989 and 1990, the numbers of recipients with PPH, Eisenmenger's syndrome, and cystic fibrosis were almost equal. Other indications for combined heart-lung transplantation have included acquired heart disease with PPH (which obviated heart transplantation alone), emphysema, pulmonary fibrosis, pulmonary thromboembolic disease, sarcoidosis, histiocytosis X, bronchiectasis, lupus, scleroderma, hemosiderosis, lymphangioleiomyomatosis, acute respiratory distress syndrome (ARDS), and leiomyosarcoma of the pulmonary artery.

Grouped according to indication for transplantation, as shown in Table 38-5, operative risk has been higher in patients with PPH. Thirteen of 34 (38%) PPH patients over 45 years of age died within 30 days. The deleterious effects of cardiopulmonary bypass and cyclosporine on pre-existing renal and hepatic dys-

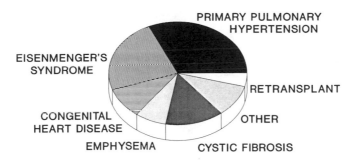

Fig. 38-6. Indications for combined heart-lung transplantation.

function, which are more common in PPH patients, may contribute to this increased risk. Of the patients with congenital heart disease, the subgroup with Eisenmenger syndrome had a much lower operative mortality (13.4%, n = 168) than that of patients with complex congenital defects, precluding heart transplantation (32.9%, n = 76). Patients with cystic fibrosis have had a low operative mortality and a late survival comparable to other indications for heart-lung transplantation.

The available data on the effects of recipient gender and age in combined heart-lung transplantation are shown in Table 38-6. Outcome does not appear to be affected by recipient gender. The ISHT Registry has received data on heart-lung recipients ranging in age from 3 months to 60 years, with an average age of 30 years.[2] Most centers continue to limit the age of recipients to less than 45 years. In contrast to heart transplantation, operative risk in the youngest heart-lung recipients is not increased, although this includes only 18 patients under 5 years of age. Recipients over 45 years of age have had a higher operative mortality. The data for 1- and 2-year survival appear to be similar for all age groups.

As in heart transplantation, the use of triple drug therapy has been reported to improve survival in combined heart-lung transplantation.[75] Improvements in renal function[76] and a decrease in viral infections[77] have also been attributed to the reduced dosages of cyclosporine.

PROGNOSIS OF HEART-LUNG TRANSPLANTATION

The ISHT Registry actuarial survival data for combined heart-lung transplantation are shown in Figure 38-7. There has been a slight improvement in operative mortality and late survival during the past 5 years. Actuarial 5-year survival is currently 45%. Five patients have now survived over 7 years, the longest surviving patient having been transplanted in November 1982.

Causes of death and effect of survival interval on

TABLE 38-5. Effect of Recipient Gender and Age on Heart-Lung Transplantation Results Since 1980

Indication	n	Operative Deaths (%)	1 Yr (%)	1 Yr (%)[a]	2 Yr (%)
PPH	240	26.7	55.9	(75.4)	50.4
CHD/ Eisenmenger syndrome	243	19.3	61.8	(76.6)	53.5
Cystic fibrosis	109	13.8	66.9	(77.6)	60.6
Emphysema	61	19.7	63.4	(78.7)	59.8

Abbreviations: PPH, primary pulmonary hypertension; CHD, congenital heart disease.
[a] Excluding operative deaths.
(Data from Kaye MP: personal communication.)

TABLE 38-6. Effect of Type of Disease on Heart-Lung Transplantation Results Since 1980

Sex	n	Operative Deaths (%)	1 Yr (%)	1 Yr (%)[a]	2 Yr (%)
Male	360	23.3	58.3	(75.5)	50.7
Female	440	22.0	62.1	(79.0)	55.2

Age	n	Operative Deaths (%)	1 Yr (%)	1 Yr (%)[a]	2 Yr (%)
0–9	53	20.8	60.4	(76.1)	53.2
10–18	104	15.4	60.5	(71.5)	49.1
19–44	571	23.5	59.7	(77.9)	54.3
45–60	102	30.4	55.4	(78.5)	47.2)

[a] Excluding operative deaths.
(Data from Kaye MP: personal communication.)

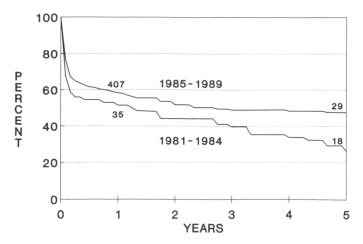

Fig. 38-7. Actuarial survival associated with combined heart-lung transplantation.

cause of death in combined heart-lung transplantation are shown in Figures 38-8 and 38-9. Technical complications, including primary graft failure, myocardial infarction, cardiac arrest, and hemorrhage, have accounted for 50% of early deaths.

Infection has been the predominant cause of early and late morbidity and mortality in heart-lung transplantation.[1,78] The significantly higher incidence of pulmonary infections in heart-lung than in heart recipients may be related to pulmonary denervation, lung preservation injury, and impairment of the mucociliary apparatus. Early mediastinal fungal infections, caused by donor or recipient tracheal contamination, have been lethal.[79]

Cytomegalovirus (CMV) seronegative recipients who receive organs from CMV-positive donors have had an extremely high risk of serious CMV infections.[80,81] CMV donor-recipient matching, antiviral prophylaxis, early diagnosis, and the availability of an effective and well-tolerated antiviral agent, gancyiclovir, has improved the outlook for CMV infection.

Rejection, usually of the lung, was reported in 10% of early and 20% of late deaths. A lower incidence of acute cardiac rejection in combined heart-lung than in heart recipients has been reported.[82] In addition, coronary atherosclerosis has been responsible for only 3% of deaths in combined heart-lung transplantation as reported to the ISHT Registry. Possible explanations are that pulmonary rejection, which tends to occur before cardiac rejection, is treated before cardiac rejection becomes established, or that the increased antigenic load associated with combined

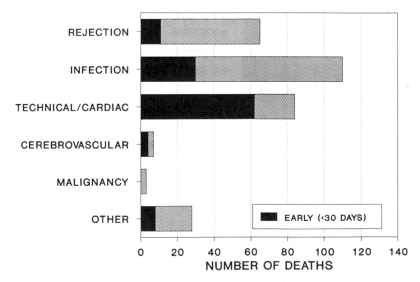

Fig. 38-8. Causes of early (<30 days) and late death in combined heart-lung recipients.

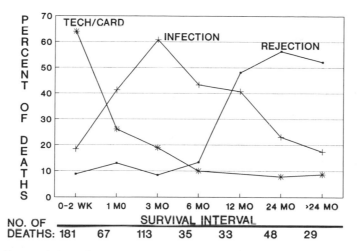

Fig. 38-9. Cause of death in combined heart-lung recipients relative to survival interval.

heart-lung transplantation results in a more favorable immune response.

As pulmonary and cardiac rejection do not necessarily occur synchronously,[83,84] surveillance endomyocardial biopsies have not proven useful in combined heart-lung recipients.[82,85,86] A deterioration in pulmonary function has been noted with both acute and chronic pulmonary rejection episodes.[82,84,86,87] Recently, the use of transbronchial biopsy[82,84,86] and bronchoalveolar lavage[88] to diagnose pulmonary rejection has been described. While these techniques may assist in early differentiation of acute rejection from infection, in almost all instances of biopsy-proven rejection requiring augmentation of immunosuppression, the patients have been symptomatic or have had acute decreases in pulmonary function tests. Therefore, it is not yet clear whether routine surveillance transbronchial biopsy in asymptomatic patients is indicated or whether it will affect long-term survival.

Bronchiolitis obliterans remains the most serious impediment to successful long-term outcome following combined heart-lung transplantation. This entity was first described in combined heart-lung transplant recipients, and affected approximately one-third of patients within one year after transplantation.[89,90] The etiology of bronchiolitis obliterans remains unclear, although it is most likely related to chronic rejection.[87,91,92] An association with CMV pulmonary infection has also been noted,[93] but it is difficult to establish which of these entities arose first. Although the rapidity of deterioration may be slowed by augmented immunosuppression during the early stages,[91,94] an unrelenting downhill course toward retransplantation or death appears inevitable.[95] A lower incidence of bronchiolitis obliterans has been reported with triple drug immunosuppression and with early diagnosis and treatment of acute rejection episodes.[75]

Heart-Lung Retransplantation

As of October 1990, the ISHT Registry has received retransplant data on 39 combined heart-lung recipients, including 34 patients with heart-lung and 5 recipients with single-lung retransplantation. The time interval to retransplantation has ranged from one day to 4 years. The indication has been primary graft failure in 20% and rejection or bronchiolitis obliterans in 80% of patients.

Survival following pulmonary retransplantation has been poor. Twenty patients [17 (50%) heart-lung and 3 (60%) single-lung retransplants] died within 30 days. In contrast to heart transplantation, a longer interval between transplant procedures does not improve operative risk. The ISHT Registry actuarial survival data for retransplantation in combined heart-lung recipients are shown in Figure 38-10. Only 13 (33%) patients survived more than 6 months. Six patients survived more than 2 years, two of whom are alive at 4 years after heart-lung retransplantation.

COST OF HEART AND HEART-LUNG TRANSPLANTATION

Many factors contribute to the costs of heart and combined heart-lung transplantation. The routine use of cyclosporine has permitted significantly shorter hospital stays and fewer hospital readmissions for rejection or infectious complications. At the University of California, San Diego, the average hospital stay after heart transplantation is 10 days and, after heart-

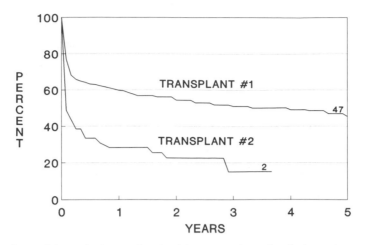

Fig. 38-10. Actuarial survival associated with retransplantation in heart-lung recipients.

lung or lung transplantation, 21 days. The costs incurred in the care of the end-stage cardiac and pulmonary patient without transplantation must be considered if a reasonable assessment of cost is to be made. Most of these patients will require recurrent hospitalizations for the treatment of exacerbations of heart and/or pulmonary failure, cardiac arrhythmias, and other complications. In 1988, Sweeney et al.[16] reported an average cost of $56,000 for status 1 (urgent) patients who died awaiting transplantation. Similar analyses of cost are not available for end-stage pulmonary failure.

Pennock et al.[56] reviewed the costs of heart transplantation at Stanford prior to 1980. The average length of in-hospital stay from 1973 to 1979 was 65 days, at a cost of $91,000. Follow-up costs in hospital averaged $10,000 for the first year and $5,000 to $7,000/year for the second and third years. Additional outpatient costs were $7,500 the first year and $5,000/year for the second and third years. The initial experience with cyclosporine at Stanford showed a decrease in hospital stay (average 45 days), with resultant lower costs ($57,000 in 5 patients). A more recent review at Stanford[38] found average charges for the first year to be $104,102 in 1985. Accounting for inflation, there was not a significant change from the previous report.

A survey of 18 transplant centers in 1987 showed that average in-hospital costs, including organ procurement and transplant team charges, varied from $52,000 to $121,000.[13] A major component was length of hospital stay. Follow-up costs appeared similar to Pennock's earlier report. In another study, Saywell et al.[97] reported an a 17-day average length of stay with total hospital costs averaging $36,000 (1987 range: $22,000 to $137,000). The total cost decreased over the 4 years of the study, again in large part due to reduction in hospital stay.

There are as yet no published reports on the costs of heart-lung or lung transplantation. In our own experience, the costs for combined heart-lung and double lung transplantation have approximated 2.5 times that for heart transplantation. The major component accounting for this increase has been a longer stay in the ICU.

SUMMARY

Much progress has been made in cardiopulmonary transplantation during the past decade. Excellent results in heart transplantation have been achieved in a wide variety of patients with end-stage heart disease. Because of the ever-increasing number of potential candidates in the face of the limited donor supply, the number of recipients requiring inotropic or additional mechanical support prior to transplantation has continued to increase. Although the risks of the procedure and of post-transplant complications have thus been increased, the results have continued to improve. The vast majority of recipients can expect a normal, unrestricted life-style.

The field of pulmonary transplantation continues to evolve rapidly. The availability of suitable lung donors is even less than for heart transplantation. Early encouraging results with single lung transplantation, recent improvements in the double lung transplant technique, and the development of alternative techniques such as single lung transplantation with repair of congenital defects will greatly affect the future role of combined heart-lung transplantation. It is hoped that future developments in immunosuppression will solve the problems of graft atherosclerosis and bronchiolitis obliterans while further decreasing the risk of infectious complications, and thus improve the long-term outlook for heart and lung transplant recipients.

REFERENCES

1. Kriett JM, Kaye MP: The Registry of the International Society for Heart Transplantation: seventh official report—1990. J Heart Transplant 9:323, 1990
2. Kriett JM, Tarazi RY, Kaye MP: The Registry of the International Society for Heart Transplantation. In Terasaki PI (ed): Clinical Transplants 1990. UCLA Tissue Typing Laboratory, Los Angeles, 1991
3. Kottke TE, Pesch DG, Frye RL et al: The potential contribution of cardiac replacement to the control of cardiovascular diseases—A population-based estimate. Arch Surg 125:1148, 1990
4. McKee PA, Casteill WP, McNamara PM, Kannel WB: The natural history of congestive heart failure: the Framingham study. N Engl J Med 285:1441, 1971
5. Fuster V, Gersh BJ, Giuliani ER et al: The natural history of idiopathic dilated cardiomyopathy. Am J Cardiol 47:525, 1981
6. Unverferth DV, Magorien RD, Moeschberger ML et al: Factors influencing the one-year mortality of dilated cardiomyopathy. Am J Cardiol 54:147, 1984
7. Franciosa JA, Wilen M, Ziesche S, Cohn JN: Survival in men with severe chronic left ventricular failure due to either coronary heart disease or idiopathic dilated cardiomyopathy. Am J Cardiol 51:831, 1983
8. Stevenson LW, Chellimsky-Fallick C, Tillisch J et al: Unacceptable risk of sudden death without transplantation if low ejection fraction is due to coronary artery disease, abstracted. J Am Coll Cardiol 15:222A, 1990
9. Morris CD, Outcalt J, Menashe VD: Hypoplastic left heart syndrome: natural history in a geographically defined population. Pediatrics 85:977, 1990
10. Bailey LL, Gundry SR: Hypoplastic left heart syndrome. Pediatr Clin North Am 37:137, 1990
11. Griffin ML, Hernandez A, Martin TC et al: Dilated cardiomyopathy in infants and children. J Am Coll Cardiol 11:139, 1988
12. Evans RW, Maier AM: Outcome of patients referred for cardiac transplantation. J Am Coll Cardiol 8:1312, 1986
13. USGAO Report: Heart transplants—Concerns about cost, access, and availability of donor organs. GAO/HRD-89-61, May 1989
14. Copeland JG, Emery RW, Levinson MM et al: The role of mechanical support and transplantation in treatment of patients with end-stage cardiomyopathy. Circulation 72:II7, 1985
15. Cabrol C, Gandjbakhch I, Pavie A et al: Total artificial heart as a bridge for transplantation: La Pitie 1986 to 1987. J Heart Transplant 7:12, 1988
16. Sweeney MS, Lammermeier DE, Frazier OH et al: Extension of donor criteria in cardiac transplantation: surgical risk versus supply-side economics. Ann Thorac Surg 50:7, 1990
17. Mayer JE, Jr, Perry S, O'Brien P et al: Orthotopic heart transplantation for complex congenital heart disease. J Thorac Cardiovasc Surg 99:484, 1990
18. Hughes JD, Rubin LJ: Primary pulmonary hypertension. An analysis of 28 cases and a review of the literature. Medicine (Baltimore) 65:56, 1986
19. Glanville AR, Burke CM, Theodore J, Robin ED: Primary pulmonary hypertension. Length of survival in patients referred for heart-lung transplantation. Chest 91:675, 1987
20. Hodgkin JE: Prognosis in chronic obstructive pulmonary disease. Clin Chest Med 11:555, 1990
21. Brantly ML, Paul LD, Miller BH et al: Clinical features and history of the destructive lung disease associated with alpha-1-antitrypsin deficiency of adults with pulmonary symptoms. Am Rev Respir Dis 138:327, 1988
22. Turner-Warwick M, Burrows B, Johnson A: Cryptogenic fibrosing alveolitis: clinical features and their influence on survival. Thorax 35:171, 1980
23. Fradet G, Smyth RL, Scott JP et al: Cystic fibrosis: a new challenge for cardiothoracic surgery. Eur J Cardiothorac Surg 4:136, 1990
24. Huang NN, Schidlow DV, Szatrowski TH et al: Clinical features, survival rate, and prognostic factors in young adults with cystic fibrosis. Am J Med 82:871, 1987
25. Smyth RL, Scott JP, Whitehead B et al: Heart-lung transplantation in children. Transplant Proc 22:1470, 1990
26. Yacoub M, Festenstein H, Doyle P et al: The influence of HLA matching in cardiac allograft recipients receiving cyclosporine and azathioprine. Transplant Proc 19:2487, 1987
27. Starnes VA, Stinson EB, Oyer PE et al: Heart transplantation in children and adolescents. Circulation, suppl. 76:V43, 1987
28. Addonizio LJ, Hsu DT, Fuzesi L et al: Optimal timing of pediatric heart transplantation. Circulation, suppl III. 80:III-84, 1989
29. Trento A, Griffith BP, Fricker FJ et al: Lessons learned in pediatric heart transplantation. Ann Thorac Surg 48:617, 1990
30. Bailey LL, Wood M, Van Arsdell G, Gundry S: Heart transplantation during the first 12 years of life. Loma Linda University Pediatric Heart Transplant Group. Arch Surg 124:1221, 1989
31. Menkis AH, McKensie FN, Novick RJ et al: Special considerations for heart transplantation in congenital heart disease. J Heart Transplant 9:602, 1990
32. Chartrand C, Guerin R, Kangah M, Stanley P: Pediatric heart transplantation: surgical considerations for congenital heart diseases. J Heart Transplant 9:608, 1990
33. Conner R, Hosenpud J, Norman D et al: Heart transplantation for cardiac amyloidosis:successful one-year outcome despite recurrence of the disease. J Heart Transplant 7:165, 1988
34. Valantine HA, Billingham ME: Recurrence of amyloid in a cardiac allograft four months after transplantation. J Heart Transplant 8:337, 1989
35. Hosenpud JD, Uretsky BF, Griffith BP et al: Successful intermediate-term outcome for patients with cardiac amyloidosis undergoing heart transplantation: results of a multicenter survey. J Heart Transplant 9:346, 1990
36. Rhenman MJ, Rhenman, B, Icenogle T et al: Diabetes and heart transplantation. J Heart Transplant 7:346, 1988

37. Armitage JM, Kormos RL, Griffith BP et al: Heart transplantation in patients with malignant disease. J Heart Transplant 9:627, 1990

38. Grattan MT, Moreno-Cabrol CE, Starnes VA et al: Eight-year results of cyclosporine-treated patients with cardiac transplants. J Thorac Cardiovasc Surg 99:500, 1990

39. Crandall BG, Renlund DG, O'Connell JB et al: Increased cardiac allograft rejection in female heart transplant recipients. J Heart Transplant 7:419, 1988

40. Olivari MT, Antolick A, Kaye M et al: Heart transplantation in elderly patients. J Heart Transplant 7:258, 1988

41. Miller CA, Pae WE, Jr, Pierce WS: Combined registry for the clinical use of mechanical ventricular assist pumps and the total artificial heart in conjunction with heart transplantation: fourth official report—1989. J Heart Transplant 9:453, 1990

42. Pennington DG, McBride LR, Kanter KR et al: Bridging to heart transplantation with circulatory support devices. J Heart Transplant 8:116, 1989

43. Cooper DKC: Clinical survey of heart transplantation between ABO blood group-incompatible recipients and donors. J Heart Transplant 9:376, 1990

44. Nakatani T, Aida A, Frazier OH, Macris MP: Effect of ABO blood type on survival of heart transplant patients treated with cyclosporine. J Heart Transplant 8:27, 1989

45. Laufer G, Miholic J, Laczkovics A et al: Independent risk factors predicting acute graft rejection in cardiac transplant recipients treated by triple drug immunosuppression. J Thorac Cardiovasc Surg 98:1113, 1989

46. DiSesa VJ, Kuo PC, Horvath KA et al: HLA histocompatability affects cardiac transplant rejection and may provide one basis for organ allocation. Ann Thorac Surg 49:220, 1990

47. Frist WH, Oyer PE, Baldwin JC et al: HLA compatibility and cardiac transplant recipient survival. Ann Thorac Surg 44:242, 1987

48. Reichenspurner H, Hildebrandt A, Boehm D et al: Heterotopic heart transplantation in 1988—recent selective indications and outcome. J Heart Transplant 8:381, 1989

49. Kirklin JK, Naftel D, Kirklin JW et al: Pulmonary vascular resistance and the risk of heart transplantation. J Heart Transplant 7:331, 1988

50. Addonizio LJ, Gersony WM, Robbins RC et al: Elevated pulmonary vascular resistance and cardiac transplantation. Circulation, suppl V. 76:V52, 1987

51. Heck CF, Shumway SJ, Kaye MP: The Registry of the International Society for Heart Transplantation: sixth official report—1989. J Heart Transplant 8:271, 1989

52. Dein J, Oyer P, Stinson EB et al: Cardiac retransplantation in the cyclosporine era. Ann Thorac Surg 48:350, 1989

53. Bristow MR, Gilbert EM, Renlund DG et al: Use of OKT3 monoclonal antibody in heart transplantation: review of the initial experience. J Heart Transplant 7:1, 1988

54. Kormos RL, Herlan DB, Armitage JM et al: Monoclonal versus polyclonal antibody therapy for prophylaxis against rejection after heart transplantation. J Heart Transplant 9:1, 1990

55. Kirklin JK, Bourge RC, White-Williams C et al: Prophylactic therapy for rejection after cardiac transplantation—a comparison of rabbit antithymocyte globulin and OKT3. J Thorac Cardiovasc Surg 99:716, 1990

56. Pennock JL, Oyer PE, Reitz BA et al: Cardiac transplantation in perspective for the future: survival, complications, rehabilitation, and cost. J Thorac Cardiovasc Surg 83:168, 1982

57. Hofflin JM, Potasman I, Baldwin JC et al: Infectious complications in heart transplant recipients receiving cyclosporine and corticosteroids. Ann Intern Med 106:209, 1987

58. Kirklin JK, Naftel DC, McGriffin DC et al: Analysis of morbid events and risk factors for death after cardiac transplantation. J Am Coll Cardiol 11:917, 1988

59. Griepp RB, Stinson EB, Bieber CP et al: Control of graft atherosclerosis in human heart transplant recipients. Surgery 81:262, 1977

60. Bieber CP, Hunt SA, Schwinn DA: Complications in long term survivors of cardiac transplantation. Transplant Proc 13:207, 1981

61. Uretsky BP, Murali S, Reddy PS et al: Development of coronary artery disease in cardiac transplant patients receiving immunosuppressive therapy with cyclosporine and prednisone. Circulation 76:827, 1987

62. Gao SZ, Schroeder JS, Alderman EL et al: Clinical and laboratory correlates of accelerated coronary artery disease in the cardiac transplant patient. Circulation, suppl V. 76:V56, 1987

63. Grattan MT, Moreno-Cabral CE, Starnes VA: Cytomegalovirus infection is associated with cardiac allograft rejection and atherosclerosis. JAMA 261:3561, 1989

64. Olivari MT, Antolick A, Ring WS: Arterial hypertension in heart transplant recipients treated with triple drug immunosuppressive therapy. J Heart Transplant 8:34, 1989

65. Ozdogan E, Banner N, Fitzgerald M et al: Factors influencing the development of hypertension after heart transplantation. J Heart Transplant 9:548, 1990

66. Ladowski J, Kormos R, Uretsky B et al: Posttransplantation diabetes mellitus in heart transplant recipients. J Heart Transplant 8:181, 1989

67. Jamieson SW, Burton NA, Bieber CP et al: Cardiac allograft survival in rats treated with cyclosporine-A. Surg Forum 30:289, 1979

68. Oyer PE, Stinson EB, Reitz BA et al: Cardiac transplantation 1980. Transplant Proc 13:199, 1981

69. Reitz BA, Wallwork JL, Hunt SA et al: Heart-lung transplantation: successful therapy for patients with pulmonary vascular disease. N Engl J Med 306:557, 1982

70. Kamholz SL, Veith FJ, Mollenkopf FP et al: Single lung transplantation with cyclosporine immunosuppression. J Thorac Cardiovasc Surg 86:537, 1983

71. Patterson GA, Cooper JD, Dark JH et al: Experimental and clinical double-lung transplantation. J Thorac Cardiovasc Surg 95:70, 1988

72. Dittrich HC, Nicod PH, Chow LC et al: Early changes of right heart geometry after pulmonary thromboendarterectomy. J Am Coll Cardiol 11:937, 1988

73. Fremes SE, Patterson GA, Williams WG et al: Single lung transplantation and closure of patent ductus arteriosus for Eisenmenger's syndrome. Toronto Lung Transplant Group. J Thorac Cardiovasc Surg 100:1, 1990

74. Trulock EP, Egan TM, Kouchoukos NT et al: Single lung transplantation for severe chronic obstructive pulmo-

nary disease. Washington University Lung Transplant Group. Chest 96:738, 1989

75. McCarthy PM, Starnes VA, Theodore J: Improved survival after heart-lung transplantation. J Thorac Cardiovasc Surg 99:54, 1990

76. Imoto EM, Glanville AR, Baldwin JC, Theodore J: Kidney function in heart-lung transplant recipients: the effect of low dosage cyclosporine therapy. J Heart Transplant 6: 204, 1987

77. Dummer JS, White LT, Ho M et al: Morbidity of cytomegalovirus infection in recipients of heart and heart-lung transplantation who received cyclosporine. J Infect Dis 152:1182, 1985

78. Brooks RG, Hofflin JM, Jamieson SW et al: Infectious complications in heart-lung transplant recipients. Am J Med 79:412, 1985

79. Dowling RD, Baladi N, Zenati M: Disruption of the aortic anastomosis after heart-lung transplantation. Ann Thorac Surg 49:118, 1990

80. Hutter JA, Scott J, Wreghitt T et al: The importance of cytomegalovirus in heart-lung recipients. Chest 95:627, 1989

81. Wreghitt T: Cytomegalovirus infections in heart and heart lung transplant recipients. J Antimicrob Chemother, suppl E 23:49, 1989

82. Higenbottam T, Hutter JA, Stewart S, Wallwork J: Transbronchial biopsy has eliminated the need for endomyocardial biopsy in heart-lung recipients. J Heart Transplant 7:435, 1988

83. McGregor CGA, Baldwin JC, Jamieson SW et al: Isolated pulmonary rejection after combined heart-lung transplantation. J Thorac Cardiovasc Surg 90.623, 1985

84. Starnes VA, Theodore J, Oyer P et al: Evaluation of heartlung transplant recipients with prospective, serial transbronchial biopsies and pulmonary function studies. J Thorac Cardiovasc Surg 98:683, 1989

85. Glanville AR, Imoto E, Baldwin JC et al: The role of right ventricular endomyocardial biopsy in the longterm management of heart-lung transplant recipients. J Heart Transplant 6:357, 1987

86. Higenbottam TW, Penketh A, Stewart S, Wallwork J: Transbronchial lung biopsy to diagnose lung rejection and infection of heart-lung transplants. Transplantation 46:532, 1988

87. Clelland C, Higenbottam T, Otulana B et al: Histologic prognostic indicators for the lung allografts of heart-lung transplants. J Heart Transplant 9:177, 1990

88. Zeevi A, Rabinowich H, Paradis I et al: Lymphocyte activation in bronchioalveolar lavages from heart-lung transplantation recipients. Transplant Proc 20:189, 1988

89. Burke CM, Theodore J, Dawkins KD et al: Post-transplant obliterative bronchiolitis and other late lung sequelae in human heart-lung transplantation. Chest 86:824, 1984

90. McGregor CG, Jamieson SW, Baldwin JC et al: Combined heart-lung transplantation for Eisenmenger's syndrome. J Thorac Cardiovasc Surg 91:443, 1986

91. Burke CM, Glanville AR, Theodore J, Robin ED: Lung immunogenicity, rejection and obliterative bronchiolitis. Chest 92:547, 1987

92. Scott JP, Fradet G, Smyth RL et al: Management following heart and lung transplantation: five years experience. Eur J Cardiothorac Surg 4:197, 1990

93. Burke CM, Glanville AR, Macoviak et al: The spectrum of cytomegalovirus infection following human heart-lung transplantation. J Heart Transplant 5:267, 1986

94. Glanville AR, Baldwin JC, Burke CM et al: Obliterative bronchiolitis after heart-lung transplantation: Apparent arrest by augmented immunosuppression. Ann Intern Med 107:300, 1987

95. Scott JP, Higenbottam TW, Clelland et al: Natural history of chronic rejection in heart-lung transplant recipients. J Heart Transplant 9:510, 1990

96. Miralles A, Kawaguchi A, Gandjbakhch I et al: Heart and unilateral lung transplantation in patients with endstage cardiopulmonary disease and previous thoracic surgery. Transplant Proc 22:1468, 1990

97. Saywell RM, Jr, Woods JR, Halbrook HG et al: Cost analysis of heart transplantation from the day of operation to the day of discharge. J Heart Transplant 8:244, 1989

Index

Page numbers followed by f *indicate figures; page numbers followed by* t *indicate tables.*